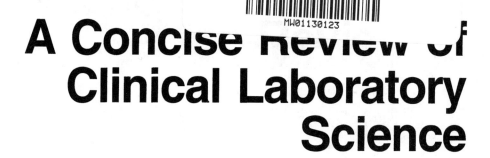

A Concise Review of Clinical Laboratory Science

A Concise Review of Clinical Laboratory Science

Joel D. Hubbard

Associate Professor
Department of Diagnostic and Primary Care
School of Allied Health
Texas Tech University Health Sciences Center
Lubbock, Texas

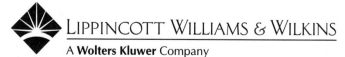

LIPPINCOTT WILLIAMS & WILKINS
A **Wolters Kluwer** Company

Philadelphia • Baltimore • New York • London
Buenos Aires • Hong Kong • Sydney • Tokyo

Editor: Elizabeth Nieginski
Managing Editor: Darrin Kiessling
Marketing Manager: Christine Kushner
Production Coordinator: Peter J. Carley
Cover Designer: Cathy Cotter
Typesetter and Digitized Illustrations: Bi-Comp, Incorporated
Printer: Port City Press, Inc.
Color Presswork: Lehigh Press
Binder: Port City Press, Inc.

Copyright © 1997 Williams & Wilkins

351 West Camden Street
Baltimore, Maryland 21201-2436 USA

Accurate indications, adverse reactions and dosage schedules for drugs are provided in this book, but it is possible that they may change. The reader is urged to review the package information data of the manufacturers of the medications mentioned.

Printed in the United States of America

Library of Congress Cataloging-in-Publication Data

Hubbard, Joel D. (Joel David), 1952–
    A concise review of clinical laboratory science / Joel D. Hubbard.
       p.   cm.
    Includes index.
    ISBN 0-683-04219-X
    1. Medical laboratory technology—Examinations, questions, etc.
  2. Medical laboratory technology—Outlines, syllabi, etc.
  I. Title.
    [DNLM: 1. Diagnosis, Laboratory—examination questions.   QY
18.2H875c 1997]
  RB38.25.H83 1997
  616.07′56—dc21
  DNLM/DLC
  for Library of Congress   96-47287
                                           CIP

04
5 6 7 8 9 0

Dedication

This book is dedicated to clinical laboratory science students everywhere. In your upcoming role as professionals, remember that your job is important to the medical world as well as to the individual patient. Be proud of the fact that you will be making a difference in people's lives. Always be excited about the unlimited opportunities available in your chosen profession and help to lead the field of Clinical Laboratory Science into the 21st century.

Preface

This text can be used as a valuable educational tool by both the novice and the experienced clinical laboratory scientist. It is designed to be a concise review of all areas of clinical laboratory science. This book will serve as a tool for students of medical technology studying for national certification examinations, such as the American Society of Clinical Pathologists (ASCP) exam, the National Certification Agency (NCA) exam, and the American Medical Technologist (AMT) exam. Practicing clinical laboratory scientists will also find this book to be a good source of review.

The text includes the most current and updated information. A concise summary of the most important facts and concepts in each subject area is presented in an outline format and is followed by sample study questions representing all taxonomic levels. This review not only covers the standard areas of clinical laboratory science, but also includes a chapter on laboratory management that addresses such topics as safety and OSHA and the most current government laboratory regulations, such as CLIA 88. A chapter with case studies is provided for practice in applied knowledge. The book concludes with a comprehensive examination of comparative length to national certification exams.

This book represents a culmination of the efforts and expertise of the faculty of the Clinical Laboratory Science program at Texas Tech University Health Sciences Center in Lubbock, Texas and reflects over 100 years of combined medical technology experience. All contributing authors reflect their professional excellence in their contributed chapters, not only as educators, but as outstanding professionals in the field of Clinical Laboratory Science.

Joel D. Hubbard

Acknowledgments

I would like to thank all of the contributing authors—Dr. Hal Larsen, Dr. Barbara Border, Dr. Sally Becker, Ms. Lori Rice-Spearman, Ms. JoAnn Tyndall Larsen, and Ms. Mary Ann Harrison—for making this book possible. Their individual expertise, willingness to present the highest quality of material, and promptness in meeting deadlines made the task of producing this text easy.

Contributors

Sally A. Becker, M.T. (A.S.C.P.), C.L.S.,
    Ph.D.
Assistant Professor
Department of Diagnostic and Primary Care
School of Allied Health
Texas Tech University Health Sciences Center
Lubbock, Texas

Barbara Border, M. T. (A.S.C.P.), Ph.D.
Cepartment of Diagnostic and Primary Care
School of Allied Health
Texas Tech University Health Sciences Center
Lubbock, Texas

Mary Ann Harrison, M.T. (A.S.C.P.), C.L.S.
    (N.C.A.)
Laboratory Manager/Coordinator, Academic
    Instructor
Department of Diagnostic and Primary Care
School of Allied Health
Texas Tech University Health Sciences Center
Lubbock, Texas

Hal S.Larsen, M. T. (A.S.C.P.), C.L.S. (N.C.A.),
    Ph.D.
Chair and Program Director
Department of Diagnostic and Primary Care
School of Allied Health
Texas Tech University Health Sciences Center
Lubbock, Texas

Jo Ann Tyndall Larsen, M.T. (A.S.C.P.), S.H.,
    C.L.S. (N.C.A.), M.S.
Adjunct Assistant Professor
Department of Diagnostic and Primary Care
School of Allied Health:
Manager, Office of Student Affairs
SOM
Lubbock, Texas

Lori Rice–Spearman, M.T. (A.S.C.P.), M.S.
Associate Professor, Assistant Program Director
Department of Diagnostic and Primary Care
School of Allied Health
Texas Tech University Health Sciences Center
Lubbock, Texas

Contents

6   Immunology and Serology   289

7   Current Issues in Laboratory Management   327

8   Clinical Microbiology   343

1

Clinical Chemistry

Barbara Border

I. CLINICAL CHEMISTRY BASICS

A. Laboratory math

1. **Concentration.** Solutions can be described in terms of the concentration of the components of the solution.

   a. A **percent solution** can be described as:

   (1) **w/w,** which is expressed as weight (mass) per 100 units of weight (g/g).

   (2) **w/v,** which is expressed as weight (mass) per 100 units of volume (g/dL).

   (3) **v/v,** which is expressed as volume (mL) per unit of volume (mL).

   b. **Molarity (M)** is expressed as mole per liter (mol/L) or millimole per milliliter (mmol/mL).

   (1) A **mole** is one formula weight, in grams, of a compound. For example, one mole of NaOH equals 40 g, because one molecule of sodium equals 23 g, one molecule of oxygen equals 16 g, and one molecule of hydrogen equals 1 g.

   (2) **Molarity** is calculated by determining what units are given in the problem, then determining the final units needed, and setting up an equation (Boxes 1-1 and 1-2).

   (3) A simple calculation for molarity problems can be performed with the following formula:

   $$\frac{\text{Grams in solution}}{\text{Volume in liters}} = \text{Formula weight} \times \text{molarity}$$

   Using the information from the first problem, the variables can be plugged in:

   $$\frac{\text{Grams in solution}}{1\,\text{L}} = 40\,\text{g (2 M)}$$

   $$\frac{x}{1} = 80\,\text{grams}$$

   $$x = 80\,\text{grams}$$

1

Box 1-1. Molarity

PROBLEM: How many grams of NaOH are needed to make 1 L of 2 M solution?

ANSWER:

Final units needed: g/L

Units of measure given: M, L

By definition, a molar solution is the number of moles per liter of solution. For a 2M solution:

$$\frac{40 \text{ g NaOH}}{1 \text{ mole}} \times \frac{2 \text{ mole}}{\text{L}} = 80 \text{ g/L} = 2 \text{ M NaOH}$$

80 g NaOH are required. To prepare the solution, 80 g NaOH are placed in a 1 L volumetric flask, and deionized water is added to make a volume of 1 L.

Using the information given in the second problem, the variables can be plugged in:

$$\frac{32 \text{ g in solution}}{0.3 \text{ L}} = 36.5 \text{ (M)}$$

$$106.7 = 36.5 \text{ (M)}$$

$$106.7/36.5 = \text{M}$$

$$2.9 = \text{M}$$

   c. Normality (N) is expressed as equivalent weight (Eq wt) per liter of volume (Eq/L or mEq/mL).

     (1) An **equivalent weight** is gram molecular weight (gmw) divided by the valence or the number of replaceable hydrogen molecules or hydroxyl groups (Box 1-3).

     (2) **Normality** is calculated by determining the units given in the problems, then determining what units are needed and setting up the equation (Boxes 1-4 and 1-5).

     (3) A simple calculation that can be used to solve normality problems involves the following formula:

$$\frac{\text{Grams in solution}}{\text{Volume in liters}} = \text{Equivalent weight} \times \text{normality}$$

Box 1-2. Determining the Molarity of a Solution

PROBLEM: What is the molarity of solution that contains 32 g of HCl in 300 mL of water?

ANSWER:

Final unit of measure needed: mol/L

Units of measure used: g/mL

Grams of HCl in 1 mole: 36.5

$$\frac{32 \text{ g HCl}}{300 \text{ ml}} \times \frac{1000 \text{ ml}}{1 \text{ L}} \times \frac{1 \text{ mole}}{36.5 \text{ g HCl}} = 2.9 \text{ mol/L}$$

Box 1-3. Determining Equivalent Weight

PROBLEM: Determine the equivalent weight of each of the following:

24 g of NaOH

65 g H_2SO_4

12 g NaCl

ANSWER:
NaOH = 40 gmw, valence = 1, Eq wt = 40
H_2SO_4 = 98 gmw, valence = 2, Eq wt = 49
NaCl = 58 gmw, valence = 1, Eq wt = 58

Using the information given in the first normality problem, the values can be plugged in:

$$\frac{80 \text{ g}}{.450 \text{ L}} = 49 \text{ (x)}$$

$$177.8 = 49 \text{ (x)}$$

$$3.62 = \text{x}$$

Using the information given in the second normality problem, the values can be plugged in:

$$\frac{49 \text{ g}}{1 \text{ L}} = 49 \text{ (x)}$$

$$49 = 49 \text{ (x)}$$

$$1 = \text{x}$$

Normality of the given solution equals 1 Eq/L.

  d. **Dilutions** are solutions formed by making a less concentrated solution from a concentrated solution. They are stated as a part (concentrate) of the concentrated substance used plus the volume of diluent used.

Box 1-4. Calculating the Normality of a Solution

PROBLEM: What is the normality of a solution containing 80 g of H_2SO_4 in 450 mL deionized water?

ANSWER:
The Eq wt of H_2SO_4: 49 g
The final units needed: Eq/L (N)
The units given: g/mL
By definition, a normal solution is the number of equivalents per liter of solution.

$$\frac{80 \text{ g } H_2SO_4}{450 \text{ ml}} \times \frac{1 \text{ Eq}}{49 \text{ g } H_2SO_4} \times \frac{1000 \text{ ml}}{1 \text{ L}} = 3.6 \text{ N}$$

Box 1-5. Calculating the Normality of a Solution

PROBLEM: Determine the N of a 0.5 M solution of H_2SO_4.

ANSWER:
Final units needed: Eq/L (N)
Units given: mol/L
Molecular weight of H_2SO_4: 98 g
The Eq wt of H_2SO_4: 49 g

$$\frac{0.5\ M\ H_2SO_4}{L} \times \frac{98\ g\ H_2SO_4}{mole\ H_2SO_4} \times \frac{1\ Eq\ H_2SO_4}{49\ g\ H_2SO_4} = 1\ N\ H_2SO_4$$

EXAMPLE: 100 μl of serum in 400 μl of saline = 100 in a total of 100 + 400 = 100/500 = 1:5 dilution.

2. **Specific gravity** is an expression of **density** (g/mL). To solve problems regarding specific gravity, it is important to know the percent purity of substance (Box 1-6).

3. **Hydration** is the process of adding water molecules to the chemical structure of a compound. It is important to consider the molecular weight of these molecules when making solutions (Box 1-7).

B. **Statistical concepts.** Statistics is the science of gathering, analyzing, interpreting, and presenting data. A statistic is a number summarizing data.

1. **Descriptive statistics** are data that can be described by their location and dispersion compared with the average. Once data are plotted on a histogram, the values typically form a symmetric curve referred to as normal or **gaussian distribution** (Figure 1-1).

2. **Common statistics** used in the clinical chemistry laboratory include mean, range, standard deviation (SD), and coefficient of variation (CV).

   a. The **mean (x)** is the arithmetic average of a set of data calculated as follows:

   $$x = x_1 + x_2 + x_3 + \ldots x_n/n$$

   where x is each individual value, and n is the number of data points or observations made.

   b. **Range (dispersion)** is the most simple statistic used to describe the spread of data about the mean. It is calculated by subtracting the smallest observation or value from the largest.

Box 1-6. Calculating Specific Gravity

PROBLEM: Determine the density in g/mL of HCl available in a stock solution of HCl, in which the purity is 53%, and specific gravity is 1.19.

ANSWER: 1.19 g/mL $\times$ 0.53 = 0.63 g/mL of HCl

Box 1-7. Calculating Molecular Weight for Hydration

PROBLEM: How much $CuSO_4 \cdot 5H_2O$ must be weighed in order to make 1 L of 0.5 M $CuSO_4$?

ANSWER: $CuSO_4 \cdot H_2O$ has five water molecules, which add 90 g to the original 160 gmw. Therefore, $CuSO_4 \cdot 5H_2O$ has a gmw = 250 g.

$$\frac{250 \text{ g } CuSO_4 \cdot 5H_2O}{\text{mol}} \times \frac{0.5 \text{ mol}}{1 \text{ L}} = 125 \text{ g/L}$$

   c. **Standard deviation (SD)** is the most commonly used statistic in the laboratory describing dispersion of groups of single observations. SD is the square root of the variance. It is calculated by adding the squares of the differences between the individual results and the mean, dividing by n-1, and calculating the square root.

   d. **Coefficient of variation (CV)** is a comparison of the relative variability in two sets of values because not all laboratory data are expressed in similar units of measure or concentrations. It is expressed as a percentage and is calculated as follows:

$$CV\% = \frac{SD}{\text{mean}} \times 100\%$$

or

$$\frac{SD(100\%)}{\text{mean}}$$

   e. **Other statistical** terms include mode (i.e., the value occurring with the greatest frequency), and median (i.e., the value that occurs in the middle of the population).

   3. The **reference range** is defined as the range of values for a given substance in healthy individuals.

C. **Quality assurance and quality control**

   1. **A quality assurance (QA) program** is a coordinated effort designed to monitor all the varied activities of the laboratory that detect, control, and prevent the occurrence of error. QA programs are required by law.

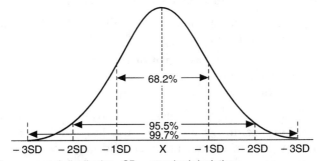

Figure 1-1. Gaussian or normal distribution. *SD* = standard deviation.

2. A **quality control (QC)** program oversees laboratory analyses to ensure accuracy and validity. It is designed to increase the probability that each result reported by the laboratory can be used with confidence by a physician making a diagnostic or therapeutic decision. QC is a subset of any laboratory QA program.

   a. **QC programs function by detecting analytic error.** The three stages of a QC program are:

      (1) The establishment of statistical limits of variation of each analytic method used

      (2) The use of statistical criteria to evaluate QC data generated per test

      (3) The implementation of remedial actions when statistical limits are exceeded

   b. QC statistical limits are set by determining the concentration of an analyte in **controls.**

      (1) Controls (e.g., serum, whole blood, urine, spinal fluid) contain known concentrations of an analyte of interest.

      (2) Controls are treated as patient samples; control results determine the validity of an analytic run.

   c. There are two **types** of QC programs.

      (1) **Internal QC programs** are necessary for the daily monitoring of the precision and accuracy of an analytic method. This program only detects changes in performance between present operation and past "stable" operations.

      (2) **External QC programs** compare the performance of different laboratories. This program maintains the long-term accuracy of analytic methods.

3. **Westgard control rules** are used to evaluate the validity of an analytic run. These rules are stated as:

   a. 1_{2s}: Use as a rejection or warning when one control observation exceeds the mean $+/-2s$ control limits.

   b. 1_{3s}: Reject a run when two consecutive control observations exceed the mean $+/-3s$ control limits.

   c. 2_{2s}: Reject a run when two consecutive control observations are on the same side of the mean and exceed the mean $+/-2s$ control limits.

   d. 4_{1s}: Reject a run when four consecutive control observations are on the same side of the mean and exceed the mean $+/-1s$ control limits.

   e. 10_x: Reject a run when 10 consecutive control observations are on the same side of the mean.

   f. R_{4s}: Reject a run if the range or difference between the maximum and minimum control observation out of the last 4–6 control observations exceeds 4s.

4. In addition to using control rules, the control data is plotted on a daily basis using a **Levy-Jennings chart or Shewhart plot.** These charts compare observed values of control materials and illustrate trends that may be occurring over a period of time.

Table 1-1. Advantages and Disadvantages of Automation

Advantages	Disadvantages
Increased work capacity per unit of time	Initial costs
Minimized variability	Discontinuity of product
Reduced errors caused by manual manipulations	Technical skill required
Reduced sample volumes	
Reduced consumable costs	

D. **Laboratory automation and computer systems**

1. **Automation** in the clinical chemistry laboratory context is the mechanization of chemical analysis to minimize manual manipulation.

   a. There are **eight major steps** typically mechanized:
      (1) Sample/reagent handling
      (2) Sample/reagent measurement
      (3) Mixing
      (4) Separation
      (5) Incubation
      (6) Reaction analysis
      (7) Derivation of results
      (8) Reporting results

   b. The **advantages and disadvantages** associated with automation are given in Table 1-1.

2. There are **three basic approaches** to automation in use today.

   a. **Continuous flow analyzers** use liquid reagents pumped through a continuous system of tubing. Each sample is introduced in a sequential manner.

   b. **Discrete analyzers** house samples and reagents in separate containers. Multiple tests can be performed on a single sample, or one test can be selected to perform on multiple samples.

   c. **Centrifugal analyzers** use centrifugal force to transfer reagents into separate analyzing chambers. These instruments are capable of running multiple samples, one test at a time, or batches.

3. **Laboratory Information System (LIS)** is a system of computer software designed to handle laboratory data.

   a. The **functions** of an LIS include:
      (1) Database of patient information
      (2) Compilation of specimen test results
      (3) Production of patient reports
      (4) Production of ancillary reports
      (5) Data storage

   b. An LIS achieves its function via a central computer, a number of input/output devices, and the computer software.

    c. **Computer hardware** is composed of the following:

        (1) **A central processing unit (CPU)** in which programmed instructions are executed

        (2) **Data storage devices** consisting of hard disks, floppy disks, and tape drives

        (3) **Input devices,** such as a keyboard, monitor, code readers, ports, and scanners

        (4) **Output devices,** such as printers, other computers, or modems

    d. **Computer software** provides the programs that instruct a computer what to do.

E. Spectrophotometry

    1. A **spectrophotometer** is an instrument that measures the transmitted light of a solution and allows the operator to read the absorbance of the solution on a meter. The components of a spectrophotometer include the following:

        a. The **light source** provides radiant energy.

            (1) **Tungsten lamps** are the typical source in most spectrophotometers.

            (2) **Deuterium (and hydrogen) lamps** are used in spectrophotometers that examine the ultraviolet (UV) spectrum.

            (3) **Mercury lamps** are used in high-performance liquid chromatography spectrophotometers.

        b. The monochromator isolates the wavelength of interest. Examples include:

            (1) Colored glass filters

            (2) Interference filters

            (3) Prisms

            (4) Diffraction gratings

        c. The **sample cell** contains the solution in:

            (1) Cuvettes

            (2) Tubing (typical in automated equipment)

            (3) Plastic packs

        d. The **photodetector** converts radiant energy to electrical energy. Three types of photodetectors are:

            (1) Photocell (barrier-layer cell)

            (2) Phototube

            (3) Photomultiplier tube

    2. **Background**

        a. **Photons.** Electromagnetic **radiant energy is described in terms of wavelike properties,** specifically as photons, which are discrete packets of energy traveling in waves.

        b. **Wavelengths.** A **wavelength (λ)** of electromagnetic energy is the **linear distance between successive wave peaks** and is usually measured in units of nanometers (10^{-9}m).

            (1) **Frequency** is the number of wave peaks per given unit of time.

            (2) **Amplitude** is the height of the peak.

        c. The **electromagnetic spectrum** has a large range of wavelengths. Gamma rays and x-rays have very long wavelengths, whereas UV rays inhabit the portion of the electromagnetic spectrum from 10–400 nm. The **visible**

spectrum lies between 400 and 800 nm. Violet light has the longest wavelength of the visible spectrum, followed by blue, green, yellow, orange, and red (VIBGYOR; ROY G. BIV). The infrared spectrum lies above 800 nm, and the shortest wavelengths are microwaves.

d. **Excitation.** Interactions of light with matter occur when a **photon intercepts an atom, ion, or molecule.** The photon is absorbed, and the energy of the photon changes the matter (excitation). Some compounds are able to dissipate the absorbed energy as radiant energy upon return to a nonexcited state. **Excitation** can involve any of the following:

(1) Movement of an electron to a higher energy state
(2) Change in covalent bond vibrations
(3) Change in covalent bond rotations

e. **Beer's law** states that the concentration of a substance is directly proportional to the amount of radiant energy absorbed:

$$A = abc \ or \ ebc$$

where, **a** (or e) is **molar absorptivity** (a constant for a given molecule); **b** is the **length of the path** traveled by the light; and **c** is the **concentration** of absorbing molecules.

f. **Standard curve.** In clinical chemistry, concentrations of unknown solutions are determined by plotting the absorbance of standard solutions (concentrations known) versus the concentrations of the standard solution, which creates a standard curve.

3. **Types of spectrophotometry**
   a. **Absorption spectrophotometry** is defined as the measurement of radiant energy absorbed by a solution. This measurement can be related to the concentration of a substance in the solution.

   (1) Every solution has an ability to absorb and transmit light, and only transmitted light can be measured. **Transmittance** is defined as the proportion of incident light that is transmitted and is usually expressed as a percentage:

$$\%T = I/I_o \times 100$$

   where **I** is the transmitted radiant energy, and I_o is the original incident radiation. Transmittance varies inversely and logarithmically with the concentration of the solution.

   (2) **Absorbance** is calculated as follows:

$$A = 2 - \log \%T$$

   The absorbance is the critical measure used in the calculation of concentration (Beer's law).

   b. **Atomic absorption spectrophotometry (AAS)** measures concentration through the detection of absorbance of electromagnetic radiation by atoms instead of molecules. It is used to measure concentration of metals that are not easily excited.

   (1) **Principle.** An element of interest is dissociated from its chemical bonds in the flame, then is in an unexcited state. At this low energy,

the atom can absorb radiation at a narrow specific bandwidth. A wavelength of light (emitted by a light source) specific for the atom is absorbed by the low-energy atoms in the flame, resulting in a decrease in the intensity of the light measured by the detector.

    (2) Components
        (a) The light source (hollow cathode lamp)
        (b) Flame (produced by a burner head)
        (c) Monochromator
        (d) Photodetector (photomultiplier tube)

  c. Nephelometry is a method of measuring concentration in terms of light energy scattered in a forward direction by small particles in solution. The intensity of the scattered light is directly proportional to the number of particles in solution.

  d. Turbidimetry is a photometric measurement of unscattered light passing through a colloidal solution of small particles. It is essentially a measurement of blocked light, and the amount of blocked light is directly proportional to the number of particles in solution.

  e. Fluorometry is the photometric measurement of light emitted by a substance that has been previously excited by a source of UV light. Once excited and driven into a higher energy state, a molecule loses energy by fluorescing. The amount of light emitted is proportional to the concentration of the substance in solution.

F. Electrochemistry and osmometry

  1. Electrochemistry is the measurement of electrical signals associated with chemical systems that are incorporated into an **electrochemical cell** (i.e., electrodes and solution in which they are immersed).

    a. In an **anode/cathode system,** electrons spontaneously flow from an electrode of high electron affinity to an electrode of low electron affinity, if the electrodes are connected via a salt bridge.

    b. Each electrode is characterized by a half-cell reaction and a half-cell potential (voltage). The electrode from which electrons flow is called the **anode.** The electrode accepting the electrons is the **cathode.**

  2. Potentiometric methods. The measurement of voltage potentials is based on the measurement of a potential (voltage) difference between two electrodes immersed in solution under the condition of zero current **electrochemical measurements.** There are various systems used for measuring these potentials.

    a. A **pH meter** is a potentiometric apparatus used to measure the concentration of hydrogen ions in solution. It measures the potential difference between one half-cell and a reference electrode.

        (1) One of the electrodes (one half-cell), the **indicator electrode,** is sensitive to and responds to changes in concentration of a particular ion species in the solution in which the electrode is immersed.

        (2) A second electrode (another half-cell), the **reference electrode,** has A potential that does not change (i.e., is not influenced by the activity of the ion being measured). It is an electrochemical half-cell that is

used as a fixed reference for the measurement of cell potentials. Examples include:
- **(a)** Standard hydrogen electrode
- **(b)** Saturate calomel electrode
- **(c)** Silver/silver chloride

(3) The **indicator electrode is** in an electrochemical half-cell that interacts with the analyte of interest. Examples include:
- **(a) Ion-selective** electrodes (ISE) measure a potential across a membrane specific for a certain analyte.
- **(b) Glass-membrane** electrodes are a type of ISE most commonly used for pH measurement.

b. Coulometry is the measurement of the amount of electricity passing between two electrodes in an electrochemical cell. The amount of electricity is proportional to the amount of a substance produced or consumed by oxidation/reduction at the electrodes.

c. Amperometry is the measurement of the current flowing through an electrochemical cell when a potential is applied to the electrodes.

3. Osmometry is the measurement of particle concentration that is related to the osmotic pressure of the solution. **Osmotic pressure** regulates the movement of a solvent across a membrane.

4. Osmolality describes the number of moles of particle per kilogram of water and depends only on the number of particles, not on what kind of particles are present.

a. The **colligative properties** of a solution are related to the number of solute particles per kilogram of solvent. Colligative properties include:
- **(1)** Osmotic pressure
- **(2)** Boiling point
- **(3)** Vapor pressure
- **(4)** Freezing point

b. Colligative properties change as the number of particles in the solution change. In the clinical chemistry laboratory, **vapor pressure** and **freezing point** are the colligative properties of interest. These can be measured in an osmometer.
- **(1) Freezing point depression.** The more particles in solution, the lower the freezing point of the solution.
- **(2) Vapor pressure depression.** Increased particles in a solution prevent solvent evaporation.

c. Osmolal gap is the difference between the calculated osmolality and the actual measured osmolality.
- **(1)** The **formula** for calculated plasma osmolality is:

$$2 \times \text{Na (mEq/L)} + \frac{\text{Glucose (mg/dL)}}{18} + \frac{\text{BUN (mg/dL)}}{2.8} = \text{mOsm/kg}$$

- **(2) If the osmolal gap is >0,** there is an indication of an abnormal concentration of unmeasured substances (typically, ethanol) in the blood.

II. SPECIAL METHODS IN CLINICAL CHEMISTRY

A. **Electrophoresis** is the **migration of charged particles in some medium** (either liquid or solid) **when an electrical field is applied.** Depending on the charge of the molecules, negatively charged particles migrate toward the positive electrode (anode), and positively charged particles migrate toward the negative electrode (cathode).

1. **Migration rate** depends on:

   a. **Charge of the molecule,** which is directly proportional to rate of movement

   b. **Size of the molecule,** which is inversely proportional to rate of movement

   c. **Electrical field,** in which increased current increases migration rate

   d. **Ionic strength of buffer,** in which increased ionic strength decreases migration rate

   e. **pH of buffer,** in which decreased pH slows migration

   f. **Viscosity of supporting medium,** which is inversely proportional to migration rate

   g. **System temperature,** in which high temperature can denature protein and slow migration

2. **Analytic electrophoretic procedures** include protein electrophoresis and isoenzyme electrophoresis.

   a. **Protein electrophoresis**

      (1) The **principle** of protein electrophoresis

         (a) **Proteins are amphoteric** (i.e., they can have positive or negative charge because of their acidic and basic side chains).

         (b) The **isoelectric point** of protein is the pH at which a protein has no net charge.

         (c) At **pH 8.6,** proteins are negatively charged and migrate toward the anode.

         (d) If the **buffer pH** is higher than the isoelectric point of protein, the protein carries a negative charge and migrates toward the anode.

      (2) The **methodology** of electrophoresis

         (a) A **support medium** (agarose gel or cellulose acetate) is put in contact with the buffer.

         (b) A **sample** is applied to the medium.

         (c) A **constant current or voltage** is applied, and particles are allowed to migrate and separate.

         (d) The **support** is fixed and stained to visualize protein bands.

   b. **Isoenzyme electrophoresis** is typically performed to visualize the isoenzymes of creatine kinase and lactate dehydrogenase.

      (1) The **principle** of isoenzyme electrophoresis is similar to that of protein electrophoresis because isoenzymes are proteins. The procedure is performed at a pH of 8.6, and the most negatively charged particles migrate toward the anode.

      (2) The **methodology** involved in isoenzyme electrophoresis is similar to that used for protein electrophoresis.

B. Immunoassay is a chemical assay based on the highly specific and tight, noncovalent binding of antibodies to target molecules (antigens). Immunoassay is typically useful when the endogenous concentration of an analyte is very low.

   1. Components in the immunoassay system include antigens and antibodies.

   a. An **antigen (ag)** is a substance that can elicit an immune response (production of a specific antibody) when injected into an animal. The antigen is typically the analyte of interest.

   b. An **antibody (ab)** is an immunoglobulin formed in response to a foreign substance (antigen). The antibody is the most important component of this system, because it determines the **sensitivity** (ability to detect small amounts) and **specificity** (the degree of uniqueness of the ag–ab reaction) of the procedure.

   (1) Polyclonal antibodies are developed by injecting an antigen into a rabbit or sheep, bleeding the animal, then purifying the antibody. Polyclonal antibodies have **high affinity** (a measure of the tightness of the ag–ab binding) and general specificity. A disadvantage is that death of the rabbit or sheep limits the availability of antibody.

   (2) Monoclonal antibodies are developed by injecting an antigen into mice and removing the antibody-producing spleen cells, which are fused with a tumor cell. These cultured tumor cells can produce unlimited amounts of antibody that are pure and specific but have lower affinity than polyclonal antibodies. Monoclonal antibodies cannot be used in nephelometric methods.

   2. Immunochemical labels are necessary to detect the ag–ab reaction.

   a. Enzyme labels are attached to the antibody. With the addition of a chromagen, they allow the immunoassay results to be quantitated colorimetrically.

   b. Fluorescent labels are attached to the antibody and are detected when a photon is released from a fluorescent molecule that is excited from its ground state to a higher state and then returns to ground. A drawback of this system lies with the autofluorescence of serum.

   c. Chemiluminescent labels are compounds that undergo a chemical reaction and form an unstable derivative. Upon return to ground state, they release energy in the form of visible light. The light is measured by a luminometer, and light intensity is related directly to the concentration of the reactants.

   d. Radioisotope labels are compounds that have the same atomic number but different weights than the parent nuclide (e.g., ^{125}I, ^{14}C). Radioisotopes decay to form a more stable isotope. In the process, they emit energy in the form of radiation (electromagnetic gamma rays) that can be detected and quantitated. The gamma rays are absorbed by a sodium iodide tube, which gives off brief flashes of light when excited. The label is usually attached to an analyte similar to that being tested.

   3. Methodologies are based on the label of the antigen or antibody (Table 1-2).

C. Chromatography is a technique used to separate complex mixtures on the basis of different physical interactions between the individual compounds and the

Table 1-2. Methods of Immunoassay

Method	Basis	What is Labeled	Use
Enzyme-linked immunosorbent assay (ELISA)	Enzyme-based	Antigen in some methods; antibody in others	Hormone testing
Enzyme-multiplied immunoassay technique (EIA, EMIT)	Enzyme-based	Antigen	Drug monitoring
Fluorescence-polarized immunoassay (FPIA)	Fluorescence-based	Antigen	Hormone testing
Fluorescent immunoassay (FIA)	Fluorescence-based	Antigen (fluorescence is proportional to concentration of analyte)	Catecholamine testing
Radioimmunoassay (RIA)	Radiation-based	Antigen	Hormone testing; drug monitoring
Immunoradiometric assay (IRMA)	Radiation-based	Antibody	Hormone testing; drug monitoring

stationary phase of the system (a solid or a liquid-coated solid). The **goal** of this technique is to produce **"fractions" for quantitation.**

1. **Mechanisms of separation** are based on the interactions of solutes with mobile and stationary phases.

   a. **Adsorption chromatography (liquid-solid chromatography)** is based on the competition between the sample and the mobile phase for binding sites on the solid (stationary) phase. Molecules that are most soluble in the mobile phase move fastest.

   b. **Partition chromatography (liquid-liquid)** depends on the solubility of the solute in nonpolar (organic) or polar (aqueous) solvents.

   c. **Ion-exchange chromatography** involves the separation of solutes by their size and the charge of the ionic species present. The stationary phase is a resin (can be cationic with free hydrogen ions or anionic with free hydroxyl ions present). Anion- and cation-exchange resins mixed together are used to deionize water.

2. **Chromatographic procedures**

   a. **Thin-layer chromatography (TLC)** is used as a **semi-quantitative** screening test. A layer of absorbent material is coated on a plate of glass, and spots of samples are applied. The solvent is placed in a container and migrates up the thin layer by capillary action. Separation is achieved by any of the previously discussed modes (see II C 1). Sample movement is compared with the standard, and **fractions are calculated using retention factor (R_f),** which is unique for specific compounds:

$$\text{Retention factor } (R_f) = \frac{\text{distance component moves}}{\text{total distance} - \text{distance solvent front moves}}$$

   b. High-performance liquid chromatography (HPLC) provides **quantitative** results. It is highly sensitive and specific. Apparatus consists of a pressure pump; a gel-filled column; a sample injector; a detector that monitors each component (e.g., spectrophotometers, amperometric detectors); and a recorder. Sample and solvent are pushed through the column, and the resulting eluent is read by the detector. The peaks that are detected and printed are specific and distinctive for each compound that is analyzed by HPLC.

   c. Gas chromatography (GC) separates mixtures of volatile compounds. It can have a solid or liquid stationary phase. The setup is very similar to HPLC, except the solvent is a gas, the sample is vaporized, and detectors are thermal conductivity or flame ionization. A special detector can be a **mass spectrometer (MS),** which measures the fragmentation patterns of ions (GCMS) and is used in drug identification. Gas chromatography is divided into two categories:

   (1) Gas–solid chromatography, in which the absorbent is a solid material

   (2) Gas–liquid chromatography (most common method used in clinical laboratories), in which the absorbing material is a liquid coated on a solid

III. BASIC ANATOMY AND PHYSIOLOGY

A. Kidney

1. **Renal structure** can be viewed both macroscopically and microscopically.

   a. The **macroscopic** structure of the kidney consists of the:

   (1) Cortex (outer layer of the kidney; filled with glomeruli)

   (2) Medulla (inner portion of the kidney; contains the duct system)

   (3) Pelvis (innermost portion of the kidney; contains ends of collecting ducts and empties into the ureter, which empties into the bladder)

   b. The **microscopic** structure of the kidney includes the **nephron,** which is considered to be the functional unit of the kidney and consists of the:

   (1) Glomerulus (made of arterioles surrounded by the distended end of a renal tubule in the renal cortex)

   (2) Proximal tubules (located in the cortex)

   (3) Henle's loop (descending and ascending limbs in the renal medulla)

   (4) Distal tubules (in the cortex)

   (5) Collecting tubules (collect urine from distal tubules to drain into the renal pelvis)

2. **Renal physiology** is based on the function of each microscopic component.

   a. Glomerular function is to strain proteins from the plasma and produce a "protein-free" filtrate that becomes urine.

   (1) The **glomerular filtration rate (GFR)** equals 125–130 mL protein-free fluid formed per minute.

   (2) Clearance indicates the number of milliliters of plasma from which the kidney can remove all of a given substance in 1 minute.

   (3) Plasma renal flow is the number of milliliters of plasma passing through the kidney in 1 minute; normal is 625 mL/min.

  b. **Tubular function** is to resorb certain substances back into the body. The **proximal tubule** resorbs 75% of water, sodium, much of glucose, amino acids, certain ions, and small molecules. Some substances have a maximum concentration in plasma, so the tubule cannot resorb it all. Excess substance spills over into urine (e.g., glucose). The proximal tubule allows for the elimination of urea and creatinine.

  c. The **Loop of Henle** adjusts urine osmolality to keep the urine watery.

  d. The **distal tubule** resorbs some salt, water, and bicarbonate, but eliminates uric acid, ammonia, and hydrogen ions. The distal tubule is under hormonal control.

  e. The **collecting ducts** are under hormonal control for resorption of water and sodium.

3. The **renal system functions** to maintain a balance of water, ions, and pH; to eliminate nonprotein nitrogens; and to synthesize certain hormones.

  a. **Water balance** is maintained by ingestion of water (controlled by the brain thirst center) and excretion/resorption of water in the renal tubules under hormonal control by antidiuretic hormone (ADH).

  b. **Ionic balance** of sodium, potassium, phosphate, calcium, and magnesium is maintained by tubule resorption under hormonal control (aldosterone). Chloride is passively resorbed with sodium.

  c. **Acid-base balance** is controlled by kidney conservation of bicarbonate ions and removal of metabolic acids (H^+) to conserve blood pH level.

  d. **Nonprotein nitrogen** (e.g., urea, creatinine, uric acid) is eliminated or filtered by the glomerulus. Some urea and uric acid is reabsorbed into the blood.

  e. The **kidneys synthesize three hormones.** In addition, the kidneys serve as a site for the hormonal action of aldosterone and ADH.

   (1) **Renin** is a vasoconstrictor synthesized in the renal medulla.

   (2) **Prostaglandins** are synthesized in the kidney and affect renal blood flow.

   (3) **Erythropoietin** increases heme production and iron insertion into red blood cells (RBCs) and is formed in conjunction with an enzyme made in the kidney.

4. **Renal system disorders** affect the glomerulus, the tubules, or other components of the system.

  a. **Glomerular diseases** affect portions of the glomerular structure.

   (1) **Glomerulonephritis** is related to group A β-hemolytic streptococcal infections. Immune complexes damage the structure of the glomerulus, leading to anemia, uremia, and edema.

   (2) **Nephrotic syndrome** refers to the increased permeability of the glomerular cell basement membrane, which leads to proteinuria and edema.

  b. **Tubular diseases** occur in all renal diseases as GFR falls and **affects acid-base balance.**

  c. **Urinary tract infections** are bacterial infections that produce bacteriuria and pyuria.

    d. Renal calculi (kidney stones) are deposits of calcium and uric acid that follow urinary tract infections and lead to hematuria.

    e. Renal failure can be acute or chronic in nature.

        (1) Acute renal failure is typically caused by cardiovascular system failure (prerenal), necrosis of the tubular system (renal), or obstruction of the lower urinary tract (postrenal). This condition leads to oliguria, proteinuria, and hematuria.

        (2) Chronic renal failure results from the chronic loss of excretory and regulatory functions. Causes vary from chronic glomerulonephritis to obstructive uropathy to renal vascular disease.

B. Liver

    1. Hepatic structure can be viewed both macroscopically and microscopically.

        a. The **macroscopic view** of the liver reveals a bilobed organ richly vascularized with two main supply vessels: the hepatic artery and the portal vein.

        b. The **microscopic** structural and functional unit of the liver is the **lobule,** which consists of:

            (1) Cords, or hepatocytes, that surround a central vein

            (2) Sinusoids consisting of blood spaces lined with endothelial cells and Kupffer's cells that surround the cords, which drain into a central vein

            (3) Bile canaliculi, or small channels between hepatocytes that carry bile formed by the hepatocytes to the bile ducts

    2. Hepatic physiology depends on the components of the liver.

        a. The **excretory/secretory function** serves to process substances that have been absorbed from the gut and then transferred to the blood for use by other cells of the body.

            (1) Bile is involved with processing of lipids. It is composed of bile acids, salts, pigments, and cholesterol. Bile salts are formed in the hepatocytes, excreted into the bile canaliculi, and stored in the gallbladder. Eventually, they are dumped into the duodenum to aid in the digestion of fats. Bile salts are then reabsorbed and re-excreted.

            (2) Bilirubin is the major bile pigment formed from the breakdown of hemoglobin when aged RBCs are phagocytized. The following steps occur: Hemoglobin is broken down into globin (reused) + iron (reused) + porphyrin (excreted) + biliverdin (reduced to bilirubin).

                (a) In the liver, bilirubin is conjugated (esterified) and becomes water soluble. This substance floats out of the bile canaliculi and into the gut, where it is eventually broken down to form **urobilinogen,** which is oxidized to produce urobilin and excreted in the stool.

                (b) Some urobilinogen is excreted by the kidney. There is some unconjugated bilirubin in the serum; increased bilirubin in the blood produces **jaundice.**

        b. Synthetic function. Albumin, alpha- and beta-globins, blood-clotting factors, glycogen, carbohydrates, fat, some lipids, ketones, and some enzymes are synthesized in the hepatocytes.

        c. Detoxification function. Hepatocytes have the capability to conjugate (and thus inactivate) a substance or to modify it chemically.

    d. Storage function. Iron, glycogen, amino acids, and some lipids are stored in hepatocytes.

  3. Hepatic disorders are conditions observed during a disease state.

    a. Jaundice, which causes yellowish discoloration of skin, is caused by abnormal bilirubin metabolism or by retention of bilirubin.

      (1) Prehepatic jaundice is the result of excessive bilirubin presented to the liver. It can occur in newborns and in people with hemolytic anemia or ineffective erythropoiesis. This condition produces increased serum unconjugated bilirubin.

      (2) Hepatic jaundice is present in people with hepatobiliary disease. This disorder exhibits increases in both unconjugated and conjugated bilirubin levels.

      (3) Posthepatic jaundice is produced by obstruction of the flow of bile into the gut either by gallstones or a tumor, which causes increased conjugated bilirubin levels in serum and urine but low urobilinogen levels in urine and colorless stool.

    b. Cirrhosis is defined as destruction of the liver's architecture. The leading cause of this condition is alcohol abuse.

    c. Reye's syndrome is liver destruction caused by viral infection, although the etiology of this disease is unknown. Ammonia accumulates in the liver and blood.

    d. Hepatitis is defined as inflammation of the liver and subsequent hepatocellular damage caused by bacterial infection, drugs, toxins, or viral infections. **Types of viral hepatitis** include:

      (1) Hepatitis A ("infectious" hepatitis), also known as hepatitis A virus (HAV), is transmitted by contamination of food and water.

      (2) Hepatitis B ("serum" hepatitis), or hepatitis B virus (HBV), has an outer coat called the HBV surface antigen (HBsAg) that covers the HBV core antigen (HBcAg). Hepatitis B is transmitted through parenteral injection or through exchange of bodily secretions, as occurs during sexual intercourse.

      (3) Hepatitis C (HCV) is a non-A, non-B hepatitis that is transmitted parenterally and is relatively rare.

      (4) Delta hepatitis can cause infection only in patients infected with hepatitis B.

C. Gastrointestinal (GI) tract. Anatomically, the GI tract is composed of five regions: the mouth, stomach, duodenum, jejunum-ileum, and large intestine.

  1. Gastric and GI functions are important to consider in the diagnosis of digestive disorders.

    a. Digestion is the chemical processing of food into an absorbable substance. It begins in the mouth and continues in the stomach and duodenum.

      (1) Gastric fluid in the stomach is composed of hydrochloric acid, pepsin, intrinsic factor, and mucus. The pH of this fluid is lower than 3.

        (a) Stimulation of gastric fluid secretion is induced by:

          (i) Brain-stomach connections that stimulate secretion in response to sight, smell, and taste of food

        (ii) Filling of stomach

        (iii) Contact of stomach lining with protein products

        (iv) The secretion of the hormone gastrin by gastric cells in response to stomach filling or to the sight, smell, or taste of food

    (b) **Inhibition of gastric fluid secretion** is caused by high gastric acidity and intestinal peptides.

  (2) **Intrinsic factor,** produced in the parietal cells of the stomach, is required for the transport of vitamin B_{12} across the intestinal wall.

b. **Absorption** is the process that allows digested food to enter the body. This process occurs in the small intestine.

2. **GI function tests** evaluate the level of function and determine the primary cause of malabsorption syndrome.

  a. **Gastric fluid analysis** serves to:

    (1) Determine pH of gastric fluid, with low pH (achlorhydria) indicative of pernicious anemia

    (2) Detect hypersecretion of gastric fluid caused by a secreting tumor (e.g., Zollinger-Ellison syndrome)

    (3) Check acid secretion in treatment of ulcers

    (4) Verify vagotomy (i.e., severing nerves to stomach for treatment of ulcers)

  b. **Lactose intolerance test** examines whether lactose is formed normally in gastric cells. The procedure involves ingestion of a lactose cocktail followed by glucose analysis. Little or no increase in serum glucose indicates lactase deficiency.

D. **The pancreas** is a highly vascularized organ connected to the small intestine by the ampulla of Vater. It is considered both an endocrine gland that synthesizes hormones and an exocrine gland that provides digestive enzymes to aid in digestion. The endocrine function is performed by cells in small groups called **islets of Langerhans.** The exocrine function is performed by cells surrounding the islets, called **acinar cells.**

1. **Pancreatic functions**

  a. **Endocrine function** is performed in the islets of Langerhans. These cell groups are composed of three types of cells.

    (1) **Alpha cells** produce **glucagon,** which stimulates the conversion of glycogen into glucose (glycogenolysis).

    (2) **Beta cells** are responsible for making **insulin,** which functions to promote glycogenesis and thereby lowers glucose levels.

    (3) **Delta cells** produce **gastrin** and **somatostatin.**

  b. **Exocrine function** is performed by the acinar cells. These cells produce the following enzymes.

    (1) **Amylase** breaks down starch and glycogen and is used to diagnose acute pancreatitis.

    (2) **Lipase** hydrolyzes fats to produce alcohols and fatty acids, with elevated levels present in people who have acute pancreatitis.

    (3) **Trypsin** is a proteolytic enzyme (functions in protein breakdown).

2. **Pancreatic disorders** typically result in decreased secretion of enzymes or hormones.

   a. **Cystic fibrosis** is a genetic disorder that leads to dysfunction of exocrine glands throughout the body, including the pancreas, liver, lungs, and salivary glands. This disorder is characterized by pulmonary disease and intestinal malabsorption caused by lack of pancreatic enzyme secretion.

   b. **Pancreatitis** (inflammation of the pancreas) is associated with alcohol abuse or gallbladder disease and also occurs in patients with lipid disorders. It can occur acutely or chronically. It is caused by the release of pancreatic enzymes from cells into the surrounding pancreatic tissue.

   c. **Diabetes mellitus** is most likely a genetic disorder that occurs when the pancreas can no longer produce insulin, which leads to hyperglycemia. This disorder almost always destroys the beta cells in the islets.

   d. **Pancreatic cancer** is a fatal disease that affects the ducts in the pancreas. Insulinoma is a tumor of the beta cells in the islets that leads to increased circulating insulin and hypoglycemia.

3. **Tests of exocrine pancreatic function**

   a. **Secretin test** determines the secretory capacity of the pancreas. It involves intubation and gathering of pancreatic fluid after stimulation with secretin, followed by measurement of fluid volume.

   b. **Quantitative fecal fat examination** determines the presence of increased fats in feces (steatorrhea), which is a disorder almost always associated with exocrine pancreatic insufficiency. A 72-hour fecal specimen is collected, and the fats extracted with ether and weighed. A screening procedure involves mixing a small amount of fecal specimen with a fat-soluble stain and examining the specimen microscopically for lipid droplets.

   c. **Sweat electrolytes** are measured to diagnose cystic fibrosis. Pilocarpine nitrate is used to stimulate sweating on skin, followed by analysis of the sweat for chloride and sodium content.

   d. **Enzyme testing** for amylase and lipase is performed using a variety of methodologies. These are listed in detail in section V.

IV. ANALYTES AND PATHOPHYSIOLOGY

A. **Amino acids** are defined as organic compounds containing both an amino (NH_2) group and a carboxyl (COO) group. Alpha-amino acids are present in proteins; they differ in their side chains, which give individual amino acids their special properties.

1. **Essential amino acids** must be supplied by dietary intake. These include valine, leucine, isoleucine, methionine, tryptophan, phenylalanine, threonine, lysine, and histidine.

2. **Ketoacids** are produced by removal of an amino group from an amino acid. Ketoacids can be either:

   a. **Glycogenic** to generate glucose precursors

   b. **Ketogenic** to generate ketone bodies

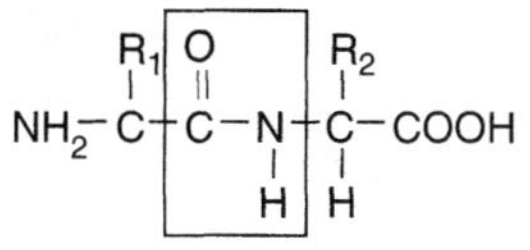

$$NH_2 - \overset{\overset{\displaystyle R_1}{|}}{C} - \overset{\overset{\displaystyle O}{\|}}{C} - \overset{}{\underset{\underset{\displaystyle H}{|}}{N}} - \overset{\overset{\displaystyle R_2}{|}}{\underset{\underset{\displaystyle H}{|}}{C}} - COOH$$

Figure 1-2. Peptide bond.

    3. Aminoacidopathies are disorders that involve faulty amino acid metabolism.

        a. Phenylketonuria (PKU) is an inherited disorder causing lack of phenylalanine hydroxylase and the inability to convert phenylalanine to tyrosine, which results in the formation of phenylpyruvate. PKU causes mental retardation in children.

        b. Maple syrup urine disease (MSUD) is a disorder of decarboxylation of the ketoacids of leucine, isoleucine, and valine, which results in accumulation of ketoacids in blood, urine, and spinal fluid. MSUD causes mental retardation or death in infants.

        c. Homocystinuria is caused by impaired enzyme activity, which results in elevated levels of homocysteine and methionine in plasma and urine.

B. Proteins are macromolecules composed of covalently linked polymers of amino acids linked by **peptide bonds** in a head-to-tail fashion (Figure 1-2). Proteins are composed of carbon, oxygen, hydrogen, nitrogen, and sulfur.

    1. Structure. The principal **plasma proteins** include albumin and the globulins. Other protein fractions include fibrinogen and complement.

        a. Albumin is responsible for the osmotic pressure of plasma and serves as a transport protein. **Prealbumin** migrates ahead of albumin during electrophoresis and transports thyroid hormones.

        b. The **globulins** are insoluble in water. There are several globulin fractions, based on their electrophoretic mobility. These include:

            (1) Alpha$_1$-globulins (α_1-fetoprotein, α_1-antitrypsin)

            (2) Alpha$_2$-globulins (haptoglobin, ceruloplasmin, and α_2-macroglobulin)

            (3) Beta-globulins (transferrin, C-reactive protein)

            (4) Gamma-globulins [immunoglobulins (Ig) G,A,M,D,E]

    2. Synthesis. Proteins are synthesized in the liver (serum proteins) or by plasma cells (immunoglobulins). Protein formation is specified by the DNA in each type of cell (hepatic or plasma).

    3. Protein catabolism takes place in the gastrointestinal tract, kidneys, and liver. Protein disintegrates into constituent amino acids, which are further deaminated into ketoacids and ammonia. Ammonia is used in the formation of urea.

    4. Classification. Proteins are classified as simple or conjugated.

        a. Simple proteins are peptide chains that hydrolyze to amino acids.

        b. Conjugated proteins are composed of protein (apoprotein) and a nonprotein substance, such as lipid (forms lipoproteins), carbohydrate (forms glycoproteins), or metals (form metalloproteins).

5. **Functions** of protein include tissue nutrition, water distribution, plasma buffer, substance transport, and structural support.

6. **Protein analysis** determines either the total nitrogen content of the sample or the total protein. The normal reference range of serum protein is 6.5–8.3 g/dL.

   a. **Total nitrogen determination** analyzes both protein and nonprotein nitrogen.

   b. **Kjeldahl's method** involves the conversion of protein nitrogen into ammonium ion. This classic method is not practical for routine use.

   c. **Refractometry** methods use the refractive index of a solution in the determination of solute concentration.

      (1) The **principle** states that the velocity of light changes when it passes between air and water, causing light to bend (refract). Therefore, the refractive index of water increases proportionally to the concentration of a solute in solution.

      (2) The solutes present in greatest concentration in serum are proteins. Therefore, this method provides an approximation useful as a rapid test, but error can occur in patients with hyperglycemia, lipemia, or azotemia.

   d. The **biuret method** is the most widely used method of protein determination. Analysis depends on the presence of peptide bonds.

      (1) The **principle** states that cupric (Cu^{2+}) ions react with peptide bonds to form a violet color proportional to the number of peptide bonds present.

      (2) This method is widely used and easily automated.

   e. The **dye-binding method** is based on the ability of proteins to bind dyes.

      (1) The **principle** of this method is that dye binds to protonated amine groups of amino acids, with absorption at 595 nm.

      (2) Dye-binding methods are used chiefly for **albumin analysis.** When albumin is positively charged, it binds to certain dyes, causing a shift in absorbance from free dye. **Brom-cresol green** is the most widely used dye, although **brom-cresol purple** is considered more specific in binding albumin.

   f. **UV absorption** is based on absorption of UV light by peptide bonds at 210 and 280 nm.

   g. **Serum protein electrophoresis (SPE)** relies on the separation of proteins based on their net electrical charges, size, properties of the support medium, and temperature of operation. Different disease states produce different electrophoretic patterns. This is a semi-quantitative method.

      (1) The **principle** of SPE states that when an electric field is applied to a medium containing charged particles, the negatively charged particles migrate toward the positive electrode (anode), and the positively charged particles migrate toward the cathode. At pH 8.6, most serum proteins have a negative charge. This separates the protein fractions in serum when an electrical field is applied.

      (2) On the support medium (cellulose acetate or agarose gel), the **pattern of migration** is as follows: Albumin is most anodic (because of its

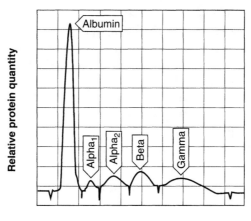

Figure 1-3. Normal serum protein electrophoretic pattern.

small size and large number of negative charges), then α_1-globulins, α_2-globulins, β-globulins; γ-globulins are most cathodic (Figure 1-3).

h. Radial immunodiffusion (RID) is a quantitative method of immunoglobulin determination.

    (1) The **principle** of RID states that an agarose gel is saturated with a specific antibody solution. Antigen (serum) is applied and diffuses radially into the medium. At the point where antigen and antibody concentration are equal, a precipitin ring forms. Measurement of the diameter of the precipitin ring squared is compared with a standard curve of antigen concentration.

    (2) RID is also referred to as the **Mancini technique.**

i. Nephelometry is used as a quantitative method for immunoglobulin analysis.

    (1) The **principle** states that immunoglobulins react with a specific antibody to produce an immunoprecipitate. Forward light scatter is measured.

    (2) Nephelometry is used for protein analysis of all body fluids.

j. Immunofixation electrophoresis (IFE) is a qualitative method for evaluation of immunoglobulins.

    (1) The **principle** of IFE states that proteins are electrophoresed into five zones as in SPE. Then, monospecific antiserum is added, and the support medium is stained for visual interpretation of bands.

    (2) IFE is used to analyze protein concentration in serum, urine, and other fluids.

k. Immunoelectrophoresis (IEP) is a qualitative method for the evaluation of immunoglobulins.

    (1) The **principle** of IEP states that proteins are electrophoresed into five zones similar to SPE, then antibody is added to produce precipitin arcs that are visually interpreted.

    (2) IEP is used to analyze serum, cerebrospinal fluid (CSF), and urine.

l. Other methods

(1) **Urinary proteins** are analyzed by:

(a) **Qualitative dipstick tests** for proteinuria, glycosuria, and other abnormal substances in the urine that rely on color change for interpretation.

(b) **Quantitative turbidimetric methods** require that a protein precipitant is added to urine. The resulting turbidity is measured photometrically.

7. **Protein disorders** are the result of high or low serum protein levels or a dysfunction of the immunoglobulins.

a. **Hypoproteinemia** can be caused by kidney disease, blood loss, malnutrition, and liver disease.

b. **Hyperproteinemia** is observed in people with dehydration or excess production of gamma globulins.

c. **Decreased serum albumin** is caused by a variety of disorders, including poor diet, liver dysfunction, GI inflammation, and renal disease.

d. **Specific globulin disorders** include the following:

(1) **Alpha$_1$-antitrypsin deficiency** is caused by pulmonary disease, and increased levels are caused by inflammation or pregnancy.

(2) **Elevated levels of α_1-fetoprotein** during pregnancy may indicate neural tube defects, spina bifida in the fetus, or twins. Very high levels are found in individuals with liver cancer. Decreased levels during pregnancy indicate a risk of fetal Down syndrome.

(3) **Haptoglobin,** an α_2-macroglobulin, is increased in inflammatory conditions, burns, and rheumatic disease. Decreased levels are seen in people with transfusion reactions or hemolytic disease.

(4) **Ceruloplasmin,** an α_2-macroglobulin, is decreased in people with Wilson's disease and malnutritive states.

(5) **Transferrin** levels are increased during iron deficiency anemia.

(6) **Immunoglobulin** increases indicate infection, liver disease, Waldenström's macroglobulinemia (IgM), multiple myeloma, or autoimmune reactions. These increases appear as a spike, either monoclonal or polyclonal, in the gamma region of SPE.

C. **Acid-base balance** assures the maintenance of a constant blood pH (7.4) through physiologic buffers, the respiratory system, and the renal system.

1. **Buffer systems** protect the body against changes in hydrogen ion concentration. Three physiologic buffers act to maintain a constant pH:

a. **The carbonic acid-bicarbonate** system

b. **Hemoglobin**

c. **The phosphoric acid-phosphate** system

2. **The respiratory system** acts to maintain acid-base balance. Oxygen is removed from oxyhemoglobin in the tissues. This allows for the acceptance of hydrogen ions, forming carboxyhemoglobin. In the lungs, carboxyhemoglobin recombines with bicarbonate to form carbonic acid, which breaks down to form carbon dioxide and water. The carbon dioxide is then expired by

respiration. Thus, **ventilation affects the pH of the blood;** this system is called the **"respiratory" component of acid-base balance.**

3. **The renal system** controls **bicarbonate concentration.** The overall reaction results in the reabsorption of sodium and bicarbonate in the kidney tubules. These substances pick up excess hydrogen ions. This system is called the **"nonrespiratory" or "metabolic" component of acid-base balance.**

4. Acid-base disorders are considered in terms of the **Henderson-Hasselbalch equation,** which states acid-base relationships:

$$pH = pK + \log \left(\frac{cA}{cHA} \right)$$

where A is the proton acceptor (base) and HA is the proton donor (acid).

5. **Blood gas analyzers** determine acid-base balance through the measurement of partial pressure of oxygen, carbon dioxide, and pH. Analyzers use electrodes as sensing devices, and bicarbonate and other parameters are calculated from the previously mentioned measurements using the Henderson-Hasselbalch equation. Oxygen saturation is calculated as well. Analyzers typically measure arterial blood gases (ABG).

   a. **pO_2 is measured amperometrically.** Oxygen diffuses across an electrode tip through an electrolyte solution to the cathode at a rate that is directly proportional to the amount of oxygen present.

   b. **pCO_2 is measured potentiometrically.** Carbon dioxide diffuses across a membrane through bicarbonate buffer, eventually forming hydrogen ions that are measured by an electrode.

   c. **pH is measured by a typical pH electrode.** Hydrogen ions diffuse into a glass membrane, developing a potential that is proportional to the difference in the concentration of hydrogen ions between the sample and the buffer within the electrode.

   d. **Bicarbonate values are calculated using the Henderson-Hasselbalch equation.**

   e. **Oxygen saturation** is the percentage of total hemoglobin that has bound oxygen and **is calculated from pO_2 and pH measurements.**

   f. **Specimen requirements** for blood gas analysis include the following.
      (1) **Arterial blood** is collected in a glass or plastic syringe. Capillary specimens can also be used (blood must be "arterialized").
      (2) **Lyophilized or liquid heparin** is the preferred anticoagulant.
      (3) **No air bubbles** should exist in the sample because they lower the pCO_2 value.
      (4) **The specimen must be placed on ice** and transported to the laboratory in 15 minutes at 4°C and tested immediately. Otherwise, pH values decrease, and pCO_2 values increase.
      (5) **Blood clots are unacceptable.**

6. **Acid-base disorders** are classified according to their cause. Compensation occurs when pH becomes abnormal.

    a. Respiratory acidosis results from hypoventilation, which causes a decrease in carbon dioxide elimination. Compensation occurs by the kidneys increasing the resorption of bicarbonate.

    b. Respiratory alkalosis results from an increase in ventilation, resulting in excessive elimination of carbon dioxide. Compensation occurs by the kidneys excreting more bicarbonate.

    c. Nonrespiratory acidosis occurs in many disorders and results in a decrease in bicarbonate levels. The lungs compensate by hyperventilating.

    d. Nonrespiratory alkalosis is produced in many disorders and results in an increase in bicarbonate levels. The lungs compensate by hypoventilation.

7. The clinical significance of blood gas levels is as follows.

    a. pCO_2 levels increase with administration of 100% oxygen or following exercise. Decreases (hypoxemia) indicate pulmonary difficulties, exposure to carbon monoxide, or improper anesthesia. Hypoxemia also may occur at high altitudes.

    b. pCO_2 levels increase with respiratory acidosis. Decreased levels indicate respiration that is too rapid.

D. Electrolytes are ions capable of carrying an electric charge. They can be either anions (negatively charged) or cations (positively charged).

1. Sodium is the most abundant extracellular cation. It contributes to the osmolality of extracellular fluid and maintains cell size and shape. Sodium is essential for transmitting nerve impulses.

    a. Regulation of sodium is performed by the renal system in two ways.

        (1) The renin-ADH system. Low blood volume (as in cardiac failure) induces secretion of renin, a vasoconstrictor, from the kidney, which raises blood pressure and causes production of ADH. In turn, fluid volume is increased by the retention of sodium.

        (2) The renin-aldosterone system. Low blood volume induces secretion of renin, which induces production of aldosterone by the adrenal glands. In turn, kidney reabsorption of sodium and retention of water increase.

    b. Sodium disorders

        (1) Hyponatremia is low serum sodium caused by gastrointestinal loss, burns, or renal problems. Dilutional hyponatremia is a relative decrease of sodium caused by excess body water, as in nephrosis or cirrhosis.

        (2) Hypernatremia is increased sodium caused by excess water loss, as in sweating or diarrhea.

2. Potassium is the major intracellular cation that regulates activity at the neuromuscular junction, as well as cardiac muscle contraction and pH.

    a. Regulation of potassium occurs in two ways:

        (1) Dietary intake, which controls the amount of potassium in the circulation

      (2) The renal system, which controls potassium by:

        (a) Aldosterone induces potassium reabsorption and secretion by the renal tubules by exchanging it for sodium.

        (b) A high concentration of hydrogen ions keeps potassium out of cells and induces its renal retention. Low hydrogen ion concentration allows more potassium ions to enter cells, which lowers serum potassium. Low hydrogen ion concentration also allows more potassium to be excreted by the kidney.

  b. Potassium disorders include:

    (1) Hypokalemia (low serum potassium), which is a result of decreased dietary intake, gastrointestinal loss, or renal dysfunction, can produce irregular heartbeat.

    (2) Hyperkalemia (high serum potassium) is rare. It occurs following excessive dietary intake, adrenal failure, blood transfusions, or crush injuries.

3. Chloride is the major extracellular anion that acts to maintain osmotic pressure, keeps the body hydrated, and maintains electric neutrality via interaction with sodium or carbon dioxide.

  a. Regulation of chloride depends on dietary intake, sodium concentration, and the chloride shift, which moves chloride into RBCs as bicarbonate diffuses out to electroneutrality.

  b. Chloride disorders include:

    (1) Hypochloremia (low serum chloride) is caused by salt loss during renal disease, diabetic ketoacidosis, or prolonged vomiting.

    (2) Hyperchloremia (elevated serum chloride) is caused by dehydration, acute renal failure, prolonged diarrhea with loss of sodium bicarbonate, and salicylate intoxication.

4. Bicarbonate is the second most abundant anion in the extracellular fluid. It is a major component of the blood buffering system, accounts for 90% of total blood carbon dioxide, and maintains charge neutrality in the cell.

  a. Regulation of bicarbonate is achieved by the kidneys, which are responsible for reabsorbing all bicarbonate as carbon dioxide.

  b. Bicarbonate (or total carbon dioxide) disorders include decreased levels observed during metabolic acidosis, renal failure, or diarrhea, and elevated levels due to carbon dioxide retention, as is observed during respiratory acidosis.

5. Primary methods of electrolyte determination include:

  a. Ion-selective electrodes that use a semipermeable membrane to develop a potential between two different ion concentrations

  b. Amperometric-coulometric titration for chloride determination, in which silver ions are combined with chloride; when excess free silver ions are noted, elapsed time is relative to the chloride concentration

  c. Atomic absorption spectrophotometry

6. Anion gap is the difference between unmeasured anions and unmeasured cations. The normal reference range for the anion gap is 6–18 mmol or mEq/L. It is useful in determining increases in unmeasured anions and is calculated as follows:

$$\textbf{Anion gap} = (\textbf{Na}^+ + \textbf{K}^+) - (\textbf{Cl}^- + \textbf{HCO}_3^-)$$

E. Nonprotein nitrogen measurements monitor and assess renal function. These substances arise from the breakdown of proteins and nucleic acids.

1. **Urea** is the major excretory product of protein metabolism and is synthesized in the liver from carbon dioxide and ammonia arising from the deamination of amino acids. It is excreted by the kidney.

   a. All **analytic methods** include, in the initial step, the hydrolysis of urea by urease and subsequent production of ammonium. Most techniques are sensitive to excess ammonia contamination.

      (1) The **coupled enzymatic assay** is a kinetic assay that involves a second enzyme.

      (2) A **pH indicator dye** detects the presence of ammonium and causes a color change, which is read by a spectrophotometer.

      (3) The **direct method** does not use urease. It measures urea directly using diacetyl monoxime.

   b. **Urea disorders** typically involve an elevated level of urea in blood, referred to as azotemia. Disorders are named in association with the location of the dysfunction.

      (1) **Prerenal azotemia** is typically caused by decreased renal blood flow to the kidneys from congestive heart failure, shock, dehydration, decrease in blood volume, greater protein breakdown (as in major illness), or high-protein diet.

      (2) **Renal azotemia** is produced by renal failure.

      (3) **Postrenal azotemia** is caused by an obstruction anywhere in the renal system (e.g., tubules, ureter).

      (4) **Uremia** is a toxic condition involving a very high serum level of urea accompanied by renal failure.

2. **Creatine** is made in the liver from amino acids and used in muscle as an energy source. In its anhydrous state, it is called **creatinine**, which is excreted into the plasma in an amount proportional to muscle mass and then excreted in the urine. Because the level of creatinine is unaffected by diet, its level reflects the GFR.

   a. **Analytic methods** for creatinine

      (1) The **Jaffé reaction** involves the reaction of creatinine with picric acid to form a reddish chromagen. The absorbance is measured colorimetrically.

      (2) The **kinetic reaction** uses various enzymes and hydrogen peroxide to form a colored product.

      (3) **Creatinine clearance** is an estimate of the GFR obtained by measuring plasma creatinine and its rate of excretion into urine. This test requires a 24-hour urine specimen and blood sample for serum creatinine determination. The formula for calculation is:

$$\frac{\text{UV}}{\text{P}} \times \frac{1.73}{\text{A}}$$

with urinary creatinine as U (mg/L), V as volume of urine (mL/min), P as plasma creatinine (mg/L), and $\dfrac{1.73}{A}$ as normalization factor for body surface area.

    b. Abnormal creatinine levels are typically elevated because of abnormal renal function, such as reduced GFR. Creatinine levels are examined in conjunction with urea to determine the cause of azotemia. The normal blood urea nitrogen (BUN):creatinine ratio is 10 to 20:1. Higher ratios indicate that the elevation of BUN is caused by prerenal rather than renal causes.

3. Uric acid is synthesized in the liver from the breakdown of nucleic acids (DNA and RNA) and transported to the kidney for resorption.

    a. Analytic methods are based on the same initial reaction involving the oxidation of uric acid by uricase to allantoin and hydrogen peroxide. There are two **coupled enzymatic methods** that involve either:

        (1) The measurement of peroxide production following reaction with phenol and 4-amino phenazone (4-AP)

        (2) The measurement of peroxide production by the catalyzed oxidation of ethanol coupled to the production of acetate

    b. Abnormal uric acid levels are either:

        (1) Elevated because of gout; increased nuclear breakdown (due to increased cell destruction, as in chemotherapy); renal disease; or toxemia of pregnancy

        (2) Decreased primarily because of severe liver or kidney disease

4. Ammonia is formed by the deamination of amino acids. It is used by the liver to produce urea and is not excreted by the kidney.

    a. Analytic methods include:

        (1) The **coupled enzymatic method,** in which ammonium reacts with alpha-ketoglutarate and reduced nicotinamide adenine dinucleotide phosphate (NADPH) to form L-glutamate and nicotinamide adenine dinucleotide phosphate (NADP), with changes in absorbance measured spectrophotometrically

        (2) The **ammonia electrode,** which is based on diffusion of NH_3 through a selective membrane

    b. Increased ammonia levels are typically caused by severe liver dysfunction (e.g., Reye's syndrome) or inadequate blood circulation through the liver.

F. Carbohydrates are polyhydroxyl aldehydes or ketones that, on hydrolysis, yield one of these compounds. Carbohydrates are a **major source of energy for the body,** and starch is the major source of carbohydrate.

    1. Classification is based on the structure of carbohydrates.

        a. Monosaccharides are simple sugars that contain 4–8 carbons and only one aldehyde or ketone group. These are **reducing sugars** (i.e., they can give up electrons). Examples include glucose and fructose.

b. **Oligosaccharides** are formed by the interaction of two monosaccharides with the loss of a water molecule and are sometimes referred to as **disaccharides.** Examples include maltose, lactose, and sucrose.

c. **Polysaccharides** are formed by interactions between many units of simple sugars. Examples are starch and glycogen.

2. **Carbohydrate metabolism** begins in the mouth.

a. **Salivary amylase** breaks down ingested starches into disaccharides, and these are further broken down into monosaccharides by disaccharides and absorbed into intestinal cells.

b. Monosaccharides are then transported to the liver and converted to glucose. Some glucose is released into the blood, and the rest is stored as glycogen in the liver and skeletal muscle.

c. **Glycogenesis** is the process of glycogen formation by enzyme action on glucose to eventually form glycogen.

d. **Glycogenolysis** is the breakdown of glycogen, with the eventual formation of glucose-6-phosphate or free glucose that can be used for energy production.

e. **Glycolysis** is the catabolism of glucose to pyruvate or lactate for adenosine triphosphate (ATP) production (Embden-Meyerhof pathway and Krebs' cycle).

f. **Gluconeogenesis** is the formation of glucose from amino acids and lipids that occurs when carbohydrate intake decreases.

3. **Factors that affect glucose levels** include:

a. **Insulin,** which is a pancreatic hormone that decreases glucose levels by increasing cellular uptake of glucose and promoting glycogenesis and lipogenesis (formation of fat from carbohydrates)

b. **Glucagon,** which is a pancreatic hormone that increases glucose levels by stimulating glycogenolysis and gluconeogenesis

c. **Epinephrine,** which is an adrenal hormone that elevates glucose levels

d. **Growth hormone and adrenocorticotropic hormone (ACTH),** which are pituitary hormones that increase glucose levels

e. **Glucocorticoids** (e.g., cortisol), which are adrenal hormones that increase gluconeogenesis and eventually elevate blood glucose

f. **Thyroid hormones,** which stimulate glycogenolysis and increase blood glucose levels

4. **Glucose disorders** depend on serum glucose levels.

a. **Hyperglycemia** occurs when the fasting blood sugar level rises higher than 110 mg/dL due to a pathologic disorder, such as diabetes mellitus or liver failure.

b. **Hypoglycemia** occurs when the fasting blood glucose level is lower than 70 mg/dL. This typically occurs as a result of hormone deficiency, drug reaction, insulin excess (as in insulinoma), or a genetic disorder.

c. **Glycosuria** (sugar in the urine) occurs when the renal threshold for glucose is exceeded (160–180 mg/dL) during hyperglycemia.

    d. Diabetes mellitus is a genetic disorder of glucose metabolism that results in insulin deficiency and lack of carbohydrate tolerance. There are **two classifications:**

        (1) Type 1, insulin-dependent diabetes mellitus. The patient presents in an acute state with hyperglycemia and ketosis. This type is caused by an autoimmune destruction of pancreatic beta cells and is usually **juvenile onset.**

        (2) Type 2, non–insulin-dependent diabetes mellitus. The patient has a level of insulin that is too low to maintain normal blood glucose levels. Most patients are obese, and onset is typically during adulthood.

5. Methods of glucose analysis include:

    a. Glucose oxidase methods. Glucose is oxidized to gluconic acid and hydrogen peroxide to eventually form a colored product. Falsely low results are caused by high serum levels of uric acid, bilirubin, or ascorbic acid.

    b. Hexokinase methods. Glucose becomes phosphorylated and dehydrogenated to eventually form NADPH.

    c. o-Toluidine (nonenzymatic method). o-Toluidine reacts with glucose in acetic acid to form a colored product. Falsely elevated glucose values are obtained by interference of mannose and galactose, whereas bilirubin induces a false decrease in glucose values.

    d. Glycosylated hemoglobin methods. The presence of glycosylated hemoglobins is examined in diabetic patients. This test examines a patient's compliance with an insulin therapy regimen over a period of 8–10 weeks.

6. Glucose metabolism tests examine a patient's ability to metabolize glucose.

    a. Glucose tolerance test (GTT) evaluates the insulin response challenge. It is useful in evaluating pregnancy-induced diabetes and involves drawing a fasting blood specimen, followed by patient ingestion of a 75-g oral dose of glucose in liquid within a 5-minute period. Blood samples are then taken at 30-, 60-, 120-, and 180-minute intervals and tested for glucose. Urine is tested as well.

        (1) Nondiabetics have negative urine tests and show highest glucose levels at 30–60 minutes, with low and normal levels following.

        (2) Severe diabetics reach peak glucose levels after 30–60 minutes, and the levels remain elevated.

    b. A 2-hour postprandial blood glucose test evaluates diabetes. A fasting blood specimen and a specimen taken 2 hours after breakfast are taken. Normal patients have no increase in serum glucose after 2 hours.

G. Lipids are substances that are insoluble in water and can be extracted from cells only by organic solvents (e.g., ether or chloroform). Lipids include fats (most abundant), steroids, and terpenes. Fats are carboxylic esters derived from glycerol and are also known as glycerides.

1. Lipid composition of food

    a. Triglycerides comprise 98% of fat found in food and are made up of 95% fatty acid and 5% glycerol. Fatty acids are long carbon chains joined by single (saturated) or double bonds (unsaturated) and a terminal carboxyl group.

b. The remaining 2% of fat in food is composed of cholesterol, phospholipids, diglycerides, fat-soluble vitamins, steroids, and terpenes.

2. The physiology of lipids involves three phases.

   a. Digestive phase begins with chewing and swallowing. Triglycerides are digested by lipase, other enzymes, bile salts, and acid in the gut to form monoglycerides and diglycerides. Cholesterol becomes surrounded by bile to form a micelle package that is absorbed by the small intestine.

   b. Absorptive phase occurs in the small intestine as triglycerides and cholesterol in the micelles are absorbed and broken down into fatty acids.

   c. Transport phase occurs as long fatty acids reassemble into chylomicrons (water-soluble macromolecules) and enter the lymphatic system. Short fatty acids enter the blood bound to albumin, and these head to all tissues, including adipose tissue.

3. Specific lipid physiology determines the function of each lipid.

   a. Cholesterol is a sterol (steroid with long side chains), which is a four-ringed structure made in liver hepatocytes from two acetate units. The process is long, and 3-hydroxy-3-methylglutaryl coenzyme A (HMG-CoA) reductase is the committed step. Cholesterol is an important constituent of cell membranes and a precursor of many hormones. Most serum cholesterol is in the form of cholesterol esters, which are **transported through the blood by low-density lipoproteins (LDL)** and **high-density lipoproteins (HDL).**

   b. Triglyceride is made up of fatty acids and glycerol and is partly synthesized in the liver hepatocyte. It is **transported through the bloodstream by chylomicrons** and **very low-density lipoproteins (VLDLs).** Triglyceride provides energy to cells as it loses its fatty acid and forms ATP, thus acting as an energy store in the form of fat, and it insulates organs through fat deposits.

   c. Phospholipids make up the bilayer of cell membranes and also form a coating that surrounds cholesterol and triglyceride and "glues" them to the lipoprotein core.

   d. Sphingolipids are important in cell membrane composition and in nerve transmission.

4. Lipoproteins are transport vehicles for lipids that contain varying amounts of specific lipid, phospholipid, and apoprotein.

   a. Chylomicrons are large molecules that contain mostly triglyceride. They originate in the intestinal tract and travel through the blood and lymph to various tissues. They are degraded in the liver.

   b. VLDLs are smaller than chylomicrons. They contain mostly endogenous triglyceride, are made in the liver, contain equal amounts of phospholipids and cholesterol, and degrade to LDLs in the circulation.

   c. LDLs contain mostly cholesterol, with equal amounts of phospholipid and protein and some triglyceride. They are taken into cells via a special cell-

Table 1-3.   Fredrickson's Classification of Hyperlipoproteinemias

Type	Plasma Appearance	Cholesterol Level	Triglyceride Level	Lipoprotein Abnormality
I (rare)	Creamy	↔, ↑	↑ ↑ ↑	High chylomicrons
IIA (common)	Clear	↑ ↑ ↑	↔	High LDL
IIB (common)	Clear	↑ ↑ ↑	↑	High LDL, VLDL
III (rare)	Cloudy	↑ ↑	↑ ↑	Abnormal LDL, VLDL
IV (common)	Milky	↔, ↑	↑ ↑ ↑	High VLDL
V (rare)	Creamy; Milky	↑	↑ ↑	High chylomicrons, VLDL

↑ = slight increase; ↑ ↑ = moderate increase; ↑ ↑ ↑ = extreme increase; ↔ = no change; LDL = low-density lipoproteins; VLDL = very low-density lipoproteins.

surface receptor—the apoprotein B (apoB) receptor—and are degraded into component parts. This is considered **"bad"** cholesterol.

    d. HDLs contain mostly protein, some cholesterol, and a little triglyceride. They are made in the liver, and they remove excess cholesterol from cells. HDL is considered the **"good"** lipoprotein.

  5. Lipid disorders usually lead to abnormal lipid deposits on walls of vasculature (**atherosclerosis**) and skin (**xanthomas**). Hyperlipidemia obstruction leads to lack of bile, so cholesterol cannot be adequately absorbed by the small intestine.

    a. Hyperlipidemia

      (1) Triglyceride levels are most affected by diet, but high triglyceride levels are often caused by diabetes or pancreatitis. Lipoprotein lipase (LPL), present in the capillary wall, hydrolyzes triglycerides for use in the tissues and can be affected by various hormones. If LPL does not function properly, serum triglyceride levels rise.

      (2) Cholesterol levels are affected mostly by genetic defects in the liver or by lack of apoB receptors on cell surfaces, which leads to elevated cholesterol levels.

    b. Hyperlipoproteinemia involves an increase in certain lipoproteins because of improper synthesis or breakdown of lipoprotein fractions. Hyperlipidemia can also induce overproduction of the lipoproteins. **Fredrickson's classification Types I to V** (Table 1-3) is based on the appearance of plasma after 24 hours at 4°C and on triglyceride and cholesterol values.

    c. Hypolipoproteinemia is caused by a genetic defect leading to absent or decreased LDL and HDL.

      (1) Absent LDL and low serum cholesterol leads to a failure to thrive, steatorrhea, central nervous system degeneration, and malabsorption of fat and vitamins.

(2) **Decreased LDL** leads to an increased life expectancy and decreased risk of myocardial infarction.

(3) **Reduced HDL** leads to an increased risk of atherosclerosis.

(4) **Absent HDL** (Tangier disease) leads to an accumulation of cholesterol esters in tonsils, adenoids, and spleen. It is considered a benign disease.

6. **Methods of lipid analysis**

   a. **Total cholesterol analysis** involves either:

      (1) **Formation of free cholesterol,** which is oxidized to form hydrogen peroxide, which then reacts with a dye to form a colored product

      (2) **Selective oxygen electrode,** which measures the rate of oxygen consumption when an enzyme specific for cholesterol is added to serum

   b. **HDL cholesterol analysis** involves precipitation of LDL and VLDL, followed by measurement of HDL in the supernatant.

   c. **LDL cholesterol analysis** involves one of the following:

      (1) **Calculation** by the following formula:

      $$\text{LDL} = \text{total cholesterol} - \left(\frac{\text{HDL} + \text{triglyceride}}{5}\right)$$

      (2) **Ultracentrifugation**

      (3) **Immunoseparation** using an ag–ab reaction

   d. **Triglyceride analysis** uses either an:

      (1) **Enzymatic method** that involves three enzymes—lipase, glycerol kinase, and glucose-6-phosphate-dehydrogenase (G6PD)—to form NADH

      (2) **Colorimetric method** involving the formation of hydrogen peroxide

H. **Vitamins** are organic molecules required by the body in small amounts for normal metabolism. Most are obtained from the diet; some are formed endogenously; others are produced by the intestine.

   1. **Fat-soluble vitamins** include A, D, E, and K.

      a. **Vitamin A** has various forms: retinal, retinol, and retinoic acid. Most carotenoids found in vegetables are precursors of vitamin A. Most vitamin A is stored in the liver, and some is transferred to cells to promote mRNA synthesis. The best understood physiology of vitamin A is in the **visual system;** a lack of vitamin A leads to night blindness.

      b. **Vitamin D** is a sterol derivative known as **cholecalciferol.** It is produced in the skin by absorption of UV light or obtained by dietary intake and stored in adipose tissue. Vitamin D is essential for **bone mineralization and neuromuscular activity,** and some forms act to regulate uptake of calcium and phosphate. Lack of vitamin D leads to rickets (failure of bones to calcify) or osteomalacia (abnormal bone synthesis).

      c. **Vitamin E (alpha-tocopherol)** is available only from dietary intake and accumulates in the liver, adipose tissue, and muscle. Vitamin E is critical for **normal neurologic structure and function,** and also functions as an **antioxidant** by preventing formation of free radicals. A deficiency of vitamin E produces a normocytic normochromic anemia.

  d. **Vitamin K** is supplied partly by diet and partly by flora in the bowel. Vitamin K is known as **phylloquinone** and is essential in the formation of **coagulation** factors, particularly prothrombin (see Chapter 2, III D).

 2. **Water-soluble vitamins** include vitamin C and the vitamin B complex.

  a. **Vitamin C (ascorbic acid)** is absorbed in the stomach and distributed to all tissues. It is a **potent reducing agent,** functions in the **synthesis of collagen,** and aids in the biosynthesis of some neurotransmitters. It is considered important in reducing the risk of certain cancers and the common cold.

  b. **The B complex vitamins** are grouped together because of their isolation from the same sources. Most B vitamins are known to serve as **enzyme cofactors,** functioning to transport atoms between molecules in enzyme-coupled reactions. Deficiency of any B vitamin affects the body's metabolism. The B vitamins include **thiamine, riboflavin, niacin, pantothenic acid, biotin, pyridoxine (B_6), the folates,** and **cyanocobalamin (B_{12}).** Lack of vitamin B_{12} produces pernicious anemia because of its function in erythropoiesis. Deficient folate leads to a megaloblastic anemia, and in pregnant women, the possibility of fetal neural tube defects.

I. Tumor markers are substances that are synthesized and released by cancer cells or made by other tissues in response to the presence of cancer cells. These markers may be present in the blood, in other fluids, on cells, or within cells.

 1. **Clinically relevant (diagnostically accessible) tumor markers** must have high disease sensitivity and specificity, and levels should reflect the status of the disease process. These analytes are typically examined by some form of immunoassay.

  a. **Oncofetal antigens** exist as normal proteins in the embryo and fetus and are also found in certain tumors.

   (1) **Carcinoembryonic antigen (CEA)** is an oncofetal antigen used to assess tumors of the colon. It is not as specific as once thought, and not all colon cancers have elevated CEA levels.

   (2) **Alpha-fetoprotein (AFP)** is an oncofetal antigen used to determine the presence of hepatic tumors (hepatoma) and testicular tumors.

   (3) **Cancer antigen (CA-125)** is a glycoprotein oncofetal antigen that appears in the serum of patients with ovarian cancer.

   (4) **CA-19** is another glycoprotein oncofetal antigen associated with gastrointestinal tumors.

   (5) **Prostate-specific antigen (PSA)** is an oncofetal antigen that is important in screening and monitoring patients with prostate carcinoma.

  b. **Placental proteins** are synthesized by placental trophoblasts and certain tumors.

   (1) **β-Human chorionic gonadotropin (β-hCG)** is typically used to determine pregnancy. However, high levels can indicate tumors of the testes or ovaries, as well as trophoblastic neoplasia.

(2) **Human placental lactogen (hPL)** is used to monitor fetal well-being, but its levels also can be elevated in patients with trophoblastic neoplasms.

c. Certain **enzymes** indicate the presence of cancer cells: **acid kinase** for stomach cancer and **alkaline phosphatase** for bone cancer.

d. Increased levels of some **hormones** indicate malignancy of the organ that produces the hormone.

2. **DNA analysis** is currently used to determine the proliferative capacity of tumor cells and is typically done by flow cytometry. Molecular diagnosis is also used to identify oncogenes, the genes that transform normal cells into malignant cells. This type of testing is becoming more widespread with the advent of simplified molecular techniques.

J. **Porphyrin** is a chemical intermediate in the synthesis of hemoglobin, myoglobin, and other respiratory pigments called cytochromes. Porphyrin measurement is important for the determination of porphyria (a disturbance of heme synthesis). Heme synthesis begins in the mitochondria.

1. **Porphyrin chemistry** involves the following principles.

a. **Synthesis.** Porphyrin is synthesized from porphin (four pyrrole rings), but side chains are substituted for the eight hydrogen atoms. A variety of substances make up the side chains (magnesium makes up part of the side chains in chlorophyll, which is a porphyrin).

(1) The **main sites** of porphyrin synthesis are bone marrow cells and liver cells.

(2) The **rate of synthesis** is controlled through regulation of the enzyme **δ-aminolevulinic acid (ALA) synthase** by the hemoproteins in the liver.

b. **Isomers.** There are four possible isomers of porphyrin, but only Types I and III occur in nature. Type III forms heme, and Type I is functionless but may be present in excess in some disorders.

c. **Clinical importance**

(1) Three porphyrin compounds are clinically important: **protoporphyrin** (excreted in feces), **uroporphyrin** (excreted in urine), and **coproporphyrin** (excreted in both). All are intermediate products in the synthesis of heme that can be assessed clinically.

(2) **Porphobilinogen and ALA** are precursors of porphyrin and can accumulate in certain porphyrin disorders. These substances are typically found in the urine of patients with acute porphyria.

(3) **Free erythrocyte porphyrins (FEP)** are porphyrins that can be extracted from RBCs, the primary one being protoporphyrin. FEP concentration is increased in persons with lead poisoning and iron deficiency anemia.

2. **Porphyrias** are inherited or acquired disorders of heme synthesis in which overproduction of heme precursors in the bone marrow or the liver cause characteristic symptoms. The porphyrias are classified based on the signs and symptoms manifested by the patient (neurologic versus cutaneous). The primary cause of porphyrias is a specific enzyme deficiency.

a. **The neurologic porphyrias** include the symptoms of abdominal pain, psychotic behavior, and neuromuscular difficulties. Clinically, the three neurologic porphyrias have in common increased urinary ALA and porphobilinogen levels.

   (1) **Acute intermittent porphyria** (most common) has a clinical presentation of increased uroporphyrin levels.

   (2) **Variegate porphyria** (rare) has a presentation of increased protoporphyrin and coproporphyrin levels.

   (3) **Coproporphyria** (rare) has a presentation of increased coproporphyrin levels.

b. **The cutaneous porphyrias** are induced by the presence of excess porphyrins in the skin, which generate oxygen radicals that attack cells and produce photosensitivity and skin lesions. The three cutaneous porphyrias have in common normal urinary ALA and porphobilinogen levels.

   (1) **Congenital erythropoietic porphyria** (the rarest of the inherited porphyrin disorders) is a severe disorder that has a presentation of increased uroporphyrin and coproporphyrin levels.

   (2) **Protoporphyria** (somewhat rare) has a presentation of increased protoporphyrin and increased free erythrocyte protoporphyrin levels.

   (3) **Porphyria cutanea tarda** (most common) appears in adults following liver disease or excessive alcohol intake. It has a clinical presentation of increased levels of uroporphyrin.

c. **Porphyrinuria** is a moderate elevation of urine coproporphyrin secondary to a number of disorders, including pregnancy, neoplasia, intoxication, and liver disease.

d. **Porphyrinemia** is a moderate elevation in erythrocyte protoporphyrin secondary to a number of disorders, including:

   (1) **Iron deficiency states,** caused by poor nutrition, malabsorption, poor iron transport, or blood loss

   (2) **Anemia** (hemolytic, iron-deficiency, sideroblastic)

   (3) **Lead poisoning**

3. **Methods of porphyrin analysis** include qualitative and quantitative procedures.

   a. **Qualitative tests** include those for:

      (1) **Urine porphobilinogen,** which is a screening test whereby normal results are negative (e.g., the Watson-Schwartz test, the Hoesch test)

      (2) **Urine porphyrins**, which is a screening test performed to measure uroporphyrin and coproporphyrin

   b. **Quantitative tests** include a variety of procedures:

      (1) **Urine tests** for presence of porphobilinogen, uroporphyrin, coproporphyrin, and ALA

      (2) **Blood tests** for ALA dehydratase (an enzyme in the blood that breaks down ALA) and protoporphyrin

      (3) **Fecal tests** for coproporphyrin and protoporphyrin

K. **Iron** is contained in the porphyrin ring of heme in hemoglobin, myoglobin, catalase, and cytochromes. The reversible interaction of iron with oxygen and the ability of iron to function in electron transfer reactions makes iron physiologically important.

1. **Iron metabolism** is controlled by its absorption in the intestine. Approximately 1 mg of iron is lost by adults daily. This loss is due to loss of RBCs and shedding of intestinal mucosal cells. In women, the menstrual cycle drains 30 mg of iron. Most circulating iron is derived from the release of iron following RBC destruction.

   a. **Absorption** of iron occurs mainly in the duodenum and includes only 5%–10% of daily iron intake. The body's iron supply is controlled by intestinal absorption.

   b. Iron **transport** involves a transport protein, **transferrin,** which binds ferric iron. The bound iron either moves to the mitochondria for heme synthesis or is stored in cells as ferritin.

   c. Iron **storage** includes storage as soluble **ferritin** (found in most cells) or relatively insoluble hemosiderin. One third of iron is stored in the liver, one third in the bone marrow, and one third in the spleen.

2. **Iron disease states** include:

   a. **Iron deficiency anemia,** which is usually caused by blood loss (menstrual cycle, ulcer, tumor)

   b. **Iron overload,** including:
      (1) **Hemosiderosis** (no tissue injury)
      (2) **Hemochromatosis**
         (a) **Hereditary hemochromatosis** is an autosomal recessive disease in which iron is deposited directly in the liver, heart, and kidney, leading to organ failure.
         (b) **Sideroblastic anemia** is caused by iron overload of unknown cause.
         (c) **Acquired hemochromatosis** follows thalassemias or lead poisoning. This disorder also occurs with chronic excessive absorption of normal iron intake.

3. **Iron analysis** involves the examination of three iron compartments: blood cells (hemoglobin), stored iron (ferritin), and circulating iron [i.e., serum iron, transferrin, iron-binding capacity (IBC)].

   a. The assay for measuring **serum iron** is based on the release of iron from transferrin and the subsequent reduction of ferric iron to ferrous iron. Serum iron is decreased during iron deficiency states, chronic inflammation, and menstruation; following blood loss; and following myocardial infarction. Iron is increased following overload, iron poisoning, and hepatitis, and during the use of oral contraceptives.

   b. **IBC** is a measurement of the maximum concentration of iron that transferrin can bind.

Table 1-4. Iron-Binding Capacity (IBC) and Transferrin Levels in Specific Disease States

Disease	Transferrin Level	Total IBC
Iron deficiency anemia	High	High
Failure to incorporate iron into red blood cells	Normal	Low
Iron overload	Normal	Low

       c. Transferrin levels are analyzed by immunoassay techniques or radial immunodiffusion. Table 1-4 presents the IBC and transferrin results that occur in specific disease states.

       d. Plasma ferritin is the most sensitive indicator of iron deficiency. Ferritin levels decline early in anemia and increase early in chronic diseases.

V. ENZYMOLOGY

  A. Enzymes are proteins that catalyze biochemical reactions but do not alter the equilibrium point of the reaction. They are not consumed or altered. Enzymes are specific to each physiologic reaction of which they are a part.

    1. Composition. Each enzyme is composed of a **specific amino acid sequence** (primary structure), which results in a stearic arrangement (secondary structure) that becomes folded (tertiary structure).

    2. Structure. Each enzyme contains an active site that binds a substrate and an allosteric site.

    3. Isoenzymes are multiple forms of the same enzyme.

    4. Cofactors may be necessary for enzyme activity and can be **activators** (inorganic) or **coenzymes** (organic). If the cofactor is bound to the enzyme, it is called a prosthetic group, and the enzyme portion is called an **apoenzyme.** The entire enzyme-cofactor molecule is called a **holoenzyme.**

    5. Classification is based on the action of the enzyme.

      a. Oxidoreductases catalyze an oxidation-reduction reaction. Examples include lactate dehydrogenase and G6PD.

      b. Transferases catalyze the transfer of a group other than hydrogen. Examples are aspartate transaminase, alanine transaminase, creatine kinase, and gamma glutamyl transferase.

      c. Hydrolases catalyze the hydrolysis of ether and ester. Examples are alkaline phosphatase, acid phosphatase, amylase, and cholinesterase.

      d. Lyases catalyze the removal of groups without hydrolysis (loss of hydroxide ion).

      e. Isomerases catalyze the interconversion of geometric or optical isomers.

      f. Ligases catalyze the joining of two substrate molecules.

    6. Enzyme kinetics deal with the relationship between the enzyme, the substrate, and the product.

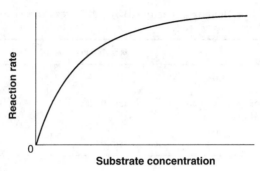

Figure 1-4. Michaelis-Menten curve.

    a. The **catalytic mechanism** is stated as:

$$E + S = ES = E + P$$

    The transition state for the ES complex has a lower energy of activation than S alone, so the reaction proceeds after the ES complex is formed.

    b. Michaelis-Menten constant (K_m) expresses the relationship between the velocity of any enzymatic reaction and the substrate concentration (Figure 1-4). K_m is the substrate concentration at which the enzyme yields half the possible maximum velocity of the reaction.

      (1) The Michaelis-Menten hypothesis of the relationship between reaction velocity and substance concentration is **expressed as a formula:**

$$V = \frac{V_{max}[S]}{K_m + [S]}$$

      (2) A **Lineweaver-Burk plot** expresses K_m as a straight line, in which V_{max} is the reciprocal of the y intercept of the straight line, and K_m is the negative reciprocal of the x intercept of the same line (Figure 1-5).

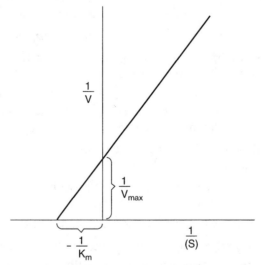

Figure 1-5. Lineweaver-Burk plot. K_m = Michaelis-Menten constant; [S] = concentration of substrate; V_{max} = maximum velocity.

   c. Factors that influence enzymatic reactions include:

     (1) Substrate concentration, by following either:

       (a) First-order kinetics, in which the reaction rate is directly proportional to the substrate concentration. With enzyme excess, the reaction rate steadily increases as more substrate is added until the substrate saturates all available enzyme.

       (b) Zero-order kinetics, in which the reaction rate is dependent on enzyme concentration only. When product forms, the excess enzyme combines with excess free substrate.

     (2) Enzyme concentration, when exceeded by substrate concentration, causes the velocity of the reaction to be proportional to the enzyme concentration.

     (3) pH. Each enzyme operates maximally at a specific pH.

     (4) Temperature. Increased temperature increases the rate of a chemical reaction by increasing the movement of molecules.

     (5) Cofactor concentration. Increasing the cofactor concentration increases the velocity of an enzymatic reaction similar to substrate concentration.

     (6) Inhibitors

       (a) Competitive inhibitors bind to the active site of the enzyme, causing K_m to increase.

       (b) Noncompetitive inhibitors bind at a place other than the active site, causing V_{max} to decrease.

       (c) Uncompetitive inhibitors bind to the ES complex; both V_{max} and K_m decrease.

   d. Enzyme activity can be measured as either an increase in product concentration, a decrease in substrate concentration, a decrease in coenzyme concentration, or an increase in concentration of altered coenzyme.

     (1) Endpoint measurements are performed after a reaction proceeds for a designated length of time, then is stopped. Measurement is made of the amount of reaction that has occurred.

     (2) Kinetic measurements are multiple measurements of absorbance change made at specific time intervals.

     (3) An **international unit (U) of enzyme activity** is the amount of enzyme that catalyzes the reaction of 1 μmol of substrate per minute under specific conditions (e.g., temperature, pH).

B. Phosphatases promote the hydrolysis of phosphate esters.

  1. Acid phosphatase (ACP) promotes the hydrolysis of orthophosphate esters, although the physiologic function of ACP is unknown.

   a. Almost every body tissue contains ACP, but significant levels are found in RBCs and platelets. In adult men, 50% of ACP is found in the prostate gland. High levels of ACP are found in semen as well.

   b. In the **measurement of total activity,** typical substrates acted upon by ACP include p-nitrophenylphosphate or thymolphthalein monophosphate. All reactions to measure ACP are carried out at a pH lower than 6.0.

     (1) Isoenzyme tests include:

       (a) Inhibition of prostate ACP by tartrate, followed by the determination of the serum level of other ACP fractions

        (b) Immunoassay with antibodies specific to certain isoenzymes

        (c) Electrophoretic procedures

    (2) Falsely low values are produced by improper anticoagulant (e.g., fluoride, oxalate, heparin) use, whereas hemolysis produces false elevations.

  c. The **major diagnostic significance** of ACP is its aid in detecting metastatic carcinoma. Other types of cancer and bone disease exhibit increases of enzyme. The presence of ACP is sometimes used as evidence of rape.

2. Alkaline phosphatase (ALP) hydrolyzes phosphate esters, but the function of this enzyme is relatively unknown.

  a. ALP exists in a wide variety of tissues, with significant amounts found in liver, bone, intestine, kidney, and placenta.

  b. In the **measurement of total activity,** the Bessey-Lowry-Brock reaction using *p*-nitrophenylphosphate as the substrate for ALP is most commonly used with pH or reaction greater than 8.0.

  c. Improper anticoagulant use produces decreased values of ALP, and a hemolyzed specimen demonstrates a false increase in ALP value.

  d. The **diagnostic significance** of ALP is its elevation during the third trimester of pregnancy and in persons with liver disease (hepatitis, cirrhosis); bone disease; hyperthyroidism; or diabetes mellitus.

  e. There are **four isoenzymes of ALP:** bone, liver, intestinal, and placental fractions. In disease states, the fractions are affected as follows:

    (1) The **bone fraction** levels are elevated in persons with bone disease (osteomalacia, rickets, Paget's disease) and high in children.

    (2) The **liver fraction** level is greatly elevated in persons with hepatobiliary obstruction.

    (3) The **placental fraction level** becomes elevated between the 16th and 20th weeks of pregnancy.

C. Transaminases catalyze the transfer of amino groups and acids. This is an important reaction in the synthesis and degradation of amino acids.

1. Distribution. Aspartate transaminase (AST) transfers an amino group between aspartate and keto acids (aspartate + α-ketoglutarate $\xrightarrow{AST}$ oxaloacetate + glutamate). Pyridoxal phosphate (vitamin B_6) is the coenzyme in this reaction.

  a. AST exists in cardiac tissue, liver, skeletal muscle, and RBCs.

  b. Three major approaches are taken in the **measurement of total activity.**

    (1) The reaction with **dinitrophenylhydrazine** couples color reagent with keto acid product.

    (2) The reaction with **diazonium salts** couples the salt with the keto acid product and forms a color.

    (3) The **coupled enzyme assay** (Karmen method) involves NADH and malate dehydrogenase and keto acid to form NAD.

      c. The **clinical significance** of AST elevations is that the elevations occur in patients with myocardial infarction, viral hepatitis, and skeletal muscle disease.

    2. Alanine transaminase (ALT) catalyzes the transfer of an amino group from alanine to α-ketoglutarate with the formation of glutamate and pyruvate.

      a. **Distribution.** ALT is localized in the liver, with some in the heart, skeletal muscle, and RBCs.

      b. The **measurement of total activity** is similar to the reactions of AST, except that the **coupled enzyme assay** uses lactate dehydrogenase to reduce pyruvate to lactate and oxidize NADH.

      c. The **clinical significance** of ALT is in the evaluation of hepatocellular disorders.

D. Creatine kinase (CK) catalyzes a reaction responsible for the formation of ATP in tissues, especially contractile systems. When muscle contraction occurs, ATP is hydrolyzed to ADP to produce chemical energy for the concentration process. CK is involved in the storage of high-energy creatine phosphate (creatine + ATP $\xrightarrow{CK}$ creatine phosphate + ADP).

    1. Distribution. CK is localized in skeletal muscle, brain, and cardiac muscle in addition to many other tissues.

    2. The **measurement of total activity** includes the following assays.

      a. The **Tanzer-Gilvarg assay** involves the reaction stated previously coupled with other enzymes (pyruvate kinase and lactate dehydrogenase) to produce a change in absorbance when measured spectrophotometrically.

      b. The **Oliver-Rosalki assay** is the reverse reaction of the one stated previously, in which creatine is produced from creatine phosphate. The enzymes used include hexokinase and G6PD.

      c. Hemolysis must be avoided when analyzing because of the presence of **adenylate kinase (AK)** in RBCs. AK induces false elevations in CK assays. Because CK activity is unstable due to the oxidation of its sulfhydryl groups, cysteine is added to both of the previously mentioned assays.

    3. The **clinical significance** of CK is in its elevation in muscle disorders. CK and one of its isoenzymes is a sensitive indicator of acute myocardial infarction and muscular dystrophy. High levels also are detected in CNS disorders, such as stroke, seizures, and malignant neoplasms.

    4. The structure of CK allows for the formation of three **isoenzymes.**

      a. **CK-MM** is the major form found in striated and cardiac muscle and normal serum. Hypothyroidism and intramuscular injections result in CK-MM elevations.

      b. **CK-MB** is localized in cardiac muscle. Elevated levels are indicative of ischemic heart disease. If the serum level of CK-MB is >6% of total CK, it is a highly specific indicator of myocardial damage. Following **acute myocardial infarction,** CK-MB levels rise within 48–72 hours, peak at 12–24 hours, and return to normal within 48–72 hours.

      c. **CK-BB** is present in small quantities in normal serum and appears if extensive damage to the brain occurs, but is present in many other tissues.

    d. Assays used for measurement of isoforms include electrophoresis, ion-exchange chromatography, and immunoassay.

        (1) CK electrophoresis is a semi-quantitative procedure. Following electrophoresis, CK-BB moves the farthest (most anodal), followed by CK-MB, then CK-MM.

        (2) CK chromatography involves an **anion exchange resin** at a pH of 8.0. The isoenzymes have different charges and can be selectively eluted.

        (3) CK immunoassay involves antisera employed against certain subunits of each isoenzyme.

E. Lactate dehydrogenase (LD) catalyzes the interconversion of lactic and pyruvic acids. It is a hydrogen-transfer enzyme that uses the coenzyme NAD.

    1. Distribution. LD is widely distributed in all tissues, with high concentrations found in the heart and liver, and low levels in RBCs, skeletal muscle, and kidneys.

    2. Measurement of total activity is based on the detection of NADH in the assay approaches.

        a. The **Wacker method** uses the lactate-to-pyruvate reaction with formation of NADH.

        b. The **Wroblewski-Ladue method** employs the reverse reaction of the Wacker method and measures the decrease in absorbance as NADH is consumed.

    3. The **diagnostic significance of LD** is in the diagnosis of cardiac, hepatic, skeletal muscle, and renal disease. Highest LD levels are seen in persons with pernicious anemia, viral hepatitis, cirrhosis, and crush injuries. An elevated LD means little without isoenzyme studies.

    4. There are, in normal serum, five different **isoforms** of LD (LD_1 to LD_5), with each isoenzyme being composed of four protein subunits.

        a. LD_1 is localized predominantly in heart muscle and RBCs and constitutes approximately 25% of total LD.

        b. LD_2 localization is similar to LD_1, but it also is found in the kidneys and comprises approximately 35% of total LD.

        c. LD_3 is found in lung, lymphocytes, spleen, and pancreas. It constitutes approximately 22% of total LD.

        d. LD_4 is found mostly in liver and skeletal muscle and comprises approximately 10% of total LD.

        e. LD_5 is similar to LD_4 in both localization and portion of total.

        f. Testing methodologies for isoforms include:

            (1) Electrophoresis. LD_1 migrates most quickly toward the anode, followed by the others in numerical order. After **myocardial infarction,** LD_1 concentration is greater than LD_2, which presents as a "flipped pattern" in electrophoresis. This pattern is also observed with hemolyzed specimens.

(2) **Immunoinhibition for the measurement of LD$_1$ activity.** This procedure involves an antibody that binds all other isoforms, leaving LD$_1$ to be assayed by chemical reaction.

F. **Miscellaneous enzymes** that are clinically significant include gamma glutamyl-transferase (GGT), amylase, cholinesterase, pseudocholinesterase, and 5'-nucleotidase.

1. **GGT** transfers a gamma-glutamyl residue to an amino acid (transpeptidation). This function is involved in peptide and protein synthesis.

   a. **Distribution.** Tissue sources of GGT include kidney, brain, prostate, pancreas, and liver. Urine contains significant amounts of GGT.

   b. **Measurement of total activity** is by the **Szasz assay.** In this reaction, the substrate is gamma-glutamyl-*p*-nitroanilide, with the release of *p*-nitro-aniline.

   c. The **clinical significance** of GGT is as follows.

      (1) GGT levels are elevated in almost all hepatobiliary disorders or biliary tract obstructions as well as in patients taking enzyme-inducing drugs like warfarin, phenobarbital, and dilantin.

      (2) GGT levels are often examined with ALP levels. If both GGT levels and ALP values are high, some type of liver disorder is suspected. If GGT is normal, and ALP is high, bone disease is likely present.

      (3) Patients with acute pancreatitis exhibit increased GGT levels. In persons with diabetes, GGT is typically increased as triglyceride levels rise.

      (4) Because alcohol has enzyme-inducing properties, the most useful application for GGT is in the **detection of alcoholism** and the monitoring of alcohol intake by patients during treatment.

2. **Amylase (AMS)** is a hydrolase that catalyzes the breakdown of starch and glycogen and produces products consisting of glucose, maltose, and dextrins. AMS is the smallest in size of all enzymes.

   a. **Distribution.** Tissue sources of AMS include the pancreas and salivary glands, as well as skeletal muscle.

   b. The **measurement of total activity** includes:

      (1) **Amyloclastic methods.** AMS acts on a starch substrate that has an iodine attached. When the starch molecule is degraded, iodine is released and measured colorimetrically.

      (2) **Saccharogenic methods.** A starch substrate is hydrolyzed by AMS to produce sugars, which are measured.

      (3) **Chromogenic methods.** A starch substrate has colored dye attached that is released upon starch hydrolysis.

      (4) **Coupled-enzyme methods** measure change in absorbance of NAD. Typically, AMS acts on maltopentose to produce maltose that is then reduced to form ATP. This reaction is then coupled with NAD.

   c. The **clinical significance** of AMS is its use in the diagnosis of acute pancreatitis. AMS levels rise 2–12 hours after onset of an attack and peak at 24 hours. Salivary gland lesions (e.g., mumps, parotiditis) also produce high levels of AMS. Patients with hyperlipidemia have low-to-normal AMS levels. Opiates constrict the pancreatic sphincters, which causes false elevations of AMS.

3. **Cholinesterase** is an enzyme that hydrolyzes the esters of choline. There are two types: **acetylcholinesterase (AChe)** and **pseudocholinesterase (PChe)**. The substrate for AChe is acetylcholine (a neurotransmitter). PChe acts on many different substrates, but mainly butyryl esters.

   a. **Distribution.** AChe is found in RBCs, brain, and nerve cells. PChe is found mostly in the serum, liver, pancreas, heart, and white matter of the nervous system.

   b. The **measurement of total activity** includes:

      (1) **Manometric techniques** measure liberated carbon dioxide from the formation of acetic acid.

      (2) **Electrometric measures** determine enzyme activity by measuring the pH decrease resulting from the liberation of acetic acid.

      (3) **Photometric method (Ellman technique).** The substrate is a thiol ester that produces a thiol, which reacts with a disulfide to form a colored compound.

   c. Regarding the **diagnostic significance** of the cholinesterases, PChe is of greatest interest. When the rate of protein synthesis declines, PChe levels decline; this indicates developing hepatocellular disease, starvation, or burn injuries. Low levels of PChe can also indicate insecticide poisoning.

4. **G6PD** is an oxidoreductase that catalyzes the oxidation of G6P to 6-phosphogluconate, which is an important first step in the pentose-phosphate shunt of glucose metabolism.

   a. **Distribution.** Tissue sources of G6PD include the adrenal glands, spleen, thymus, RBCs, and lymph nodes. In the RBC, G6PD functions to maintain NADPH in a reduced form to protect hemoglobin from oxidation and to prevent red cell hemolysis.

   b. In the **measurement of total activity,** the formation of NADPH is measured colorimetrically.

   c. **Diagnostic significance.** Clinically, deficiency of G6PD is an inherited sex-linked trait most common in African-Americans. Increases of G6PD are seen in persons with myocardial infarction and megaloblastic anemia.

5. **5'-nucleotidase (5'-NT)** originates in the liver or diseased bone. 5'-NT becomes elevated in liver disease, as does ALP, but 5'-NT does not increase in patients with bone disease. Serum levels of 5'-NT are more sensitive to liver cancer.

VI. ENDOCRINOLOGY

A. A **hormone** is a chemical substance that is produced and secreted into the blood by an organ or tissue and has a specific effect on a target tissue located away from the site of hormone production. The collection of hormones, carrier proteins, and other components of these processes forms the **endocrine system;** hormones act in conjunction with the CNS to maintain the internal chemical conditions necessary for cellular function and emergency demands.

   1. **Hormone classification.** Hormones are classified either by their tissue of origin or their structure.

Table 1-5. Tissues and the Hormones They Produce

Tissue of Origin	Hormone(s) Produced
Hypothalamus	Thyrotropin-releasing hormone, corticotropin-releasing factor, other releasing factors
Anterior pituitary	Thyroid-stimulating hormone, adrenocorticotropic hormone (ACTH), follicle-stimulating hormone, luteinizing hormone, prolactin, growth hormone
Posterior pituitary	Vasopressin, oxytocin
Adrenal medulla	Epinephrine, norepinephrine
Adrenal cortex	Cortisol, aldosterone, 11-deoxycortisol
Thyroid	Triiodothyronine, thyroxine, calcitonin
Parathyroids	Parathyroid hormone
Pancreas	Insulin, glucagon
Gastrointestinal tract	Gastrin, others
Ovaries	Estrogens, progesterone
Placenta	Progesterone, human chorionic gonadotropin, human placental lactogen
Testes	Testosterone, other androgens
Kidneys	$1,25\text{-}(OH)_2$, vitamin D, erythropoietin
Unknown	Prostaglandins

a. Hormone **classification by tissue of origin** involves the production of hormones by certain tissues (Table 1-5). Some tissues produce "releasing factors" that act on another tissue to release certain hormones.

b. Hormone **classification by structure** involves the specific chemical makeup of hormones. Hormones of the same basic structure appear to produce the same fundamental biochemical changes.

   (1) **Peptide hormones** make up the majority of hormones. **Releasing factors** are peptides. The hormones are water-soluble and do not require transport proteins to move through the blood. They are synthesized and stored within the cell and have a short half-life (5–60 minutes) in the circulation.

   (2) **Steroid hormones** are involved in the regulation of sexual development and characteristics. All steroid hormones are synthesized from **cholesterol** as the basic molecule. They are not water soluble, and they require a transport protein to travel through the blood. Steroid hormones are synthesized in the adrenal gland, gonads, or placenta and have a long half-life (60–100 minutes) in the circulation.

   (3) **Amino acid derivatives** (amines) have properties similar to those of both steroid and peptide hormones.

(4) Fatty acid derivatives include the prostaglandins.

2. **Mechanisms of hormone action** typically depend on the type of hormone.

   a. **Hormone/receptor interaction** involves the binding of hormone to a specific receptor molecule on or within a cell.

   b. **Hormone binding** occurs on or within a cell.

      (1) Binding at the cell surface produces a conformational change in the receptor complex that leads to release of proteins and formation of AMP from ATP within the cell. **Cyclic AMP (AMP-c)** then causes cellular enzymes to be phosphorylated, and these enzymes can exert regulatory control on biochemical reactions within the cell. Most peptide hormones interact with cells in this manner. However, insulin phosphorylates without AMP.

      (2) Internal binding typically involves steroid hormones. Diffusion into the cell occurs before attachment to a specific receptor within the cell. The steroid/receptor complex then migrates to the DNA in the nucleus and exerts control over the type and amount of **RNA** produced and ultimately over what proteins are synthesized.

3. **Hormone release** is controlled by a number of factors.

   a. **Regulation by releasing factors** involves a complex system of "factors" produced by tissues that induce synthesis of a specific hormone. For example, a decline in blood pressure causes corticotropin-releasing factor to be released, which in turn induces the release of adrenocorticotropic hormone and constriction of blood vessels.

   b. **Prohormones** are precursors of peptide hormones. Following hydrolysis of a portion of its peptide chain, a prohormone becomes an active hormone. The hydrolysis is controlled by the cell containing the prohormone.

   c. **Feedback control** involves the release of a hormone that regulated prior steps in the releasing process. For example, thyroid hormones feed back to the hypothalamus to "shut off" thyrotropin-releasing hormone so excess thyroid hormone will not be produced.

4. **Hormone transport proteins** affect both the concentration of a hormone and its influence on the system. Peptide hormones are transported in the unbound state.

   a. **Types** of transport proteins are specific for each hormone. The attachment of hormone to protein is through noncovalent linkages.

      (1) Steroid and thyroid hormones are bound to albumin, sex hormone-binding protein, or cortisol-binding globulin.

      (2) Amines are transported by serum proteins and thyroxine-binding globulin.

   b. **Transport protein level can affect hormone action.** Relative amounts of bound and free hormone determine the degree of stimulus provided by the hormone. Only the free (unbound) fraction of a hormone exhibits activity, so any situation that affects the transport protein level or degree of binding has an impact on the concentration of the free hormone. The measurement of the transport protein concentration is sometimes an integral part of the hormone assay.

Box 1-8. Hormones of the Anterior
Pituitary Gland

Prolactin (PRL)
Growth hormone (GH)
Luteinizing hormone (LH)
Follicle-stimulating hormone (FSH)
Thyroid-stimulating hormone (TSH)
Adrenocorticotropic hormone (ACTH)

B. The **hypothalamus and pituitary gland** are integral components of the endocrine system.

   1. The **pituitary gland** is made up of two parts—the anterior lobe (adenohypophysis) and the posterior lobe (neurohypophysis)—and is located in a bony cavity at the base of the skull.

      a. The **anterior pituitary** cells are responsible for hormone production (Box 1-8).

      b. The **posterior pituitary** does not synthesize any known hormone but serves as a storage area for certain hormones (e.g., oxytocin, vasopressin) produced by the hypothalamus.

   2. The **hypothalamus** is a part of the CNS that lies at the base of the brain above the pituitary. The hypothalamus is connected to the pituitary gland via a cluster of nerves and blood vessels called the pituitary stalk. Neurons in the hypothalamus produce a number of **releasing and inhibiting factors** that affect a number of other endocrine glands (Box 1-9).

   3. The **regulation of production and secretion** of hormones that are produced or housed in the endocrine glands is explained by the concept of the feedback loop.

      a. The **feedback loop** is composed of two endocrine organs: the pituitary gland and the target endocrine gland.

      b. Two types of feedback exist.

Box 1-9. Hormones of the Hypothalamus

Corticotropin-releasing factor (CRF)
Gonadotropin-releasing hormone (Gn-RH)
Growth hormone-releasing factor (GH-RF)
Luteinizing hormone-releasing hormone (LH-RH)
Oxytocin
Prolactin release-inhibiting factor (PIF)
Prolactin releasing factor (PRF)
Somatostatin (somatotropin-release inhibiting factor, SRIF)
Thyrotropin-releasing hormone (TRH)
Vasopressin [antidiuretic hormone (ADH)]

(1) **Negative feedback** occurs when the stimulating hormone induces production of a hormone, elevated levels of which turn off pituitary release of the stimulating hormone. For example, high levels of thyroid hormones stop the release of thyrotropin-releasing hormone (TRH) from the hypothalamus and thyroid-stimulating hormone (TSH) from the pituitary gland, which in turn halts production of the thyroid hormones.

(2) **Positive feedback** occurs when a structure secretes a hormone in response to a stimulating hormone released from the pituitary gland. The released hormone induces more stimulating hormone to be released from the pituitary gland. For example, follicle-stimulating hormone (FSH) and luteinizing hormone (LH) induce the release of the hormone estradiol from the ovary, which then feeds back on the pituitary gland to release more FSH and LH.

4. **Pathologic conditions** involving the pituitary or hypothalamus manifest themselves in a variety of symptoms.

   a. The clinical manifestions of **anterior pituitary disorders** result either from hypersecretion or hyposecretion of hormones.

      (1) **Hypersecretion** usually involves one hormone. It is not uncommon for hypersecretion to be associated with the hyposecretion of another tropic hormone.

         (a) **Primary factors** center on disorders of the pituitary gland: either pituitary adenomas or pituitary hyperplasia.

         (b) **Secondary factors** center on disorders of the hypothalamus or may relate to ectopic production of pituitary hormones by nonendocrine tumors or to the hyposecretion of hormone by the target tissue.

      (2) **Hyposecretion** can be decreased secretion of one hormone, a group of hormones, or all hormones. The latter condition is referred to as "panhypopituitarism."

         (a) Single hormone hyposecretion results from lesions on the hypothalamus.

         (b) **Pituitary adenoma,** causing hypersecretion of one hormone, is commonly the cause of hyposecretion of remaining pituitary hormones because of the destruction of the pituitary gland by the growing tumor.

   b. **Specifics of pathologic conditions** associated with dysfunction of the anterior pituitary gland.

      (1) **Growth hormone (GH)**

         (a) The effects of **hypersecretion** are age dependent. In adults, the resulting condition is called **acromegaly,** which is the progressive enlargement of the distal parts of the extremities. In children, the resulting condition is **gigantism.** Both conditions usually result from pituitary adenomas secreting GH and compression of adjacent tissues of the pituitary gland, causing hyposecretion of other tropic hormones.

         (b) **Hyposecretion** in children leads to pituitary **dwarfism** (small stature but proportionally built).

(2) Prolactin (PRL)

(a) **Hypersecretion** causes **galactorrhea** or lactation and is associated with infertility and amenorrhea in women and impotence in men. It usually is induced by pituitary adenoma.

(b) **Hyposecretion** leads to the lack of lactation in postpartum women.

(3) ACTH

(a) **Hypersecretion** is referred to as **Cushing's disease,** with symptoms including truncal obesity, hyperglycemia, hypertension, and protein wasting. It is caused by pituitary adenoma, adrenal hyperplasia, or excess production by a nonendocrine tumor.

(b) **Hyposecretion** causes weight loss, weakness, and gastrointestinal problems.

(4) TSH

(a) **Hypersecretion** causes **thyrotoxicosis** and is the result of either hyperactivity of the thyroid or hyperactivity of the pituitary gland, leading to increased TSH release.

(b) **Hyposecretion** is difficult to differentiate from primary hypothyroidism.

(5) Gonadotropins (FSH and LH)

(a) **Hypersecretion** results in sexual precocity and is usually a result of brain tumors in the region of the hypothalamus.

(b) **Hyposecretion** results in sexual underdevelopment and infertility.

c. The clinical manifestations of **posterior pituitary** dysfunction involve either vasopressin or oxytocin. These disorders result from either hypothalamic dysfunction or some peripheral disease.

(1) Vasopressin (ADH) regulates water reabsorption and blood pressure by affecting the renal tubules and the arterioles.

(a) **Hypersecretion** of ADH results in a condition referred to as **syndrome of inappropriate ADH secretion (SIADH).** The disorder occurs in a wide variety of conditions, including meningitis, head injury, tuberculosis, hypoadrenalism, hypothyroidism, and cirrhosis. SIADH is associated with hyponatremia (low blood sodium) and hypertonic urine, despite normal renal and adrenal function. Symptoms include weakness, malaise, poor mental status, convulsions, and coma. It is typically caused by release of ADH from ectopic tumors.

(b) **Hyposecretion** of ADH is associated with **diabetes insipidus.** Symptoms include insatiable thirst, polydipsia (excessive drinking), and polyuria (excessive urine volume). This disorder results from destruction of the posterior pituitary gland or the hypothalamus.

(2) No known disorders are associated with excess or deficient secretion of **oxytocin.**

C. Adrenal glands. One **adrenal gland** is situated on top of each kidney. Each adrenal gland is composed of two distinct layers: the **adrenal cortex** (the outermost region) and the **adrenal medulla** (the innermost region).

1. The **adrenal cortex** is composed of three distinct tissues:
   a. Zona glomerulosa
   b. Zona fasciculata
   c. Zona reticularis

2. The **adrenal medulla** is composed of sheets of irregular cells with small nuclei called **chromaffin cells.**

3. **Adrenal hormones**
   a. **Glucocorticoids** are steroid hormones produced in the zona fasciculata and reticularis of the adrenal cortex.
   b. **Mineralocorticosteroids** are steroid hormones produced in the zona glomerulosa.
   c. **Catecholamines** are amine hormones produced in the adrenal medulla.

4. **Adrenal endocrine function** includes regulation of proteins, carbohydrates, and many other metabolic functions.
   a. **Glucocorticoids** are synthesized from cholesterol. They are transported bound to plasma proteins [albumin and corticosteroid-binding protein (CBP)], are catabolized by the liver and kidneys, and are regulated by the hypothalamus-pituitary-adrenal axis. The primary action of the glucocorticoids is catabolic (i.e., promoting protein and lipid breakdown, inhibiting protein synthesis).
      (1) **Cortisol** is the primary glucocorticoid produced and secreted by the adrenal cortex. Its functions include:
         (a) Affecting carbohydrate metabolism
         (b) Having a role in protein and lipid metabolism
         (c) Suppressing the inflammatory response
         (d) Increasing blood glucose levels by stimulating gluconeogenesis in the liver
         (e) Maintaining normal blood pressure
         (f) Stimulating the GFR and thus increasing urine production
         (g) Stimulating erythropoiesis
      (2) **Target tissues** of glucocorticoid action include the kidney glomerulus and renal tubules, bone marrow stem cells, hepatocytes, and adipose tissue.
   b. **Mineralocorticosteroids** are synthesized from cholesterol, transported bound to CBP and albumin, and are catabolized by the liver and the kidney. The primary action is regulation of electrolytes. They are regulated by three factors: the renin-angiotensin system, potassium, and ACTH.
      (1) **Aldosterone** is the primary mineralocorticoid produced and secreted by the adrenal cortex. Its functions include:
         (a) Stimulating sodium resorption in the distal convoluted tubules in exchange for potassium or hydrogen
         (b) Increasing blood volume (via renin/angiotensin system) and pressure
         (c) Regulating extracellular fluid volume
      (2) **Target tissues** of mineralocorticoid action include the distal renal tubules and the large intestine.

(3) Regulation of aldosterone secretion via the **renin/angiotensin system** is achieved as follows. Decreased blood volume or blood pressure induces the release of kidney renin, which induces the production of angiotensin I and II. Angiotensin II affects release of aldosterone from the adrenal gland, which ultimately causes the kidney distal tubule to retain sodium, thereby raising blood volume and blood pressure.

c. Catecholamine production is not limited to the adrenal medulla. Norepinephrine is predominantly synthesized in the CNS, whereas epinephrine is predominantly synthesized by the adrenal medulla. Catecholamines are products of the hydroxylation of the amino acid tyrosine. They are transported free in the blood and regulated by feedback inhibition of synthesis.

(1) Catecholamine **functions** include:

  (a) Mobilization of energy stores by increasing blood pressure, heart rate, blood sugar level (by stimulating glycogenolysis)

  (b) Neurotransmitter actions

  (c) Release in response to pain and emotional disturbance (stress) to mobilize organs

(2) Tissue targets include the liver and adipose tissue.

(3) Approximately 20% of catecholamines are excreted into the urine as **metanephrine** and **normetanephrine;** approximately 80% are converted to **vanillylmandelic acid (VMA)** by the enzyme monoamine oxidase (MAO).

5. Diseases associated with the **adrenal cortex** center on hyperfunction (excess production of bioactive molecules) or hypofunction. Etiology of these diseases may be neoplastic, hyperplastic, vascular, inflammatory, autoimmune, infectious, hereditary, or idiopathic (cause unknown).

a. Hyperadrenalism involves three basic conditions.

  (1) Cushing's syndrome involves excess cortisol production, either at the level of the adrenal gland or by increased release of ACTH.

  (2) Hyperaldosteronism involves excess aldosterone production with symptoms of hypertension. There are two causes.

  (a) Conn's syndrome is induced by an aldosterone-secreting adrenal adenoma or adrenal hyperplasia and is a rare cause of hypertension.

  (b) Excess renin production leads to elevated aldosterone levels.

  (3) Congenital adrenal hyperplasia is a genetic disorder causing a deficiency of enzymes in the synthetic pathways that lead to cortisol and aldosterone production. ACTH levels are increased, and steroid hormones are hypersecreted. A common cause of this condition is a **21-hydroxylase deficiency.**

b. Hypoadrenalism is caused by adrenal hypofunction or insufficiency and can be induced by three conditions:

  (1) Primary disease involving the adrenal cortex (known as **Addison's disease**), which is relatively rare

  (2) Secondary adrenal insufficiency precipitated by decreased levels of corticotropin-releasing hormone (CRH) or ACTH

(3) Long-term suppression of the hypothalamic-pituitary-adrenal axis by glucocorticoids

6. The major **disorder** of the **adrenal medulla** is pheochromocytoma. **Pheochromocytoma** is a relatively rare, usually benign tumor arising in the chromaffin cells of the adrenal medulla that results in hypersecretion of catecholamines. Pheochromocytomas occur as an inheritable disorder.

7. **Laboratory analysis of adrenal function** involves several different testing methodologies.

   a. The laboratory investigation of **Cushing's syndrome** proceeds in two stages.
      (1) The fact that the patient has autonomous cortisol production must be established by using the **dexamethasone suppression test.** This test involves the injection of a synthetic steroid that acts like cortisol (dexamethasone) to induce feedback inhibition of cortisol release at the level of the pituitary.
      (2) The cause of the disease must be differentiated.

   b. **Plasma cortisol** values normally display diurnal variation, with the highest levels occurring in the morning and the lowest levels in the early evening. Evening values are lower than 50% of the early morning concentrations. Classically, samples are drawn at 8 A.M. and 4 P.M. Three general methods are used for the estimation of cortisol:
      (1) Porter-Silber color reaction (obsolete)
      (2) Sulfuric acid-induced fluorometry, which induces fluorescence in a sample with sulfuric acid but overestimates plasma cortisol
      (3) Immunoassay

   c. **Primary hyperaldosteronism** is analyzed by examining serum and urine potassium. Values of serum potassium lower than 3.5 mmol/L, coupled with a urine potassium excretion rate greater than 30 mmol/24 h, are commonly seen in persons with primary hyperaldosteronism. The definitive test for primary hyperaldosteronism, however, is the measurement of serum or urine aldosterone following a **high salt challenge.** Primary hyperaldosteronism caused by an aldosterone-producing tumor demonstrates no change in plasma aldosterone levels following salt challenge, whereas primary aldosteronism caused by adrenal hyperplasia demonstrates a rise in plasma aldosterone. A simple method for investigating **Conn's syndrome** is to measure serum and urine potassium when a patient is not receiving diuretics.

   d. **Congenital adrenal hyperplasia** is analyzed by investigating the possibility of adrenal insufficiency. The patient may also suffer biochemical consequences of excess androgen, and measurements of testosterone in serum and pregnanetriol in urine may be requested.

   e. In the analysis of **Addison's disease,** patients typically exhibit postural hypotension, hyponatremia, and hyperkalemia. The ACTH stimulation test is given; it involves injection of synthetic ACTH and subsequent measurement of ACTH and cortisol at 30 and 60 minutes. High ACTH with no cortisol response indicates Addison's disease.

f. There are many ways to investigate **pheochromocytoma.** Urinary metabolites (e.g., VMA, metanephrines) can be quantitated, or plasma epinephrine and norepinephrine can be measured. In difficult cases, when the patient has episodic hypertension of short duration, a **clonidine suppression test** combined with plasma catecholamine measurements is performed. Clonidine suppresses catecholamine release from the CNS but not from the adrenal gland.

D. The **thyroid gland** is a bilobed endocrine gland located in the lower part of the neck that is composed of groups of cells called follicles. This gland contains two cell types: **Follicular cells** produce the hormones thyroxine (T_4) and triiodothyronine (T_3), and **parafollicular cells** (lying adjacent to the follicles) produce the hormone calcitonin.

   1. Thyroid hormones require iodine for their **synthesis.** The iodine combines with the protein thyroglobulin to form hormone precursors that in turn combine to form T_3 and T_4.

      a. The hormones are either stored within the follicle or released into the bloodstream. In the blood, most T_4 eventually gives up an iodine molecule and forms T_3. There is much more circulating T_3 than T_4.

      b. Approximately 98% of circulating T_3 and T_4 is bound to protein, including **thyroxine-binding globulin (TBG)** and thyroxine-binding albumin. Some hormone remains unbound or free, and this is the physiologically active fraction.

      c. Thyroid hormone **function** includes action at the cellular level to regulate carbohydrate, lipid, and protein metabolism. The hormones also act on the CNS, stimulate the heart, and have a role in physical growth and development.

      d. The **regulation** of T_3 and T_4 occurs in the following manner.
         (1) Thyroid-releasing hormone (TRH) is released by the brain and stimulates the release of **TSH (thyrotropin)** from the pituitary gland.
         (2) TSH stimulates iodine uptake by the thyroid gland and also causes the release of T_3 and T_4 from the thyroid gland.
         (3) High serum levels of free T_3 and T_4 "shut off" the release of TSH from the pituitary gland, whereas decreased levels induce TSH release.

   2. Thyroid disorders are caused by increased or decreased levels of the circulating hormones T_3 and T_4. A wide variety of physical diseases can be traced back to a dysfunctional thyroid gland.

      a. Hypothyroidism is a serum level of thyroid hormone that is insufficient to provide for the metabolic needs of cells. This disorder affects women four times more than men between the ages of 30 and 60 years. Hypothyroidism is usually referred to as primary, secondary, or tertiary, depending on the site of the dysfunction.

         (1) The **symptoms** of hypothyroidism include an enlarged thyroid gland (goiter), fatigue, impairment of mental processes, and loss of appetite. Myxedema (loss of hair, swelling of the hands and face, course skin) occurs as the disease progresses.

(2) The **causes** of hypothyroidism relate to the area of tissue damage. In addition, hypothyroidism can be caused by lack of dietary iodine.

 (a) **Primary hypothyroidism** involves the inadequate secretion of thyroid hormones caused by a damaged or surgically removed thyroid gland. Congenital hypothyroidism is caused by the absence of the thyroid gland. Laboratory results indicate decreased T_3, T_4, free thyroxine index (FT_4I), T_3 uptake (T_3U), and increased TSH.

 (b) **Secondary hypothyroidism** involves decreased production of TSH caused by pituitary disorder leading to low serum levels of the thyroid hormones. Laboratory results indicate all thyroid test values are decreased.

 (c) **Tertiary hypothyroidism** is caused by hypothalamic failure leading to a lack of TRH production.

(3) In the **laboratory evaluation** of hypothyroidism, the earliest abnormality is increased TSH, followed by decreased serum levels of T_4, T_3, and a low T_3 resin uptake result.

b. **Chronic immune thyroiditis (Hashimoto's disease)** is caused by a genetic abnormality in the immune system and involves massive infiltration of the thyroid gland by lymphocytes. The symptoms match those of hypothyroidism.

c. **Hyperthyroidism** is caused by excessive thyroid hormone in the circulation. This causes cells to become overactive. The disorder is sometimes referred to as **thyrotoxicosis.**

(1) The **symptoms** of hyperthyroidism include weight loss, loss of muscle mass, hyperactivity yet quick fatigability, insomnia, increased sweating, nervousness, palpitations, goiter, and bulging eyes.

(2) The **causes** of this disorder include pituitary tumors that cause excessive TSH secretion, thyroid carcinoma, or toxic multinodular goiter (gland produces excess hormones).

(3) The **laboratory evaluation** of hyperthyroidism in the initial evaluation reveals elevated thyroid hormone serum levels and decreased serum TSH.

d. **Graves' disease** is an autoimmune disorder that occurs six times more frequently in women than in men. In this disorder, immunoglobulins stimulate the thyroid gland by binding to TSH receptors. Symptoms are similar to those of hyperthyroidism. Laboratory results indicate increased T_3, T_4, FT_4I, and T_3U, and decreased or normal TSH.

e. **Thyroiditis** is an inflammation of the thyroid gland caused by either bacterial or viral infection.

3. **Assays** for thyroid function include testing for serum level of total (both bound and free) or free T_3, total or free T_4, TSH, and TBG. These tests are typically immunoassays. Other thyroid tests include the following:

a. **T_3 resin uptake** analyzes the capacity of TBG to bind thyroid hormones. It is an indirect measurement of the number of free binding sites on the TBG molecule.

b. Free thyroxine index (FT$_4$I) indirectly assesses the concentration of circulating free T$_4$. It is calculated by multiplying the value of the total T$_4$ by the percentage value of the T$_3$ resin uptake.

c. Thyroid antibody screens assay for the presence of thyroid-stimulating immunoglobulins, such as those in Graves' disease and Hashimoto's thyroiditis.

d. TRH stimulation test measures pituitary TSH stores and is considered conclusive for hyperthyroidism, although it is not needed in most hyperthyroid patients. In patients with slightly elevated hormone levels (but other symptoms of hyperthyroidism), TRH is injected, and blood samples are assayed for TSH. TSH levels rise rapidly in a normal person but will not rise in a hyperthyroid patient.

E. Parathyroid hormone is produced by the **parathyroid glands,** which are small, paired structures located in the posterior thyroid capsule. They may, however, be located in other parts of the neck or upper chest cavity. The sole function of the parathyroid gland is the production of parathyroid hormone.

1. Parathyroid hormone (PTH) synthesis begins with the precursor proparathyroid hormone. Successive cleavages of the pre- and the pro-amino acid sections yields 84-amino acid PTH molecule that is packaged in granules for storage, secretion, or degradation.

a. The **major physiologic action** of PTH is mineral homeostasis. Specifically, PTH is involved in the metabolism of both calcium and phosphorus by the kidney and bone. A complex interrelationship exists between PTH, cholecalciferol (vitamin D), and calcitonin.

b. Transport. Parathyroid hormone, unlike many other proteins, is transported as a freely circulating, intact, active molecule. The biologically inactive amino acid fragments can be detected in the serum as well.

c. The primary determinant of PTH **release** is the serum concentration of ionized calcium, considered to be the biologically active form of serum calcium. Other substances that impact PTH secretion rates include:

(1) Magnesium, which has an effect on PTH that both parallels and modulates the effect of calcium on PTH release
(2) Biogenic amines like epinephrine, dopamine, and serotonin
(3) Vitamin D

2. PTH has an important **role in calcium and phosphorus metabolism.**

a. Calcium is a mineral proved to be essential for heart muscle contraction, hemostasis, and cell responsiveness. Calcium homeostasis is regulated not only by PTH but also by cholecalciferol (vitamin D) and the thyroid hormone calcitonin. The overall effect of PTH is to raise blood calcium levels through its action on bone and kidney.

(1) In **bone,** PTH increases bone resorption of calcium into serum.
(2) In the **kidney,** PTH increases the renal reabsorption of calcium.

b. Phosphorus, or rather compounds of phosphate, are in all living cells and participate in many important biochemical processes. The overall effect of PTH is to lower phosphorus concentrations, whereas vitamin D acts to increase blood phosphate.

    c. Calcitonin is produced by parafollicular cells in the thyroid. In general, the overall effect of calcitonin is to decrease blood calcium because of its effect on both bone and renal calcium processing, which is just the opposite of PTH.

        (1) In **bone,** calcitonin inhibits bone resorption of calcium.

        (2) In the **kidneys,** calcitonin decreases the renal reabsorption of calcium, phosphorus, sodium, potassium, and magnesium.

3. Pathologic conditions involving a dysfunctional parathyroid gland most often manifest as hypocalcemic or hypercalcemic states.

    a. Hypocalcemia is classified as either being associated with deficient PTH concentration or being independent of PTH activity (vitamin D-deficient states). In general, the PTH-dependent hypocalcemic disorders fall into **two categories:** those related to hyposecretion of PTH and those related to tissue resistance to PTH (known as pseudohypoparathyroidism).

        (1) Primary hypoparathyroidism is synonymous with hyposecretion of PTH. It is caused by surgical removal of the parathyroid glands, trauma following surgery, or radiotherapy directed toward the thyroid gland. The clinical manifestations are those of hypocalcemia and include tetany (muscle spasms), skin changes (especially drying), brittle hair, hypotension, and GI upset. Low serum calcium and high phosphorus are hallmarks of this disorder.

        (2) Idiopathic hypoparathyroidism is rare and can be hereditary or seen in conjunction with other endocrine disorders. A very low serum calcium level and a very high phosphorus level are indicative of this condition.

        (3) Pseudohypoparathyroidism (PHP) is characterized by a lack of responsiveness to PTH by the renal system or other organ systems, not by a decrease in PTH. Serum PTH levels are typically normal to increased in this condition.

    b. Hypercalcemia is diagnosed when serum calcium levels rise higher than 102 mg/L or are sustained at levels greater than 100 mg/L. Symptoms range from no symptoms to manifestations of polyuria, polydipsia, kidney stones, acid-base disorders, nausea, stupor, or coma. Malignancy (e.g., multiple myeloma, leukemia, lymphoma) and hyperparathyroidism account for most cases of hypercalcemia. Although symptoms associated with hyperparathyroidism vary, symptomatic hyperparathyroidism is seen predominantly in association with bone disease or kidney stones.

        (1) Primary hyperparathyroidism most often results from parathyroid adenoma or hyperplasia. Adenomas tend to involve one gland, whereas hyperplasia involves multiple glands. Additionally, hyperparathyroidism can be associated with other endocrine disorders, collectively referred to as multiple endocrine neoplasia (MEN), which involve the pituitary, pancreas, thyroid, and adrenal glands. Serum calcium is increased, PTH is increased, and phosphorus is normal to decreased.

        (2) Secondary hyperparathyroidism is a condition associated with an attempt for the body to compensate for hypocalcemic states. It is commonly seen in patients with renal failure who cannot excrete

Table 1-6. Reproductive Hormones

Endocrine Gland	Hormone Produced/Released	Target Tissue	Response
Hypothalamus	LH-releasing hormone	Anterior pituitary	LH secretion; FSH secretion
Anterior pituitary gland	LH	Ovarian follicle	Ovulation
		Luteal cell	Progesterone produced
		Leydig cell	Testosterone produced
	FSH	Ovary	Follicular maturation; estradiol produced
		Sertoli cells	Spermatogenesis
Ovary (follicles)	Estrogens	Hypothalamus	FSH inhibited
		Pituitary	FSH inhibited; LH secretion
		Gonads	Secondary sex characteristics develop
		Uterus	Preparation of endometrium
Corpus luteum	Progesterone	Uterus	Maintenance of endometrium
		Mammary gland	Lactation
Testes	Androgens (testosterone)	Male prostate, genitalia, larynx, skeleton	Growth and development; maturation

FSH = follicle-stimulating hormone; LH = luteinizing hormone.

phosphorus, resulting in a decrease in calcium, which stimulates the secretion of PTH. Serum calcium is low, PTH is increased, and phosphorus is increased.

4. **Laboratory analysis** of parathyroid function involves determination of various hormone and electrolyte levels.

   a. **The primary analytes of interest** in parathyroid function evaluation are **calcium** (total and ionized), **phosphorus** (inorganic), and **PTH** (C-terminal, N-terminal). PTH levels should always be considered along with serum calcium levels.

      (1) **PTH C-terminal analysis** examines the intact PTH molecule and is highly specific for detecting hyperparathyroidism.

      (2) **PTH N-terminal analysis** measures both the whole PTH molecule and the amino-terminal fragments in the serum.

   b. **Additional analytes of secondary interest** include calcitonin, vitamin D, magnesium, bicarbonate, and nephrogenous cyclic adenosine monophosphate(cAMP). **Nephrogenous cAMP** is under direct influence of PTH and is a measure of the urinary portion of cAMP produced by the kidneys and excreted by the renal tubules.

F. **Reproductive hormones** (Table 1-6). A complex interrelationship exists between the hypothalamus, pituitary gland, and the gonads (ovaries and testes).

The reproductive hormones produced by these glands are primarily responsible for the growth and maturation of the gonads in women and men. Men and women produce and secrete the same sex hormones, but the differentiating factor is the quantity of hormones produced and the genetic makeup of the individual.

1. **FSH and LH** are glycoprotein hormones synthesized in the anterior pituitary gland and transported unbound via the systemic circulation to target tissues. These hormones are metabolized in a manner similar to proteins.

   a. **In the woman,** FSH induces the growth of the ovum inside the follicle, and LH triggers release of the ovum.

   b. **In the man,** FSH induces spermatogenesis in the Sertoli's cells of the testes, and LH [referred to as interstitial cell-stimulating hormone (ICSH) in the man] stimulates the production of testosterone by the Leydig's cells.

2. **Progesterone, testosterone, androgens, estrone, and estradiol** are steroid hormones synthesized either in the testes, ovaries, or adrenal glands. Each of these steroid hormones has cholesterol as its precursor. The synthesis of each specific hormone depends on the activation of genes in the endocrine gland in which it is produced. These compounds are transported in the bloodstream bound to specific plasma proteins [sex hormone-binding globulin (SHBG), albumin, corticosteroid-binding globulin (CBG)]. They are catabolized mainly in the liver by reductive processes, then excreted in the urine as glucuronide or sulfate conjugates.

   a. **The ovaries** produce estrogens (i.e., estrone, estradiol), androgens, and progesterone. The estrogens are responsible for development of the uterus, fallopian tubes, and female sex characteristics. Estrogens also prepare the uterine endometrium (lining) for pregnancy. Progesterone prepares the breast for lactation and maintains the endometrium.

      (1) **Estradiol** is the chief estrogen produced specifically by the maturing follicle within the ovary.

      (2) **Estrone,** the other major biologically important estrogen, is produced either in the peripheral tissues via conversion of prohormone androstanedione or in the ovary from the conversion of estradiol.

      (3) **Another estrogen, estriol,** is produced in the placenta. Therefore, little is present in nonpregnant women.

      (4) **Progesterone** is produced by the corpus luteum (the structure that forms in a follicle that has released its ovum). It is present in significant amounts following ovulation.

      (5) **Androstanedione** is the chief female androgen.

   b. **The testes** in adult men produce testosterone and small amounts of androstanedione, dehydroepiandrosterone, and estradiol. Testosterone induces growth of the male reproductive system, prostate gland, and development of male sex characteristics, including hypertrophy of the larynx and initiation of spermatogenesis. The other androgens are also responsible for the secondary sex characteristics in men.

   c. **Adrenal gland** androstanedione is converted to testosterone in the peripheral tissues and accounts for approximately 5% of the total testosterone in men.

3. The **regulation** of all reproductive processes involves a complex series of interrelated events and endocrine systems, including the hypothalamus, the pituitary gland, and the gonads.

   a. **In women,** the **menstrual cycle** controls reproductive events. High serum levels of FSH induce follicular development and estrogen release. The increased level of estrogen causes a decrease in the release of FSH at the level of the pituitary gland and also causes an increase in serum LH. LH initially causes estrogen levels to decline, then induces maturation and rupture of the follicle, which releases ovum. Estrogen levels increase following this release, the ruptured follicle becomes the corpus luteum, and progesterone is produced. Progesterone inhibits LH release from the pituitary gland. Serum FSH and LH levels continue to decline, and regression of the corpus luteum induces decreased serum levels of estrogen and progesterone, initiating menstruation. The estrogen-induced inhibition of FSH release by the pituitary gland is removed, and FSH levels begin to increase, beginning the cycle again.

   b. **In men,** increased levels of serum testosterone inhibit the release of ICSH from the pituitary, thereby decreasing the production of testosterone by Leydig's cells.

4. **Abnormalities of testicular function** focus on the lack of or excessive production of androgens. Both increased and decreased androgen production can be a primary condition resulting from testicular dysfunction, or it may be a secondary condition resulting from hypothalamus-pituitary dysfunction.

   a. **The symptoms of hypogonadism** are directly dependent on the time of the development of androgen deficiency. Prepubertal hypogonadism is caused by the absence of androgen production. Infantile genitalia persists; growth continues but is decreased. This condition is often not apparent until the adolescent period when normal adolescent development does not occur. Postpubertal hypogonadism results in minimal changes.

      (1) **Primary hypogonadism** is caused by a lack of androgenic feedback by FSH/LH on the hypothalamus-pituitary axis, which is typically caused by a genetic defect in testicular development. Laboratory results indicate increased serum and urine gonadotropins (LH/FSH), decreased serum androgens (testosterone), and decreased urinary 17-ketosteroids.

      (2) **Secondary hypogonadism** is caused by primary hypopituitarism or a hypothalamic dysfunction that results in decreased production of LH and FSH by the pituitary gland. Absence of serum and urine gonadotropins and decreased serum androgens are indicated by laboratory results.

   b. **Hypergonadism** is most often a condition resulting from excessive androgen production by a testicular tumor. It can also occur secondary to hypothalamus-pituitary dysfunction, with a resulting increase in FSH/LH secretion. In the adult, there is little physical change with these disorders. However, increased androgen levels in children result in precocious puberty.

      (1) **Primary hypergonadism** is indicated by high serum androgen levels, high urinary 17-ketosteroid levels, and low serum gonadotropin levels.

(2) **Secondary hypergonadism** can be differentially diagnosed by the presence of high serum androgen levels, high urinary 17-ketosteroid levels, and elevated gonadotropin levels.

5. **Abnormalities of ovarian function** present as either hypo- or hyperfunction, both of which are considered as either primarily caused by ovarian disease or secondarily caused by hypothalamus and pituitary dysfunction.

   a. Ovarian **hypofunction** is also a time-dependent condition. If it occurs before the onset of puberty, it induces delayed or absent menstruation. If it occurs after the onset of puberty, it will result in secondary amenorrhea (lack of menstruation).

   (1) **Primary ovarian hypofunction** is caused by a lack of estrogenic feedback on the hypothalamus-pituitary system, which results in increased release of FSH and LH from the pituitary gland. Characterized by increased serum levels of gonadotropins and decreased estrogen levels, there are **two common causes** of this condition.
   (a) **Menopause,** the termination of reproduction in women
   (b) **Turner's syndrome,** a congenital endocrine disorder in which the ovaries cannot secrete estrogen

   (2) **Secondary ovarian hypofunction** results from hypothalamic-pituitary dysfunction or serious illness. Laboratory results indicate decreased serum gonadotropins, estrogen, and progesterone. The three most common causes of this condition are:
   (a) Tumors and necrosis of the pituitary gland (e.g., Sheehan's syndrome)
   (b) Congenital hypothalamic disorders
   (c) Illnesses such as congenital heart disease, chronic renal disease, rheumatoid arthritis, rapid weight loss, anorexia nervosa, or hyperthyroidism

   b. Ovarian **hyperfunction** is usually caused by estrogen-secreting tumors or may be idiopathic in origin.

   (1) **Primary ovarian hyperfunction** is the result of the presence of an estrogen-secreting tumor, which results in decreased serum FSH/LH levels. Irregular uterine bleeding is a typical symptom.
   (2) **Secondary ovarian hyperfunction** is idiopathic and results in increased estrogen secretion caused by the presence of increased FSH/LH levels. Sexual precocity (early development of secondary sex characteristics) is the primary condition associated with this disorder.

6. **Other conditions** involving female reproductive hormones include:

   a. **Hirsutism,** or excess hair along the midline of the female body (i.e., lip, chin, chest), is typically caused by excess androgen production by the ovaries or adrenal glands.

   b. **Polycystic ovary syndrome,** or enlarged ovaries, is associated with infertility and other menstrual irregularities.

   c. **Infertility** is caused by lack of ovulation in women and inappropriate sperm production in men.

7. **Laboratory analysis** of reproductive endocrinology involves serum and urine testing of a variety of hormones and their metabolites or function tests that

involve stimulation or suppression of various hormones. The measurement of hormones—particularly FSH, LH, progesterone, estradiol, testosterone, and progesterone—is necessary before carrying out the numerous stimulation or suppression test protocols used to establish the cause of the endocrine disorder. Most endocrine components are examined by immunoassay.

VII. TOXIC AND THERAPEUTIC DRUGS

A. Toxicology is the study of toxic drugs or poisons. A **toxicant** (poison) is any substance that, when taken in sufficient quantity, causes sickness or death. **Toxicity** is a relative term used to compare one substance with another; a toxic substance is one with a toxicity defined as "extremely" or "super" toxic.

B. Factors that influence toxicity include the following:

1. The nature of the toxicant regarding its solubility and physical state (i.e., gas, liquid, solid)

2. The exposure variables of the toxicant, including its dose dependency, route, rate of administration, and duration of exposure

3. The biologic variables of the individual ingesting the toxicant, including age, genetic makeup, and the ability to acetylate certain drugs

4. The toxicokinetics of the toxicant regarding its transformation by metabolic processes before exerting an effect on the ingestor

C. Specific drugs considered to be toxicants are composed of several categories. Some of these drugs are also considered to be therapeutic in nature.

1. **Analgesics** are anti-inflammatory agents and painkillers. There are a variety of substances that are considered to be analgesics. These drugs are also considered to be therapeutic.

   a. **Salicylate (aspirin)** is considered toxic at a serum level of >90 mg/dL 6 hours following ingestion. The time since ingestion must be known to determine severity of toxicity.

      (1) **Salicylate intoxication** results in the following: stimulation of the respiratory system with initial respiratory alkalosis, conversion of pyruvate to lactate, inhibition of oxidative phosphorylation, and breakdown of fatty acids to produce ketoacids. Eventually, metabolic acidosis occurs.

      (2) Renal clearance of salicylate can be increased by **forced alkaline diuresis.**

   b. **Acetaminophen,** if present in serum at 300 μg/mL 2 hours after ingestion, induces hepatic toxicity. Again, time since ingestion is critical in determining acetaminophen intoxication.

      (1) **Intoxication** results in hepatocystic necrosis 3–4 days after overdose because of the inability of the liver to adequately conjugate the metabolite of acetaminophen (i.e., actamidoquinone) to glutathione. High levels of acetamidoquinone in the liver induce hepatocyte death.

      (2) **Antidote.** The effective antidote for acetaminophen overdose is **N-acetylcysteine,** which is thought to act as a glutathione substitute and binds to the metabolite.

2. **Barbiturates** are **short-acting** (pento-, secobarbital); **intermediate-acting** (amo-, beta-, butalbarbital); and **long-acting** (phenobarbital) sedatives that exert a tranquilizing effect through their depressant effect on the CNS. Because these substances have a tendency to become habit-forming, they have been replaced by other drugs, such as fluorazepam. However, phenobarbital still is used to control epilepsy. The barbiturates can be considered as substances of abuse or as analgesics.

   a. Barbiturate **intoxication** results in cardiac arrest and respiratory depression through its effect on the CNS.

   b. There are **no real antidotes** for barbiturate overdose except the establishment of an open airway, aiding respiration, and maintaining cardiac output.

3. **Narcotics (opioids)** are compounds that produce sleep and pain relief (or stupor in overdose amounts) by acting to depress the CNS. This group includes heroin, morphine, codeine, and methadone. Most of these drugs are habit-forming and can be considered drugs of abuse.

   a. **Intoxication.** The toxic effects of overdose include depression of respiration caused by a decreased sensitivity to carbon dioxide and coma. Heroin is metabolized by the liver to form morphine and is excreted by the kidney as morphine glucuronide.

   b. **Antidote.** The effective antidote for narcotic overdose is **naloxone,** a narcotic antagonist.

4. **Pesticides** are compounds designed to kill specific organisms. Many forms exist, including organic complexes, organophosphates (largest single group of pesticides), and carbamates. These compounds inhibit AChE, which results in specific effects on the heart and respiratory centers, muscle cramps, and certain CNS effects.

   a. **Intoxication.** The method used for the determination of pesticide poisoning is the examination of PChE (an isoenzyme of AChE found in serum).

   b. **Antidote.** The effective antidote for pesticide poisoning is **atropine sulfate.**

5. **Carbon monoxide** is a tasteless gas with 200-fold greater affinity for hemoglobin than oxygen.

   a. **Intoxication.** During carbon monoxide poisoning, hemoglobin cannot adequately exchange carbon dioxide for oxygen because of the increased amount of carboxyhemoglobin present. Suffocation and death follow.

   b. **Antidote.** The effective antidote for carbon monoxide poisoning is **removal of the source** of carbon monoxide or **removal of the victim** from the source.

6. **Metal poisoning** includes intoxication by the heavy metals lead, arsenic, and mercury.

   a. **Lead poisoning** is most typically caused by lead paint ingestion or continuous exposure to lead in the soil.

      (1) **Intoxication.** Lead is found primarily in RBCs in intoxicated victims but produces widespread effects, such as gastrointestinal irritation, weight loss, kidney damage, convulsions, and in children, altered cognition and encephalopathy. Death occurs because of peripheral vascular collapse or brain involvement.

      (2) **Antidote.** Administration of ethylenediaminetetraacetic acid (EDTA), penicillamine, and other **lead chelates** that bind the lead and allow it to be excreted by the kidney. Examination of urinary ALA levels and RBC protoporphyrins can determine the occurrence of lead poisoning after serum and urine lead levels have returned to normal.

   b. **Mercury (mercury salts)** is found in antibacterial agents, photographic reagents, pesticides, and batteries. Poisoning by these agents is typically the result of overexposure or ingestion.

      (1) **Intoxication.** Effects of mercury poisoning include gastrointestinal irritation, severe kidney damage, or neurologic symptoms.

      (2) **Antidote.** As with lead poisoning, **chelates,** such as EDTA, penicillamine, or dimercaprol [also referred to as British antilewisite (BAL)] bind the mercury and render it excretable.

   c. **Arsenic** is found in pesticides, weed killer, and some paints.

      (1) **Intoxication.** Arsenic induces purging gastroenteritis, shredding of the stomach lining, and causes Mees' lines in the fingernails because of keratin binding. Death typically occurs because of hemorrhagic gastroenteritis. Because arsenic is cleared rapidly from the blood, urine is the specimen of choice for analysis.

      (2) **Antidote. Chelation therapy** with penicillamine or BAL is effective.

7. **Substances of abuse** include a variety of compounds that, when found in high levels in the urine or serum, can incriminate an individual. It is mandatory in substance-of-abuse analysis to obtain a satisfactory specimen and to process the specimen in a secure part of the laboratory.

   a. **Ethanol** is the most common toxicant and substance of abuse seen in patients in emergency departments in the United States. It acts by depressing the CNS and increasing the heart rate and blood pressure. Ethanol **metabolism** occurs in the liver by alcohol dehydrogenase, which converts alcohol to acetaldehyde, which is then excreted to acetate. A blood level of 0.1 g/dL is defined as intoxicating.

   b. **Methanol** is widely used in paints, solvents, antifreeze, and solid canned fuels. Poisoning with methanol is typically caused by ingestion.

      (1) **Intoxication** by methanol is considered more dangerous than ethanol poisoning because of the formation in humans of formaldehyde and formic acid as metabolites. Formic acid formation results in metabolic acidosis, pancreatic necrosis, and visual system impairment.

(2) Antidotes for methanol poisoning include the administration of sodium bicarbonate to treat the acidosis and ethanol to bind alcohol dehydrogenase and block the formation of the metabolites.

c. **Amphetamines** are CNS stimulants that block dopamine receptors in the brain. Amphetamine **metabolism** occurs in the liver and produces benzoic acid.

   (1) Intoxication by amphetamines can produce severe depression, respiratory difficulties, and episodes of paranoia.

   (2) Antidote. The antidote for amphetamine overdose is forced acid diuresis.

d. **Cocaine** is a CNS stimulant that is metabolized by cholinesterase to form benzoylcognine, which is excreted by the kidney.

   (1) Intoxication. Cocaine overdose produces hypertension, myocardial infarction, or seizure. Cardiotoxicity can occur and result in sudden death following cocaine use.

   (2) Antidote. There is no antidote for cocaine overdose except the passage of time and urinary excretion.

e. **Cannabinoid compounds [tetrahydrocannabinol (THC), marijuana]** produce psychologic effects and are stored in fat cells. THC is excreted in the urine for an extended period of time depending on use (i.e., infrequent users excrete THC for shorter periods than do chronic users). Overdose of this drug is rare and is not severe enough to be life-threatening.

f. **Phencyclidine (PCP, angel dust)** is an abused anesthetic that is illegally used as a hallucinogen.

   (1) Intoxication. This drug can produce violence, seizures, respiratory depression, or death.

   (2) Antidote. Treatment for PCP overdose is diazepam. PCP is unmetabolized and excreted in the urine as phencyclidine.

D. **The drug screen** rapidly identifies a drug or drugs present in the blood, urine, or gastric contents of a patient suffering from toxicity. Neutral and basic drugs as well as drug metabolites are best detected in urine, whereas acidic drugs are best found in detectable concentrations in blood and serum. Following a positive drug screen, confirmatory methods must be used to quantitatively analyze drug levels in a patient.

1. **TLC** is one method of drug detection used as a drug screen. It detects a wide variety of drugs but cannot separate closely related compounds. Blood and urine can both be analyzed with this method. The presence of a substance is determined by its rate of migration on silica gel–coated plates compared with the rate of migration of a standard.

2. **Gas-liquid chromatography** allows for clearer identification and greater sensitivity in the identification of drugs. It can be used as a confirmatory technique for drugs detected by TLC.

3. **Colorimetric "spot" tests** are rapid qualitative tests that rely on the analyst's eye as the detection instrument. These tests can analyze both urine and serum. Some of these tests involve a simple chemical color change, and some involve a handheld immunoassay system.

  E. Confirmatory drug tests are required to confirm and quantify those drugs
     found in a patient's serum or urine using drug-screening methods.

   1. Gas chromatography/mass spectrometry is a sensitive technique used to
      confirm drugs detected by screening techniques. Typically, urine samples
      are initially analyzed by gas chromatography to determine the presence of
      compounds, then reanalyzed by mass spectrometry to examine the fragments
      of these compounds for relative abundance in the sample.

   2. Immunoassay techniques use antibodies to detect drugs. These methods
      are usually automated and in the form of enzyme immunoassays.

   3. Ethanol testing is typically performed using gas chromatography. However,
      an enzyme assay using alcohol dehydrogenase and measuring the increase in
      NADH formation following the reaction is widely used and can be automated.

   4. Heavy metal testing is most often performed by atomic absorption spectro-
      photometry.

  F. Therapeutic drugs are prescribed agents that aid in the alleviation of specific
     symptoms in a patient. These drugs must be monitored to determine what doses
     are inadequate or excessive in the treatment of the patient. Accurate and precise
     timing, both in administering the drug and obtaining blood samples, are important
     in therapeutic drug monitoring (TDM). Therapeutic drugs are classified based on
     their action. Often, the ingested drug (called the "parent" drug) is metabolized to
     form an active metabolite that produces an effect similar to the parent drug.

   1. Cardioactive drugs are divided into two categories; the cardiac glycosides
      and the antiarrhythmic drugs. These agents serve to maintain normal heart
      function.

      a. Digoxin is the major cardiac glycoside and is derived from the digitalis
         plant. It improves cardiac contractility by altering the force of contraction
         through its effect on the ATPase pump in heart muscle. This affects sodium,
         potassium, and calcium transport in the heart. Blood specimens must be
         collected 8 hours after a dose of digoxin is administered because its peak
         concentration in tissue occurs 6–10 hours after administration. Digoxin
         toxicity produces symptoms of nausea, rapid heart rate, and visual impair-
         ment. Digoxin is excreted as **digoxigenin** in the urine.

      b. The **antiarrhythmic drugs** are prescribed to treat irregular heartbeat that
         produces inappropriate ventricular contraction or tachycardia (increased
         heart rate).
         (1) Lidocaine is used for the treatment of faulty ventricular contractions
            and arrhythmias. It binds to α_1-acid glycoprotein and is metabolized in
            the liver, producing two active **metabolites,** monoethylglycinexylide
            and glycinexylide. Lidocaine **toxicity** produces disorientation and
            possible respiratory arrest.
         (2) Procainamide is used to treat inappropriate ventricular contractions
            and tachycardia. This drug is metabolized in the liver to form an
            active **metabolite,** N-acetylprocainamide, which produces the same
            effect as its parent drug. Therefore, serum levels of both drugs must
            be analyzed. Procainamide **toxicity** results in bradycardia (slow
            heartbeat), nausea, and arrhythmia.

(3) **Disopyramide** stabilizes the heartbeat. It is both excreted by the renal system as the unchanged drug and is metabolized in the liver to form an inactive metabolite. Symptoms of **toxicity** are bradycardia, nausea, and anticholinergic effects (e.g., dry mouth, constipation).

(4) **Quinidine** is a myocardial depressant that decreases the heart's ability to conduct current. It is metabolized in the liver to produce several active **metabolites,** including 3-hydroxyquinidine. If quinidine is added to a digoxin therapy regimen, an interaction occurs that induces an increase in digoxin concentration.

(5) **Propranolol** is prescribed for atrial and ventricular arrhythmias and hypertension. It is considered to be a beta-blocker because of its effect on certain adrenergic nerve endings in the nervous system, and it modifies the metabolism of lipids and carbohydrates. It is metabolized in the liver to form several **metabolites.** One metabolite, 4-hydroxypropranolol, has high activity. Toxic effects include fatigue and weakness.

2. **Anticonvulsants** function to alter transmission of nerve impulses within the brain to minimize the seizures of epilepsy. It is difficult to evaluate the effectiveness of these drugs because of the unpredictability of seizure occurrence.

a. **Phenobarbital** is used to treat all types of seizures except absence seizures. It is effective in children and neonates. It is metabolized in the liver, and serum concentrations increase during the administration of valproic acid or salicylic acid. Phenobarbital can produce toxic effects, such as confusion or irritability.

b. **Phenytoin** corrects grand mal seizures. It is metabolized by the liver and can interact with several drugs that induce increased serum concentration or increased metabolism of phenytoin. Overdosage of this drug can cause ataxia, coma, and vitamin D deficiency.

c. **Valproic acid** is prescribed for absence (petit mal) seizures. As with most drugs, it is metabolized in the liver. Valproic acid affects many other anticonvulsants by inhibiting their metabolism in the liver, thus increasing serum concentration.

d. **Primidone** is metabolized in the liver to form phenobarbital. Therefore, dual analyses must be performed to determine the proper dosage of this drug. It is used to treat both grand mal and complex-partial seizures. Toxicity produces nausea, ataxia, and anemia.

e. **Carbamazepine** is typically used for treatment of various seizures and facial pain. The liver produces an active metabolite called carbamazepine-10,11-epoxide. Toxicity is characterized by ataxia, seizures, and leukopenia.

f. **Ethosuximide** is prescribed for the treatment of petit mal seizures. There are no active metabolites produced in the liver. Toxic effects include nausea, lethargy, or increased frequency of petit mal seizures.

3. **Bronchodilators** act to relax bronchial smooth muscle for relief or prevention of asthma. **Theophylline** is the most common in this category of therapeutic drugs and is metabolized in the liver to produce several metabolites,

including caffeine. Overdosage of theophylline produces nausea, nervousness, and seizures.

4. **Psychotropic or antipsychotic drugs** are used to treat psychotic patients. They can be categorized in two classes: lithium and the antidepressants. Other psychoactive drugs include fluoxetine and traizolam.

   a. **Lithium** treats manic-depressive illness. The mechanism of action of lithium as a mood stabilizer remains unknown, although effects on synaptic neurotransmission are thought to be the cause. Lithium is filtered by the renal glomerulus and eliminated as the unchanged drug. Acute intoxication by lithium is characterized by vomiting, diarrhea, tremor, ataxia, and convulsions.

   b. **Antidepressants,** or tricyclic antidepressants, are used to treat depression that has no apparent organic or social cause. These drugs act to block uptake of neurotransmitters in the CNS. Antidepressants include imipramine, nortriptyline, amitriptyline, and desipramine, all of which are metabolized by the liver to form active **metabolites.** The active metabolites include desipramine (parent is imipramine), nortriptyline (parent is amitriptyline), and 2-hydroxy-desipramine (parent is desipramine). Toxic reactions to these drugs include cardiac depression, tremor, dry mouth, and manic excitement.

   c. **Fluoxetine** is not chemically related to the tricyclic antidepressants, but has a similar effect by blocking serotonin uptake by nerve terminals in the CNS and by platelets. The active metabolite of this agent is norfluoxetine.

5. **Antineoplastic drugs** are used in the management of certain tumors, including cancer of the breast(s), teste(s), pharynx, and sometimes the lung(s). These agents work by inhibiting DNA synthesis.

G. **Therapeutic drug monitoring (TDM).** To achieve a specific pharmacologic effect (e.g., lowering blood pressure, pain relief), a certain concentration of drug must be reached at the site of interaction between the drug molecule and the receptor (e.g., cell membrane) to elicit the clinical effect. Any dose that does not result in a measurable or quantifiable effect is subtherapeutic. Therefore, TDM must be performed to determine proper timing and dose. TDM is also performed to determine patient compliance to the drug-taking regimen, to monitor drug interactions, and to monitor drugs that are used for a preventive effect.

1. **Changes in drug concentrations** in the body, which occur with time, are related to the course of the pharmacologic effects. The change in drug concentration **over time** is described by the following steps.

   a. The active ingredient of any dose must be released from the dose form (tablet, capsule, suspension). **Liberation** is the release of this ingredient, followed by the process of the drug passing into solution.

   b. **Absorption** is the process by which the drug molecule is taken up into systemic circulation. **Mechanisms** of absorption include passive diffusion, active transport, and pinocytosis. Following absorption through the intestinal mucosa, a drug traverses the hepatic system, where some drugs undergo substantial metabolism and elimination. This is called **first-pass elimination or metabolism.**

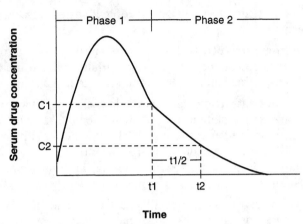

Figure 1-6. Single dose-response curve. C = concentration; $t_{1/2}$ = half-life.

c. Drug molecules can be confined to the blood, leave the bloodstream, and enter the extravascular space, or they can migrate into various tissues. This is referred to as **distribution,** a process that typically occurs between a period of 30 minutes and 2 hours. The **bioavailability** of a drug is the amount of drug that is absorbed into the system and is available for distribution.

d. **Metabolism** is the process of transformation of the parent drug molecule to its metabolite(s). Metabolites are usually water soluble and can be easily excreted. Most metabolism occurs in the liver, where enzymes catalyze oxidation, reduction, or hydrolysis of the drug.

e. **Elimination** is the process of excretion of the drug from the body. Drugs are typically excreted in the urine but also can be eliminated in the feces, sweat, expired air, and saliva.

2. **Basic principles.** TDM measures drug concentrations during therapy with pharmaceutical agents.

a. **A steady-state drug level** (complete with peaks and troughs) exists for each drug. When a single dose of a drug is administered orally, the blood level changes markedly over time and, at some time, the concentration in the plasma reaches its **peak** (highest point) and then declines. Immediately before the next dose of medication, a **trough** level occurs.

(1) **For single-dose administration,** the rate of decline in concentration is expressed in terms of **half-life,** which is the time required for the concentration of the drug to decrease by 50% (Figure 1-6). The half-life is different for each drug.

(2) At steady-state levels, the rate of administration of the drug is equal to the rates of metabolism and excretion, allowing the drug level to remain constant.

b. **Therapeutic range.** Drug concentration in blood can be subtherapeutic, therapeutic, or toxic. No clinical improvement can be expected after a single administration of a drug, so the goal is to achieve the therapeutic range, which is the amount of available drug that provides the optimum amount of medication for treatment of the clinical disorder. Obviously, multiple dosing is required to reach this level.

H. **Pharmacokinetics** is the mathematical interpretation of drug disposition over time to determine proper dosing amounts of a therapeutic drug. Pharmacokinetic responses are typically graphic plots of blood concentration of the drug versus time, such as a dose-response curve (see Figure 1-6). Three kinetic processes are used to describe the fate of drugs in the body over a period of time and can be illustrated in a dose-response curve.

   1. **First-order kinetics** describe absorption, distribution, and elimination of drugs. This means that the rate of change of concentration of a drug is dependent on the drug concentration. It is represented by the first phase of the dose-response curve.

   2. **Zero-order kinetics** describe the rate of change of concentration of a drug that is independent of the concentration of the drug. That is, a constant amount of drug is eliminated per unit of time. This typically depends on the ability of the liver to metabolize the drug. This is illustrated by the second phase of the curve.

   3. **Michaelis-Menten kinetics** state that if a drug concentration in a system exceeds the capacity of the system, the rate of change of concentration proceeds according to the Michaelis-Menten equation.

I. **Laboratory analysis** of therapeutic drugs includes enzyme immunoassays and fluorescence-polarized immunoassays. Gas chromatography and high-pressure liquid chromatography are also used. Serum is typically the specimen of choice for drug analysis, although urine metabolites are measured in some cases.

Study Questions

Directions: Each of the numbered items or incomplete statements in this section is followed by answers or by completions of the statement. Select the ONE lettered answer or completion that is BEST in each case.

1. What is the molarity (M) of a solution containing 50 g NaCl (formula weight = 58 g) in 500 mL deionized water?

a. 0.58 M
b. 1.27 M
c. 1.72 M
d. 2.50 M
e. 8.42 M

2. The Westgard rules for quality control were designed to decrease subjectivity in data analysis and to aid in troubleshooting in the chemistry laboratory. One of the rules is listed as 4_{1s}. This rule is described by which one of the following statements?

a. the numeric difference between the maximum and minimum control values exceeds 4s
b. two consecutive control values exceed either +2s or −2s
c. one control value exceeds either +4s or −4s from the mean
d. four consecutive control values are on the same side of the mean and exceed either +1s or −1s from the mean
e. control values from 4 consecutive days varied more than +1s or −1s from the mean

3. In regard to spectrometry, Beer's law states that

a. the frequency of a wave is inversely proportional to the wavelength
b. every solution has the ability to absorb and transmit light
c. the concentration of a substance in solution is directly proportional to the amount of light absorbed by that substance
d. light scattered by small particles in solution is of the same frequency as the incident light
e. the amount of transmitted light varies directly with the concentration of the solution

4. Which one of the following formulae is correct regarding the retention factor (R_f) of solutes in thin-layer chromatography?

a. R_f is equal to the total distance a component migrates
b. R_f is equal to the total distance the solvent front moves divided by the distance a component moves
c. R_f is equal to the distance a component moves divided by the total distance the solvent front moves
d. R_f is equal to the total distance the solvent migrates multiplied by the distance a component moves
e. R_f is equal to the total distance the solvent front moves

5. An increase in only the conjugated fraction of bilirubin indicates which one of the following conditions?

a. biliary obstruction
b. hemolysis
c. hepatitis
d. a newborn blood sample
e. nephrotic syndrome

6. Pulmonary disease is one of the primary causes for a deficiency of which one of the following globulins?

a. ceruloplasmin
b. haptoglobin
c. transferrin
d. α_1-fetoprotein
e. α_1-antitrypsin

7. When performing serum protein electrophoresis at pH 8.6 on agarose gel, which one of the following fractions migrates the farthest toward the anode?

a. α_1-globulin
b. α_2-globulin
c. gamma globulin
d. beta globulin
e. albumin

8. The biuret method of protein determination involves which one of the following actions?

a. the complexing of cupric ions with peptide bonds
b. the binding of a dye to an amino group of the protein
c. the complexing of cuprous ions with peptide bonds
d. the binding of a dye to a carboxyl group of the protein
e. the ability of proteins to carry both positive and negative charges

9. The kidney exercises its metabolic control over blood pH by altering the retention of which one of the following substances?

a. water
b. bicarbonate
c. carbon dioxide
d. oxygen
e. phosphorus

10. The Henderson-Hasselbalch equation is stated as

a. $pK = pH + \dfrac{\log [HCO_3]}{[H_2CO_3]}$

b. $pK = pH + \dfrac{\log [H_2CO_3]}{[HCO_3]}$

c. $pH = pK + \dfrac{\log [HCO_3]}{[H_2CO_3]}$

d. $pH = pK + \dfrac{\log [H_2CO_3]}{[HCO_3]}$

e. $pH = pK + \dfrac{H_2CO_3}{HCO_3}$

11. A decrease in blood carbon dioxide levels inducing the increased resorption of bicarbonate is classified as which one of the following acid-base disorders?

a. respiratory acidosis
b. respiratory alkalosis
c. metabolic acidosis
d. metabolic alkalosis
e. compensation

12. Creatinine clearance is calculated by which one of the following formulae?

a. $\dfrac{\text{urinary creatinine}}{\text{total volume} \times \text{plasma creatinine}} \times \dfrac{1.73}{A}$

b. $\text{plasma creatinine} \times \text{urinary creatinine}$ $\times \text{total volume} \times \dfrac{1.73}{A}$

c. $\dfrac{\text{urinary creatinine} \times \text{total volume}}{\text{plasma creatine} \times \dfrac{mL}{min}} \times \dfrac{1.73}{A}$

d. $\dfrac{\text{plasma creatinine} \times \dfrac{mL}{min}}{\text{urinary creatinine} \times \text{total volume}} \times \dfrac{1.73}{A}$

e. $\dfrac{\text{total volume}}{\text{urinary creatinine} \times \text{plasma creatinine}} \times \dfrac{1.73}{A}$

13. A patient being evaluated for diabetes is given oral liquid glucose and has blood samples drawn at 30-, 60-, 120-, and 180-minute intervals following ingestion of the liquid to be analyzed for serum glucose. This patient will be diagnosed as having severe diabetes if the serum glucose

a. becomes elevated 180 minutes after ingestion of glucose
b. remains normal at all times following ingestion of the glucose
c. becomes elevated 120 minutes following glucose ingestion
d. becomes elevated 60–120 minutes after glucose ingestion and remains elevated
e. becomes elevated 30–60 minutes following glucose ingestion and then rapidly returns to normal

14. A milky appearing plasma specimen is analyzed for lipid content. An extremely elevated serum triglyceride, normal to slightly elevated cholesterol, and an elevated level of very low-density lipoproteins (VLDL) were observed. These results most likely indicate

a. type I hyperlipoproteinemia
b. type IIA hyperlipoproteinemia
c. type IIB hyperlipoproteinemia
d. type III hyperlipoproteinemia
e. type IV hyperlipoproteinemia

15. A distinguishing laboratory finding related to the cutaneous porphyrias is

a. increased urine aminolevulinic acid (ALA) and porphobilinogen (PBG)
b. normal urine ALA and PBG
c. increased uroporphyrin only
d. normal blood porphyrins
e. increased protoporphyrin only

16. The Michaelis-Menten formula expressing the relationship between reaction velocity and substrate concentration is stated as

a. $V = \dfrac{V_{max}[S]}{K_m + [S]}$

b. $V = \dfrac{K_m[S]}{V_{max} + [S]}$

c. $V = \dfrac{K_m + [S]}{V_{max}[S]}$

d. $V = \dfrac{V_{max} + [S]}{K_m[S]}$

e. $V = \dfrac{V_{max} + K_m[S]}{[S]}$

17. An elevated serum creatine kinase (CK)-MM fraction was determined in conjunction with a greatly elevated CK-MB fraction. This pattern is typical of which one of the following disorders?

a. brain trauma
b. hypothyroidism
c. stroke
d. acute myocardial infarction
e. muscular dystrophy

18. Laboratory results obtained following serum analysis indicate the following results: decreased T_3, decreased T_4, decreased TSH, decreased free thyroxine index, and decreased T_3 uptake. What is the most likely diagnosis?

a. thryotoxicosis due to pituitary tumor
b. Graves' disease, an autoimmune disorder
c. primary hypothyroidism due to damaged thyroid gland
d. secondary hypothyroidism due to pituitary damage
e. tertiary hypothyroidism due to hypothalamic failure

19. Primary hypergonadism caused by a testicular tumor typically results in precocious puberty in the prepubertal male. A laboratory workup of a patient with this disorder would show

a. low serum androgen, low 17-ketosteroids (17-KS), low serum follicle-stimulating hormone (FSH) and interstitial cell-stimulating hormone (ICSH)
b. high serum androgen, low 17-KS, high serum FSH and ICSH
c. high serum androgen, high 17-KS, low serum FSH and ICSH
d. low serum androgen, high 17-KS, high serum FSH and ICSH
e. low serum androgen, high 17-KS, low serum FSH and ICSH

20. Which one of the following explanations could account for drug toxicity after ingestion of a normally prescribed dose?

a. decreased renal clearance caused by kidney disease
b. administration of another, possibly interactive, drug at the same time
c. altered serum protein binding caused by liver disease
d. inappropriate timing of a blood draw to check therapeutic levels leading to overdosing
e. all of the preceding

21. In regard to pharmacokinetics, zero-order kinetics state which one of the following principles?

a. the rate of change of drug concentration is dependent on the drug concentration itself
b. the rate of change of drug concentration is dependent on the distribution of the drug
c. the rate of change of drug concentration is independent of drug concentration and is dependent on the metabolism of the drug
d. the rate of change of drug concentration is dependent on the substrate on which the drug acts
e. the rate of change of drug concentration is dependent on the distribution of the drug

Directions: Each of the numbered items or incomplete statements in this section is negatively phrased, as indicated by a capitalized word such as NOT, LEAST, or EXCEPT. Select the ONE lettered answer or completion that is BEST in each case.

22. All of the following therapeutic drugs have an active metabolite EXCEPT

a. lidocaine
b. digoxin
c. procainamide
d. quinidine
e. imipramine

23. A tumor involving the anterior pituitary gland could cause hypersecretion of all of the following hormones EXCEPT

a. follicle-stimulating hormone (FSH)
b. growth hormone (GH)
c. vasopressin
d. thyroid-stimulating hormone (TSH)
e. prolactin

24. All of the following statements concerning ammonia are correct EXCEPT

a. ammonia is formed by the deamination of amino acids in the liver
b. severe liver dysfunction, as seen in Reye's syndrome, produces a decrease in serum ammonia levels
c. ammonia is used in the formation of urea and is therefore not excreted by the kidney
d. increased serum ammonia levels can be observed when there is inadequate blood circulation through the liver
e. the reaction of ammonia with α-ketoglutarate is used to determine serum ammonia levels

Answers and Explanations

1. The answer is c [I A 1 b (2)]. Molarity is calculated by first determining the units given in the problem, then the units required in the solution of the problem, and finally setting up the equation. In this problem, the units given are grams and milliliters, and the required final unit is mol/L. The number of grams in 1 mole of NaCL is 58. Therefore,

$$\frac{50 \text{ g NaCl}}{500 \text{ ml}} \times \frac{1000 \text{ ml}}{1 \text{ L}} \times \frac{1 \text{ mole}}{58 \text{ g}} = 1.72 \text{ mol/L}$$

2. The answer is d [I C 3]. The Westgard control rules determine whether an analytic run should be rejected or accepted on the basis of the control values, thereby increasing objectivity. The rule 4_{1s} states that an analytic run should be rejected when four consecutive control observations are on the same side of the mean and exceed either $+1s$ from the mean or $-1s$ from the mean.

3. The answer is c [I C 7 a]. Beer's law is stated as follows: $A = abc$, where measured absorbance (A) is equal to the constant absorptivity of a substance (a) multiplied by the length of the light path (b) multiplied by the concentration of the solution (c). Because absorbance is usually measured, and the concentration is calculated, the equation can be rearranged to give $c = A/ab$. Because a and b are constant, there is a linear relationship between the absorbance of a material and the concentration of that material in a solution.

4. The answer is c [II C 2 a]. In thin-layer chromatography (TLC), spots of samples and standards are applied to a coated glass plate and exposed to a solvent. Following migration of these substances, the relative mobility of each located spot can be calculated by dividing the distance the analyte travels from the origin by the distance traveled by the solvent front. This calculated factor (i.e., retention factor [R_f]) allows comparison with the standards, as well as reasonable identification of specific drugs.

5. The answer is a [III B 3 a (2), 4 a (3)]. Bilirubin is conjugated in the liver. Conjugated bilirubin increases in serum because of an obstructive process that hinders the excretion of this water-soluble form of bilirubin. The obstruction typically occurs in the bile duct as a result of stones or a tumor. In patients with hepatitis, both conjugated and unconjugated components increase because of damage to the liver's cytoarchitecture. Hemolysis and lack of certain enzymes in the newborn induces an increase in the unconjugated bilirubin fraction.

6. The answer is e [IV A 4 a]. Alpha$_1$-antitrypsin acts to inhibit the proteolytic enzyme trypsin. A hereditary defect in the production of this globulin leads to a deficiency associated with emphysema and related pulmonary problems, perhaps caused by increased destruction of pulmonary tissue by trypsin.

7. The answer is e [IV B 6 g (1), (2)]. In an electrical field, negatively charged particles (anions) travel in the direction of the positive pole (anode). The rate of migration depends on the amount of charge on the molecule, the size of the molecule, and the support medium used in the electrophoresis. At pH 8.6, most proteins are negatively charged, and albumin, because of its small size and large number of negative charges, migrates the most quickly and the farthest toward the anode.

8. The answer is a [IV A 6 d (a)]. The reagent most widely used for quantitation of serum total protein is called biuret reagent, which is prepared by dissolving copper sulfate in water. When used in a protein assay, the cupric ions (Cu^{2+}) form a complex with peptide bonds, particularly the amide linkage of the protein. The intensity of the purplish blue complex is related to the concentration of the protein in the sample.

9. The answer is b [IV B 3]. The renal tubules can increase or decrease the formation of bicarbonate from the glomerular filtrate. When the urine in the proximal tubule becomes more acidic, the bicarbon-

76

ate concentration decreases as the pCO_2 concentration increases, which causes carbon dioxide to enter the tubular cells and eventually converts to bicarbonate. This process maintains or restores a normal physiologic pH.

10. The answer is c [IV B 4]. The Henderson-Hasselbalch equation states the relationship between pH and the acid-base concentration in the blood. The pH of plasma at physiologic temperature is 6.1. Because the normal ratio of bicarbonate concentration to carbonic acid is approximately 20:1 and the log_{10} of 20 is 1.3, the equation applied to normal plasma produces a pH value of 7.4. Thus, any change in bicarbonate or carbonic acid concentrations cause a change in plasma pH.

11. The answer is b [IV B 6 b]. An excessive loss of carbon dioxide through hyperventilation is the primary cause of respiratory alkalosis. The increase in exhalation of carbon dioxide shifts the bicarbonate equilibrium toward the formation of carbon dioxide and water by decreasing the hydrogen ion concentration, which results in an increase in blood pH.

12. The answer is c [IV D 2 a (3)]. A sensitive assessment of the renal system is obtained through measurement of creatinine clearance. Calculation of creatinine clearance is done after measurement of serum creatinine and the creatinine in a timed urine specimen (usually a 24-hour specimen). The formula is abbreviated as UV/P, but it is more accurately stated as urinary creatinine in mg/dL multiplied by the total urine volume in milliliters divided by plasma creatinine in mg/dL multiplied by 1440 (the number of minutes in 24 hours).

13. The answer is d [IV E 3 d (1)]. The glucose tolerance test is used to determine how the body uses glucose after it has been absorbed into the circulation. Following measurement of fasting blood sugar, oral glucose is administered, and blood samples are collected every 30 minutes for 2 hours. If the initial fasting sample is greater than 140 mg/dL of glucose, the testing is terminated. If diabetes mellitus is present, the 2-hour blood sugar value will increase greater than 200 mg/dL, and one other sample will increase to this level as well. Values will remain elevated throughout the testing period.

14. The answer is e [IV F 5; Table 1-3]. Frederickson's classification of hyperlipoproteinemia is used in the diagnosis of hyperlipoproteinemia based on the appearance of plasma at 4°C and on lipid values. In Type IV, the most common hyperlipoproteinemia, cholesterol values are slightly increased, triglycerides are greatly increased, and very low density lipoproteins (VLDLs), which are responsible for transporting triglycerides, are increased. Disorders producing Type IV hyperlipoproteinemia include diabetes mellitus, pancreatitis, and thyroid disorders.

15. The answer is b [IV I 2 b]. Porphyrin accumulation in the skin leads to chronic inflammation and blistering of the skin on exposure to sunlight. In these cutaneous porphyrias, several enzyme deficiencies are thought to cause the photosensitivity, although the disorder may be acquired following excessive alcohol consumption, excess iron accumulation, or exposure to estrogen. Aminolevulinic acid (ALA) and porphobilinogen (PBG) are not excreted in excess in patients with cutaneous porphyrias. The urine level of ALA and PBG is normal because the enzymes that synthesize them are unaffected.

16. The answer is a [V A 6 b (1); Figure 1-4]. Several factors are involved in the rate of enzymatic reactions, including substrate concentration, enzyme concentration, and the presence of cofactors. The Michaelis-Menten equation describes the effect substrate concentration has on the rate of the reaction. If the enzyme is present in high enough amounts, the rate of the reaction is determined by the concentration of the substrate itself. As substrate level increases, the enzyme reaction rate also increases. However, there is a point when a further increase in substrate does not induce any increase in reaction rate, as evidenced by the Michaelis-Menten curve.

17. The answer is d [V D 4 a, b]. Creatine kinase (CK) is distributed in skeletal muscle, brain, and cardiac muscle. In acute myocardial infarction, both CK-MM and CK-MB fractions are elevated. The MB fraction is specific for cardiac muscle, and the MM fraction is specific for skeletal muscle.

18. The answer is d [VI D 2 a (2) (b)]. Most cases of hypothyroidism present with an increased thyroid-stimulating hormone (TSH) level. However, if the primary defect is in the pituitary gland, the TSH level decreases with the thyroxine (T_4) and triiodothyronine (T_3) uptake. A deficiency of TSH leads to loss of stimulation of the thyroid gland and diminished production of thyroid hormones.

19. The answer is c [VI F 5 b (1)]. The major androgens synthesized by the testes are testosterone, androstanedione, and dehydroepiandrosterone (DHEA). A testicular tumor leads to overproduction of these steroid hormones. The 17-ketosteroids are metabolites of andosterone and DHEA and would be increased in this type of disorder as well because of the elevated levels of these steroids. Elevated testosterone levels inhibit the production of follicle-stimulating hormone (FSH) and interstitial cell-stimulating hormone (ICSH), which are anterior pituitary hormones produced in men.

20. The answer is e [VII G 1, 2]. The goal of drug administration is to achieve the therapeutic range, which is the level of drug concentration in the bloodstream that provides optimum medication for improvement of the disorder being treated. Information regarding protein status, liver function, renal impairment, other medicaments being administered, and time since last dose must be taken into account when therapeutic drugs are administered. All of these can affect the toxic or the therapeutic effect of the drug.

21. The answer is c [VI H 2]. Pharmacokinetics describe the disposition of a therapeutic drug over a period of time. First-order pharmacokinetics, which are similar to enzyme kinetics, state that a drug's physiologic concentration affects the rate at which the concentration of that drug changes. This change is caused by absorption, distribution, and elimination of that drug, all of which are dependent on drug concentration. Zero-order kinetics state that the rate of change of a drug's physiologic concentration does not depend on the concentration of the drug, but instead on how the drug is metabolized by the liver per unit of time.

22. The answer is b [VII F 1 a]. The excretion product of digoxin is digoxigenin, a substance that has no known activity as a cardioactive drug. The remaining therapeutic drugs have metabolites that have activity similar to the parent drug.

23. The answer is c [VI B 1 b]. Vasopressin, or antidiuretic hormone, and oxytocin are hormones synthesized in the hypothalamus, a specialized portion of the brain. Once synthesized, vasopressin and oxytocin are stored in the posterior portion of the pituitary gland and released on appropriate stimulation.

24. The answer is b [IV D 4 d]. Reye's syndrome is a rare disease that affects primarily small children. The cause is unknown, but appears to begin with a viral infection of the respiratory tract or chickenpox. When the fever accompanying the disease is treated with aspirin, it is thought to contribute to the pathology of liver disease. Because of hepatic involvement, certain hepatic enzymes increase. A hallmark of Reye's syndrome is increased serum ammonia.

2
Hemostasis and Coagulation

Joel Hubbard

I. PLATELET PHYSIOLOGY

A. General considerations. Platelets, which exist in whole blood in concentrations of 150,000–440,000/mm^3, are disk-shaped cells **necessary for hemostasis.** Platelets are formed from the cytoplasm of **megakaryocyte** in the marrow.

1. **A Wright's-stained blood film** provides an estimation of platelet numbers, size, and distribution.

2. **Platelet number** can be obtained by manual platelet count (**hemacytometer**) or an electronic cell counter.

B. Platelet ultrastructure (Figure 2-1)

1. **Glycocalyx is the outer membrane surface.** It is rich in glycoproteins, which serve as membrane receptors.

   a. **Glycoprotein Ib** is the receptor for **von Willebrand's factor** (vWF) in the presence of **ristocetin.**

   b. **Glycoproteins IIb and IIIa** are receptors for **vWF** and **fibrinogen,** and are exposed by stimulation of thrombin or adenosine diphosphate (ADP).

   c. **Glycoprotein Va** is the receptor for **thrombin.**

2. **Microtubule and micro filaments.** These provide an **active means of platelet contraction** to squeeze out the contents of the cytoplasmic granules.

   a. **Microtubules** form the submembranous band around the circumference of the cell and structurally support the normal discoid-shaped platelets.

   b. The **contractile microfilaments** (thrombasthenin) contain actin and are closely related to the microtubule.

3. **The open canalicular system** provides direct communication between intracellular and extracellular compartments.

4. **A dense tubular system** forms a circle within the microtubule.

   a. This system serves as a site for arachidonic acid metabolism.

   b. This system also functions as a calcium-sequestering pump that maintains platelet cytoplasmic calcium levels.

5. **Mitochondria** are responsible for energy production.

79

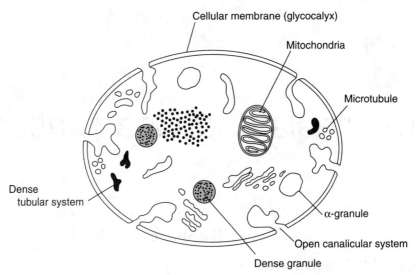

Figure 2-1. Diagram of platelet ultrastructure showing the major intracellular morphologic features. (Reprinted with permission from Besa EC: *Hematology.* Baltimore, Williams & Wilkins, 1992, p. 202.)

6. **Glycogen granules** provide energy substrate.

7. **Alpha (α) granules** contain contact-promoting factors, including:
   a. Platelet fibrinogen
   b. Platelet-derived growth factor (PDGF)
   c. von Willebrand's factor (factor VIII:R)
   d. β-Thromboglobulin (BTG)
   e. Platelet factor 4 (heparin-neutralizing)
   f. Fibronectin

8. **Dense granules** contain nonprotein factors, including:
   a. Adenosine diphosphate (ADP)
   b. Adenosine triphosphate (ATP)
   c. 5-Hydroxytryptamine (5-HT; or serotonin)
   d. Calcium

C. **Platelet function**
   1. **Damaged subendothelium** releases factors that **activate the platelet, transform its shape,** and **evolve a "sticky" platelet aggregate to plug the leak.** These factors include:
      a. Collagen
      b. Fibronectin
      c. vWF (factor VIII:R)
      d. Thrombin
      e. ADP

2. **Tissue platelet activators** cause the platelet to change shape from discoid to spherical. **Alpha and dense granules** undergo internal contraction and centralization. The complete process is **calcium dependent.**

   a. The exposure of surface membrane receptors to vWF and fibrinogen results in cytoplasmic calcium ionization, stimulation of ATP generation, and activation of the actin monomers in the micro filaments.

   b. Contractions result in a centralization of the cytoplasmic granules and a release of their contents through the canalicular system.

3. **Plug formation,** or secondary aggregation, is primarily stimulated by **thrombin and thromboxane A$_2$ (TXA$_2$).**

   a. Membrane-binding of vWF and collagen to platelet receptors unmasks membrane **phospholipid A$_2$,** which is the precursor of arachidonic acid, and is important for the production of TXA$_2$ and other prostaglandins. **Phospholipid A$_2$** is unmasked by the binding of vWF and collagen to platelet receptors on the membrane.

   b. TXA$_2$ inhibits adenylate cyclase [thus, it inhibits the formation of cyclic adenosine monophosphate (cAMP)] and liberates sequestered calcium into cytoplasm. Calcium causes further cytoplasmic contraction, release of granule contents, and platelet aggregation.

   c. **Thrombin** enzymatically cleaves fibrinogen to form **fibrin,** which is necessary to stabilize the platelet plug.

4. **Growth-limiting factors of the platelet aggregate** include:

   a. **Blood flow,** which washes away coagulation-promoting factors

   b. Release of prostaglandin **PGI$_2$ (prostacyclin)** by the surrounding vascular tissues

5. **Granular release** of substances from dense granules, such as serotonin, prostaglandins (except for TXA$_2$), and lysozymes causes local inflammation and vasodilation, which increases blood flow.

D. **Kinetics**

1. **Megakaryocytopoiesis development occurs by endomitosis** (i.e., nuclear splitting without cell division).

   a. A single megakaryoblast nucleus may contain 2–64 times the normal number of chromosomes.

   b. **Nuclear chromatin** is densely staining, dispersed early, and more compact at later stages.

   c. **Nucleoli** are small at all development stages.

2. **Stages of megakaryocytic maturation** (Figure 2-2)

   a. **Megakaryoblasts** descend from a unipotential stem cell **(CFU-Meg).** They are characterized by overlapping nuclear lobes and basophilic staining cytoplasm; their size ranges from 6–24 μm.

   b. **Promegakaryocytes** are larger than megakaryoblasts (14–30 μm in diameter) and have more cytoplasm.

      (1) The nucleus becomes increasingly lobulated and spreads out into a horseshoe shape.

      (2) Red-pink granules are visible in the center of the cell.

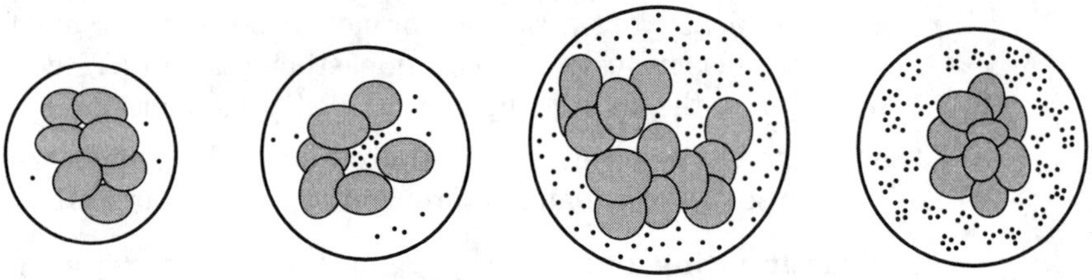

	Megakaryoblast	Promegakaryocyte	Granular megakaryocyte	Mature
Size range	0 – 24 μm	14 – 30 μm	15 – 56 μm	20 – 50 μm
Cytoplasmic staining	Deep blue (basophilic)	Basophilic with pink center	Mostly pink	Totally pink
Granules	Rare	Few	Extensive	Organized into platelet fields
Nuclear morphology	Few compacted lobes	Lobes spread out in horseshoe shape	Many lobes spread out	Many compacted lobes
N:C ratio	High	Moderate	Moderate	Low

Figure 2-2. Morphologic characteristics of stages of megakaryocytic maturation comparing the nuclear and cytoplasmic variations of each stage. *N:C* = nuclear-cytoplasmic ratio.

    c. Granular megakaryocyte (16–56 μm) are characterized by increased spreading of nuclear lobes and spreading of pink granules throughout the cytoplasm.

    d. Mature megakaryocyte (20–50 μm) have a compact nucleus, and the basophilia of cytoplasm has disappeared.

      (1) Platelet fields are clusters of pink granules in the cytoplasm.

        (a) Platelet fields are produced by an invagination of surface membrane, separating the cytoplasm into individual platelets.

        (b) Individual platelets are shed from the megakaryocyte cytoplasm into the marrow sinuses, and then are released into the vascular lumen.

      (2) Each mature megakaryocyte produces from 2000–7000 platelets that each range in size from 2–3 μm.

3. Maturation time from the blast stage to platelet formation is typically 5 days.

4. Normal marrow contains approximately 15 million megakaryocyte. This equates to approximately 5–10 megakaryocyte per 10X power field when bone marrow smears are microscopically examined.

5. Normal circulation life of a platelet is 8–10 days.

6. Platelets are removed by macrophage in the liver and spleen or by active use in daily coagulation mechanisms.

7. Circulating platelets are distributed between the spleen and blood.

    a. One third of the circulating platelets are always **in the spleen.**

b. The platelet count is **higher** in patients **without a spleen** and **lower** in patients with **splenomegaly** (enlarged spleen).

8. Regulation of the platelet count

a. Under **normal conditions** the platelet count (or mass) is constant, even with active use. This indicates a feedback system that adjusts production to consumption.

(1) Rebound thrombocytopenia occurs after platelet transfusion.

(2) Rebound thrombocytosis occurs after platelet depletion.

b. Feedback stimulus results in an increased megakaryoblast endomitosis, which increases platelet volume and number. It also affects committed unipotential stem cells, which results in more megakaryoblast.

E. Laboratory measurements of platelet activities

1. Initial evaluation includes a platelet count and slide estimate, with a reference value of **150,000–440,000/mm³.**

2. Bleeding time is an effective screening test of platelet function.

a. Reference values are approximately **3–8 minutes.**

b. Increased bleeding times are seen in:

(1) Patients taking drugs with antiplatelet action (e.g., aspirin)

(2) Patients with von Willebrand's disease (vWD)

(3) Patients who suffer from congenital platelet abnormalities

(4) Patients with platelet counts lower than 100,000/mm³

3. Platelet aggregation is measured with a **platelet aggregometer.**

a. Basic principle. Citrated, platelet-rich plasma is stirred in the aggregometer while a light beam is passed through the suspension.

b. A **chemical stimulus is added** [e.g., collagen, epinephrine, ADP, ristocetin, A23187 (calcium ionifier), arachidonic acid, γ-thrombin (partially trypsinized thrombin)].

c. γ-**Thrombin** retains aggregating properties but lacks clotting ability.

d. The shape change from discoid to spheroid is monitored as an **initial decrease** in light transmittance.

e. Subsequent aggregation allows an increase of light to pass through the suspension to the photodetector and to be recorded as an **increase in light transmittance.**

II. PLATELET PATHOPHYSIOLOGY

A. Quantitative platelet disorders (Figure 2-3)

1. Thrombocytopenia is characterized by a decrease in the number of circulating platelets (i.e., less than 100,000/mm³). Clinical evidence of thrombocytopenia includes an increased number of petechiae, hemorrhages, prolonged bleeding time, and impaired clot retraction. Decreased circulating platelet counts result from the following conditions:

a. Low platelet counts can result from **defective production in the bone marrow.**

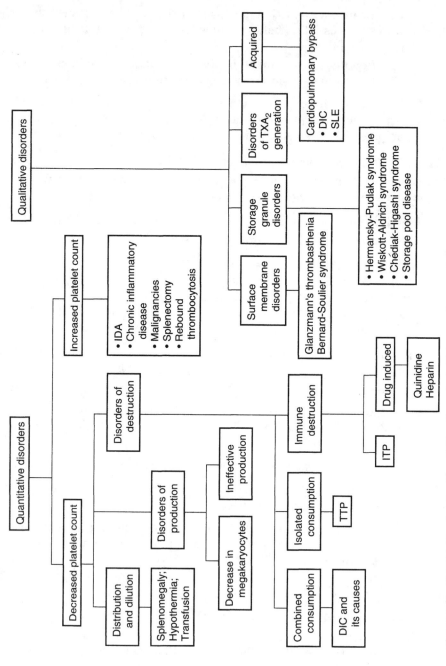

Figure 2-3. Platelet disorder algorithm. DIC = disseminated intravascular coagulation; IDA = iron deficiency anemia; ITP = idiopathic thrombocytopenic purpura; TTP = thrombotic thrombocytopenic purpura; TXA_2 = thromboxane A_2; SLE = systemic lupus erythematosus.

84

(1) Decreased numbers of megakaryocyte are seen in the following disorders:

   (a) Congenital disorders (e.g., Fanconi's anemia, maternal infection)

   (b) Acquired disorders seen with the use of radiation, alcohol, thiazide diuretics, chloramphenicol, and cancer chemotherapy

   (c) Marrow replacement by malignant cells, which occurs with metastatic carcinoma, leukemia, lymphoma, myeloma, and myelofibrosis

(2) Ineffective platelet production in the marrow is seen with all of the following conditions:

   (a) Hereditary thrombocytopenia

   (b) Vitamin B_{12} or folate deficiency **(megaloblastic anemia)**

   (c) Di Guglielmo's syndrome (also known as erythroleukemia)

   (d) Proximal nocturnal hemoglobinuria (PNH)

b. Thrombocytopenia can result from **disorders of distribution and dilution** of platelets in the circulation. These conditions include:

   (1) Splenic pooling, which is commonly seen with splenomegaly and hypersplenism

   (2) Hypothermia, which results in vascular shunting

   (3) Dilution in the circulation by transfused stored blood

c. Thrombocytopenia can result from disorders that result in the **destruction of platelets.**

   (1) Combined consumption of both platelet and coagulation factors is seen with:

      (a) Toxicity due to snake venoms

      (b) Tissue injury

      (c) Obstetric complications (e.g., aborted fetus, toxemia of pregnancy)

      (d) Neoplasms (e.g., promyelocytic leukemia, carcinoma)

      (e) Bacterial and viral infections

      (f) Intravascular hemolysis

   (2) Isolated consumption of platelets results from the following disorders:

      (a) Thrombotic thrombocytopenia purpura (TTP) is caused by excessive deposition of platelet aggregates in renal and cerebral vessels. Physiologically, TTP is believed to be **caused by vascular wall dysfunction,** disrupting the inert basement membrane.

         (i) Clinical diagnosis. TTP is three times more prevalent in women than men at an average age of 35 years. The majority of patients are seen with microangiopathic hemolytic anemia; thrombocytopenia; neurologic symptoms (e.g., headaches, seizures); fever; and renal disease.

         (ii) Laboratory diagnosis of TTP includes a prothrombin time (PT) that is normal in 88% of patients, an activated partial thromboplastin time (APTT) that is normal in 94% of patients, and a fibrinogen level that is normal in 79% of patients. Fibrin-degradation products (FDP) are normal

Table 2-1. Acute and Chronic Idiopathic Thrombocytopenia Purpura (ITP): A Comparison

	Acute ITP	Chronic ITP
Onset	Children aged 2–6 years; sudden onset, often after viral infections	Adults aged 20–40 years; women three times more than men; slow, asymptomatic onset
Duration	2–6 weeks; spontaneous remission in 80%	Months to years
Platelet count	$<20,000/mm^3$	$30,000/mm^3$ to $80,000/mm^3$
Pathophysiology	Altered platelet-membrane proteins cause formation of platelet autoantibodies	Associated with systemic lupus erythematosus (SLE)
Therapy	Corticosteroids	Splenectomy; immunosuppressive chemotherapy (vincristine, vinblastine)

in 53% of patients, weakly positive in 23%, and positive in 24%.

      (iii) Pathophysiology of TTP possibly results from vascular endothelial cell damage, an increase in a platelet-aggregating factor, a possible deficiency of platelet-aggregating factor inhibitor, a decrease in prostacyclin (PGI_2), an increase in PGI_2 degradation, or an absence of a plasminogen activator.

   (b) Hemolytic uremic syndrome

   (c) Vasculitis [as seen with systemic lupus erythematosus (SLE)]

   (d) Disseminated intravascular coagulation (DIC)

(3) Immune destruction of platelets occurs in the following disorders:

   (a) Idiopathic (immunologic) thrombocytopenia purpura (ITP) is an autoimmune disorder (Table 2-1). Common laboratory findings include an increase in mean platelet volume (MPV), decreased platelet count, increased bone marrow platelet production, increased marrow megakaryocyte, a normal bleeding time, and platelet-associated IgG.

   (b) Acute ITP occurs in children 2–6 years of age. There is a sudden onset of thrombocytopenia, which often follows viral infections such as rubella, chickenpox, cytomegalovirus (CMV), and toxoplasmosis.

      (i) Duration. Acute ITP usually lasts for 2–6 weeks, with a spontaneous remission in 80% of patients.

      (ii) Platelet count is usually lower than $20,000/mm^3$ in patients with acute ITP.

      (iii) Pathophysiology. Acute ITP is caused by viral attachment and antigenic alteration of platelet membrane proteins, which result in formation of platelet autoantibodies, most often IgG. IgG-coated platelets are removed by macrophages in the spleen.

        (iv) Therapy. Because acute ITP is usually self-limited, corticosteroids are the treatment of choice when therapy is instituted. Steroids suppress macrophage phagocytic activity, decrease Fc-receptor function, and decrease antibody-platelet binding. Splenectomy is rarely needed, and platelet transfusion is ineffective.

    (c) Chronic ITP occurs in adults 20–40 years of age. It is found in women three times more than in men and has a slow, asymptomatic onset of thrombocytopenia.

        (i) Duration. Chronic ITP can last from months to years.

        (ii) Platelet count usually ranges from 30,000–80,000/mm^3.

        (iii) Pathophysiology. Chronic ITP is often associated with SLE.

        (iv) Therapy. Splenectomy is the most common treatment because it decreases the number of macrophage with Fc receptors. Immunosuppressive chemotherapy with vincristine or vinblastine is used in severely affected patients.

    (d) Post-transfusion purpura occurs in 1%–2% of persons who receive blood transfusions. Production of **antiplatelet antibodies** by the recipient of platelet transfusions results in the destruction of platelets.

    (e) Isoimmune neonatal purpura is caused by maternal viremia (e.g., CMV or rubella) or maternal drug ingestion.

    (f) Drug-induced antibody formation is most commonly seen with the use of **quinidine and heparin.** The drugs function as haptens, combining with a serum protein and causing an antibody response. The drug-antibody complex attaches to platelets, which results in agglutination, complement fixation, and destruction by macrophages.

  d. Thrombocytopenia can result from a **combination of mechanisms** (e.g., alcoholism, lymphoproliferative disorders).

  e. Heparin-induced thrombocytopenia is observed in more than 10% of patients who undergo heparin therapy.

    (1) Risk from thrombosis without heparin therapy is greater than the risk of bleeding from heparin-induced thrombocytopenia.

    (2) The **mechanism** of thrombocytopenia is due to a direct platelet-aggregating effect, as well as immune destruction by antiplatelet antibodies.

    (3) Laboratory diagnosis. A normal aggregation pattern in platelet aggregometer studies is found, **except** that adding heparin as a stimulant will **increase aggregation** instead of blunting the aggregation reaction.

  f. Thrombocytopenia associated with human immunodeficiency virus (HIV) infection is severe but rarely hemorrhagic.

    (1) Characteristics similar to classic ITP include:

        (a) Abundant megakaryocytes

        (b) Occasional giant platelets

        (c) Immune origin

        (d) Absence of splenomegaly

(2) **Characteristics different** from ITP include:
  (a) Greater levels of bound antibody
  (b) Involvement of immune complexes

2. **Thrombocytosis** is characterized by an increase in circulating platelet counts greater than $450,000/mm^3$.

  a. **Essential thrombocytosis** is the result of a primary bone marrow disorder. Although it is characterized by an increased number of platelets, it is caused by a clonal proliferation that affects all hemopoietic cells. Often, patients with a thrombocytosis will have increased bleeding tendencies because of possible accompanying functional abnormalities. Essential thrombocytosis is most commonly seen in patients with the following disorders:

  (1) Hodgkin's disease
  (2) Polycythemia vera
  (3) Myelofibrosis
  (4) Chronic myelogenous leukemia
  (5) Thrombocythemia

  b. **Secondary thrombocytosis** is a secondary response most commonly associated with the following disorders:

  (1) **Iron deficiency anemia** associated with chronic blood loss
  (2) **Chronic inflammatory disease** may be associated with high platelet counts
  (3) **Splenectomy-associated thrombocytosis**
  (4) **Rebound thrombocytosis,** which may occur after a platelet depletion through a massive blood loss

B. **Causes of qualitative platelet abnormalities**

  1. **Surface membrane defects** that are genetically acquired

  a. **Glanzmann's thrombasthenia** is a functional abnormality in which the platelets are normal in number and appearance.

  (1) **Laboratory diagnosis** is based on an **abnormal pattern of aggregation** observed in response to the majority of aggregating agents. Only **ristocetin** induces the initial phase of aggregation, followed by a wave of **disagglutination** rather than a second wave of true agglutination.

  (2) **Genetic defects** result in a decrease in platelet surface **glycoproteins IIb and IIIa** and in a reduction in the number of available **fibrinogen-binding** sites.

  b. **Bernard-Soulier disease** is a functional platelet disorder that may appear similar to ITP.

  (1) **Laboratory diagnosis** is based on the aggregation pattern and the platelet count.

  (a) The aggregation pattern seen in Bernard-Soulier disease is the reverse of that seen in Glanzmann's. Aggregation and granular content release are **normal** with the majority of aggregating agents, **except ristocetin.**

  (b) Granular release induced by thrombin is reduced.

(2) **Genetic defects** result in a decrease in the platelet membrane **vWF receptor (glycoproteins Ib and V).**

(3) Bernard-Soulier disease **must be differentiated from vWD,** in which there is a decrease in vWF (VIII:R) **not** in the binding site. Exogenous vWF added to plasma cryoprecipitate corrects this bleeding disorder for vWD patients but will not reverse the symptoms of those patients with Bernard-Soulier disease.

2. **Abnormalities in the granular fraction of the platelet**

   a. **Congenital deficiencies in dense granules,** which contain ADP, ATP, serotonin, and calcium, show diminished platelet aggregation in the second wave of aggregation.

      (1) **Hermansky-Pudlak syndrome** is caused by decreased numbers of platelet-dense granules.

      (2) **Chédiak-Higashi syndrome** is an autosomal disorder resulting in giant lysosomes in the cytoplasm of all precursor blood cells in the marrow. Giant lysosomes are also found in megakaryocyte, which results in dense granule destruction.

      (3) **Wiskott-Aldrich syndrome** is a sex-linked decrease in the number of dense granules.

      (4) **Storage pool disease** is a platelet disorder in which there is an **increase in the ratio of ATP to ADP** based on total cellular content.

   b. **Alpha-granule deficiencies** are rare platelet functional abnormalities in which both aggregation and release properties are diminished. This disorder is also known as **gray platelet syndrome** because of the staining characteristics of the platelet.

3. **Deficiencies of thromboxane generation** can occur because of a genetic deficiency of the cyclo-oxygenase enzyme. Platelet aggregation tests are **unresponsive to arachidonic acid** as a stimulator.

4. **Acquired** disorders of platelet function exist that are **secondary** to the following conditions:

   a. **Thrombocytopenia** and platelet function defects, caused by a depletion of α-granules, are seen in some patients after **cardiopulmonary bypass.**

   b. **Acquired storage pool deficiency** is seen in patients with SLE, chronic ITP, and DIC.

   c. **Uremia due to kidney failure** sometimes causes platelet aggregation abnormalities because of prostacyclin production and decreased platelet TXA_2 production.

III. BLOOD COAGULATION AND FIBRINOLYSIS (Figure 2-4)

A. **Initiating reactions (contact activation)**

   1. **The intrinsic system** refers to the path of the coagulation cascade in which **prekallikrein, heavy molecular weight kininogen (HMWK), and factors XII, XI, X, IX, VIII, V, II, and I** are involved in the formation of a fibrin clot. In the laboratory, the APTT is used to test the coagulation cascade.

      a. **Initiation** of the intrinsic system coagulation cascade is by the **activation of factor XII (Hageman factor).**

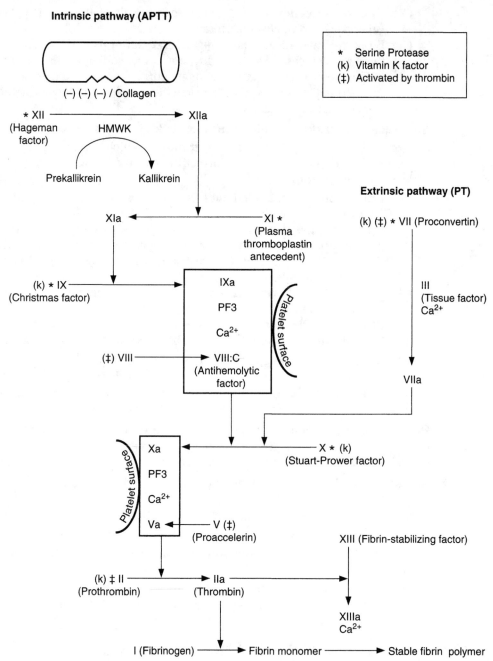

Figure 2-4. The coagulation cascade. Each enzymatic factor represented by roman numerals is converted in turn to an activated form designated by the letter "a." The intrinsic pathway consists of high molecular weight kininogen (HMWK); prekallikrein; and factors I, II, V, VIII, IX, X, XI, and XII. The intrinsic pathway is screened by the activated partial thromboplastin time (APTT). The extrinsic pathway consists of factors I, II, V, VII, and X. It is screened by the prothrombin time (PT) test. Ca^{2+} = calcium ion; PF3 = platelet factor 3; (−) = negative surface charge of exposed subendothelium.

       (1) Vascular damage exposes **negatively charged** subendothelial tissue.

       (2) The inactive **zymogen** form of factor XII is attracted to the negatively charged endothelial surface of the damaged blood vessel. The negative polarity activates factor XII by causing the molecule to expose its active serine center. The activated form of factor XII is then denoted as factor XIIa.

    b. There are **three products of factor XIIa reactions.**

       (1) **Prekallikrein** is enzymatically cleaved by factor XIIa to produce kallikrein, which in turn produces **bradykinin.**

         (a) Bradykinin functions to increase local vasodilatation and membrane permeability to increase local blood flow.

         (b) The reaction requires **HMWK as a cofactor** (see Figure 2-4).

       (2) **Plasminogen** is enzymatically cleaved by factor XIIa to functional **plasmin,** which initiates clot dissolution reactions.

       (3) Factor XIIa enzymatically activates **factor XI** (plasma thromboplastin antecedent) to yield **factor XIa.** The activation of factor XIa will continue the coagulation cascade.

  2. The **extrinsic system**

    a. Initiation. Contact activation of the extrinsic system begins with the **activation of factor VII.**

       (1) **Factor III,** known as **tissue factor,** is the primary activator of VII to VIIa, which is a potent serine protease.

       (2) Tissue factor consists of **lipoproteins,** which are produced in many tissues.

       (3) Minor activation of factor VII can occur by proteolytic attack from factors XIIa, Xa, IXa, or thrombin.

    b. In **laboratory testing** of the **extrinsic system, lipoprotein-rich extracts** are added to citrated plasma as the **prothrombin (PT) reagent** to support the activation of factor VII by tissue factor.

B. Intermediate reactions

  1. Factor VIIa in the **extrinsic pathway** enzymatically alters factor X to yield Xa in the presence of factor III. Factor VIIa has limited ability to activate the conversion of IX to its activated form (IXa).

  2. Factor IX in the **intrinsic pathway** is most strongly activated by the direct enzymatic action of XIa.

    a. Initiation. This reaction does **not** require tissue factor lipoprotein as extrinsic pathway activation. It **does** require negatively charged membrane phospholipids and ionized calcium. **Platelets are the main source of in vivo phospholipid surfaces.**

    b. In **laboratory testing** of the **intrinsic system,** phospholipid extracts are added to citrated plasma as part of the APTT reagent to provide the activation for platelet-supported reactions.

  3. Factor X (Stuart-Prower factor) is activated by two different pathways.

    a. In the **extrinsic pathway,** factor X is enzymatically activated by **VIIa,** with **factor III** and **calcium** as cofactors.

    b. In the **intrinsic pathway,** factor X is activated by **factor IXa.** Factor IXa forms a complex with a platelet phospholipid membrane surface and **factor VIII (antihemolytic factor)** in the presence of calcium.

4. The **factor VIII complex** is a high molecular weight (MW) complex formed of two subunits.

    a. **VIII:C (antihemolytic factor)** is synthesized in the liver and is genetically controlled on the X-chromosome **(sex-linked transmission).**

        (1) Function. Factor VIII:C serves as a **cofactor in the activation of factor X by factor IXa.** The presence of VIII:C accelerates the reaction rate by 500–1000 times.

        (2) Activator. Factor VIII:C is activated by **thrombin.**

        (3) Inactivator. Coagulation inhibitor **protein C (PC)** breaks down factor VIII:C enzymatically.

        (4) Pathology. An inherited deficiency of factor VIII:C is known as **hemophilia A.**

    b. **Factor VIII:R (vWF)** is synthesized by endothelial cells, megakaryocyte, and platelet and demonstrates autosomal genetic expression.

        (1) Function. vWF supports the adhesion of platelets to the exposed subendothelial surface of the blood vessel.

        (2) Activator. vWF activation occurs through the release of **platelet aggregators** from damaged subendothelial tissue, and from the release of **platelet α-granule contents.**

        (3) Pathology. An inherited deficiency of factor VIII:R is known clinically as **von Willebrand's disease (vWD).**

5. **Factor Xa activation** begins the **common pathway,** because the following enzymatic reactions are shared by both the intrinsic and the extrinsic pathways.

    a. Factor Xa enzymatically cleaves the zymogen **prothrombin** (factor II) to its activated form, **thrombin.**

    b. The activated form of **factor V (proaccelerin)** acts as a cofactor for factor Xa activation of prothrombin. Factor V is converted to its active form by thrombin.

    c. The combination of phospholipid membrane surface, factor Xa, factor Va, and calcium forms the receptor complex known as **thrombomodulin,** which supports the enzymatic conversion of prothrombin to the active enzyme thrombin (see Figure 2-4).

6. **Thrombin (IIa)** is a powerful enzyme with many functions, including:

    a. Enzymatic conversion of **fibrinogen to fibrin monomer**

    b. Activation of **factor XIII (fibrin stabilizing factor)**

    c. Activation of **platelet aggregation**

    d. Activation of factor V and factor VIII:C

    e. Activation of PC

    f. Weak activation of **factor VII to factor VIIa**

C. **Fibrin clot formation** is the last step in the coagulation cascade.

1. **Thrombin** enzymatically converts **fibrinogen** (factor I) to **fibrin.**

2. **Fibrinogen** has the highest plasma concentration of any clotting factor, with a normal range of **150–400 mg/dL.** The molecule is produced in the liver and has a unique molecular structure.

   a. The fibrinogen monomer consists of two identical subunits bound together to produce a symmetric structure.

   b. **Three nodular domains** in the fibrinogen molecule have been identified as two **identical D regions** at either carboxy-terminal end and a **central E domain** at the N-terminal end.

3. Thrombin enzymatically activates the fibrinogen monomer by splitting off the **fibrinopeptides Aα and Bβ** from the N-terminals in the E domain.

4. The **thrombin-exposed N-terminal peptides** in the E domain react noncovalently by electrostatic forces with polar D domain regions of adjacent fibrin molecules to form a polymer structure.

5. **Formation of a fibrin polymer** is the endpoint detected in the majority of in vitro clotting time tests.

6. **Clot stabilization** is achieved by **factor XIIIa (fibrin stabilizing factor),** from the formation of covalent bonds between chains of adjacent fibrin molecules.

   a. The inactive circulating zymogen form of factor XIII is activated by the proteolytic action of thrombin, with calcium and fibrinogen serving as cofactors.

   b. Factor XIIIa also covalently cross-links α_2-antiplasmin to the fibrin clot, rendering the clot less susceptible to lysis by **plasmin.**

D. **Vitamin K–dependent factors** are coagulation factors (i.e., factors II, VII, IX, X) and inhibitors [i.e., PC, protein S (PS)] that depend on vitamin K metabolism to be completely functional.

   1. **Without vitamin K,** the coagulation factors and inhibitors are nonfunctioning, even when present in normal concentrations.

   2. **Coumarin anticoagulants** inhibit vitamin K reduction from the epoxide form. The end result is that factors II, VII, IX, and X are rendered inactive.

      a. Unlike heparin, coumarin is inactive as an in vitro anticoagulant and functions only as a therapeutic in vivo anticoagulant.

      b. The **PT** test is the best screening method for **coumarin therapy** because factor VII has the shortest half-life and is the most sensitive to levels of coumarin therapy.

E. **Natural inhibitors of coagulation** function to counterbalance the effects of coagulation factors, provide limitations for the forming fibrin clot, and prevent systemic thrombus formation.

   1. **Antithrombin III** is the principal inhibitor of **thrombin and factor Xa,** with limited inhibitory activity against factors IXa, XIa, and XIIa.

      a. **Antithrombin III** functions by binding with thrombin to form a 1:1 inactive complex.

      b. **Heparin** serves as a cofactor in the inactivation, thereby increasing the reaction rate by more than 2000 times.

2. **α_2-macroglobulin** is a minor inhibitor of thrombin.

3. **Complement C_1 inhibitor** is a minor inhibitor of factors XIa and XIIa.

4. **α_1-antitrypsin** has limited inhibition of thrombin, kallikrein, and factor XIa.

5. **PC** is a vitamin K–dependent inhibitor that circulates as an inactive zymogen.
   a. **Activator.** PC is activated by thrombin as part of the thrombomodulin platelet receptor complex.
   b. **Function.** PC **inactivates** factors VIII:C and Va in the presence of cofactor **PS**. PS also depends on vitamin K, functions to enhance binding of PC to phospholipid surfaces, and increases the rate of Va and VIIIa inactivation by PC.

F. **Laboratory testing of coagulation depends on the quality and freshness of the plasma specimen obtained.** Whole blood anticoagulated with **sodium citrate** is the specimen of choice. A **9:1 blood:citrate ratio** is required for accurate coagulation testing, because a ratio of less than 9:1 may falsely increase results. Conditions that can interfere with obtaining the required 9:1 ratio are an abnormally high hematocrit, traumatic blood drawing, or a hemolyzed specimen. **EDTA contamination** can falsely increase PT and APTT results. Specimens must be assayed as soon as possible, and the plasma must be kept cold to avoid factor deterioration.

1. **PT** tests for **extrinsic pathway** deficiencies in factors **VII, X, V, II, and I** (fibrinogen).
   a. **Reagent.** A **lipoprotein tissue extract** from brain or lung tissue serves as the reagent source of tissue factor. An excess of calcium is also added to the PT reagent.
   b. **Principle.** Citrated plasma is added to the lipoprotein reagent with calcium, and the time required for fibrin clot formation is measured.
   c. **Reference range.** Although the PT assay has an approximate normal range of **11–13 seconds**, it is important for each laboratory to establish its own range.
   d. **Variation.** The addition of **Russell's viper venom (Stypven)** instead of lipoprotein reagent activates factor X directly, bypassing factor VII as a necessary component variable. This variation of the common PT is known as the **Stypven time.**

2. **APTT** tests for **intrinsic pathway** deficiencies in factors **prekallikrein, HMWK, and factors XII, XI, IX, X, VIII, V, II, and I.**
   a. **Reagents.** A phospholipid-rich preparation is used as a platelet-membrane substitute. An **activator** such as kaolin, ellagic acid, or celite is also added to the APTT reagent to provide the negative surface charge required to activate factor XII and prekallikrein. Calcium chloride is used as an additional reagent to initiate clotting.
   b. **Principle.** A citrated plasma sample is preincubated with the phospholipid reagent to initiate contact activation factors in the intrinsic pathway. Following incubation, calcium chloride reagent is added as a separate reagent to initiate the clotting cascade. The time required for fibrin clot formation to occur is measured.

    c. **Reference range.** The APTT assay has an approximate normal range of **25–40 seconds,** but it is important for each laboratory to establish its own range.

3. **Thrombin time (TT)** tests for a **deficiency or inhibition of fibrinogen.**

    a. **Principle.** Commercially prepared thrombin reagent is added to citrated plasma, and the time required for clot formation is measured.

    b. **Reference range.** The range is generally **10–20 seconds,** but each laboratory should establish its own range.

    c. **A prolonged TT** can occur in patients receiving therapeutic heparin, patients with increased fibrin degradation products, and patients with any disorder of hypofibrinogenemia.

    d. **TT Variation. The reptilase-R test** is an alternate method to test for fibrinogen activity.

        (1) The **methodology** of the reptilase-R test is similar to the TT test, except that the reptilase reagent is added to plasma instead of thrombin to activate the proteolytic conversion of fibrinogen to fibrin.

        (2) The reptilase time is **not** inhibited by heparin and demonstrates only minimum inhibition by FDP.

4. **Quantitative fibrinogen** assay is an expansion of the TT methodology.

    a. **Principle.** A measured amount of commercially prepared thrombin reagent is added to citrated plasma. The clotting time is measured and compared with the clotting times of plasma **fibrinogen standards** containing **known** amounts of fibrinogen.

    b. A standard curve is constructed, and the clotting time in seconds is plotted against milligrams per deciliter of fibrinogen. Patient unknown data can be quantitated for fibrinogen from a standard curve.

    c. **Reference range.** The normal range for a quantitative fibrinogen is **200–400 mg/dL.**

5. **Substitution tests** (Table 2-2) can be adapted if primary tests like the PT or APTT are abnormally prolonged and indicate a factor deficiency. The patient's deficient plasma is diluted 1:1 with a plasma or serum substitute, and the APTT or PT is repeated. A correction of the original prolonged APTT or PT indicates that the deficient factor had been added to the patient's plasma by the substitution solution. The prepared substitution solutions are as follows.

    a. **Aged plasma** lacks labile factors **V and VIII** but retains normal activity of all other coagulation factors. **Normal plasma** retains normal activity of all coagulation factors.

    b. **Fresh absorbed plasma** lacks vitamin K factors (i.e., factors II, VII, IX, X), but retains normal activity of all other coagulation factors.

    c. **Aged serum** lacks factors I, II, V, and VIII but retains normal activity of all other coagulation factors.

6. **Final confirmation and quantitation of a factor deficiency** is done with specific factor assays. These methods use a test plasma with a known defi-

Table 2-2. Substitution Testing with Mixing Studies*

Extrinsic Pathway PT	Intrinsic Pathway APTT	Factor-deficient Plasma or Serum		
		Normal Plasma	Adsorbed Plasma	Aged Serum
I	I	+	+	(−)
II	II	+	(−)	(−)
V	V	+	+	(−)
VII		+	(−)	+
	VIII	+	+	(−)
	IX	+	(−)	+
X	X	+	(−)	+
	XI	+	+	+
	XII	+	+	+

APTT = activated partial thromboplastin time; (−) = factor missing; + = factor present; PT = prothrombin time.
*By using the PT and APTT screening tests and mixing patient plasma samples with known factor deficient plasma, the majority of coagulation factor deficiencies can be determined. Each factor deficiency will result in a specific testing pattern.

ciency, which is titrated and tested against the patient's plasma unknown factor deficiencies. Factors can also be immunologically assayed with enzyme-linked immunosorbent assay (ELISA) methodology.

7. **Chromogenic assays** constitute methods that use a synthetic substrate targeted to be enzymatically altered by a specific serine protease or serine protease inhibitor in a patient's plasma specimen.

  a. **Principle.** The specific substrate is cleaved by the targeted serine protease factor in the plasma sample to yield a chromogenic (colored) or a fluorogenic compound.

  b. **Measurement.** An endpoint reaction yields a color whose intensity is directly proportional to the activity of the serine protease. The color intensity can be measured on a spectrophotometer and quantitated with a standard curve.

G. **Normal fibrinolysis** refers to the enzymatic pathway of clot dissolution in which **plasmin** is the key enzyme responsible for breaking down bonds in the fibrin polymer and releasing **fibrin degradation products (FDP)**.

1. **Plasmin activation** results from proteolytic cleavage of a circulating inactive zymogen known as **plasminogen** by either of two pathways:

  a. **Extrinsic pathway activation** in vivo involves a tissue proteolytic enzyme and fibrin as a cofactor.

(1) Urokinase can also convert plasminogen to plasmin and is used as a thrombolytic agent.

(2) Streptokinase is a streptococcal-derived protein used as a therapeutic thrombolytic drug.

b. Intrinsic pathway activation of plasmin involves factors XIIa, kallikrein, or HMWK.

2. **Plasmin degradation of fibrin** begins by the breaking down of the fibrin polymer into a monomer form known as **fragment X.** This fragment is identical to a fibrin monomer, consists of one E domain and two D domains, and retains clotting properties.

   a. Fragment X is **further cleaved to produce FDP,** which consists of:

   (1) Fragment Y, which consists of one E domain and one D domain

   (2) Fragment E, which consists of the E domain only

   (3) Fragment D, which consists of the D domain only

   (4) D dimer, which consists of two D fragments of linked monomers

   b. The FDPs produced during fibrinolysis have anticoagulating effects of their own because they **inhibit** the process of **fibrin polymerization,** demonstrate competitive **inhibition of thrombin,** and **prolong the TT test.**

3. **Other functions of plasmin** in addition to fibrin degradation include:

   a. Fibrinogen degradation

   b. The inactivation of factor VIII:C

   c. The inactivation of factor V

   d. Direct anti-aggregation effect on platelets

4. α_2-**Antiplasmin** inhibits the actions of plasmin by forming a 1:1 complex with plasmin, which prevents fibrin binding.

   a. α_2-Antiplasmin is bound to the fibrin by factor **XIIIa.**

   b. α_2-**Macroglobulin** also has weak antiplasmin activity.

H. Laboratory tests for fibrinolysis

1. **Latex agglutination** can measure freely circulating FDP in the patient's serum. Latex coated with anti-fibrinogen detects the presence of increased levels of FDP. **Only serum can be used** to avoid interference with endogenous fibrinogen.

2. **Whole blood clot lysis time** tests for increased plasmin activity.

3. **Plasminogen or α_2-antiplasmin can be measured** serologically or with chromagenics.

4. **D dimer test** is based on a highly specific, monoclonal antibody directed against a unique neoantigen of covalently crosslinked D fragments resulting from fibrinolysis. The D dimer has several advantages in detecting degradation fragments when compared with the standard FDP assay.

   a. The FDP assay can be run on **plasma,** eliminating the risk of false positives.

b. D dimer is **superior in sensitivity and specificity** as compared with the conventional FDP assay (i.e., sensitive to as little as 20 ng/mL, as compared with 10 μ/mL for conventional latex FDP).

5. **Protamine sulfate turbidity test** assays for an increase in fibrin monomers. Fibrin-split products, if present in the plasma in increased amounts, precipitate out to produce turbidity in a weak solution of protamine sulfate. The effects of heparin are also antagonized.

6. **Prothrombin fragment 1.2 (F-1.2)** is a new assay that tests for the presence of the fragment generated when prothrombin is activated to thrombin (factor IIa).

   a. Prothrombin fragment serves as a sensitive biologic **marker of thrombin generation and Xa activity** because generation of F-1.2 precedes thrombus formation.

   b. Levels are elevated in persons predisposed to **thrombotic risk** (e.g., cancer, heart disease, orthopedic surgery).

   c. Levels are depressed in persons undergoing anticoagulant therapy.

I. **Vascular factors in coagulation**

1. **Blood vessels are lined** with a continuous monolayer of endothelial cells anchored to inert basement membrane by a subendothelial matrix.

2. **In arteries and arterioles,** the subendothelial layer is surrounded by layers of smooth muscle cells and adventitia with fibroblasts.

3. When **vascular subendothelium** is exposed by vessel damage, platelet aggregation and coagulation can be directly initiated by **collagen release** and indirectly by **tissue-released vWF.**

   a. **Platelet factor 4 (PF4)** is then released by activated platelets and functions to inactivate heparin-like compounds secreted by mast cells in the exposed subendothelium.

   b. PGI_2, released by vascular endothelial cells that surround the damaged area, **inhibits** platelet aggregation and limits the spread of the thrombus formation.

   c. The **thrombomodulin** receptor on endothelial cell surfaces is formed to provide a site for Xa activation of prothrombin to thrombin.

4. **Platelet-derived growth factor (PDGF)** released from platelet granules stimulates the growth and migration of smooth muscle cells, endothelium, and fibroblasts to heal the wound.

5. **Tears in larger vessels** with surrounding smooth muscle cells have enhanced coagulatory effects.

   a. Both clotting pathways are activated by the release of tissue factor III (extrinsic pathway) and the activation of Hageman factor XIIa (intrinsic pathway) by exposed endothelium.

   b. PGI_2 is released from smooth muscle cells to limit and localize clotting.

6. **Capillaries** do not have a smooth muscle layer, and veins have very little, so clotting occurs primarily by platelet aggregation and activation of the extrinsic

pathway. Tissue factor III is present, but activators from subendothelium and smooth muscle are minimal.

IV. COAGULATION DISORDERS (Figure 2-5)

A. Disorders of fibrinogen and related disorders

1. **Hereditary disorders of fibrinogen** can be caused by quantitative or qualitative abnormalities of either fibrinogen or **fibrin-stabilizing factor (factor XIII).** In most of the disorders, the APTT, PT, and TT tests **are prolonged.**

    a. **Afibrinogenemia** is a **quantitative deficiency** of fibrinogen caused by a lack of **synthesis by the liver.**

    (1) Severe hemorrhages predominate in the umbilical, mucosal, gastrointestinal (GI), and intracranial regions.

    (2) The most common treatment is replacement therapy with **cryoprecipitate** or **fresh frozen plasma (FFP)** to raise the blood fibrinogen level higher than 60 mg/dL.

    b. **Dysfibrinogenemia** is a **qualitative abnormality** in the **structure and function** of the fibrinogen molecule.

    (1) Fibrinogen levels may be normal, and the **bleeding time is usually normal.**

    (2) Post-traumatic or postoperative **bleeding of mucosal tissues** is common.

    c. **Factor XIII deficiency** can be clinically severe with moderate-to-severe bleeding. Delayed bleeding and wound healing is often observed after trauma.

    (1) The APTT, PT, and TT tests are **normal.**

    (2) Low factor XIII concentrations are detected by incubation of a fibrin clot in a **5M urea solution.** A normal fibrin clot will not be dissolved in 5M urea after 24 hours, but a clot deficient in factor XIII will be dissolved after 24 hours.

2. **Acquired disorders of fibrinogen** occur secondary to other pathologic events.

    a. **DIC** refers to a deposition of large amounts of fibrin throughout the microcirculation that results in a pathologic activation of coagulation pathways. DIC can be fatal, self-limiting, acute, or chronic.

    (1) **Classification.** DIC is classified as a **consumption coagulopathy** because it results in a depletion of platelets as well as plasma coagulation factors.

    (2) **Physiologic effects.** Plasminogen is activated systemically to plasmin, resulting in an increase in FDP in the plasma. There is possible red blood cell (RBC) fragmentation caused by damage from multiple thromboemboli.

    (3) **Common coagulation test results** include:

    (a) A decreased platelet count

    (b) A prolonged PT, APTT, and TT

    (c) An elevated FDP or D dimer

    (d) A decreased fibrinogen

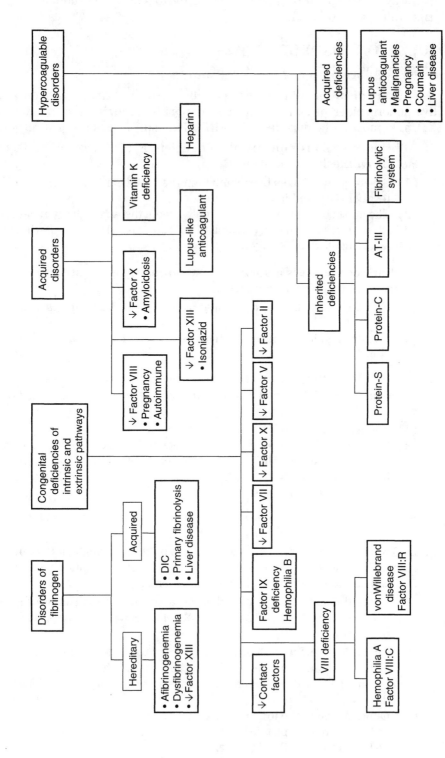

Figure 2-5. Coagulation disorder algorithm AT-III = antithrombin III; DIC = disseminated intravascular coagulation.

        (4) The **causes of DIC are widespread** and can occur from intrinsic or extrinsic pathway activation.

           (a) Extrinsic system activation occurs by large amounts of tissue factor entering the circulation, and can result from **hypofibrinogenemic states of pregnancy, metastatic carcinoma, or promyelocytic leukemia.**

           (b) Intrinsic system activation results from events that damage or alter the vascular endothelium, thereby exposing collagen (e.g., **infectious diseases, antigen-antibody complexes, liver disease, snake venom poisoning, massive trauma, or surgery**).

        (5) Treatment for DIC varies with the cause, but most often FFP-pooled platelet, cryoprecipitate, or low molecular weight heparin is used to treat the symptoms and break the cycle.

    b. Primary fibrinolysis is symptomatically similar to DIC but results from **increased levels of plasmin.**

        (1) Common causes include **cirrhosis, shock, metastatic carcinoma of the prostate, injury to the genitourinary tract,** and leaking of **urokinase** from the urine into tissues.

        (2) Common coagulation test results include decreased fibrinogen, prolonged PT or APTT, and increased FDP or D dimer. In contrast to DIC, primary fibrinolysis usually demonstrates a **normal platelet count,** and the RBC morphology **does not show fragmentation.**

        (3) A test tube sample from a patient with primary fibrinolysis will initially form a clot that dissolves in 1–2 hours.

    c. Liver disease can be associated with coagulation disorders because the majority of the coagulation factors are synthesized in the liver.

        (1) A decrease in factor VII occurs first because factor VII has the shortest half-life of the coagulation factors.

        (2) In patients with severe liver disease, the PT usually is prolonged; in later stages, the APTT will also be prolonged.

        (3) Severe liver disease often causes **decreased fibrinogen production (hypofibrinogenemia)** or an **abnormal fibrinogen molecule (dysfibrinogemia).**

    d. Therapeutic heparin administration, commonly used in postsurgical and cardiac patients, can prolong the APTT and TT acutely and can prolong the PT with chronic use. In a patient receiving heparin, abnormal coagulation results must be distinguished from similar coagulopathies if the patient history is unknown. This can be done with the reptilase-R time test (Table 2-3).

B. Inherited deficiencies of other factors in the intrinsic and extrinsic pathways

    1. Hemophilia A is an inherited deficiency or dysfunction of factor **VIII:C** (antihemolytic factor).

        a. Inheritance pattern is sex-linked (i.e., on the X chromosome), and female homozygotes with a hemophiliac father and carrier mother are very rare.

        b. There are **three patterns of severity.**

Table 2-3. Comparison of the Thrombin and Reptilase* Times to Distinguish
Inherited Fibrin-Related Disorders from Acquired Fibrinogen Disorders

Thrombin Time	Reptilase Time	Defect
Infinitely prolonged	Infinitely prolonged	Dysfibrinogenemia
Infinitely prolonged	Infinitely prolonged	Afibrinogenemia
Prolonged	Equally prolonged	Hypofibrinogenemia
Prolonged	Normal	Heparin
Prolonged	Slight to moderate	Fibrin degradation product (FDP)

*Reptilase activates fibrinogen in a manner similar to thrombin but is not sensitive to heparin and FDP inhibition.

(1) **Severe** hemophilia A is diagnosed in patients with spontaneous hemorrhages and a factor **VIII:C level less than 1%** of the normal level.

(2) **Moderate** hemophilia A is diagnosed in patients who have VIII:C levels **lower than 5%** of the normal level.

(3) **Mild** hemophilia A is seen in patients with **6%–30%** of the normal VIII:C levels. Typically, these patients only bleed excessively in association with trauma or surgical procedures.

c. **Human alloantibodies** to VIII:C are produced in a minority of severe hemophilia A cases.

(1) Approximately **10%** of severe hemophiliacs are positive for cross-reacting material (CRM+). CRM is an antigen that neutralizes anti-VIII:C antibodies.

(2) Approximately 90% of hemophiliacs are negative for CRM.

d. Patients with moderate-to-severe hemophilia A demonstrate a **clinical bleeding pattern** of spontaneous bleeding **into joints or muscles,** excessive postoperative hemorrhage, and easy bruising.

e. Predicted **coagulation profile results** include:

(1) Normal bleeding time (usually)

(2) Normal PT and TT

(3) Prolonged APTT if VIII:C levels are less than 0.2 U/mL (i.e., less than 20% activity)

(4) Female heterozygote carriers will have 25%–75% VIII:C activity that will not usually show up on laboratory testing.

f. **Treatment** of hemophilia A is based on **replacement therapy.**

(1) **Cryoprecipitate** is a plasma-fraction preparation prepared by thawing FFP at 4°C. It contains a concentrated portion of fibrinogen and VIII complex.

(2) **Preparations rich in factor VIII:C** are more costly, but are effective.

2. **Hemophilia B** (Christmas disease) is an inherited **deficiency in factor IX** resulting from a **sex-linked** (X-chromosome) mutation.

   a. Diagnosis. Hemophilia B is less common than hemophilia A. However, clinical symptoms are virtually indistinguishable, and laboratory differential diagnosis is necessary.

   b. Treatment. A correct laboratory diagnosis must be made because treatment of hemophilia B is different than treatment of hemophilia A.

     (1) Cryoprecipitate is deficient in factor IX but rich in the factor VIII complex.

     (2) FFP replacement therapy is the treatment of choice for hemophilia B, because FFP contains active factor IX. However, it is deficient in factor VIII.

     (3) The half-life of factor IX (24 hours) is longer than that for factor VIII (12 hours), so the administration of treatment for a factor IX deficiency is less frequent.

   c. Coagulation profile results initially may not produce results that differ from a patient with hemophilia A because the bleeding time, PT, and TT will also be normal, and the APTT will be prolonged. If hemophilia is suspected, and the APTT is prolonged, substitution tests or assay for factors IX and VIII activity should be performed.

3. vWD occurs almost as frequently as hemophilia A.

   a. Genetically, vWD is inherited as an autosomal dominant condition.

   b. The mutation is generally a defect in the **VIII:R** component of factor VIII, but partial deficiencies in the VIII:C portion often occur.

   c. Patients with vWD characteristically **bleed from mucous membranes and subcutaneous tissues.**

     (1) Easy bruising and GI bleeding is common.

     (2) Muscle hematomas and deep vessel hemorrhages are not as common as in hemophilia A.

   d. Production of VIII:R and VIII:C are controlled by different tissues but circulate as a **VIII:C/VIII:R complex.**

   e. The vWF molecule consists of a basic monomer form, but it also combines with additional monomers to produce a series of multimers of increasing molecular weight.

     (1) Largest **MW multimers** possess the functional activities contributing to **platelet-mediated homeostatic events.**

     (2) Antigenically, there appears to be a plasma vWF that is synthesized from a tissue source and a platelet-derived vWF based on multimer size.

     (3) The variation of vWF size results in several clinical **subclassifications** of this disorder.

       (a) Clinical **Type I vWD** is the most common "classic" form of vWD, in which a partial decrease of all sizes of vWF MW multimers occurs.

       (b) Clinical **Type II vWD** patients have a selective absence of higher MW multimers.

         (i) In patients with **Type IIa vWD,** ristocetin-induced activity is decreased because both platelet and plasma vWF are absent.

(ii) In patients with **Type IIb vWD,** the ristocetin-induced activity is normal or increased because only plasma high-MW multimers are decreased.

(c) Patients with **Type III vWD** suffer from the most rare and severe type, because factor VIII:C is almost nondetectable.

(d) Some patients are classified as having a **platelet-type variant,** which is similar to Type IIb, but is accompanied by a **thrombocytopenia.**

f. The **common laboratory coagulation results** for patients with vWD include:

(1) **Prolonged bleeding time** and increased **petechiae** because platelet adhesion to capillaries is impaired

(2) Normal PT time

(3) Prolonged APTT test, **only if VIII:C activity is less than 20%**

(4) Platelet aggregation reactions that are normal with ADP, epinephrine, collagen, or thrombin activation, but impaired **ristocetin-induced aggregation**

g. **Treatment.** Factor VIII concentrations are not useful because they contain primarily factor VIII:C and are deficient in high MW multimers of vWF. The treatment of choice, therefore, is **cryoprecipitate.**

(1) The clinical response to treatment in a patient with vWD differs from treatment of a patient with hemophilia A.

(2) The increase in VIII:C levels following treatment in hemophilia A patients is directly proportional to the amount of cryoprecipitate infused. This relationship is not found with the treatment of patients with vWD.

(a) Cryoprecipitate infusion given to patients with vWD **stimulates production of VIII:C** because the defect is not in VIII:C, but in VIII:R.

(b) Blood levels of VIII:C activity slowly peak 4–24 hours after treatment to blood levels **greater than the amount contained in the infused cryoprecipitate.**

4. **Deficiencies of factor XII, HMWK, prekallikrein, or factor XI** are rare and genetically **autosomal recessive.**

a. **Factor XI deficiencies** have the highest incidence in the Jewish population.

b. These bleeding disorders are clinically mild, and severe bleeding is not usually observed. Bleeding is more commonly noted, however, with factor XI deficiencies.

c. **Common laboratory coagulation results** reflected by these deficiencies include:

(1) Prolonged APTT

(2) Normal PT, TT, and bleeding time

(3) Normalization of the APTT results following a prolonged incubation of the patient's plasma with an activating factor such as kaolin (observed with a **prekallikrein deficiency**)

Table 2-4. Laboratory Diagnosis Matrix for Coagulation Disorders

	PT Normal	PT Abnormal
APTT normal	Factor XIII deficiency (H)	**Extrinsic pathway disorder** Factor VII deficiency (H) **Early liver disease** (Ac) **Coumarin drugs** (Ac)
APTT abnormal	**Intrinsic pathway disorders** (H) With clinical bleeding: Factor VIII, IX, XI deficiencies Without clinical bleeding: Deficiencies of contact activation factors **Lupus anticoagulant** (Ac) **Heparin** (Ac) **Factor VIII inhibitors** (Ac)	**Common pathway disorders** (H) Deficiencies of factors I, II, V, X **Liver disease** (Ac) **Disseminated intravascular coagulation** (Ac) **Vitamin K deficiency** (Ac) **Coumarin drugs** (Ac)

Ac = acquired; APTT = activated partial thromboplastin time; H = hereditary; PT = prothombin time.

5. **Factor VII deficiencies** are rare autosomal recessive disorders that are not usually associated with a serious clinical bleeding history. Common laboratory **coagulation results** from a patient with a factor VII deficiency include:

   a. Normal APTT, TT, and bleeding time

   b. Prolonged PT but a **normal** Stypven time

6. **Factor X deficiencies** are rare autosomal recessive disorders that can be caused by quantitative and qualitative abnormalities of the factor X molecule. The expected laboratory **coagulation profile** includes:

   a. Prolonged PT and APTT

   b. Normal TT and bleeding time

7. **Factor V deficiencies** are rare autosomal recessive disorders.

   a. The level of factor V activity in the patient's plasma does not directly correlate to the patient's clinical severity.

   b. Approximately one third of patients with factor V deficiency have an increased bleeding time because of the platelet-related function of factor V of binding factor X to the platelet surface.

   c. The **common laboratory coagulation results** include:

      (1) Prolonged APTT and PT times
      (2) Normal TT

8. **Prothrombin (factor II) deficiencies** are extremely rare. The **common laboratory coagulation profile** includes:

   a. **Prolonged PT and APTT,** which can be corrected in substitution testing only by **fresh normal plasma**

   b. Normal fibrinogen assay

C. **Acquired coagulation disorders** (Table 2-4)

   1. **Acquired disorders of factor VIII** are primarily caused by the presence of **autoimmune inhibitors** of factor VIII.

   a. Inhibitors to VIII:C occasionally develop in normally healthy women **after childbirth** and disappear after a few months.

   b. Acquired VIII:R (vWD) is seen in people with **autoimmune disease or lymphoproliferative disorders.**

2. **Acquired inhibition of factor XIII** occurs following drug therapy with a tuberculosis drug known as **isoniazid.**

3. Factor X deficiencies occur rarely in persons with an autoimmune disease known as **amyloidosis.**

4. **Lupus-like anticoagulant** is developed in 10%–20% of persons with **SLE,** in a significant number of patients taking **phenothiazine,** and occasionally in individuals with **lymphoproliferative disorders.**

   a. Inhibitors most commonly used are **immunoglobulin G (IgG)** and occasionally **IgM.** Autoantibodies found in the patient's plasma are directed against the phospholipid portion of **phospholipoprotein** components found in **APTT reagent.**

   b. Patients with lupus-like anticoagulant occasionally have a **mild thrombocytopenia.**

   c. The presence of clinical bleeding with lupus-like anticoagulant is found only in patients with high titers of anticoagulant.

   d. The antibody is first detected by a slightly prolonged APTT, with a normal PT and TT.

   (1) The APTT will **not** be corrected with a 1:1 dilution of patient plasma and normal plasma as in a typical factor deficiency.

   (2) Increasing prolonged times are directly proportional to extended incubation times with the APTT phospholipid reagent.

   e. Further testing for a specific factor deficiency proves to be normal.

5. **A vitamin K deficiency** results in impaired synthesis of factors **II, VII, IX, X, PC, and PS.**

   a. Causes of vitamin K deficiency are varied and include:

   (1) Inadequate diet
   (2) Biliary obstruction
   (3) Intestinal malabsorption diseases
   (4) Gut sterilization by chronic antibiotic therapy
   (5) Hemorrhagic disease of the newborn, which is caused by a slowly developing liver function and corrected by administration of vitamin K_1
   (6) Coumarin therapy, which inhibits vitamin K metabolism and therefore the vitamin K–dependent coagulation factors

   b. Expected **laboratory coagulation profile** includes:

   (1) Acute prolonged PT (and possibly APTT) with chronic deficiency
   (2) Normal TT and fibrinogen

6. **Heparin binds antithrombin III,** greatly enhancing its ability to bind and inactivate thrombin.

   a. Exogenous heparin therapy is a fast and potent form of anticoagulation.

   b. Heparin is commonly used to treat thrombosis. Many patients receive heparin for a short period to prevent emboli after major surgery.

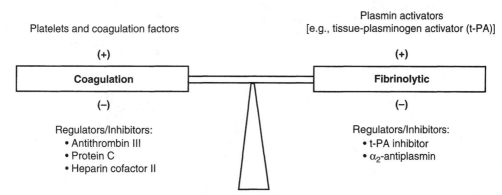

Figure 2-6. Balance of hemostasis. Coagulation and fibrinolytic systems are in perfect balance as long as positive and negative influences are equal. Platelets and coagulation factors drive the clotting process, while plasmin activators drive the opposing fibrinolytic system. Both systems are held in check by regulators and inhibitors.

    c. The APTT is the most commonly used test to monitor heparin therapy, but the TT is also prolonged.

    d. Occasionally, the PT is prolonged if the patient has received heparin for a long period.

    e. If the PT, APTT, and TT are greatly prolonged, the possibility of the presence of heparin should be considered before investigating a factor deficiency.

    f. The unconfirmed presence of heparin in the patient's plasma can be confirmed by the addition of **protamine sulfate** to the plasma sample to inhibit the action of heparin and normalize all prolonged tests.

D. Hypercoagulability disorders are distinguished by **pathologic thrombosis** in the coronary circulation, cerebral circulation, or the deep veins of the legs.

    1. Hypercoagulability resulting from hereditary deficiency is seen mainly in patients younger than 40 years and is often fatal. The most common deficiencies are in antithrombin III, PC, and plasminogen.

        a. Genetically induced deficiencies of **natural inhibitors,** including **PS, PC, and antithrombin III,** are found in 25% of persons with this disorder.

        b. **Disorders of the fibrinolytic system** comprise 30% of reported genetic deficiencies and result from:

            (1) Decrease in plasminogen or defective function
            (2) Decrease in **tissue-plasminogen activator (t-PA)**
            (3) Abnormal fibrinogen molecule
            (4) Factor XII/prekallikrein deficiency

        c. **Miscellaneous causes** of genetic hypercoagulability involve **blood vessel and platelet damage.**

    2. Acquired disorders of hypercoagulability are usually seen in patients older than 40 years and usually occur secondary to a primary pathology, such as **lupus anticoagulant, malignancies, or pregnancy.**

    3. Regulation of systems of hemostasis is kept in balance by inhibitors of coagulation and fibrinolysis (Figure 2-6).

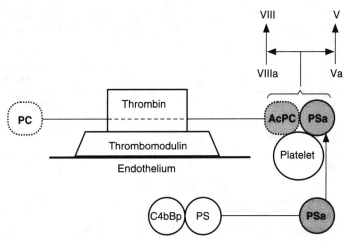

Figure 2-7. Inhibition of coagulation by protein S (PS) and protein C (PC). PS serves as a cofactor in PC inactivation of coagulation factors V and VIII. PS exists as in inactive protein-bound (C4bBp) form and an active nonbound form (Psa). PC is activated by thrombin, and activated PC (AcPC) combines with Psa on the platelet surface to inactivate factors V and VIII.

4. **Antithrombin III deficiencies** affect 1 in 5000 people.
   a. **Inherited deficiencies** can be classified as either a **Type I or Type II** deficiency.
      (1) A **Type I deficiency** is characterized by a **decrease in activity and a decrease in the antithrombin III molecule.**
      (2) A **Type II deficiency** is characterized by a **decrease in activity,** but a normal amount of antithrombin III molecule.
   b. **Acquired antithrombin III deficiencies** result from the following primary disorders:
      (1) **DIC,** which results in consumption of the molecule
      (2) **Cirrhosis,** which results in decreased production
      (3) **Nephrotic syndrome,** which results from a loss of the molecule in the urine
      (4) **Medications** (e.g., heparin, estrogen, L-asparaginase)

5. **PC deficiencies** (Figure 2-7) are one of the most common causes of hypercoagulability disorders and can be either inherited or acquired.
   a. **Inherited deficiencies** are genetically heterozygous in 6%–12% of cases. The majority of PC deficiencies are severe (homozygous). Patients exhibit low or absent PC levels. Low levels result in serious clinical symptoms, such as ecchymotic areas of skin with purpura and tissue necrosis, blindness, and CNS thrombosis.
   b. **Acquired deficiencies** are caused by chronic oral anticoagulant therapy with coumarin (vitamin K blocker). The result is **coumarin necrosis,** which is caused by a rapid functional decrease of PC.

6. **PS deficiencies** can be inherited or acquired. PS is a vitamin K–dependent glycoprotein that is synthesized in the liver.

Table 2-5. Clinical Subtypes of Protein S Deficiencies

Subtype	Free PS (Nonbound)	Functional Activity	Total PS
Type I	Low	Low	Low
Type IIa	Low	Low	Normal
Type IIb	Normal	Low	Normal

PS = protein S.

a. PS circulates in two forms: an inactive form bound to a protein known as **C4b-BP,** and as freely circulating PS with full functional activity. The **active form of PS functions as a cofactor for PC** inactivation of factors V and VIII (see Figure 2-7).

b. Inherited deficiencies of PS comprise 8%–11% of the thrombotic population and have been classified into three clinical subtypes (Table 2-5).

c. **Acquired PS deficiencies** can occur secondary to the following conditions:
   (1) Oral coagulants (e.g., coumarin)
   (2) Pregnancy
   (3) Oral contraceptives
   (4) Low vitamin K levels
   (5) Liver disease
   (6) Acute inflammation
   (7) Newborn

Study Questions

Directions: Each of the numbered items or incomplete statements in this section is followed by answers or by completions of the statement. Select the ONE lettered answer or completion that is BEST in each case.

1. Which one of the following sets correctly lists the vitamin K–dependent factors?

a. I, II, VII, VIII, X, XII
b. III, V, IX, XII
c. VII, X, XI
d. II, VII, IX, X

2. Fresh adsorbed plasma is deficient in which one of the following?

a. factors V and VII
b. factors II, VII, IX, and X
c. factors I, II, V, and VIII
d. vitamin K

3. The one-stage prothrombin time (PT) test is the classic test of the extrinsic pathway. The reagents used in this determination include

a. thromboplastin and sodium chloride
b. thromboplastin and calcium oxalate
c. thromboplastin and calcium chloride
d. platelet factor III and calcium chloride

4. The normal range for the prothrombin time (PT) test is

a. 11–13 seconds
b. 15–20 seconds
c. 25–40 seconds
d. 40–60 seconds

5. The following results were obtained on a patient:

PT 12 seconds (normal, 11–13 seconds)
APTT 55 seconds (normal, < 40 seconds)
TT 12 seconds (normal, 10–20 seconds)

APTT plus aged serum not corrected
APTT plus adsorbed plasma not corrected
APTT plus normal plasma not corrected

Which one of the following is the most probable coagulation problem to investigate first?

a. disseminated intravascular coagulation (DIC)
b. factor VIII:C deficiency
c. lupus anticoagulant
d. factor XI deficiency

6. An activated partial thromboplastin time (APTT) in a 79-year-old female patient admitted for minor surgery was 55 seconds, but the prothrombin time (PT) and thrombin time (TT) were within normal range. The patient had no clinical manifestations of a bleeding problem, and she had no family or personal history of bleeding problems. The APTT was corrected with normal plasma, aged serum, and adsorbed plasma. These laboratory results and the medical history are consistent with which one of the following disorders?

a. lupus anticoagulant
b. deficiency in factor II
c. deficiency in factor XII
d. deficiency in factor IX

110

Directions: Each of the numbered items or incomplete statements in this section is negatively phrased, as indicated by a capitalized word such as NOT, LEAST, or EXCEPT. Select the ONE lettered answer or completion that is BEST in each case.

7. Contact activation products directly resulting from factor XIIa activation include all of the following products EXCEPT

a. activation of prothrombin to thrombin
b. activation of prekallikrein to kallikrein
c. activation of plasminogen to plasmin
d. activation of plasma thromboplastin antecedent to its activated form

8. All of the following statements regarding protein C (PC) are correct EXCEPT

a. it depends on proper vitamin K metabolism for activity
b. it has protein S (PS) as a cofactor
c. it is activated by thrombin
d. it activates factors VIII:C and V

9. An increase in fibrin monomers or fibrin degradation products (FDP) can cause an abnormal result with each of the following EXCEPT

a. FDP test
b. thrombin time (TT)
c. protamine sulfate test
d. the addition of 5M urea to the fibrin clot

10. All of the following are functions of thrombin EXCEPT

a. converts fibrinogen to fibrin monomer
b. activates fibrin stabilizing factor
c. induces platelet aggregation
d. inactivates protein C (PC)

11. Platelet function and activity can be measured in the laboratory using a platelet aggregometer by adding all of the following stimulators to platelet-rich plasma EXCEPT

a. adenosine diphosphate (ADP)/adenosine triphosphate (ATP)
b. ristocetin
c. arachidonic acid
d. proaccelerin

12. Hypercoagulability resulting from genetically induced deficiency includes all of the following disorders EXCEPT

a. decrease in protein S (PS)
b. decrease in tissue-plasminogen activator
c. blood vessel damage
d. factor IX deficiency

13. Fibrin degradation products (FDP) consist of all of the following components EXCEPT

a. fragment E
b. protein S (PS)
c. fragment X
d. fragment D

14. The prothrombin time (PT) is most commonly used for all of the following EXCEPT

a. testing deficiencies of factors I and II
b. monitoring heparin therapy
c. monitoring coumarin therapy
d. testing factor VII deficiencies

15. Platelet activation and aggregation depends on all of the following EXCEPT

a. prostacyclin (PGI$_2$)
b. release of activating factors from damaged subendothelium (e.g., collagen)
c. calcium
d. thromboxane A$_2$ (TXA$_2$)

16. All of the following statements are true of hemophilia B EXCEPT

a. it exhibits a prolonged activated partial thromboplastin time (APTT) and a normal prothrombin time (PT)
b. it is an inherited deficiency of factor IX
c. it can be easily differentiated from hemophilia A with a routine coagulation profile
d. it is best treated by fresh frozen plasma (FFP) replacement therapy

Directions: Each set of matching questions in this section consists of a list of four to twenty-six lettered options (some of which may be in figures) followed by several numbered items. For each numbered item, select the ONE lettered option that is most closely associated with it. To avoid spending too much time on matching sets with large numbers of options, it is generally advisable to begin each set by reading the list of options. Then, for each item in the set, try to generate the correct answer and locate it in the option list, rather than evaluating each option individually. Each lettered option may be selected once, more than once, or not at all.

Questions 17–20

For each description of a qualitative platelet disorder that follows, select the disorder with which it is most closely associated.

a. storage pool disease
b. Wiskott-Aldrich syndrome
c. Bernard-Soulier syndrome
d. Glanzmann's thrombasthenia

17. An autosomal recessive inherited disorder characterized by a thrombocytopenia, giant platelet, and an abnormal aggregation pattern with restitution stimulation caused by a decrease in platelet membrane receptors I and V

18. A sex-linked inherited disorder caused by a decrease in number of platelet-dense granules

19. An inherited autosomal recessive disorder caused by a decrease in platelet membrane glycoproteins IIb and IIIa, characterized by a normal platelet count and a failure to initiate platelet in vitro aggregation with all aggregating agents

20. An autosomal recessive inherited disorder caused by decreased adenosine triphosphate (ATP):adenosine diphosphate (ADP) amounts in the platelet-dense granular fraction

Answers and Explanations

1. The answer is d [III D]. Factors II, VII, IX, and X are all serine proteases produced in the liver that depend on functional vitamin K metabolism for their activation.

2. The answer is b [III F 5 b]. The vitamin K factors (i.e., II, VII, IX, X) are selectively removed in the process of creating adsorbed plasma.

3. The answer is c [III F 2]. The prothrombin time (PT) reagent consists of a lipoprotein extract (i.e., thromboplastin), which mimics endogenous tissue factor, and calcium chloride.

4. The answer is a [III F 2 c]. The normal range for the prothrombin time (PT) test is 11–13 seconds. However, times may vary slightly among laboratories. Each laboratory should establish its own normal range.

5. The answer is c [IV C 4]. The patient presented with a prolonged activated partial thromboplastin time (APTT) and a normal thrombin time (TT), neither of which were corrected by any serum or plasma substitutions. In fact, normal plasma did not correct prolonged times. These results would eliminate any fibrinogen disorder because normal and adsorbed plasma contain fibrinogen. An inhibitor appears to be present; therefore, lupus anticoagulant would logically be investigated first. Prolonged APTTs and TTs caused by disseminated intravascular coagulation (DIC) would most likely correct with normal plasma. A factor XI deficiency would correct with all substitutions. Factor VIII:C deficiency is eliminated because normal plasma and adsorbed plasma substitution correction did not correct the prolonged APTT. Both substitutions would correct a prolonged APTT in a patient with factor VIII:C deficiency.

6. The answer is c [IV B 4; Table 2-1]. The prolonged activated partial thromboplastin time (APTT) in combination with a normal prothrombin time (PT) and thrombin time (TT) indicates that the deficiency lies in the intrinsic pathway, not the common or extrinsic pathways. All substitution agents contain factor XII and demonstrate correction of the prolonged APTT result. The patient did not have a history of clinical bleeding, which is commonly seen in factor XII deficiencies. A factor IX deficiency would also exhibit a prolonged PT result. Lupus anticoagulant would result in an absence of correction with normal plasma, adsorbed plasma, or aged serum. A deficiency of factor II can be eliminated because the PT was in the normal range.

7. The answer is a [III A 1 d]. Activated factor XII participates in three important activation reactions: prekallikrein to produce bradykinin; plasminogen to plasmin; and factor XI (i.e., plasma thromboplastin antecedent) to factor XIa. Factor X complex activates prothrombin (factor II).

8. The answer is d [III E 5]. Protein C (PC) inactivates coagulation factors VIII:C and V. PC is vitamin K dependent, requires cofactor protein S (PS) for optimal activity, is activated by thrombin, and is associated with the thrombomodulin complex.

9. The answer is d [III G 2 b; III H 5]. The urea solubility test (i.e., addition of 5M urea to the fibrin clot) is used to test for factor XIII deficiency. Fibrin degradation products (FDP) produced in fibrinolysis have anticoagulating effects of their own. An increase of degradation products inhibits the process of fibrin polymerization and demonstrates the competitive inhibition of thrombin, thereby prolonging the thrombin time (TT). The protamine sulfate test produces a turbid solution in the presence of increased fibrin-split products, which provides a positive test result.

10. The answer is d [III B 6]. Thrombin is a very versatile enzyme that has many functions. It converts fibrinogen to fibrin monomer; it activates factor XIII; it induces platelet aggregation; it provides a positive feedback to activate factors V and VIII:C; and it activates protein C (PC). Thrombin also plays a minor catalytic role in the activation of factor VII.

11. The answer is d [I E 3 b]. Proacelerin is the same as coagulation factor V; it is not used as a commercial platelet stimulator. Adenosine diphosphate (ADP)/adenosine triphosphate (ATP), ristocetin, and arachidonic acid are all examples of stimulators that can be used. Additional stimulators are collagen, A23187 (calcium ionophore), epinephrine, and partially trypsinized γ-thrombin.

12. The answer is d [IV D 1]. The latest research has indicated that thrombotic episodes can result from several genetically induced deficiencies caused by a variety of factors. These types of thrombotic disorders are seen primarily in people younger than 40 years of age. A deficiency in factor IX would result in hemophilia B, which is a bleeding disorder.

13. The answer is b [III G 2]. The fibrin polymer is first broken down into a monomer called fragment X, which consists of an E domain and two D domains (same structure as a fibrin monomer). Fragment X is further cleaved to produce fragment Y (E and D domains), fragment E (E domain only), fragment D (D domain only), and D dimer. Protein S (PS) is the cofactor of protein C (PC), which is a coagulation inhibitor.

14. The answer is b [III D 2, F 2 a]. The prothrombin time (PT) tests for deficiencies of factors belonging to the extrinsic pathway. Coumarin anticoagulants have their resulting effect by inhibiting vitamin K reduction from the epoxide form. This renders factors II, VII, IX, and X inactive. The PT test is the best screening method for coumarin therapy. Factor VII has the shortest half-life and is the most sensitive to levels of coumarin therapy. The activated partial thromboplastin time (APTT) is the coagulating screening test that is most sensitive to the anticoagulating effects of heparin.

15. The answer is a [I C 1, 2, 5]. The damaged subendothelium releases activators from the tissue that transform the shape of the platelet and initiate aggregation. Collagen, fibronectin, factor VIII:R, calcium, and adenosine diphosphate (ADP)/adenosine triphosphate (ATP) are all powerful aggregators. Thromboxane A_2 (TXA_2) is released from the platelet to amplify the aggregation response. Prostacyclin (PGI_2) acts to limit and antagonize the aggregation process.

16. The answer is c [IV B 2]. Hemophilia B (Christmas disease) is a genetic deficiency of factor IX. A factor IX deficiency shares identical screening results [i.e., activated partial thromboplastin time (APTT) and prothrombin time (PT)] with a factor VIII:C deficiency. Both hemophilias exhibit a prolonged APTT and a normal PT. Fresh frozen plasma (FFP) is rich in factor IX and, economically, is a choice treatment.

17–20. The answers are 17-c, 18-b, 19-d, 20-a [II B 1 a–b, 2 a]. Bernard-Soulier platelet disorder results from a genetic deficiency in the platelet membrane von Willebrand factor (vWF) receptor (i.e., glycoproteins Ib and V). The blood film may look similar to that of an idiopathic thrombocytopenia purpura (ITP) patient with thrombocytopenia and giant platelet. This qualitative disorder demonstrates a platelet aggregation pattern that is the reverse of the pattern seen with Glanzmann's thrombasthenia. The aggregation and granular content release are normal with all agents except restitution. Wiskott-Aldrich syndrome is a congenital deficiency in dense granules that is distinguished by its X chromosome inheritance. Glanzmann's thrombasthenia is a genetically induced abnormality in platelet membrane receptors. Platelets are typically present in normal number and appearance. The defect is a decrease in platelet surface glycoproteins IIb and IIIa, which results in a reduction in the number of available fibrinogen binding sites and demonstrates an abnormal pattern of aggregation in response to all aggregating agents except restitution. Storage pool disease is a genetic anomaly affecting platelet-dense granules with an abnormal adenosine triphosphate (ATP):adenosine diphosphate (ADP) granular ratio.

3
Routine Hematology

Joel Hubbard

I. LABORATORY ANALYSIS

A. Electronic cell counting. Because of manufacturer diversity and the complexity (i.e., performance characteristics) of cell counters that exists among laboratories, individual laboratory instrumentation is not presented here.

1. **Multiparameter cell counters** provide 10 or more common parameters, including count of red blood cells (RBCs), white blood cells (WBCs), and platelets, with a totally automatic diluting system. The most common parameters provided by current cell counters include:

   a. RBC count

   b. WBC count

   c. Hemoglobin (Hb)

   d. Hematocrit (HCT)

   e. Mean corpuscular volume (MCV)

   f. Mean corpuscular hemoglobin (MCH)

   g. Mean corpuscular hemoglobin concentration (MCHC)

   h. Platelet count

   i. **Mean platelet volume (MPV)** is determined from the platelet histogram curve. The reference range is **6.5–12 fL.**

   j. **Red cell distribution width (RDW)** provides an estimate of RBC **anisocytosis** (size variation).

115

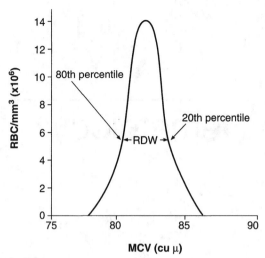

Figure 3-1. Normal red cell distribution curve from a red blood cell (RBC) histogram. MCV = mean corpuscular volume; RDW = red blood cell distribution width.

(1) Calculation. The RDW (Figure 3-1) is calculated from the following formula:

$$\textbf{RDW} = (\textbf{A} - \textbf{B}) \div (\textbf{A} + \textbf{B}) \times \textbf{k}$$

where A = the MCV, in which 20% of the RBCs are larger than the rest; B = the MCV, in which 80% of the RBCs are larger than the rest; and k = a constant that represents the number that is required to give a normal value of 10.

(2) The **normal reference range** for the RDW is **8.5–14.5.** Samples showing values greater than 14.5 should be carefully checked for anisocytosis.

(3) Diagnostic use. When considered with the MCV, the RDW can be of use diagnostically, as illustrated in Table 3-1.

Table 3-1. Diagnostic Use of Red Cell Distribution Width (RDW) and Mean Corpuscular Volume (MCV)

MCV	RDW	Clinical Importance
Normal	Normal	Acute bleeding, anemia of chronic disorders, RBC molecular deficiencies
Normal	High	Early stages of a nutritional deficiency (including iron deficiency anemia), myelofibrosis, sideroblastic anemia, cytotoxic chemotherapy
Low	Normal	Thalassemia minor, anemia of chronic disorders
Low	High	Iron deficiency anemia, hemoglobinopathies, thalassemia major
High	Normal	Aplastic anemia
High	High	Autoimmune hemolytic anemia, folate or vitamin B_{12} deficiency

RBC = red blood cell.

2. Electrical impedance

a. Particles (most often cells) are forced to flow through small openings (i.e., apertures) between two electrodes in an ionic solution.

(1) Electrical resistance (R). As each cell passes through the opening, the electrical resistance between the two electrodes increases, because cells are poor conductors of electricity.

(2) Voltage (V). As R increases, V increases. A **voltage pulse of short duration is produced for each cell that passes through the aperture.** The magnitude of voltage is proportional to the cell volume or size, and the number of voltage pulses is proportional to the frequency of particles passing through the aperture.

b. Methods

(1) RBCs and WBCs are counted in duplicate or triplicate. Each of the duplicated counts must agree within a standardized range of deviation from each other.

(2) The MCV is often determined directly **from the voltage-pulse heights** from the RBC count or histogram curve (see I B).

(3) The Hb of the sample is **obtained spectrophotometrically from the WBC dilution.**

(4) Platelets are counted in duplicate or triplicate **in the RBC aperture bath.** Particles ranging from **2–20 fL** [1 **femtoliter** (fL) $= 10^{-15}$ L = 1 cubic micrometer (mm^3)] in the RBC bath are sorted as platelets and plotted as a platelet histogram.

(5) RBC indices are computed parameters commonly obtained from automated cell counters.

(a) The HCT is computed **from the RBC count and the MCV** and calculated from the following formula:

$$\text{HCT\%} = [\text{RBC} \times \text{MCV}] \div 10$$

(b) The MCH is computed **from the MCV and the MCHC** and calculated from the following formula (note that $1\ \mu\mu g = 1$ pg):

$$\text{MCH pg} = [\text{MCV} \times \text{MCHC}] \div 100$$

or

$$\text{MCH} = [\text{Hb} \times 10] \div \text{RBC count}$$

(c) The MCHC is computed **from the Hb and HCT** and calculated from the following formula:

$$\text{MCHC\%} = [\text{Hb} \div \text{HCT}] \times 100$$

c. Common errors

(1) Missing parameter(s)

(a) Any WBC or RBC count grossly out of the normal range must be treated with suspicion, and the sample must be repeated.

(b) The **"rule of three"** (i.e., 3 times the Hb value should agree $\pm$ 3% with the HCT value). If it does not, the sample must be repeated.

(c) Any one of the indices being "singly" out of range must be considered suspicious.

(2) **Carryover** from high to low WBC counts is a problem with some cell counters because it can amount to a 2%–3% error. Carryover results from incomplete removal of all WBCs from the counting chamber between counts.

   (a) If the ratio of successive counts exceeds 3:1, then the second count may be in error by as much as 5%.

   (b) It may be necessary to **repeat any low WBC count** that follows a high count.

(3) **Increased WBC counts** greater than 50,000/mm^3 may produce a proportional **elevation in Hb values** because of increased cellular turbidity in the WBC counting baths. In addition, the **MCV and HCT may also be increased** because the number of WBCs is high enough to produce error when sized and counted in the RBC aperture bath.

(4) **Extremely microcytic** MCVs may be overestimated by the instrument.

(5) **High patient glucose concentrations** greater than 400 mg/dL result in intracellular hyperosmolality in RBCs and may cause **a high MCV and HCT, with a low MCHC.**

(6) **Cold agglutinins** in high titer give a **falsely high MCV, low RBC counts, and very high MCHCs.**

   (a) A good clue for this problem is to look for **RBC clumping** in a thin area on the blood smear.

   (b) Warming the blood or diluent to 37°C may eliminate this problem.

(7) **Very high plasma lipid levels** resulting in lipemic plasma may produce turbidity in the WBC aperture bath and falsely **increase the Hb, MCH, and MCHC.**

B. **Blood cell histograms** are provided by many high-volume instruments to **provide size distributions** of the different cell populations. The volume, given in mm^3 or fL, is plotted against the relative frequency for platelets, WBCs, and RBCs (Figure 3-2).

1. The **WBC histogram** provides a count and plot of **cells in the WBC aperture bath larger than 45 fL.**

   a. **Normal WBC histograms** have **three distribution peaks:**

      (1) The first peak, ranging **from 45–90 fL,** represents a small mononuclear population of cells (i.e., **lymphocytes**).

      (2) The second peak, ranging **from 90–160 fL,** represents a minor population of large mononuclear cells (i.e., **monocytes**). An increase in the number of cells in this size range can also represent abnormal cell types, such as the **immature precursor cell types found in patients with leukemia.**

      (3) **The major population and third peak, which ranges from 160–450 fL,** represents normal mature types of **granulocytes.**

   b. **Calculated values**

      (1) A **percentage value** for granulocytes, lymphocytes, and monocytes is calculated combining the distribution values and the total WBC distribution spread. Newer cell counters (e.g., Coulter Stack-S) also give values for eosinophils and basophils.

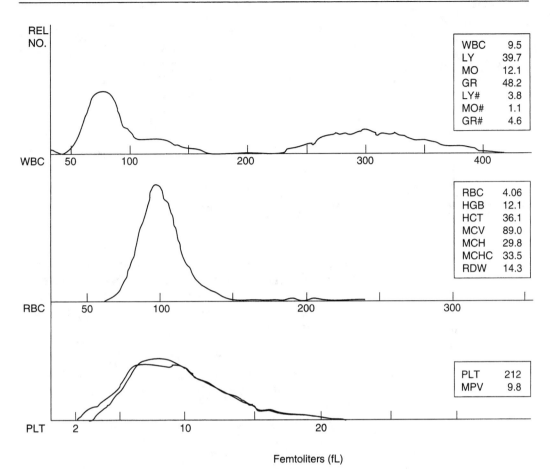

Figure 3-2. Typical cell histogram of normal blood. Note the normal distribution curves of the white blood cell (WBC), red blood cell (RBC), and platelet (PLT) cell populations. The histogram was created by a Coulter model S-Plus IV cell counter. GR = granulocyte; HCT = hematocrit; HGB = hemoglobin; LY = lymphocyte; MCH = mean corpuscular hemoglobin; MCHC = mean corpuscular hemoglobin count; MCV = mean cell volume; MO = monocyte; MPV = mean platelet volume; RDW = red cell distribution width.

(2) An **absolute value** of each cell fraction (in cells/mm^3) is calculated from the product of the total WBC count and the percent fraction of each cell type.

c. Abnormal WBC histogram patterns can alert the technologist and physician to possible pathology and alert the technologist to include a manual differential count.

   (1) The **lower threshold is 45 fL,** but the histogram will extend lower to detect abnormalities, as shown in Figure 3-3.

   (2) Error flags

   (a) Region code (R) flags signal irregularities in the WBC distribution and will appear next to the differential parameters that are in error. The "R" stands for the region. The following numerals indicate the location in the WBC histogram where the interference was detected:

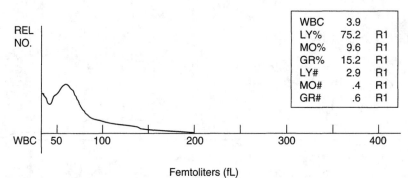

Figure 3-3. Abnormal white blood cell (WBC) histogram representing an R1 distribution. Note the high takeof: from the Y axis. GR = granulocyte; LY = lymphocyte; MO = monocyte.

   (i) **R1** warns of increased **interference** in the area **left of the lymphocyte peak** (approximately 35 fL), which is typically caused by **sickled RBCs, nucleated RBCs, or clumped and giant platelets** being counted in the WBC aperture bath (see Figure 3-3).
   (ii) **R2** warns of excessive overlap of cell populations at the **lymphocyte/mononuclear cell boundary** (approximately 90 fL) caused by the presence of abnormal cell types, such as **atypical lymph, blast, or plasma cells** (Figure 3-4).
   (iii) An **R3** warning (Figure 3-5) is caused by excessive overlap of cell populations at the **mononuclear/granulocyte boundary** (approximately 160 fL), which is due to the **increased presence of immature granulocytes** (i.e., bands, metamyelocytes).
   (iv) An **R4** warning (Figure 3-6) is caused by the extension of the cell distribution past the upper end of the WBC threshold (approximately 450 fL). This most commonly occurs when the granulocyte population is very high.
   (v) **RM** is the error code for **multiple region overlap.**

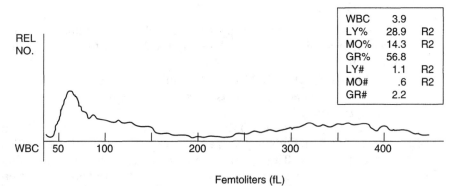

Figure 3-4. Abnormal white blood cell (WBC) histogram representing an R2 distribution. GR = granulocyte; LY = lymphocyte; MO = monocyte.

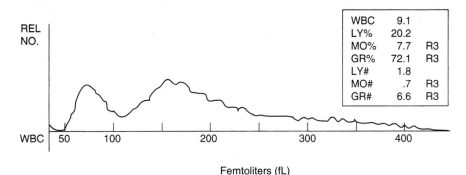

Figure 3-5. Abnormal white blood cell (WBC) histogram representing an R3 distribution. GR = granulocyte; LY = lymphocyte; MO = monocyte.

    (b) Other signal flags include **H,** which occurs when a parameter value is higher than the set normal limit, and **L,** which occurs when a parameter value is lower than the set normal limit.

  2. RBC histograms represent the cells counted in the RBC dilution, **in the size range of 36–360 fL,** which are sorted and plotted as frequency against cellular volume.

    a. Normal RBC histogram. A single peak should be found normally **between 70 fL and 110 fL,** and the peak should coincide with the MCV (Figure 3-7).

    b. Abnormal RBC histograms result when the MCV of the curve falls outside of the normal range of 80–100 fL, or when the RDW is greater than 14.5.

      (1) An **increased MCV** shifts the curve to the right, and a decreased MCV shifts the curve to the left.

      (2) An **increased RDW** is reflected by an increase in the "width" of the area beneath the curve (Figure 3-8).

      (3) In some disorders there may be **two populations of RBCs** [i.e., a microcytic population and a macrocytic population of cells (see Figure 3-8)].

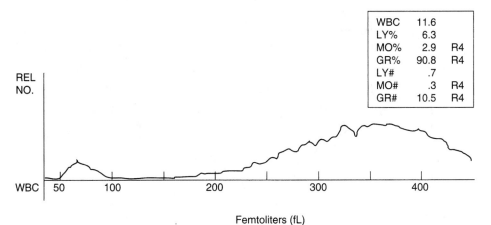

Figure 3-6. Abnormal white blood cell (WBC) histogram representing an R4 distribution. GR = granulocyte; LY = lymphocyte; MO = monocyte.

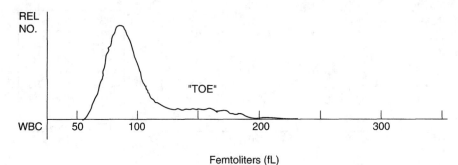

Figure 3-7. Normal red blood cell (RBC) distribution of an RBC histogram. Note that the extended distribution between 100 fL and 200 fL, which is called the toe, is normal. This area represents RBC duplicates, triplicates, agglutinated RBCs, aperture artifacts, and an occasional white blood cell (WBC).

   3. **Platelet histograms** represent cells in the RBC counting baths that are in the **size range of 2–20 fL.** Cells in this range are counted, and their frequency is plotted against cellular volume. **Atypical platelet histograms** can result in some disorders when large platelets are present (see Figure 3-2).

C. **X-Bar-B ($\overline{X}_B$) statistical analysis**

   1. **Background.** Research has shown that RBC indices (i.e., MCV, MCH, MCHC) of patient populations are stable over time. This stability is the basis of a hematology quality control technique known as $\overline{X}_B$ analysis.

   2. **Function.** Use of this statistical tool quickly determines the direction and amount of daily change caused by the instrument, reagents, or sample handling.

   3. **Establishment**

      a. **Target values of MCV, MCH, and MCHC** are determined by calculating the mean of 250–1000 samples for each of the three parameters.

      b. Once target values are determined, **ongoing analysis** can be applied using small "batches" of 20 samples.

      c. The **mean and standard deviation** of each batch is compared with the target value of each parameter and averaged with the mean and standard deviation of the previous batches.

   4. **The hematology system is considered "in control"** when the batch means are within established standard deviation limits of the target values.

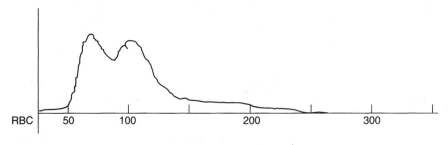

Figure 3-8. Abnormal red blood cell (RBC) histogram distribution illustrating dual RBC populations.

      5. The percent difference between each batch mean and its corresponding target value can be calculated and displayed on a **Levy-Jennings graph.**

D. Laser scatter counting and flow cytometry

    1. A wide range of diagnostic applications can be found from using the principles of laser scatter and flow cytometry.

      a. Routine cell counting and **differential separation** of the white cells can be routinely performed.

      b. These techniques can be used to help **presumptively characterize acute and chronic leukemias and lymphomas.**

      c. Specialized flow cytometry instrumentation can differentially **separate types of leukemic cells, tumor cells, or subtype lymphocyte functional types** (e.g., B lymphocytes, T lymphocytes, T-lymphocyte subtypes).

      d. These types of cell counters can be adapted to perform **reticulocyte counts.**

      e. One of the most far-reaching applications of flow cytometry technology is the **DNA analysis** of rapidly growing tumor tissue.

    2. Principles of operation combine chemistry and flow cytometry for the evaluation of individual blood-cell populations in each of several flow cells or "channels."

      a. General steps of flow cytometry include:

        (1) Preparation and staining of cell populations with cytochemical marking for further analysis

        (2) Flow cell measures of cell size, cytochemical staining properties, and frequency of each cell type

        (3) Computer conversion of measurements into common hematologic parameters

      b. In the **RBC channel,** RBCs are diluted and passed through a flow cell for counting with the technology of **laser scatter.**

        (1) RBC indices and RDW are computed and reported from the total RBC count.

        (2) Many flow cytometry instruments provide **RBC morphology measurements.**

      c. The **WBC/myeloperoxidase (MPO) channel** consists of a specialized flow cell in which leukocytes are counted and differentiated.

        (1) The blood is diluted, the RBCs are lysed, and the WBCs are stained for **MPO activity.** MPO is found in the **greatest amount in granulocytes.** Slight-to-moderate amounts of MPO exist in monocytes; very little exists in lymphocytes and immature leukocyte precursor cells (i.e., blasts).

        (2) The WBCs enter a flow cell where two-dimensional light-scatter and light-absorption properties are determined for each cell.

        (3) Stained cells absorb more light and scatter light at a different angle than unstained cells. The end result is a **two-dimensional leukocyte cytogram.**

        (4) The **peroxidase (MPO) channel** gives a total WBC count and absolute numbers of neutrophils, lymphocytes, monocytes, and **large un-**

stained cells (LUC). The mean peroxidase activity is expressed as the **mean peroxidase index (MPXI)** and scaled from $-10-+10$.

d. **Basophils.** In some flow cytometry instruments, basophils are not classified in the peroxidase channel because they appear in the same area on the scattergram as lymphocytes. Basophils, therefore, require separate analysis in a separate channel.

(1) RBCs are fully lysed, and WBCs are partially lysed, leaving only anucleated leukocytes.

(2) Cells in this channel enter a flow cell and are analyzed by two-angle light scatter from a laser source.

(3) Basophils are more resistant to lysis than other leukocytes. They are counted and sorted separately.

(4) Due to variations in nuclear texture, segmented nuclei have a higher component of wide-angle scatter.

(5) Based on their properties of wide-angle light scatter (Figure 3-9), a ratio of segmented nuclei to nonsegmented nuclei (i.e., immature myeloid cells) is reported as a **lobularity index (LI).**

(a) **A high LI indicates a large population of segmented nuclei.**

(b) **A low LI indicates a morphologic shift to the left,** with more bands and immature neutrophil forms.

II. HEMATOPOIETIC TISSUES are organs and tissue areas in which **blood cell production or regulation** occurs. These tissues include areas of fetal hematopoiesis, the spleen, lymphatic tissues, and the bone marrow.

A. **Embryonic and fetal hematopoiesis**

1. **Primitive erythroblasts are the first blood cells** formed by the first month of embryonic life. These cells are formed outside the embryo in the mesenchyme of the **yolk sac.**

2. **By the sixth week** of embryonic life, the **liver** becomes the primary hematopoietic organ for producing definitive **erythroblasts, which mature to nonnucleated RBCs.**

3. **In midfetal life,** the **spleen** and **lymph nodes** begin a limited role as secondary lymphoid organs.

4. **In the last half** of fetal life, **bone marrow hematopoiesis begins** and becomes progressively more important. Hematopoiesis in the liver begins to slowly diminish by the last trimester.

5. **Shortly after birth,** hematopoiesis ceases in the liver, and the **marrow** becomes the **only site** for production of **erythrocytes, granulocytes, monocytes, platelets, and B lymphocytes.**

a. Hematopoietic **primitive stem cells** and **committed progenitor cells** are located in the marrow.

b. In an infant, most bone marrow is actively hematopoietic.

c. With increasing age, marrow for hematopoiesis becomes progressively limited.

d. The spleen and lymph nodes serve as **secondary lymphoid tissue for lymphocyte development and differentiation.**

Peroxidase channel

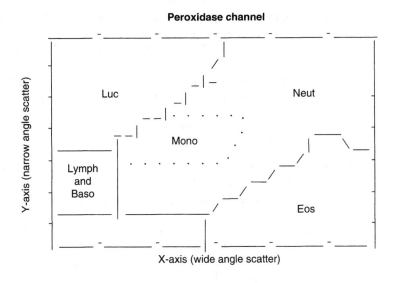

Basophil – leukocyte channel

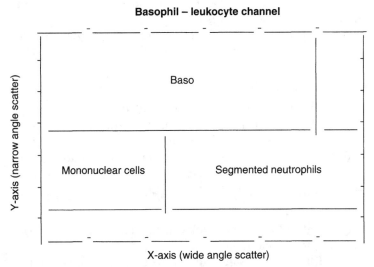

Figure 3-9. Typical format of a scattergram cell distribution report of a flow cytometer cell-counting instrument. Large unstained cells (Luc), basophils (Baso), eosinophils (Eos), neutrophils (Neut), and monocytes (Mono) are represented.

B. Spleen

    1. Internal structure is divided into **white pulp** and **red pulp.**

        a. The pulp is divided by **fibrous trabeculae,** which contain:

            (1) Arteries that emerge from the trabeculae, giving off right-angle branches into the white pulp and terminating in lymphatic nodules

            (2) Veins that drain the venous sinuses of the red pulp into the hepatic-portal blood vessels

            (3) Lymphatics that are scattered throughout the spleen and pass through lymphatic nodules

        b. White pulp is so named because it contains concentrations of WBCs (i.e., lymphocytes and macrophages) in anatomically select areas of the spleen.

    (1) **A periarterial lymphatic sheath** consisting of **T lymphocytes** is wrapped around the central artery.

    (2) **Lymphatic nodules,** located throughout the white pulp, contain a **germinal center.**

      (a) The **marginal zone,** which surrounds the germinal centers and separates the red and white pulp, is rich in **T lymphocytes and macrophages.**

      (b) The nodules are held together by a network of fibrous reticular cells.

  c. **Red pulp** is so named because it contains venous sinuses and cords of fibrous trabeculae.

    (1) Blood from marginal zones and central arterial terminals in the white pulp drains into the red pulp.

    (2) RBCs that enter the cords must pass through a porous membrane separating the cords from venous sinuses.

      (a) **Pores** in the fibrous trabeculae are only approximately **3** μ**m in diameter.**

      (b) **RBCs, which are an average of 7** μ**m,** must be squeezed through the small pores.

      (c) **RBCs that are old or contain cytoplasmic inclusions** do not have the necessary pliability to transverse the pores, and they **are destroyed.**

2. **Functions of the spleen**

  a. **RBC filtration** occurs to eliminate cellular impurities.

    (1) The process of "squeezing" RBCs through the narrow fenestrated cord **selectively eliminates** old or abnormal RBCs.

    (2) **RBCs and platelets coated with autoimmune gamma G immunoglobulin are also destroyed** by the **macrophages** in the red pulp.

  b. **Cell grooming or restructuring** of RBCs with intracellular inclusions occurs in the red pulp.

    (1) **Reticulocytes** are delayed in transit because of small amounts of cytoplasmic RNA.

    (2) **RBC cytoplasmic inclusions** such as deoxyribonucleic acid (DNA), ribonucleic acid (RNA), iron, denatured Hb, or a remaining nucleus are squeezed from RBCs as they work their way through the tiny pores. **Cellular debris is eliminated by splenic macrophages.**

  c. In humans, the spleen serves as a **reservoir for platelets and lymphocytes.**

    (1) **Up to 30% of circulating platelets** are sequestered by the spleen through slow transit.

    (2) The spleen is rich in mature **lymphocytes** destined for antigen-dependent differentiation.

  d. The spleen serves as an important organ involved in **immunity.**

    (1) White pulp contains approximately **25%** of the peripheral **T lymphocytes in transit** between circulation and tissue.

    (2) Approximately **10%–15%** of peripheral **B lymphocytes** are found in splenic nodules.

    (3) The spleen provides a locale for immunity-induced lymphocyte differentiation and antibody production. It serves as an important organ for **immunoglobulin M (IgM) production** by B lymphocytes.

3. **Asplenia** (the absence of splenic function) can be caused by either surgical removal (e.g., splenectomy) or radiation overexposure. This condition can also occur in association with malabsorption syndromes. The hematologic results of asplenia include:

   a. Increased susceptibility to infection

   b. Acute granulocytosis

   c. Acute thrombocytosis, with occasional giant platelets

   d. Chronic and absolute lymphocytosis and monocytosis

   e. Increased appearance of immature RBCs in the circulation

   f. Increased amount of circulating RBCs with cytoplasmic inclusions or abnormal forms (e.g., Howell-Jolly bodies, target cells, and burr cells)

4. **Splenomegaly**

   a. Definitions

   (1) **Splenomegaly** describes an enlarged spleen.

   (2) **Hypersplenism** describes exaggerated inhibitory or destructive functions of the spleen, which is usually accompanied by splenomegaly.

   b. Clinical presentation. Splenomegaly results in **vascular congestion** and **portal hypertension.** RBCs, granulocytes, and as many as 90% of circulating platelets may be trapped, which results in **anemia, leukocytopenia,** and **thrombocytopenia.** A **hypercellular marrow** results in response to a chronic pancytopenia.

C. **Lymphatic tissues**

   1. **Lymphopoiesis** is anatomically divided between two areas.

      a. Primary lymphatic tissues include the **bone marrow** for B lymphocytes, the **thymus** for T lymphocytes, and sites of active hematopoiesis in the fetus.

      b. Secondary lymphatic tissues serve as reservoirs for already differentiated lymphocytes. These tissues include the **lymph nodes, spleen, and gut-associated lymphatic tissue.**

   2. **The thymus** is a primary tissue for T-lymphocyte development.

      a. The cortex, or outer part of the organ, consists of several cell types.

      (1) Small and medium **primitive T cells** (i.e., **thymocytes**) are the youngest cells found in the thymus.

      (2) **Epithelial cells** serve as important effectors of T-cell differentiation.

      (3) The corticomedullary junction is rich in **macrophages.**

      b. The medulla, or interior of the organ, is rich in **maturing T lymphocytes, epithelial cells,** and concentric swirls of squamous epithelial cells known as **Hassall's corpuscles.** Mature immunocompetent T lymphocytes leave the medulla and enter the circulation to migrate to secondary lymphoid tissues to await "specific" immune differentiation.

   3. **Lymph nodes,** spread throughout the body in a "second" vascular system, comprise part of the **secondary lymphatic system.**

      a. All lymph empties and is recirculated into the bloodstream via the right thoracic duct and the left thoracic duct, which is the major lymphatic vessel.

b. All nodes are separated from each other by thin-walled vessels known as **lymph ducts.** The normal **anatomic structure** of each node includes a cortex, paracortex, and medulla.

(1) The cortex contains **lymphocyte follicles (nodules)** with germinal centers. These follicles are unique to lymph nodes and the spleen.

(a) All follicles are arranged in a row beneath the surface capsular lining.

(b) These follicles contain a concentration of **macrophages and B lymphocytes.**

(c) The germinal centers are surrounded by a high concentration of **T lymphocytes.**

(2) The paracortex is defined as the area between the cortex and medulla. This area of the node is **rich in macrophages,** as well as **B and T lymphocytes** in transit.

(3) The medulla, or inside of the node, is arranged in parallel cords of **small lymph and plasma cells.**

4. Lymphopoiesis is defined as lymphocyte production or regulation in primary or secondary lymphatic tissues.

a. Lymphocyte production in primary tissues is continuous and **independent of antigen stimulation.**

(1) The production rate is in excess of demand.

(2) Only a fraction of newly formed lymphocytes in the primary tissues survive to gain access to secondary lymphoid organs.

b. Lymphocyte proliferation in secondary tissues is **antigenic stimulation-dependent,** resulting in the proliferation of specific clonal populations of lymphocytes to carry out the immunologic response.

c. Of circulating lymphocytes, **75%–85% are T lymphocytes, and 10%–15% are B lymphocytes.**

d. T lymphocytes are more actively motile and recirculate more than B lymphocytes.

(1) T cells migrate among the blood (30 minutes), spleen (6 hours), and lymph nodes (15–20 hours).

(2) B lymphocytes do not freely circulate and may stay in a lymph node for as long as 30 hours.

D. Bone marrow

1. Structure and development

a. Fat-cell occupation of the bone marrow space begins by 4 years of age, at which time the growth of bone cavities has exceeded the body's need, and the available space in bone cavities has grown faster than the needed circulation blood mass.

(1) Fat-cell growth occurs first at the diaphysis of long bones and slowly extends to the center of the bone.

(2) By 18 years of age, fatty replacement has limited active **hematopoietic**

marrow to the vertebrae, ribs, skull, sternum, proximal epi-
physes of long bones, and the iliac crest of the pelvis.

(3) Because of this available fatty bone marrow reserve, reactivation of
extramedullary organs rarely takes place.

b. **Organization.** The marrow is organized in a spokelike pattern of venous
sinuses and cords of hematopoietic tissue.

(1) **Venous sinuses** are covered on the marrow side by **endothelial
cells** and on the sinus side by a basement membrane and **reticular
adventitial cells,** which put out projections or "nests" to support
hematopoietic cells.

(2) **Megakaryocytes** lie within the cords close to the sinus wall. Strings
of platelets peel directly into the venous sinus.

(3) **Erythroblasts** lie close to venous sinuses in clusters or colonies.

(a) Each cluster consists of a central macrophage (**i.e., nurse cell**)
surrounded by erythroblasts in various stages of maturation.

(b) When mature, the reticulocyte squeezes through the basement
membrane and endothelial layer to be released into the venous
sinus.

c. **Nerve supply.** The marrow has an extensive supply of nerves, which may
play an important autoregulatory role to adjust blood flow to the rate of
cellular maturation and proliferation.

2. **Bone marrow functions**

a. **Minor.** The marrow has a minor function in the **antigen processing** of
cellular and humoral immunity.

b. **Major.** The major function of the marrow is the **production and proliferation of blood cells (hematopoiesis).** Marrow hematopoiesis is divided
into **three major compartments or cell types** (Figure 3-10).

(1) **Stem cells,** known as **pluripotential or multipotential** cells, retain
the ability to differentiate into any cell line.

(a) The stem cells are referred to as **colony-forming units–spleen
(CFU-S).**

(b) CFU-S differentiate in either of two pathways, giving rise to either
secondary multipotential stem cells, which give rise to primitive B or T lymphocytes, or **multipotential stem cells,** which
give rise to the nonlymphocytes.

(2) **Progenitor (committed) cells** are also known as **unipotential stem
cells,** because they differentiate into only one cell line. Committed
stem cells include **BFU-E, CFU-E, CFU-MEG,** and **CFU-GM** (see
Figure 3-10 for descriptions of abbreviations).

(3) **Precursor cells** comprise the third marrow compartment. Each type
of unipotential stem cell matures into a blast form (e.g., myeloblast,
megakaryoblast, erythroblast).

3. **Bone marrow examination** can be performed with an aspirate and a biopsy,
both of which are nonsurgically obtained by a pathologist from either the
sternum or the **pelvic iliac crest.**

a. **Background.** The weight of the marrow in an adult is 1300–1500 g. Marrow
can undergo complete transformation within hours to days. A marrow
examination is vital to the diagnosis of many diseases, such as myeloprolif-

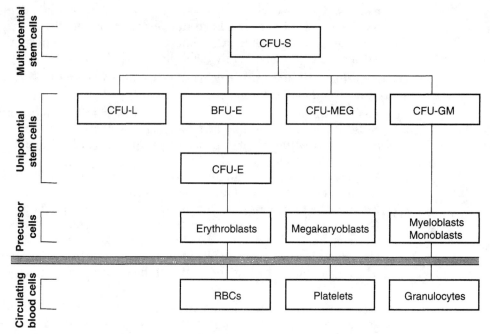

Figure 3-10. Hematokinetics in the bone marrow. Hematopoiesis in the marrow consists of three compartments: multipotential stem cells, unipotential stem cells, and precursor cells. Cell types include the following: Colony-forming unit (CFU) in the spleen (CFU-S), lymph (CFU-L), erythroid cells (CFU-E), megakaryocytes (CFU-MEG), and granulocytes/monocytes (CFU-GM); burst-forming unit erythroid (BFU-E).

erative diseases, lymphoproliferative diseases, and some severe anemias of unknown origin.

b. **Preparation of aspirate.** A marrow aspirate must be prepared with speed and quick drying to prevent clotting of the specimen. The types of preparations made with an aspirate include:

(1) **Marrow films** stained with Wright's stain

(2) **Direct films** stained with Wright's stain

(3) **Marrow imprint** stained with Wright's stain

(4) **Crush preparations** stained with Wright's stain

(5) **Histologic study** of marrow particles

(6) **Gross quantitative study** of marrow

c. **Marrow preparations from aspiration or biopsy are stained** for cell morphology or iron content.

(1) The **Wright's stain** is most commonly used.

(2) **Prussian blue stain** is used for the quantitation of iron in the macrophages of the marrow.

(a) **Hemosiderin or ferritin** are stained, and the staining intensity is graded from 1+–4+ (2+–4+ is normal for adults).

(b) **Sideroblasts** (i.e., normoblasts containing one or more particles of stainable iron) can be examined and quantitated.

(i) Normally, 20%–60% of the late normoblasts are sideroblasts.

(ii) Sideroblasts are decreased with various iron storage anemias.

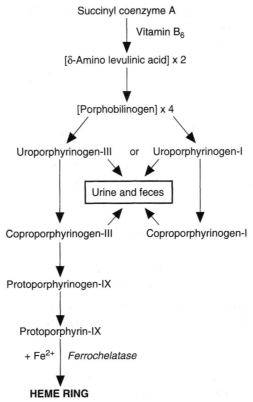

Figure 3-11. Formation of heme from succinylcoenzyme A (SCA). The III isomer is the biologically active form. The enzyme ferrochelatase inserts the iron into the pyrrole ring.

    d. Examination of cellularity is expressed as the ratio of the volume of hematopoietic cells to the volume of marrow space for the patient's age.

        (1) A current peripheral blood cell count, platelet count, and reticulocyte count [see IV F 5 c (2)] should be included with a marrow examination.

        (2) Cellularity is estimated from gross quantitative study and histologic sections of marrow biopsy.

        (3) Irregularities of cellular distribution are first examined with a low-power scan of the slide, then examined at 500X or 1000X for cellular characteristics.

           (a) A **differential count** of 300–1000 cells is completed.

           (b) A **myeloid/erythroid (M:E) ratio** is estimated by comparing the percent of total granulocytes with total normoblasts. The **normal** M:E ratio in the adult is **2:1 to 4:1.**

III. HEMOGLOBIN SYNTHESIS, STRUCTURE, AND FUNCTION

    A. Heme synthesis (Figure 3-11)

        1. Synthesis occurs on the mitochondria of normoblasts and begins with succinylcoenzyme A (SCA), which is a by-product of the tricarboxylic acid (TCA) cycle.

a. SCA combines with glycine to yield an unstable intermediate known as α-amino–β-ketoadipate.

b. The intermediate is decarboxylated to form delta (δ)-**aminolevulinic acid (ALA).**

   (1) This reaction occurs in **mitochondria** and requires pyridoxal phosphate (i.e., **vitamin B$_6$**).

   (2) Trace amounts of ALA, which is normally found in urine, are increased in certain abnormalities of heme synthesis (e.g., **lead poisoning**).

c. Two molecules of ALA combine to form **porphobilinogen (PBG).**

   (1) Normally, trace amounts of PBG can be measured in urine.

   (2) **Increased** amounts of PBG are excreted in **acute intermittent porphyria** and are detected by a color reaction with **Ehrlich's aldehyde reagent.**

2. Four molecules of porphobilinogen combine to form **uroporphyrinogen I or III.**

a. The type III isomer form is converted by way of **coproporphyrinogen III,** and **protoporphyrinogen IX** to **protoporphyrin IX.**

b. Iron is inserted into protoporphyrin by the mitochondrial enzyme, **ferrochelatase,** to complete the formation of the heme moiety.

c. In certain diseases, this pathway may be partially blocked.

   (1) Type I isomers of uroporphyrinogen and coproporphyrinogen are formed and **excreted in excess urinary amounts as uroporphyrin I** and **coproporphyrin I.**

   (2) **Protoporphyrin** is normally found in mature RBCs, but concentrations are **increased in lead poisoning and iron deficiency anemia.**

B. Globin chain synthesis

1. Polypeptide chains are manufactured on ribosomes in the normoblast cytoplasm.

2. Globin chains are assembled from two pairs of polypeptide chains (i.e., four chains per hemoglobin molecule).

3. Four primary chains (i.e., α, β, γ, δ) can be produced. Each type of globin chain is different by only a few amino-acid substitutions.

4. There are many Hb forms, depending on the combination of the two pairs of globin chains.

a. An **embryonic form,** $\alpha_2\varepsilon_2$, is detected early in fetal life.

b. By 3 months of embryonic life, embryonic Hb is replaced by **fetal Hb (Hb F).**

   (1) Hb F consists of two alpha chains and two gamma chains (i.e., $\alpha_2\gamma_2$).

   (2) Hb F **is the major Hb in the fetus** and newborn infant.

   (3) Hb F has a **higher oxygen affinity** than that of adult Hb.

   (4) Beta-chain production does not begin until the 20th week of prenatal life, so adult Hb is approximately 10% between 20 and 35 weeks, and 15%–40% at birth.

   (5) **After birth, the production of Hb F slowly ceases,** and by 6 months of age, it constitutes less than 8% of the total Hb content.

    (a) By 1 year of age, infants have less than 2% Hb F.

    (b) Less than 1% Hb F is normally found in adults. Reactivation of Hb F production may occur in pregnancy and in some disorders of erythropoiesis.

  c. Adult hemoglobin (HbA) is the major adult form, consisting of two alpha chains and two beta chains (i.e., $\alpha_2\beta_2$).

  d. Hemoglobin A$_2$ (HbA$_2$) accounts for **1.5%–3.5%** of normal adult hemoglobin.

    (1) HbA$_2$ consists of two alpha chains and two delta chains (i.e., $\alpha_2\delta_2$).

    (2) Delta-chain synthesis occurs only in normoblasts and is absent in reticulocytes.

    (3) The HbA$_2$ form is **increased in some beta-thalassemias and in iron deficiency anemia.**

  e. Genetic control of globin-chain production is seen as gene separation.

    (1) The production of α-chains is coded on **chromosome 16.**

    (2) The production of all other globin chains is coded on **chromosome 11.**

C. Structure and function of hemoglobin

  1. The main function of an RBC is to contain, transport, and protect hemoglobin molecules.

  2. Each Hb molecule consists of four globin chains (most commonly, $\alpha_2\beta_2$) and four heme groups, each with a center iron molecule.

  3. Each globin chain has a hydrophobic "pocket" that contains a heme group.

    a. This arrangement protects the Fe^{2+} from oxidation to the ferric form (i.e., Fe^{3+}).

    b. The **ferric form cannot bind oxygen.**

  4. The iron of each heme is directly bonded to a nitrogen atom of a histidine side chain. This histidine is known as the **proximal histidine** and **functions to increase the oxygen affinity** of the heme ring.

  5. A second histidine, known as the **distal histidine,** is on the opposite side of the heme plane. This histidine sterically **diminishes the binding of carbon monoxide (CO)** and **inhibits the oxidation of the heme iron to the ferric state.**

  6. One molecule of Hb can bind up to eight atoms of oxygen (i.e., two oxygens per heme ring).

  7. Hemoglobin exhibits three kinds of allosteric effects (i.e., interactions that occur between spatially distinct sites within the molecule).

    a. Cooperative binding of oxygen increases the amount of oxygen that can be carried by a hemoglobin molecule.

    (1) The binding of one molecule of oxygen to a heme group **facilitates the further binding of oxygen** to other heme groups in the same molecule.

    (2) This property is responsible for the pattern seen with the sigmoid-

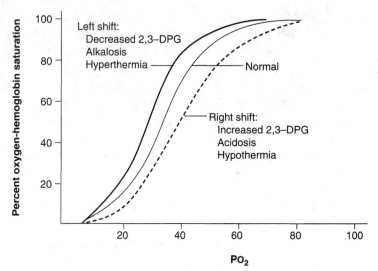

Figure 3-12. The normal dissociation curve of normal human blood shows a decreased affinity state (right shift) and an increased affinity state (left shift). PO_2 = partial pressure of blood oxygen tension. 2,3-DPG = 2,3-diphosphoglycerate.

shaped hemoglobin **oxygen dissociation curve,** as illustrated in Figure 3-12.

    b. The **Bohr effect** is the chemical phenomenon whereby protons (i.e., H^+ atoms) and carbon dioxide (CO_2) promote the release of oxygen from the Hb molecule.

        (1) This characteristic is physiologically important to **enhance the release of oxygen** in metabolically active tissues.

        (2) Each RBC contains an enzyme known as **carbonic anhydrase** (CA), which catalyzes the conversion of the CO_2 given up by tissues and water (H_2O) to produce carbonic acid (H_2CO_3), as shown by the chemical equation that follows:

$$\text{Metabolically active tissue} \xrightarrow{\text{CA}} CO_2 + H_2O \rightarrow HCO_3^- + H^+$$

        (3) The H^+ liberated by this reaction binds to sites on the globin chain, lowering the Hb oxygen affinity and releasing more oxygen to the tissues.

        (4) A small portion of the CO_2 binds to amino-end terminal groups of the globin chains and is transported to the lungs as **carboxy-hemoglobin. The binding of CO_2 further lowers Hb oxygen affinity.**

        (5) In the lungs, the binding of oxygen releases H^+ and displaces bound Hb-CO_2, as illustrated by the chemical reaction that follows:

$$HCO_3^- + H^+ \xrightarrow{\text{CA}} CO_2 + H_2O$$

    c. The third allosteric effect demonstrated by Hb is the **regulation of the oxygen affinity of Hb by 2,3-diphosphoglycerate (2,3-DPG).**

        (1) Only one molecule of 2,3-DPG can be bound per Hb molecule by cross-linking between the two β chains.

(2) 2,3-DPG binds more weakly to HbF than to HbA, which **partially explains why HbF has a higher oxygen affinity.**

  d. Allosteric properties of Hb arise from interactions between the α and β chains. Hemoglobin can exist in **two allosteric forms.**

    (1) **The T (i.e., tense) form** is the **low oxygen affinity state** of hemoglobin.

      (a) The quaternary structure of Hb is **stabilized by noncovalent electrostatic bonds between the different globin chains.**

      (b) Globin-chain bonds partially "close off" the heme pockets, making accessibility of oxygen to the heme iron more difficult.

      (c) On oxygenation in the lungs of the first heme, the iron moves into the plane of the heme and pulls the proximal histidine.

      (d) The resulting movement of the histidine breaks some of the noncovalent chain-chain bonds, opening up the reactive sites of the Hb molecule and shifting the equilibrium from the T form to a high-affinity state.

      (e) The **T form is stabilized by** any one of the following:

        (i) Binding of 2,3-DPG

        (ii) Binding of CO_2

        (iii) Binding of H^+

    (2) The **R (i.e., reactive) form** refers to the high oxygen affinity state, in which the iron in each heme ring is readily accessible to oxygen binding.

D. Oxygen transport

  1. **Regulation.** The amount of oxygen reaching the tissues can be regulated by either altering the number of circulating RBCs, which causes a change in the rate of erythropoiesis, or by altering the affinity of hemoglobin for oxygen.

  2. In a **normal steady state,** the amount of oxygen and CO_2 exchanged in the lungs is equal to the amount exchanged in the tissues.

  3. **Oxygen is carried in the blood in two forms.**

    a. Approximately 3% of oxygen is **dissolved in the plasma.**

    b. The majority of oxygen is **carried by Hb** in the RBCs. **Each gram of Hb** has the maximum capacity to bind **1.34 mL of oxygen.**

  4. **Carbon monoxide binds 210 times stronger** than oxygen to a hemoglobin molecule.

    a. If a person were breathing room air (i.e., 21% oxygen) contaminated with as little as 0.1% CO, half of the Hb-binding sites would be filled with CO.

    b. In addition to lowering Hb-oxygen saturation, CO results in a left shift of the oxygen dissociation curve, **which reflects an increased Hb-oxygen affinity state.**

E. Carbon dioxide transport

  1. **Approximately 5% of the total CO_2** in arterial blood is **physically dissolved in plasma.**

  2. **Approximately 5% of the CO_2,** known as **carbamino-CO_2,** is carried in blood bound to amino groups of **plasma proteins.**

3. **Approximately 90% of the blood CO_2 is converted to bicarbonate and H^+ ions.**

IV. ERYTHROCYTES AND ERYTHROPOIESIS

A. **Erythroid maturation**

1. **Production begins with the multipotential stem cell (CFU-S).** The differentiation of a stem cell, induced by certain microenvironmental influences, results in a committed erythroid progenitor cell.

2. **The committed unipotential cell compartment** for erythropoiesis consists of two compartments, as defined by their behavior in cell culture systems.

   a. **BFU-E stem cells** (see Figure 3-10) maintain an active cell cycle maintained by a **burst-promoting factor** released by the local microenvironment.

   (1) BFU-E cells have a **low concentration of erythropoietin (EPO)** receptors and respond only to high concentrations of EPO.

   (2) **T lymphocytes** are required for optimal BFU-E growth.

   b. Differentiation of the BFU-E cell pool gives rise to the unipotential **CFU-E stem cell pool** (see Figure 3-10).

   (1) CFU-E cells have a **high concentration of EPO membrane receptors;** hence, they respond to low EPO concentrations.

   (2) EPO stimulation transforms the CFU-E cell into the earliest recognizable erythroid precursor, the **pronormoblast.**

3. **Pronormoblasts (rubriblasts)** comprise the first recognizable erythroid precursor stage as well as the **first hemoglobin-synthesizing cell.** These blasts begin a controlled process of photoporphyrin production, globin-chain synthesis, iron uptake, and Hb assembly.

   a. **Size.** Pronormoblasts measure approximately **20 μm in diameter** (the largest of erythroid precursors).

   b. **Distinguishing morphologic and cytoplasmic characteristics** are presented in Table 3-2.

   c. This is an **actively mitotic** stage, and its division forms two **basophilic normoblasts.**

4. **Basophilic normoblasts (prorubricytes)** are slightly smaller in size than pronormoblasts.

   a. **Distinguishing morphologic and cytoplasmic characteristics** are given in Table 3-2.

   b. This is an **actively mitotic** stage, and its division gives rise to two **polychromatic erythroblasts.**

5. **Polychromatic erythroblasts (rubricytes)** are slightly smaller than prorubricytes.

   a. **Distinguishing morphologic and cytoplasmic characteristics** are given in Table 3-2.

   b. This stage undergoes one or more mitotic divisions, depending on the level of erythropoiesis.

   c. After the last mitotic division, the **nucleus becomes small and condensed (i.e., pyknotic),** which gives rise to the next stage.

Table 3-2. Morphologic and Cytoplasmic Characteristics of Erythroid Cells

Cell Type	Morphologic Characteristics	Cytoplasmic Characteristics
Pronormoblasts	Fine, uniform chromatin pattern Intensely staining chromatin Prominent nuclear membrane One to three prominent nuclei	Moderate in amount Moderately basophilic (bluish) Granules are absent
Basophilic normoblasts (prorubricytes)	Coarse, partially clumped chromatin with a wheel spoke pattern Nuclear parachromatin stains pink Nucleoli are present but not always visible Cell borders often irregular because of pseudopodia	Moderate in amount Deeply basophilic due to a high amount of cytoplasmic RNA
Polychromatic erythroblasts (rubricytes)	Nuclear volume occupies only half of the cell area Intensely staining chromatin Moderately condensed chromatin	Stains various shades of gray due to mix of RNA and hemoglobin
Orthochromic normoblasts (metarubricytes)	Smaller normoblasts than previous stage Last stage in maturation sequence with nucleus	Abundant hemoglobin Fewer polyribosomes Slight polychromasia
Reticulocytes	Nuclear material extruded Immature reticulocytes are larger than RBCs Immature reticulocytes are sticky because of a layer of transferrin on membrane	Polychromatic due to remaining RNA

RBCs = red blood cells; RNA = ribonucleic acid.

6. **Orthochromic normoblasts (metarubricytes)** are the last nucleated stage in the maturation sequence.

   a. This is the first **nonmitotic** stage, with **smaller** normoblasts than the previous stage.

   b. **Distinguishing morphologic and cytoplasmic characteristics** are given in Table 3-2.

7. **Reticulocyte.** Cytoplasmic contractions and undulations extrude the nucleus of the metarubricyte with a small rim of cytoplasm and Hb, which changes

the cell into a reticulocyte. Morphologic and cytoplasmic characteristics are given in Table 3-2. Other characteristics include:

a. Macrophages phagocytose the extruded nuclear material.

b. The reticulocyte is **released into the circulation after 2 days** of maturation in the marrow.

c. Eight reticulocytes are normally produced from one pronormoblast.

d. Reticulocytes **synthesize Hb for approximately 1 day** after leaving the marrow.

e. Residual **ribosomes, mitochondria, and other organelles are removed in the spleen** or are internally dissolved. The result is a mature RBC, which has an **average life span of 120 days.**

8. Iron incorporation is a vital part of erythroid maturation.

a. Iron is transferred from **transferrin** into the young normoblasts, where it becomes attached to specific normoblast membrane receptors.

(**1**) **Free iron** is shuttled into the normoblast, and the transferrin molecule is released for recirculation.

(**2**) **Intracellular iron** is shuttled to the mitochondria for heme-ring production, or it is temporarily deposited in the cytoplasm as ferritin.

b. A **secondary supply of iron** is provided by a central **macrophage** through cell-to-cell delivery.

9. Normoblastic and megaloblastic maturation. Megaloblasts are abnormal erythroid cells. Megaloblastic development parallels all stages of erythrocyte maturation.

a. Megaloblastosis is an **abnormal maturation** of erythroid precursors resulting from a **vitamin B_{12} or folic acid deficiency.**

b. Megaloblasts have an **impaired ability to synthesize and replicate their own nuclear DNA.** Intermitotic and mitotic **phases of mitosis** are prolonged and out of synchrony.

(**1**) As a result, nuclear maturation lags behind cytoplasmic maturation.

(**2**) The nuclear chromatin pattern of megaloblasts is more open, and breaking up of the nucleus is common (**i.e., karyorrhexis**).

(**3**) This results in an increased frequency of circulating RBCs with **Howell-Jolly bodies,** which are remnants of nuclear chromatin.

B. Regulation of erythrocyte production

1. The number of circulating RBCs may be regulated by changing the **rate of production in the marrow** or the **rate of release from the marrow.** This regulation is normally well balanced, because the rate of RBC destruction does not significantly vary.

2. Impaired oxygen transport to the tissues and low intracellular oxygen tension triggers RBC production in the marrow. Conditions that stimulate erythropoiesis include:

a. Anemia

b. Cardiac or pulmonary disorders

c. High altitudes

3. Oxygen tension in tissues is regulated, in part, by the oxygen affinity of Hb.

    a. Modulation. Hemoglobin-oxygen affinity is modulated by the concentration of **phosphates** in the RBC.

      (1) The primary phosphate is **2,3-DPG.**

      (2) 2,3-DPG combines with β chains of the reduced Hb molecule, which results in reduced Hb affinity for oxygen binding.

    b. In areas of **hypoxic tissue,** as oxygen moves from Hb into the tissue, the amount of reduced Hb decreases. This results in:

      (1) More 2,3-DPG being bound

      (2) Lower Hb oxygen affinity, which results in more oxygen being released to the tissues

    c. If tissue hypoxia persists, the depletion of 2,3-DPG leads to increased glycolysis and production of more 2,3-DPG, which further lowers Hb oxygen affinity.

  4. Reduced intracellular oxygen tension leads to the production of **EPO.**

    a. Background. EPO is a glycoprotein hormone that **controls RBC production at the level of the marrow.**

      (1) Production. EPO is produced **mainly by kidney** glomeruli, when cells in the glomerular tuft of the kidney experience a reduced oxygen tension.

      (2) Location. EPO is present in the plasma and urine of all mammals, with a biologic half-life of 4–6 hours and a normal reference range of **22–54 milli-immunochemical units per milliliter (mU/mL).**

    b. Three main EPO marrow effects include:

      (1) Stimulation of committed unipotential cells to proliferate and differentiate into pronormoblasts

      (2) Shortening the generation time of each maturation stage

      (3) Promoting **early release of reticulocytes** into the blood

    c. The **end result of EPO stimulation** is an **increased number of marrow normoblasts.**

  5. Other regulators of erythropoiesis

    a. Plasma Hb may have a feedback stimulation on RBC production or result in increased EPO production.

    b. Hemolytic anemias result in a higher reticulocyte count than other disorders that stimulate RBC production.

    c. Androgens have a synergistic effect on EPO release and are thought to be the cause of higher red cell values in men.

C. Erythrocyte structure

  1. General considerations. RBCs are biconcave disks with a **mean diameter of 7–8 μm** and a mean **volume of 90 fL.** The RBC has **no nucleus or mitochondria and cannot synthesize protein** but is packaged with enough limited metabolism to exist for **120 days.**

    a. RBCs have **more surface area than volume,** which creates a soft, pliable cell.

    b. The life span of an RBC depends on the relationship between the RBC membrane and metabolism. An RBC must have good self-healing ability.

Cell damage or injury can produce cell fragments rather than Hb leakage and cell lysis.

   c. The main mission of an RBC is to carry oxygen and carbon dioxide to and from all tissues.

   d. With cell aging, enzymatic failure leads to the loss of pliability and splenic destruction.

2. **The RBC membrane** is a lipid bilayer, two molecules thick, consisting of tightly packed phospholipid molecules.

   a. **Cholesterol** is found in the bilayer in a **1:1 molar ratio with phospholipids.**

   (1) RBC membrane cholesterol is in rapid exchange with **plasma unesterified cholesterol.**

   (2) Cholesterol content of the RBC membrane depends on the plasma concentration of cholesterol, free bile acids, and the esterifying enzyme **lecithin cholesterol acyltransferase (LCAT).**

   (3) **Changes in RBC shape and survival** can result from changes in plasma lipids.

   (a) Patients with **hepatocellular disease or biliary obstruction** have **impaired LCAT activity.**

   (b) This results in **cholesterol overloading** of the RBC membrane and **excess RBC membrane surface area.**

   (c) Red cells appear as **target cell forms** and **acanthocytes,** which have a **reduced survival** compared with normal RBCs.

   b. **Membrane proteins** are of two basic classes.

   (1) **Integral proteins provide anion channels** through the RBC membrane.

   (a) These proteins are in contact with both sides of the membrane.

   (b) Oligosaccharide chains are attached to the external surface of transmembrane proteins, providing a negative charge to the RBC surface, which **prevents autoagglutination of RBCs.**

   (2) **Peripheral proteins** provide a **structural network** on the inner surface of the membrane, giving the cell its biconcave structure. Peripheral proteins consist of **spectrin, components 4.1 and 5,** and **actin.** Abnormalities of these proteins are responsible for **cell-shape deformities and hemolytic anemias** (e.g., hereditary elliptocytosis, hereditary spherocytosis).

   c. **The outside layer** of the RBC membrane contains **numerous antigenic determinants,** which provide a genetically determined "specific map" of the RBC surface.

   (1) **More than 300 RBC antigens have been identified, comprising approximately 15 genetically distinct blood group systems.**

   (2) RBC antigens are composed largely of the **oligosaccharide groups of the integral proteins.**

   (3) **Almost all antigenic groups are intrinsic parts of the membrane** and appear during early cell development. The exception is the **Lewis group,** which is secondarily absorbed onto cell surfaces.

(4) **Common RBC antigen systems** include:
    (a) **ABO**
    (b) **Secretor and Lewis**
    (c) **Ii**
    (d) **MN and P**
    (e) **Rh, Kell, and Duffy**

D. **Erythrocyte metabolism**
   1. **The RBC has no nucleus or mitochondria** to metabolize fatty and amino acids for the provision of energy substrates.

   2. **Energy metabolism in the RBC is almost exclusively through the breakdown of glucose.**

   3. **Three basic metabolic pathways** are found in the RBC (Figure 3-13).

      a. **Embden-Meyerhof (EM) pathway** is a nonoxidative **anaerobic pathway** that handles **90% of glucose utilization in the RBC.**
         (1) The end result of the pathway is the **net production of 2 adenosine triphosphate (ATP).**
             (a) ATP is necessary for the survival of an RBC because ATP:
                 (i) Maintains cell shape and flexibility
                 (ii) Energizes the metabolic pumps that control cellular sodium, potassium, and calcium flux
                 (iii) Preserves membrane lipids
             (b) **Deficiencies in ATP,** due to an inherited or acquired defect in glycolysis, can reduce cell survival and **result in hemolytic anemia.**
         (2) The EM pathway also **plays an essential role in maintaining pyridine nucleotides in a reduced state [i.e., nicotinamide adenine dinucleotide, reduced form (NADH)]** to support the conversion of methemoglobin (HbM) to hemoglobin in the methemoglobin reductase pathway.
             (a) HbM results from the oxidation of iron (Fe) from **ferrous ion (Fe^{2+})** to **ferric ion (Fe^{3+}).**
             (b) HbM has a **very low oxygen binding affinity.**
             (c) The accumulation of HbM greatly reduces the oxygen-carrying capacity of the RBC.
             (d) The methemoglobin reductase pathway counteracts the oxidized state by reducing Fe^{3+} to Fe^{2+}.
             (e) This pathway relies on the reducing capacity of nicotinamide adenine dinucleotide (NAD).
             (f) Persons homozygous for an abnormal methemoglobin reductase gene accumulate 20%–40% Hb M in RBCs.
             (g) Persons with heterozygous enzyme deficiency maintain sufficient HbM under normal conditions but are susceptible to hemolysis by oxidizing drugs.

      b. **The Luebering-Rapaport pathway is necessary for the production of 2,3-DPG.**
         (1) The amount of 2,3-DPG produced at any one time depends on the glycolysis rate-limiting enzyme, **phosphofructokinase.**

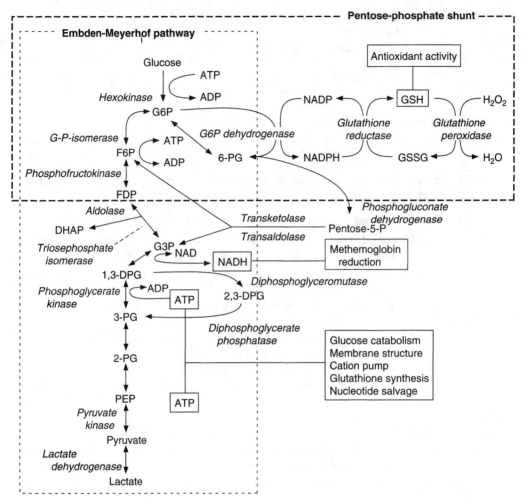

Figure 3-13. The metabolism of the red blood cell (RBC) is primarily from anaerobic glycolysis via the Embden-Myerhof (EM) pathway and the pentose-phosphate shunt. ADP = adenosine diphosphate; ATP = adenosine triphosphate; DHAP = dihydroxyacetone phosphate; 1,3-DPG = 1,3-diphosphoglycerate; 2,3-DPG = 2,3-diphosphoglycerate; FDP = fructose-1,6-diphosphate; F6P = fructose-6-phosphate; G-P-isomerase = glucose-phosphate isomerase; G3P = glucose-3-phosphate; G6P = glucose-6-phosphate; GSH = glutathione (reduced form); GSSG = glutathione (oxidized); NAD = nicotinamide-adenine dinucleotide; NADH = nicotinamide-adenine dinucleotide (reduced form); NADP = nicotinamide-adenine dinucleotide phosphate; NADPH = nicotinamide-adenine dinucleotide phosphate (reduced form); pentose-5-P = pentose-5-phosphate; PEP = phosphoenylpyruvate; 2-PG = 2-phosphoglycerate; 3-PG = 3-phosphoglycerate; 6-PG = 6-phosphogluconate. (Reprinted with permission from Besa E, Catalano PM, Kant J, et al: Hematology. Baltimore, Williams & Wilkins, 1992, p 98.)

(2) 2,3-DPG production also depends on an adequate supply of inorganic phosphate.

(3) 2,3-DPG binds to Hb and **decreases the oxygen affinity of Hb,** thereby releasing more oxygen to the tissues.

c. **Hexose monophosphate shunt** (i.e., pentose-phosphate shunt) **couples oxidative metabolism with nicotinamide-adenine dinucleotide phosphate (NADP) and glutathione reduction.**

(1) This pathway is **functionally dependent on glucose-6-phosphate dehydrogenase (G6PD).**

(2) When this pathway is functionally deficient, globin denaturation occurs, and Hb precipitates out of solution to form inclusions (i.e., **Heinz bodies**) along the inner surface of the RBC membrane. This commonly occurs in patients with **X-linked G6PD deficiency.**

E. Erythrocyte Life Cycle

1. A constant red-cell mass in the circulation is ensured by the balance between delivery of RBCs from the marrow to the blood and the removal of aged or abnormal RBCs from the circulation.

2. As RBCs age, catabolic changes occur that result from cellular **enzyme depletion,** which leads to a **decrease in cell flexibility.**

   a. Cell rigidity makes it more difficult for RBCs to get through small capillaries or splenic sinusoids. The $2–3\mu$m-fenestrations of the splenic sinusoids remove aged or abnormal RBCs that have a higher degree of rigidity.

   b. Splenic trapping results in cell lysis and monocyte/macrophage phagocytosis of debris.

3. Extravascular destruction is removal of RBCs by the spleen and liver (i.e., reticuloendothelial system). This pathway is the **most efficient method** of cell removal and recovery of essential components such as amino acids and iron.

   a. Intramacrophage RBC breakdown occurs following phagocytosis, when the RBC is attacked by lysosomal enzymes. Hb is broken down by an enzyme known as **heme-oxygenase.**

   b. Iron is released from the heme group, returned to **plasma transferrin,** and transported back to the erythroid marrow. Small amounts of iron can be stored within the reticuloendothelial macrophage as **ferritin or hemosiderin.**

   c. Amino acids from globin chains are redirected to the body's amino acid pool.

   d. The photoporphyrin pyrole ring is broken down at the α-methane bridge, and its α-carbon is exhaled as **CO.**

   (1) The opened tetrapyrole, **bilirubin,** is carried by plasma albumin in the **unconjugated** (i.e., the indirect bilirubin) form to the liver.

   (2) Bilirubin is conjugated in the liver to form **bilirubin glucuronide** (i.e., direct bilirubin).

   e. Conjugated bilirubin is excreted from the liver into the small intestine via the bile duct, where it is converted by bacterial flora to **urobilinogen.**

   (1) Most urobilinogen is **excreted in the stool as urobilin.**

   (2) Between 10% and 20% of urobilinogen is reabsorbed by the gut. The reabsorbed urobilinogen is either excreted in urine or returned to the gut via an **enterohepatic cycle.**

   (3) With **liver disease,** the enterohepatic cycle is impaired, and an **increased amount of urobilinogen is excreted in the urine.**

4. Intravascular destruction of RBCs accounts for less than 10% of RBC loss, but it can increase in certain hemolytic diseases. Free hemoglobin is disposed of in the following manner:

   a. The **free hemoglobin tetramer** is unstable in plasma; therefore, tetramers are quickly dissociated into $\alpha_1\beta_1$ **dimers.**

b. Hemoglobin dimers are quickly **bound to plasma haptoglobin.**

  (1) Haptoglobin binding stabilizes the heme-globin bond and **prevents renal excretion of Hb.**

  (2) The haptoglobin-hemoglobin complex is removed from the circulation by reticuloendothelial macrophages and is processed intracellularly in the same manner as extracellular RBC destruction.

  (3) There is a limited supply of plasma haptoglobin, so the number of haptoglobin-hemoglobin complexes that can be formed acutely is limited.

  (a) A sudden release of several grams of Hb intravascularly can exceed the haptoglobin-binding capacity.

  (b) When the haptoglobin-hemoglobin complex is processed in the macrophage, the haptoglobin itself is also catabolized.

  (c) A **decrease or absence of serum haptoglobin may be used to indicate increased intravascular hemolysis.**

c. If haptoglobin is depleted, unbound Hb dimers are free to be filtered by the renal glomerulus.

  (1) As much as 5 g/d can be **reabsorbed by renal tubular epithelial cells** and converted to **hemosiderin for storage.**

  (2) If the amount of free Hb is high, the tubular uptake capacity can be exceeded. Then, dimers are excreted in the urine as free Hb.

  (3) Large amounts of filtered Hb can be destructive to renal tubular cells.

  (4) A large amount of Hb excretion is accompanied by the excretion of hemosiderin and iron loss.

d. Part of the free Hb not bound to haptoglobin may be oxidized to **methemoglobin.**

  (1) The **heme rings dissociate from the globin chains** and are bound to another transport protein, **hemopexin.**

  (2) Heme-hemopexin complexes are cleared from the circulation by reticuloendothelial macrophages and catabolized.

  (3) A small percent of the heme groups are bound to albumin as **methemalbumin.**

F. Measurements of RBC production and destruction

  1. Anemia occurs when delivery of RBCs to the circulation is decreased or when the removal of RBCs from the blood is increased and cannot be compensated for by increased marrow production (see Chapter 4).

  a. When anemia develops, the end result is **tissue hypoxia.**

   (1) Hypoxia stimulates **increased erythropoietin** production by the kidneys.

   (2) Increased EPO levels result in a normoblastic hyperplasia, which produces more RBCs to be released into the circulation.

  b. In a normal person, **the marrow is capable of 6–8 times the normal output.**

  2. Measurement of the total erythron must take into account the balance between marrow production, survival in the circulation, and destruction in the hepatic and splenic macrophage (Figure 3-14).

  3. Measurement of total RBC production can be obtained from an absolute

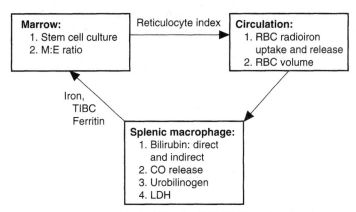

Figure 3-14. Laboratory measurement of the red blood cell (RBC) life cycle. Anemia can result from a marrow production defect or from an RBC survival disorder (e.g., hemolysis). Therefore, the correct laboratory tests can determine the source and cause of most anemias. TIBC = total iron-binding capacity; LDH = lactate dehydrogenase.

measure of the number of immature erythroid cells through the injection and tracking of **radioactive iron.**

4. **Measurements of Hb catabolism and RBC survival** can be obtained with several methods.

   a. An indication of the amount of heme breakdown can be determined by the **amount of exhaled CO.**

   b. **Urobilinogen** can be measured in the stool.

   c. **Serum bilirubin and lactate dehydrogenase (LDH)** levels can provide a quantitative indication of RBC turnover. **Hemolytic disorders can result in high levels of bilirubin and LDH.**

   d. **RBC survival** can be estimated by removing a sample of whole blood and labeling it with the radioisotope **chromium 51 (^{51}Cr-labeled).**

5. **The functional capacity of the erythroid marrow** can be measured with several methods.

   a. Relative numbers of **marrow stem cells** may be estimated using cell culture techniques.

   b. The **density of the erythroid marrow** can be estimated from a bone marrow examination and by obtaining a **M : E ratio** [see II D 3 d (3)(b)].

      (1) The **normal adult M : E ratio ranges from 2 : 1 to 4 : 1.**

      (2) A hemolytic disorder may display an M : E of 1 : 1, which indicates an erythroid hyperplastic marrow.

      (3) An erythroid **hypoplastic** marrow may demonstrate a M : E ratio greater than 4 : 1.

   c. The **reticulocyte count** is a good way to effectively measure the production rate of RBCs.

      (1) **Background.** Because RBC intracellular RNA disappears after about a day in the circulation, the reticulocyte count provides a rough measurement of the number of RBCs being delivered by the marrow to the circulation each day.

Table 3-3. Maturation Index

Hematocrit (%)	Reticulocyte Maturation Time (D)
45	1.0
35	1.5
25	2.0
15	2.5

(2) **Method.** Basically, a reticulocyte count is obtained by staining RBCs with a vital stain known as **new methylene blue.**
  (a) Blood smears of stained RBCs are made, and a set number of RBCs are counted while the total number of reticulocytes are simultaneously counted.
  (b) Reticulocytes are **reported as a percent of RBCs.**
  (c) **Normal values range from 0.5%–2.0%.**
(3) If the total RBC count is also determined, the **absolute reticulocyte count** can be determined by **multiplying the percent reticulocytes by the RBC count.**
  (a) The **normal** absolute reticulocyte count ranges from **25,000–75,000/mm³.**
  (b) The **formula** for obtaining the absolute reticulocyte count is:

$$\text{\% reticulocytes} \times (\text{RBCs} \times 10^6/\text{mm}^3) = \text{reticulocytes} \times 10^6/\text{mm}^3/\text{d}$$

(4) Because the normal maturation time for reticulocytes in the circulation is 1 day, the normal RBC production is an **average of 50,000/mm³/d.**
(5) Often, an increased **circulatory maturation** time of reticulocytes, which is caused by accelerated release from the marrow, must be taken into account.
  (a) Even with increased erythropoiesis, reticulocytes still need 2–3 days to mature.
  (b) To avoid an overestimation of daily RBC production, a correction factor is used based on the **estimated maturation time of reticulocytes in the circulation.**
    (i) The finding of **polychromatic RBCs or nucleated RBCs (NRBCs) on the blood smear indicates accelerated erythropoiesis, a shift reticulocytosis,** and a need to correct the reticulocyte count for circulating maturation time with the **maturation index.**
    (ii) The maturation index **varies inversely with HCT** (Table 3-3).
  (c) **Example.** A patient is seen with a HCT of 25%, an RBC count of $2.89 \times 10^6/\text{mm}^3$, and a reticulocyte count of 7%. The calculated absolute reticulocyte count of this patient is:

$$.07 \times (2.89 \times 10^6/\text{mm}^3) = 202 \times 10^3/\text{mm}^3$$

(i) Because the average normal reticulocyte count is 50,000, this patient has the following rate of reticulocyte production:

$$\frac{202,000}{50,000} = 4 \text{ times normal amount}$$

(ii) When corrected for maturation time using the patient's HCT of 25% (see Table 3-3), there are $4 \div 2 = 2$ times as many reticulocytes per day as normal.

(d) An **alternate method** used to correct for shift reticulocytosis is by calculating the **reticulocyte index (RI).**

(i) **Example.** Using the same patient values as before, the formula for obtaining an RI is:

$$RI = 7\% \times \frac{\text{Patient's HCT (25\%)}}{\text{Normal HCT (45\%)}} = 4\%$$

(ii) Once the RI is known, the **reticulocyte production index (RPI)** can be determined:

$$\frac{RI\ (4\%)}{\text{Maturation time (2 days)}}$$
$$= 2 \text{ times as many reticulocytes/day}$$

6. **Measurement of blood volume** might be necessary for the diagnosis of certain disorders such as anemias or polycythemia (i.e., increase in RBC volume).

   a. Substances that **combine with RBCs (e.g., chromium 51)** can be used to directly measure the total red cell volume. Then, the plasma and whole blood volumes can be calculated from the HCT value.

   b. Substances that **combine with plasma proteins** can be used to directly measure plasma volume. Then, the red cell and whole blood volumes can be calculated from the HCT value.

      (1) **Evan's blue dye** binds to plasma proteins.

      (2) **Radio-iodine saturated albumin (RISA)** mixes with native albumin to provide a measure of plasma volume.

G. **RBC morphology: normal and abnormal**

   1. **Size variations in RBCs** can have a diagnostic implication and are important to report.

      a. **Anisocytosis** is a term indicating RBC variation in size.

         (1) Anisocytosis is usually quantitated as 1+, 2+, 3+, or 4+. There must be a variation in size of more than 10% of erythrocytes per high-power field for a grading of 1+.

         (2) When possible, use the RDW to aid in recognition and quantitation of anisocytosis. **An RDW greater than 15.0 indicates anisocytosis.**

      b. **Normocytosis** of RBCs indicates relatively uniform size (i.e., less than 10% variation).

      c. **Macrocytosis** is a term used to indicate the presence of large RBCs with a mean diameter greater than 8 μm.

         (1) Macrocytosis should be **quantitated** in the following manner:

   (a) 1+ (i.e., slight) if there are approximately 25% macrocytic RBCs present per high-power field

   (b) 2+–3+ (i.e., moderate) if there are 25%–50% macrocytic RBCs present per high-power field

   (c) 4+ (i.e., marked) if there is greater than 50% macrocytic RBCs per high-power field

  (2) When possible, **use the patient's MCV** to aid in a quantitation of macrocytosis. **An MCV greater than 100 fL indicates macrocytosis.**

  (3) Macrocytosis has the following **diagnostic implications:**

   (a) Megaloblastic anemias

   (b) Shift reticulocytosis (e.g., hemolysis)

   (c) Anemia of liver disease

 d. Microcytosis should be quantitated in a manner similar to the quantitation of macrocytosis. If the MCV is not available, finding a small lymphocyte provides a comparable scale.

  (1) An MCV less than 80 fL indicates microcytosis.

  (2) Microcytosis has the following **diagnostic implications:**

   (a) Iron-related disorders

   (b) Sideroblastic anemias

   (c) Anemia of chronic disorders

   (d) Thalassemias

2. The color of the RBCs can be related to the Hb content of the cells.

 a. Normochromic RBCs have a normal red color and Hb content. If possible, the patient's **MCH and MCHC** should be used to provide guidelines for RBC color appearance.

 b. Hypochromia refers to RBCs that show a **less than normal amount of hemoglobin staining,** and the cells' central pallor is increased to more than one third of the cell diameter (Color Plate 1). The patient's **MCH and MCHC** should be used to provide guidelines for RBC color appearance. Hypochromia should be graded in the following manner:

  (1) 1+ (i.e., slight) if RBCs show a central pallor occupying one third to two thirds of the cell's diameter

  (2) 2+–3+ (i.e., moderate) if RBCs show a central pallor occupying more than two thirds of the cell's diameter

  (3) 4+ (i.e., marked) if RBCs show red hemoglobin staining that appears only as a rim on the periphery of the cell

3. Shape changes often have a diagnostic implication and should be graded as slight, moderate, or marked (i.e., 1+, 2+, or 3+) per microscopic field at a magnification of 1000X.

 a. Poikilocytosis refers to RBC variation in shape. There must be a variation in shape of more than 10% of the RBCs per high-power field for a grading of 1+.

 b. Spherocytosis indicates RBCs of spherical shape (Color Plate 2).

  (1) Spherocytes appear microcytic and hyperchromic because of their spherical form. The central pallor is absent (i.e., the typical doughnut shape is absent).

  (2) Grading. Spherocytosis should be graded as slight, moderate, or marked (i.e., 1+, 2+, 3+) using the same guidelines previously described for changes in size.

(3) Spherocytes will be normocytic with a **normal MCV.**

(4) Diagnostic implications of spherocytes are as follows:

    (a) Hereditary spherocytosis

    (b) Hemolysis

c. Ovalocytosis (i.e., elliptocytosis) indicates red cells that vary in shape from slightly oval to pencil-shaped or cigar-shaped (Color Plate 3).

  (1) Ovalocytosis is reported if more than 10% of RBCs per microscopic field are oval or elliptical in shape.

  (2) The diagnostic implications of ovalocytosis are as follows:

    (a) Hereditary elliptocytosis

    (b) Megaloblastic anemias

d. Sickle cells (i.e., drepanocytes) are flattened and elongated cells that are often curved and may have the appearance of a curved blade (i.e., sickle) with sharp points (Color Plate 4). The presence of sickle cells in any amount suggests an investigation of **sickle cell anemia.**

e. Burr cells are irregularly shaped RBCs with symmetric, knobby projections.

  (1) Burr cells are produced by a rupture of the cell membrane by enlarged cytoplasmic vacuoles.

  (2) Care must be taken to distinguish burr cells from crenated RBCs, which are produced by too rapid a drying of the blood smear.

  (3) Diagnostically, burr cells implicate **renal disease.**

f. Schistocytosis (i.e., fragmented RBCs) are pieces of RBCs that are small and triangular with pointed ends. **Schistocytes** are commonly found in patients with **hemolytic anemia and severe burns.**

g. Tear drop cells (i.e., dacryocytes) have one pointed end and a round body. Tear drop RBCs have the following **diagnostic implications:**

  (1) Megaloblastic anemias

  (2) Myelofibrosis with myeloid metaplasia

  (3) Acquired hemolytic anemias

h. Acanthocytes are irregularly shaped RBCs with asymmetric, sharp projections (Color Plate 5).

  (1) Acanthocytes are produced by **cholesterol overloading** of the membrane.

  (2) Diagnostically, acanthocytes implicate **chronic liver disease.**

4. Abnormal forms of RBCs should be graded as slight, moderate, or marked (i.e., 1+, 2+, or 3+) per microscopic field at a magnification of 1000X.

a. Target cells (i.e., leptocytes) are flattened RBCs that reveal peripheral and central zones of Hb, giving the appearance of a target (Color Plate 6).

  (1) Target cells are produced by **cholesterol overloading** of the membrane.

  (2) The **diagnostic implications** of target cells are as follows:

    (a) Chronic liver disease

    (b) Thalassemias

    (c) Hemoglobinopathies

b. **Polychromatophilia** (i.e., polychromasia) refers to an increase in the number of younger RBCs (e.g., reticulocytes) with incomplete hemoglobinization.

   (1) These cells are larger than normal RBCs, lack a central pallor, and stain a pale blue.

   (2) Polychromasia should be **quantitated** in the following manner:

       (a) **1+** if 1–3 polychromatic cells are found per microscopic field

       (b) **2+** if 3–5 polychromatic cells are found per microscopic field

       (c) **3+** if more than five polychromatic cells are found per microscopic field

c. **Basophilic stippling** describes cytoplasmic inclusions. RBCs have cytoplasm that is stippled with a number of fine blue granules, which are ribosomal-RNA remnants (Color Plate 7).

   (1) Stippled cells are **quantitated** in the following manner:

       (a) **Slight** if one stippled RBC is noted in every other microscopic field

       (b) **Moderate** if 1–2 stippled RBCs are noted in every microscopic field

       (c) **Marked** if three or more stippled RBCs are noted in every microscopic field

   (2) The **diagnostic implications** of basophilic stippling are as follows:

       (a) **Lead poisoning**

       (b) **Toxin poisoning**

       (c) **Conditions that greatly accelerate erythropoiesis**

d. **Cabot rings** are thready, blue, ring-shaped, twisted, or figure-eight RBC cytoplasmic inclusions. They are seen rarely in **severe anemia.**

e. **Howell-Jolly Bodies** are dark violet-staining DNA remnants in RBCs (Color Plate 8).

   (1) These inclusions usually occur singly and average 1 μm in diameter.

   (2) The **diagnostic implications** of Howell-Jolly bodies are as follows:

       (a) **Splenectomy**

       (b) **Hemoglobinopathies**

       (c) **Severe hemolysis**

f. **NRBCs** are usually **orthochromic normoblasts** but can represent any stage of erythroid maturation (Color Plate 9).

   (1) Their presence in the peripheral circulation is indicative of **marrow stimulation**.

   (2) NRBCs are **normally found in newborns.**

   (3) They are reported as the number of NRBCs counted per l00 WBCs.

   (4) The **diagnostic implications** of NRBCs are as follows:

       (a) **Acute hemorrhage**

       (b) **Congestive heart failure**

       (c) **Hypoxia**

       (d) **Hemolytic anemia**

       (e) **Leukemias**

       (f) **Megaloblastic anemias**

       (g) **Myelofibrosis**

    g. Pappenheimer bodies are RBC cytoplasmic inclusions measuring up to 2 μm in diameter (Color Plate 10). One to ten may be seen in a single RBC. The granules are **free iron** and stain dark violet with Wright's stain.

        (1) Particles also stain positive with an iron stain (i.e., **Prussian blue**).

        (2) The presence of Pappenheimer bodies indicates abnormal hemoglobin synthesis.

        (3) The **diagnostic implications** of Pappenheimer bodies are as follows:

            (a) Severe hemolytic anemia

            (b) Asplenia and post-splenectomy state

            (c) Sideroblastic anemia

            (d) Thalassemias

            (e) Megaloblastic anemia

    h. Rouleau formation is reported if the RBCs become aligned in aggregates resembling stacks of coins. Rouleau often is seen as an artifact in thick areas of the blood film.

        (1) Rouleau is **quantitated** in the following manner:

            (a) Slight, if 1–2 RBC chains are found per thin microscopic field

            (b) Moderate, if 3–4 RBC chains are found per thin microscopic field

            (c) Marked, if five or more RBC chains are found per thin microscopic field

        (2) The **diagnostic implication** of rouleau is often associated with **hyperproteinemia disorders such as multiple myeloma.**

Study Questions

Directions: Each of the numbered items or incomplete statements in this section is followed by answers or by completions of the statement. Select the ONE lettered answer or completion that is BEST in each case.

1. The red cell distribution width (RDW) is a parameter that measures

a. variation in white blood cell (WBC) size and morphologic type
b. variation in red blood cell (RBC) shape and provides an index for poikilocytosis
c. mean cell volume (MCV) of red cells
d. variation of RBC size and provides an index of anisocytosis

2. When the heme ring is broken down in the macrophage, the iron is either returned to the erythroid marrow by transferrin or stored in the macrophage as which one of the following?

a. haptoglobin
b. sideroblasts
c. Howell-Jolly bodies
d. ferritin

3. Two patients each have a hemoglobin (Hb) of 10.0 g/dL and a hematocrit (HCT) of 33%. Mr. Smith's red blood cell (RBC) count is 3.0×10^6/mm^3, and Mr. Jones' RBC count is 5.0×10^6/mm^3; both have a mean corpuscular hemoglobin concentration (MCHC) of 30.3 g/dL. The RBC morphologies of these two men are best described by which one of the following statements?

a. both individuals are normocytic, normochromic
b. both individuals are macrocytic, normochromic
c. Mr. Smith's RBCs are microcytic, normochromic; Mr. Jones' RBCs are macrocytic, normochromic
d. Mr. Smith's RBCs are macrocytic, hypochromic; Mr. Jones' RBCs are microcytic, hypochromic

4. An electrical impedance cell counter gave a histogram report on a patient with R1 signal flags printed by relative and absolute white blood cell (WBC) differential results. The meaning and most likely cause of these results is

a. a dual population of red blood cell (RBC) sizes in the patient's blood
b. excess interference in the valley left of the lymphocyte peak (< 35 fL) caused by the presence of sickled RBCs, many nucleated red blood cells (NRBCs), or clumped or giant platelets
c. excessive overlap of cell populations at the mononuclear/granulocyte boundary (approximately 160 fL) caused by an increased presence of more immature granulocytes
d. a substantially increased WBC count

5. To perform its function in the circulation and to survive 120 days, a red blood cell (RBC) requires a membrane that has a high

a. lipid-to-protein ratio
b. impermeability
c. rigidity
d. pliability (deformability)

6. The small, round red blood cell (RBC) inclusions that appear basophilic (dark blue or violet) with Wright's stain are nuclear remnants whose numbers increase following splenectomy. These inclusions are called

a. Howell-Jolly bodies
b. Döhle's bodies
c. Heinz bodies
d. vacuoles

7. Poikilocytosis refers to which one of the following characteristics?

a. color of red blood cells (RBCs)
b. size of RBCs
c. shape of RBCs
d. an increased number of normoblasts

8. The red cell precursor from which the nucleus is extruded is the

a. rubriblast
b. orthochromic normoblast
c. basophilic normoblast
d. polychromatic normoblast

9. The majority of hemoglobin (Hb) is synthesized in the _____, where the heme moiety is produced in the cytoplasm in the _____ of the cell, and the globin chains are produced on the _____ of the cell.

a. reticulocyte, ribosomes, membrane
b. macrophage, cytoplasm, mitochondria
c. pronormoblast, nucleus, ribosomes
d. normoblast, mitochondria, ribosomes

10. An acute increase in intravascular hemolysis results in an increase in which one of the following aspects of plasma?

a. haptoglobin
b. indirect bilirubin
c. hemopexin
d. conjugated bilirubin

11. A patient was admitted to the hospital with a suspected anemia. A CBC was performed, and the following values were reported:

RBC $3.00 \times 10^6/mm^3$
Hb   9.5 g/dL
HCT   27%
RET CT   13.4%

If, due to the anemia, the reticulocyte maturation time in the circulation is now twice as long, what is this patient's absolute reticulocyte count and reticulocyte production index (RPI)?

a. 100,000/mm³; normal reticulocytes/d
b. 1,000,000/mm³; 2x reticulocytes/d
c. 50,600/mm³; 0.5x reticulocytes/d
d. 404,000/mm³; 4x reticulocytes/d

12. The Embden-Myerhof (EM) pathway is a vital metabolism pathway in red blood cell (RBC) metabolism. Which one of the following statements about this pathway is correct?

a. this pathway handles 25% of RBC energy production
b. this pathway produces transferrin, which is needed to maintain iron in its ferrous form
c. this pathway is fueled by free fatty acids
d. this pathway has an essential role in maintaining reduced nicotinamide adenine dinucleotide (NADH) and nicotinamide-adenine dinucleotide phosphate (NADPH) in a reduced state to support the conversion of methemoglobin back to oxyhemoglobin

13. A lymph node is structurally divided into

a. a cortex containing nodules of stem cells
b. a paracortex rich in macrophages, B lymphocytes, and T lymphocytes in transit
c. follicles, each containing a germinal center of macrophages
d. a medulla arranged with nests of developing erythroid precursors

14. The flow cytometer generally counts white blood cells (WBCs) based on which one of the following principles?

a. WBCs can be stained for myeloperoxidase (MPO) activity and differentiated based on the fact that different types of WBCs have a variable amount of MPO activity and staining intensity
b. WBCs are poor conductors of electrical current and will cause a voltage pulse when passing through an aperture
c. different WBCs carry a different overall electrical charge, and the overall charge of each cell is measured and differentiated as each cell passes through the flow cell
d. a histogram can be generated separately, each for different WBC populations based on cell size or volume

15. The general clinical effects of splenomegaly include which one of the following?

a. a hypocellular bone marrow
b. increase in circulatory blood volume
c. anemia, thrombocytopenia, and granulocytopenia
d. an increase in the platelet count

Directions: Each of the numbered items or incomplete statements in this section is negatively phrased, as indicated by a capitalized word such as NOT, LEAST, or EXCEPT. Select the ONE lettered answer or completion that is BEST in each case.

16. By-products of heme catabolism include all of the following EXCEPT

a. carbon monoxide (CO)
b. haptoglobin
c. bilirubin
d. hemosiderin

17. All of the following statements regarding iron metabolism are correct EXCEPT

a. two thirds of the body's iron is found in normoblasts and red blood cells (RBCs)
b. the ferrous (Fe^{2+}) form is the active oxygen-binding valance
c. the majority of iron used in heme synthesis is recycled from degraded hemoglobin (Hb) from intravascular and extravascular hemolysis pathways
d. iron is stored in basophils as hemosiderin

18. In erythropoiesis, unipotential stem cell differentiation proceeds into a maturation series of several recognizable and distinct nucleated erythroid precursors, which are represented by all of the following EXCEPT

a. polychromatic normoblast
b. basophilic normoblast
c. reticulocyte
d. orthochromic normoblast

19. Common techniques for examining a bone marrow aspirate include all of the following EXCEPT

a. a Wright's-stained direct film to obtain a platelet estimate
b. a Wright's-stained crush preparation
c. a Prussian blue stain of a direct marrow film for sideroblasts and iron storage
d. a Wright's-stained marrow imprint

20. In the blood, carbon dioxide (CO_2) is carried from the tissues to the lungs in all of the following forms EXCEPT

a. carbamino-CO_2
b. bicarbonate (HCO_3^-)
c. dissolved in plasma
d. as carbon monoxide (CO)

Answers and Explanations

1. The answer is d [I A 1 j]. The red cell distribution width (RDW) provides an estimate of red cell size variation, or anisocytosis. It represents a coefficient of variation of the area under the red blood cell (RBC) histogram curve. The wider the spread of the RBC histogram curve, the greater the RDW value.

2. The answer is d [IV A 8 a]. The average life span of the red blood cell (RBC) is approximately 120 days. Billions of RBCs each day are broken down in the macrophages of the reticuloendothelial system (i.e., spleen and liver), and the materials are recycled. One of the most vital materials stored or recycled is hemoglobin iron. The majority of recycled iron is bound to its carrier protein—transferrin—and taken to the marrow to be transferred to maturing erythroid precursors. Iron not readily needed by marrow erythroid maturation is stored in the form of ferritin in spleen, liver, and marrow macrophages. Haptoglobin binds heme dimers in hemolysis, and Howell-Jolly bodies are intracellular deoxyribonucleic acid (DNA) inclusions in RBCs.

3. The answer is d [I A 2 b (5)(a)]. The values of hematocrit (HCT), red blood cell (RBC) count, and mean corpuscular hemoglobin concentration (MCHC) are provided for both patients. A mean corpuscular volume (MCV) must be calculated to obtain the necessary information. The formula for MCV can be derived from the formula for HCT.

$$HCT\% = [RBC \times MCV] \div 10$$

Solving for MCV,

$$MCV = [HCT\% \div RBC] \times 10$$

Therefore, for Mr. Smith,

$$MCV = [33 \div 3.00] \times 10$$
$$MCV = 110$$

And, for Mr. Jones,

$$MCV = [33 \div 5.00] \times 10$$
$$MCV = 66$$

The MCHC is lower than 32 g/dL, therefore, both patients are hypochromic. Based on their calculated MCV values, Mr. Smith is macrocytic, and Mr. Jones is microcytic.

4. The answer is b [I B 1 c (2)]. Region 1 (R1) signal flags are associated with the white blood cell (WBC) histogram curves only. The region flags refer to abnormal size distribution between populations of WBCs. They have nothing to do with cell numbers. A region 2 (R2) flag indicates overlap in cellular distribution between the lymphocyte and monocyte regions. A region 3 (R3) signal flag indicates overlap between the monocyte and granulocyte peaks. A region 4 (R4) signal flag indicates an excessive granulocyte population and extension of the curve to the right.

5. The answer is d [IV C 1]. The life span of a red blood cell (RBC) depends on the relationship between the RBC membrane and metabolism. The main mission of an RBC is to carry oxygen and carbon dioxide (CO_2) to and from the tissues. With cell aging, enzymatic failure leads to the loss of pliability and splenic destruction.

6. The answer is a [IV G 4 e]. Howell-Jolly bodies are dark violet-staining red blood cell (RBC) inclusions that consist of deoxyribonucleic acid (DNA) remnants averaging 1 μm in diameter. They are most commonly seen in the blood of splenectomized individuals or persons with hemoglobinopathies or severe hemolysis. Heinz bodies are the result of hemoglobin (Hb) precipitation and are demonstrated with a crystal violet stain. Vacuoles and Döhle's bodies are white blood cell (WBC) cytoplasmic inclusions.

7. The answer is c [IV G 3 a]. Poikilocytosis describes a variation in shape and is usually quantitated as 1+, 2+, 3+, or 4+. There must be a variation in shape of more than 10% of the red blood cells (RBCs) for a grading of 1+.

8. The answer is b [IV A 6; Table 3-2]. The rubriblast (i.e., pronormoblast) is the first morphologically recognizable stage, followed by the basophilic normoblast, then the polychromatic normoblast. The final stage of maturation to have a nucleus is the orthochromic normoblast. The condensed nucleus is extruded from the orthochromic normoblast and becomes a reticulocyte.

9. The answer is d [III A 1, B 1]. Hemoglobin (Hb) is synthesized in the cytoplasm of all stages of developing normoblasts and continues up to the early reticulocyte stage. Heme rings and globin chains are synthesized at separate locations in the cytoplasm. Heme rings are produced on the mitochondria of normoblasts, and globin chains are manufactured on cytoplasmic ribosomes.

10. The answer is b [IV E 3 d]. The opened tetrapyrrole, known as bilirubin, is carried in the unconjugated form to the liver. The unconjugated form is measured as the indirect bilirubin. Bilirubin is conjugated in the liver to be excreted via the bile duct. The conjugated form is measured as the direct bilirubin. Haptoglobin and hemopexin are binding proteins for heme-ring fragments and decrease in the plasma with hemolysis.

11. The answer is d [IV F 5 c(3),(5)]. The absolute reticulocyte count represents the actual number of reticulocytes found in the peripheral blood, and it can be calculated by multiplying the patient's red blood cell (RBC) count (in millions) by their reticulocyte count (in decimal form). This patient's absolute reticulocyte count can be calculated as shown:

$$0.134 \times 3.00 \times 10^6/mm^3 = 402,000/mm^3$$

To derive the reticulocyte production index (RPI), the reticulocyte index (RI) must first be calculated as follows:

RI = 13.4% × [27% (patient's HCT) ÷ 45% (normal HCT)]
RI = 8.04%

Once the RI has been calculated, the patient's RPI can be obtained with the following formula:

RPI = patient's RI ÷ maturation time (from Table 3-3)

Therefore,

RPI = 8.04 ÷ 2.0 = 4 times as many reticulocytes per day

12. The answer is d [IV D 3 a]. The Embden-Myerhof (EM) pathway is an anaerobic metabolic pathway that handles 90% of red blood cell (RBC) glucose utilization. The net production of this pathway is 2 adenosine triphosphate (ATP) molecules per 1 molecule of glucose. ATP is necessary for RBC survival because ATP maintains cell shape and flexibility, fuels the membrane's metabolic pumps, and preserves membrane lipids. This pathway also plays an essential role in maintaining pyridine nucleotides [i.e., reduced nicotinamide adenine dinucleotide phosphate (NADPH) and reduced nicotinamide adenine dinucleotide (NADH)] in a reduced state to support the recycling of methemoglobin back to oxyhemoglobin.

13. The answer is b [II C 3 b]. The lymph node is structurally divided into a cortex, or outside layer, which contains rows of lymphocyte follicles. Each follicle contains a germinal center rich in macrophages and B lymphocytes. The germinal center is surrounded by a high concentration of T lymphocytes. The paracortex, the area between the cortex and medulla, is rich in a mixed arrangement of macrophages, B lymphocytes, and T lymphocytes in transit into the medulla of the node. The medulla, or center of the node, is arranged in parallel cords of small lymphocytes and plasma cells.

14. The answer is a [I D 2]. Flow cytometry is generally based on the principle of separating cells into counting channels, or flow chambers. Red blood cells (RBCs) and their properties are counted and evaluated in an RBC channel based on the principle of laser light scatter. White blood cells (WBCs) are counted and analyzed in a myeloperoxidase channel. Leukocytes are first cytochemically stained with the enzyme myeloperoxidase. Laser scatter patterns are then analyzed for frequency, size, and staining characteristics through narrow and wide-angle light scatter. A scattergram is generated to depict results.

15. The answer is c [II B 4 b]. Splenomegaly results in vascular congestion and portal hypertension. Red blood cells (RBCs), granulocytes, and up to 90% of circulating platelets may be trapped. This can result in anemia, leukocytopenia, and thrombocytopenia. A hypercellular marrow results as a response to a chronic pancytopenia.

16. The answer is b [IV E 3]. Carbon monoxide (CO), bilirubin, and hemosiderin are all by-products of heme-ring catabolism. CO is split off when the heme tetrapyrrole ring is broken down. The opened tetrapyrrole is known as bilirubin. Iron is released from the heme group and stored within reticuloendothelial macrophages as ferritin or hemosiderin. Haptoglobin is not a by-product of heme catabolism, but is the heme dimer-binding protein produced in the liver.

17. The answer is d [III B 3 a; IV A 8 a, E 3 b]. Iron is stored in monocytes and macrophages but not in basophils.

18. The answer is c [IV A; Table 3-2]. The pronormoblast, basophilic normoblast, polychromatic normoblast, and orthochromic normoblast are all nucleated stages of erythroid maturation. When the orthochromic normoblast extrudes its nucleus, it becomes a reticulocyte. The reticulocyte is the first erythroid stage without a nucleus. Reticulocytes then mature into red blood cells (RBCs).

19. The answer is a [II D 3 b, c]. A marrow aspirate or biopsy can be stained with a variety of stains. Marrow films, direct films, marrow imprints, and crush preparations are stained with Wright's stain. The previous preparations can also be stained for iron using Prussian blue stain. Biopsy specimens can be stained with histologic stains for analysis. Slide platelet estimates are performed only on peripheral blood smears stained with Wright's stain.

20. The answer is d [III E; IV E 3 d]. Carbon dioxide (CO_2) is the by-product of cellular metabolism. CO_2 must be eliminated from the body to allow reoxygenation of hemoglobin (Hb). This metabolite is transported to the lungs for expiration in three forms. The majority (90%) is converted to bicarbonate and hydrogen ions to buffer blood pH. Small amounts are bound to protein groups (e.g., carbamino-CO_2) or are physically dissolved in plasma. CO_2 is never converted to carbon monoxide (CO) in the blood, because this metabolite is toxic. The only intracellular source of CO is from the catabolism of heme rings into bilirubin.

4

Hematologic Disorders

Joel Hubbard

I. **RED BLOOD CELL INDICES AND THEIR USE IN THE DIAGNOSIS OF ANEMIA**

A. **Red blood cell (RBC) indices,** known as **corpuscular constants,** are provided by the majority of automated cell counters. Indices can also be calculated individually from the RBC count, hemoglobin (Hb), and hematocrit (Hct) values.

B. **These parameters are useful in the diagnosis, classification, and differentiation of anemias,** as seen in Table 4-1. They can also provide useful guidelines in accessing blood smear RBC morphology.

C. **Individual corpuscular constants** include the mean cell volume (MCV), mean corpuscular hemoglobin (MCH), and mean corpuscular hemoglobin concentration (MCHC).

1. **MCV** is defined as the mean or average size (in cubic microns) of the individual erythrocyte.

a. The MCV may be calculated from the volume and number of erythrocytes in a given quantity of blood (Box 4-1). **The formula for calculation is as follows:**

$$\frac{Hct\% \times 10}{RBCs \times 10^6/mm^3} = mcv\ fL$$

b. **The normal MCV** for an adult is **80–100 fL.**

(1) If the cells are larger than normal, the MCV is increased, and the condition is called **macrocytosis.** If the condition is associated with an anemia, it is called a **macrocytic anemia.**

(2) If the cells are smaller than normal, the MCV is decreased, and the condition is called **microcytosis** (or **microcytic anemia** if associated with anemia).

2. **MCH** is the mean or average amount of Hb by weight per cell, expressed in micromicrograms ($\mu\mu g$) or picograms (pg).

a. **Calculation.** The MCH may be calculated from the **Hb and the Hct values**

159

Table 4-1. Morphologic Classification of Anemia and RBC Morphology by Indices Range

RBC Morphology	MCV (fL)	MCH (pg)	MCHC (%)	Anemias
Normocytic/normochromic	80–100*	27–31*	32–36*	Acute blood loss Hemolytic anemias Aplastic anemia (early stage) Myelophthisic anemia Stem cell–related anemias
Macrocytic/normochromic	High	High	Normal	Megaloblastic anemia Anemia of liver disease Chronic aplastic anemia Acute hemolytic anemia (with shift reticulocytosis)
Microcytic/normochromic	Low	Normal	Normal	Anemia of chronic inflammation
Microcytic/hypochromic	Low	Low	Low	Iron deficiency anemia Thalassemia Lead poisoning Porphyrias Sideroblastic anemia

MCH = mean corpuscular hemoglobin; MCHC = mean corpuscular hemoglobin concentration; MCV = mean cell volume; RBC = red blood cell.
*Indices shown as normal range.

(Box 4-2). The formula for calculation is as follows:

$$\frac{\text{Hb g/dL} \times 10}{\text{RBCs} \times 10^6/\text{mm}^3} = \text{MCH (pg)}$$

    b. **The normal MCH** for the adult is **29 +/− 2 pg.**

        (1) In macrocytic erythrocytes, the amount of Hb may be greater than normal. The increase in Hb parallels the increase in cell size.

        (2) The RBC is never supersaturated with Hb. **There is no such thing as a hyperchromic RBC.**

  3. MCHC is the mean or average Hb concentration (in grams) per 100 mL of packed erythrocytes.

    a. **Calculation.** The MCHC is calculated by dividing the Hb in grams per 100 mL (g/dL) of blood by the volume of packed erythrocytes per 100 mL of blood and multiplying by 100 (Box 4-3). The formula for calculation is as

Box 4-1. Calculation of Mean Cell Volume (MCV)

EXAMPLE:

Calculating the MCV of a patient with an RBC count of $5.0 \times 10^6/\text{mm}^3$ and a Hct of 45%:

$$\text{MCV} = \frac{45 \times 10}{5.0} = 90 \text{ fL}$$

Box 4-2. Calculation of Mean Corpuscular Hemoglobin (MCH)

EXAMPLE:

Calculating the MCH for a patient who has a Hb of 15 g/dL and an RBC count of $5.0 \times 10^6/mm^3$:

$$MCH = \frac{15 \times 10}{5.0} = 30 \, pg$$

follows:

$$\frac{Hb \, g/dL}{Hct \, \%} \times 100 = MCHC \, g/dL$$

    b. Normal range for adults is **34 +/− 2%.** RBCs in which the MCHC is found decreased are termed **hypochromic.** The only pathologic condition in which the MCHC may be increased is **spherocytic anemia.** The MCHC also increases in the presence of cold agglutinins and agglutinated RBCs.

II. RED BLOOD CELL (RBC) DISORDERS can be classified as either **polycythemias** or **anemias.** Polycythemias are disorders that have an increase in circulating RBCs, and therefore, an increased Hct. Anemias are disorders that have a decrease in circulating RBCs; therefore, these disorders have a decreased Hct.

    A. Polycythemias are characterized by an **increase in Hct** greater than 53% in men and 51% in women.

        1. Clinical symptoms are caused by hypervolemia or hyperviscosity.

            a. Hyperviscosity can cause sluggish flow of blood and a tendency toward **thrombosis and disseminated intravascular coagulation (DIC).**

                (1) The **decreased oxygen flow to tissues** is compensated for by the higher Hct and increased blood volume (i.e., hypervolemia), which increases vessel diameter and therefore results in increased tissue perfusion.

                (2) This is not a benefit, however, because cardiac work is increased to deliver the same amount of oxygen as normal.

            b. Hypervolemia increases blood-vessel diameter and therefore results in increased tissue perfusion. This can cause increased cardiac work, which is dangerous for an individual who is predisposed to heart problems.

        2. Types of polycythemia include relative and absolute. Absolute polycythemia must be differentiated from relative polycythemia before treatment can ensue.

            a. Relative polycythemia refers to a condition in which the total RBC mass is normal but the Hct is elevated because the plasma volume is decreased.

Box 4-3. Calculation of Mean Corpuscular Hemoglobin Concentration

EXAMPLE:

Calculating the MCHC of a patient who has a Hb of 15 g/dL and a Hct of 45%:

$$MCHC = \frac{15 \times 100}{45} = 33 \, g/dL$$

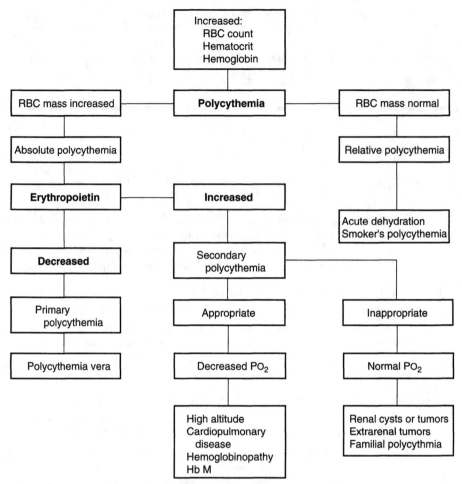

Figure 4-1. Algorithm for the differential diagnosis of the polycythemias. P_{O_2} = pressure of oxygen; RBC = red blood cell.

(1) Relative polycythemia can be **caused by acute dehydration** resulting from severe diarrhea, burns, or chronic diuretic therapy.

(2) Spurious (false) polycythemia is related to chronic **smoking.** Nicotine induces a loss of plasma volume.

b. **Absolute polycythemia** refers to an increase in the total RBC mass in the body. This is a true erythrocytosis caused by marrow erythroid hyperplasia or, secondarily, by an increase in erythropoietin (EPO), as illustrated in Figure 4-1.

B. **Anemias** are characterized by a **reduced Hb concentration** of less than 12 g/dL in men and 11 g/dL in women.

1. Clinical symptoms are caused by a **decreased oxygen-carrying capacity of the blood and tissue hypoxia.**

2. The **physiologic effects** of anemia include the following:

a. **A decreased Hb oxygen-affinity state** results in a right shift of the oxygen dissociation curve.

  b. Decreased tissue perfusion in select areas of the body is caused by redistribution of blood flow favoring the more oxygen-dependent tissues, such as the brain and myocardium.

  c. Increased cardiac output results in anemic patients to maintain adequate tissue oxygen tension.

  d. Increased RBC production by the marrow results from an increase in EPO release from the kidneys because of a decrease in oxygen tension.

   (1) A compensatory increase in marrow erythropoietic cellularity occurs 4–5 days following a decrease in Hb values.

   (2) Erythroid hyperplasia in the marrow results in increased reticulocyte count and nucleated red blood cells (NRBCs) in the circulation.

 3. Types of anemias

  a. Absolute anemias result from either impaired RBC production, blood loss, or accelerated RBC destruction **(hemolysis).**

   (1) Physiologic causes include:

    (a) Stem cell disorders

    (b) DNA disorders

    (c) Heme and globin disorders

    (d) RBC survival disorders (i.e., hemolytic disorders)

   (2) Morphologic classifications (see Table 4-1) include the following (see Chapter 3):

    (a) Macrocytic

    (b) Microcytic

    (c) Normocytic

  b. Relative anemia can result from an increase in plasma volume rather than a decrease in the number of RBCs.

   (1) A dilutional anemia can occur by the **third trimester of pregnancy.**

   (2) Macroglobulinemia and multiple myeloma are associated with an increase in plasma globulin and protein concentration. This increase in plasma protein causes a hyperosmotic plasma, and a dilutional anemia is caused by a compensatory increase in plasma volume.

III. STEM CELL DISORDERS are a group of RBC disorders that result from an **imbalance in marrow multipotential or unipotential stem cell production** and maturation. The imbalance is seen as either an increase in cellular production (i.e., polycythemia) or a decrease in cellular production, which results in an anemia.

 A. Polycythemias (see Figure 4-1)

  1. Primary absolute polycythemia is characterized by **pancytosis or pancytopenia** (i.e., all cell lines either increased or decreased). Initially, proliferation of erythroid, myeloid, and megakaryocytic bone marrow elements is uncontrolled. **Polycythemia vera** is a clonal disorder that results in **failure of the multipotential stem cell.**

  a. Laboratory characteristics of polycythemia vera include:

   (1) Increased RBC count and Hct

   (2) Increased bone marrow erythroid iron stores, which trap and deplete tissue iron stores

   (3) Decreased to absent EPO levels

(4) **Increased white blood cell (WBC)** count, which is reflected by an **increase in levels of serum and urine muramidase** and **serum vitamin B$_{12}$** and vitamin B$_{12}$ binding proteins

(5) **Thrombocytosis**

b. Patients who have polycythemia vera are commonly observed to have the **clinical characteristics** of splenomegaly and spontaneous hemorrhaging due to thrombosis and hyperviscosity.

c. **Treatments** for polycythemia vera include the following:

(1) **Therapeutic phlebotomy** is used to reduce the growing RBC volume. Therapeutic phlebotomy, however, further depletes tissue iron stores and can result in **an iron-deficient (i.e., microcytic/hypochromic) erythrocytosis.**

(2) **Splenectomy** is used to relieve symptoms caused by splenomegaly and blood pooling.

(3) **Chemotherapy** is used to treat patients who have advanced disease to kill rapidly growing malignant stem cells.

d. Polycythemia vera can evolve into **myelofibrosis** or a **myeloid metaplasia** following chemotherapeutic treatment. Between 10% and 15% of patients progress to **acute myelogenous leukemia.**

2. **Secondary absolute polycythemia** has a **normal WBC and platelet count** and can be classified as:

a. Polycythemia caused by **appropriate EPO production**

b. Polycythemia caused by **inappropriate EPO production**

c. **Familial polycythemia,** which is seen in children who have functionally normal Hb, Hb-oxygen saturation, and cardiopulmonary dysfunction

(1) These children have high EPO levels unrelated to Hb concentration.

(2) The uncontrolled EPO production is most likely caused by a **defect in the regulation of EPO production.**

(3) Another variation of this genetic disorder is an **inherited deficiency of 2,3-diphosphoglycerate phosphatase activities,** which results in polycythemia.

B. **Anemias** (Figure 4-2) caused by a **defect in stem cell erythropoiesis** most commonly result from a depression of colony-forming units-erythroid (CFU-E) and burst-forming units-erythroid (BFU-E) unipotential stem cell maturation and differentiation.

1. **Anemia of chronic disorders** is usually a mild form of anemia occurring secondary to a **chronic inflammatory disorder** such as an infection, rheumatoid arthritis (RA), or neoplastic diseases.

a. **RBC production** by the marrow is **normal but insufficient** to compensate for a decreased RBC survival.

b. The marrow CFU-E is capable of responding to EPO, **but EPO production is low.**

c. This anemia is partially caused by a **defect in iron metabolism** that results from a block in the secondary iron storage system.

(1) Monocytes and macrophages have a reduced ability to move stored intracellular iron to the erythroid marrow cells.

Confirm with RBC indices

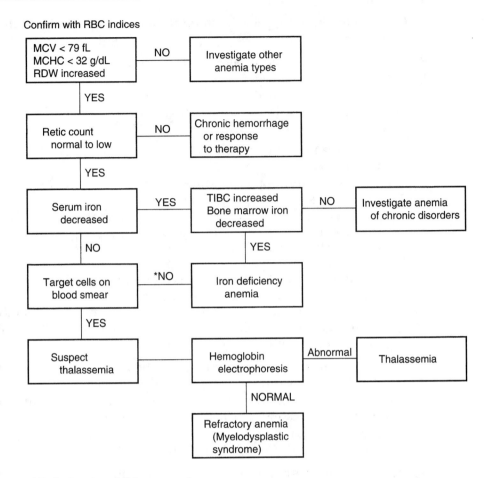

* Early stage iron deficiency anemia

Figure 4-2. Algorithm for the differential diagnosis of iron deficiency anemia from other microcytic/hypochromic anemias. MCHC = mean corpuscular hemoglobin concentration; MCV = mean cell volume; RBC = red blood cell; RDW = red cell distribution width; TIBC = total iron-binding capacity.

    (2) This recycling block results in a **low serum iron** level and an **increase in the storage iron in tissue macrophages.**

    (3) Systemic inflammation results in the release of **interleukin-1** from macrophages, which blocks macrophage iron release. This decreases the reutilization of recycled iron that is released from heme catabolism.

  d. Laboratory characteristics of anemia of chronic disorders include the following:

    (1) Typically normocytic/normochromic RBCs that can be microcytic/hypochromic in some cases

    (2) Slight anisocytosis and poikilocytosis

    (3) **Normal reticulocyte count**

    (4) Unaltered WBC and platelet counts, except alterations resulting from the causative disease

    (5) **Marrow is normocellular,** but sideroblasts are decreased

(6) **Serum iron is decreased, and total iron binding capacity (TIBC) is normal or decreased**

2. An **anemia of renal insufficiency** occurs in patients who have end-stage renal disease.

   a. There is a general correlation between the severity of the anemia and the degree of elevation of the blood urea nitrogen (BUN). When BUN is greater than 100 mg/dL, the Hct is usually lower than 30%.

   b. The primary **cause** of the anemia is a **decreased production of EPO by the damaged kidney.**

   (1) **Ineffective erythropoiesis** also results because of an impaired ability of the CFU-E to respond to EPO.

   (2) **RBC survival is also decreased** because of hemolysis that results from the **damaging effects of uremic plasma.**

   (a) Hemolysis caused by uremia results in the formation of **burr cells.**

   (b) **Burr cells and RBC fragments** are seen in the blood of a patient who has hemolytic-uremic syndrome.

   (c) Increased blood urea levels also **affect the functional ability of platelets.** Bleeding is a common problem that further amplifies the anemia.

3. **Anemia of liver disease** is characterized by **shortened RBC survival** and **inadequate RBC production** that occurs secondary to a chronic liver disease.

   a. RBC morphology is usually **macrocytic** or normocytic, with **target cells or acanthocytes** caused by increased surface membrane cholesterol.

   (1) These abnormal RBCs are removed at a higher rate by the spleen.

   (2) Their survival is reduced when compared with normal RBCs.

   b. The patient often has an accompanying splenomegaly with cirrhosis, which further decreases RBC survival.

   c. The **reticulocyte count is increased slightly,** and the **platelet count is normal or decreased.**

   d. A differential diagnosis must distinguish this anemia from other macrocytic anemias. Patients who have anemia of liver disease usually have a **normal WBC count and serum vitamin B_{12} and folate levels;** patients who have megaloblastic anemias do not.

4. **Anemias of endocrine disease** can occur with hypothyroidism and androgen-deficient states.

   a. Anemia of **hypothyroidism** involves a mild-to-moderate anemia with a normal reticulocyte count.

   (1) Thyroid hormone regulates the cellular metabolic rate, and therefore, the tissue oxygen requirement.

   (2) With a decrease in thyroid hormone (i.e., hypothyroidism), there is a smaller tissue oxygen requirement, which is interpreted by the kidneys as a more than adequate oxygen tension. The net result is a **decrease in the production of EPO.**

   (3) This type of anemia often is a macrocytic/normochromic anemia but can also be a normocytic/normochromic anemia.

        (4) The anemia may be complicated by iron deficiency or folic acid or vitamin B_{12} deficiency, and the laboratory results may reflect these forms of anemia.

   b. A **deficiency in testosterone secretion** in men results in a decrease in RBC production and a decline of approximately 2 g/dL of Hb.

5. Myelophthisic anemia is an anemia associated with bone marrow infiltration and hyperproliferation by nonerythroid cells.

   a. A **leukoerythroblastic reaction** commonly accompanies the anemia.

        (1) Normoblasts of varying degrees of maturation are typically found on the blood smear with a **reticulocytosis.**

        (2) Increased leukocytes along with their immature forms are also found on the peripheral blood smear.

        (3) RBC morphology is normocytic/normochromic but can be macrocytic.

        (4) Platelets are normal or decreased and often have abnormal forms.

   b. The usual **causes of myelophthisic anemia** include:

        (1) Metastatic carcinoma

        (2) Multiple myeloma

        (3) Leukemia

        (4) Lymphoma

        (5) Lipidoses or storage disease

6. Aplastic anemia is a marrow disorder characterized by a **reduction in the number or function of multipotential stem cells,** with a resulting pancytopenia. This disorder is more commonly found in adults.

   a. The marrow is hypocellular, with patchy areas of normal cellularity and **increased fat cell infiltration.**

   b. The **diagnosis** of severe aplastic anemia is made in pancytopenic patients when at least **two of the following three peripheral blood values** are found:

        (1) A WBC count lower than 500 cells/mm^3

        (2) A platelet count lower than 20,000/mm^3

        (3) A reticulocyte count lower than 1%

   c. Aplastic anemia can be **acute** and rapidly fatal, or it can have a slow onset and a **chronic** course.

   d. Most patients are initially seen with the following common **clinical characteristics:**

        (1) Bleeding as a result of thrombocytopenia

        (2) Increased susceptibility to infections due to leukopenia

        (3) All of the symptoms typical of anemia

        (4) The absence of splenomegaly

        (5) Iron overload from repeated transfusions

   e. In 50% of patients, no specific agent can be correlated with the disease. **Known causes** of aplasia include:

        (1) Drugs (33%)

        (2) Chemicals or toxins (4%)

        (3) Infections and infectious hepatitis (4%)

        (4) Miscellaneous causes (59%)

f. The **pathogenesis** of aplastic anemia is thought to occur from either one or a combination of several of the following physiologic mechanisms:

(1) Defective or insufficient multipotential colony-forming unit-spleen (CFU-S) stem cell population

(2) Altered microenvironment that is unable to provide for normal differentiation and development of the stem cell compartment

(3) Absent humoral and cellular stimulators for hematopoiesis

(4) Excessive suppression of hematopoiesis by T lymphocytes or macrophages

(5) Stem cells interacting among themselves, with one clone inhibiting the growth of another

(6) Immunologic mechanisms that suppress hematopoiesis

g. **Treatment** focuses on symptoms and finding the cause of suppression. Accepted courses of treatment include:

(1) Blood transfusions

(2) Stimulation of residual marrow with androgens or adrenocorticoids

(3) Controlling infections with antibiotics

(4) Controlling bleeding problems

(5) Bone marrow transplantation for acceptable candidates younger than 40 years

(6) EPO therapy to stimulate residual bone marrow

h. **Laboratory values** for a patient who has aplastic anemia include the following:

(1) RBC morphology is normocytic/normochromic but often is **macrocytic, with a normal red cell distribution width (RDW)**

(2) Slight anisocytosis and poikilocytosis

(3) **Absence of circulating normoblasts** in light of the degree of the anemia

(4) An absolute **leukopenia** with a relative lymphocytosis

(5) **Thrombocytopenia**

(6) Elevated levels of leukocyte alkaline phosphatase (LAP)

(7) Decreased marrow iron stores

(8) **High serum iron concentration**

(9) **Very high plasma and urine EPO levels**

i. **Toxins.** Aplastic anemia is often associated with toxic chemical or physical agents.

(1) **Toxic aplastic anemias** are known to occur after exposure to mustard compounds; benzene; chemotherapy drugs (e.g., busulfan, urethan); antimetabolite drugs; or ionizing radiation.

(2) **Hypersensitive aplastic anemia** has been known to occur following treatment with certain classes of therapeutic drugs or chemicals that cause an **autoimmune suppression** of the bone marrow.

(a) This effect has been noted with drugs such as antibiotics, anticonvulsants, analgesics, antithyroid drugs, antihistamines, and insecticides.

(b) **Chloramphenicol** is the most common cause of drug-induced aplasia. Up to 50% of patients who receive this drug on a long-term basis will have a resulting mild pancytopenia that is reversible with drug withdrawal.

  j. Aplastic anemia can occur **secondary to other diseases** or conditions, such as:
   (1) **Infection,** most often occurring as a sequela to **infectious hepatitis**
   (2) **Paroxysmal nocturnal hemoglobinuria (PNH)**
   (3) Pregnancy (usually remits after delivery)

  k. **Aplastic anemia (Fanconi's anemia)** refers to individuals with a **genetic predisposition to bone marrow failure.**
   (1) Detection occurs between the ages of 1 and 8 years.
   (2) Often, several family members are affected.
   (3) There is a high incidence of developmental abnormalities, which include some of the following symptoms:
     (a) Hyperpigmentation
     (b) Short stature
     (c) Hypogonadism
     (d) Malformation of the fingers and toes
     (e) Malformation of the organs
     (f) Abnormalities of the chromosome pattern of lymphocytes and marrow cells

7. **Pure red cell aplasia** is an unusual disease characterized by the **selective depletion of only the erythroid bone marrow tissue.**
  a. The disorder is **a unipotential (CFU-E) stem cell defect** that is believed to be **related to an immunologic dysfunction.**
  b. Transitory arrest of erythropoiesis may occur in the course of a **hemolytic anemia that is preceded by an infection.**
  c. **Congenital RBC aplasia (Blackfan-Diamond anemia)** is a rare disorder diagnosed between the ages of 1 and 6 years.
   (1) **CFU-E and colony-forming burst (CFU-B) stem cells are decreased.**
   (2) Patients have a severe normocytic or slightly macrocytic anemia and a **low reticulocyte count.**
   (3) Leukocytes and platelets are usually normal in numbers.
   (4) The marrow shows a reduction in all developing erythroid cells, except pronormoblasts.
   (5) **Hemoglobin F (HbF) is elevated as high as 5%–25%.**
   (6) The **RBC fetal antigen is present.**
  d. **Acquired pure red cell aplasia** is rare but occurs more **in adults** than in children.
   (1) **Typical laboratory findings** include a decreased reticulocyte count and marrow erythroid precursor depletion.
   (2) Up to **50%** of patients have an associated cancer of the thymus (i.e., **thymoma**).
   (3) Remission of the anemia after surgical removal of the thymus occurs in 25% of patients.
   (4) Acquired red cell aplasia is thought to occur through the production

of a **cytotoxic autoantibody against erythroid precursors and a plasma inhibitor of heme synthesis.**

8. **Refractory anemia** is an ill-defined group of chronic anemias occurring **in persons older than 50 years.**

   a. **Laboratory features** commonly include a normocytic or macrocytic anemia, **decreased reticulocyte count, pancytopenia, and a hypercellular marrow with erythroid hypoplasia.**

   b. Refractory anemia is now classified with the myeloproliferative disorders as one of five **myelodysplastic syndromes.**

   c. The anemia can **develop into an acute leukemia** with the presence of blast cells in the peripheral circulation.

C. **Heme disorders** represent a group of anemias that result from a defect in the synthesis of the heme ring in the mitochondria of developing normoblasts (Figure 4-3).

1. **General considerations**

   a. Disorders of heme synthesis result in a **microcytic/hypochromic** anemia.

      (1) Microcytosis is accompanied by an MCV lower than 80 fL (normal = 80–100 fL).

      (2) Hypochromia is accompanied by an **MCH less than 25 pg** (normal = 27–33 pg) and by an MCHC less than 32 g/dL (normal = 32–36 g/dL).

   b. Heme disorders can be **caused by** either enzyme deficiencies in the heme biosynthetic pathway (i.e., **porphyrias**), or by **iron-related disorders.**

2. **Porphyrias are a group of inherited or acquired disorders** that can occur from the deficiency of one or several biosynthetic enzymes. These disorders result in **ineffective hematopoiesis** and a **hemolytic anemia.**

   a. The **rate of biosynthesis** of the heme ring is controlled to a large extent by the reaction rate of the beginning enzyme, **δ-aminolevulinic acid (ALA) synthetase.**

      (1) The activity of this enzyme is reducible by some drugs and steroids.

      (2) The enzyme is **inhibited by negative feedback of the completed heme ring.** If the production of heme is inhibited somewhere along the pathway, there is a resultant decrease in heme rings and **an increase in the activity of ALA synthetase,** which drives the pathway up to the point of the block and results in an increase in the intermediate compounds behind the block.

   b. **Acute porphyrias** are inherited enzyme deficiencies that begin with acute hemolytic episodes.

      (1) **Acute intermittent porphyria (AIP)** is a hereditary autosomal dominant condition.

         (a) **Clinical symptoms** include:
             (i) Abdominal pain with vomiting
             (ii) Constipation
             (iii) Hypertension
             (iv) Peripheral neuritis
             (v) Behavioral changes and psychosis

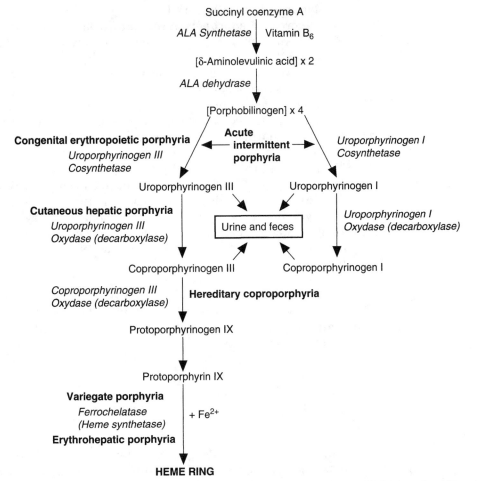

Succinyl coenzyme A

ALA Synthetase | Vitamin B$_6$

[δ-Aminolevulinic acid] x 2

ALA dehydrase

[Porphobilinogen] x 4

Congenital erythropoietic porphyria   **Acute**   *Uroporphyrinogen I*
Uroporphyrinogen III   ← intermittent →   *Cosynthetase*
Cosynthetase   **porphyria**

Uroporphyrinogen III   Uroporphyrinogen I

Cutaneous hepatic porphyria   *Uroporphyrinogen I*
Uroporphyrinogen III   Urine and feces   *Oxydase (decarboxylase)*
Oxydase (decarboxylase)

Coproporphyrinogen III   Coproporphyrinogen I

Coproporphyrinogen III   **Hereditary coproporphyria**
Oxydase (decarboxylase)

Protoporphyrinogen IX

Protoporphyrin IX

Variegate porphyria
Ferrochelatase   + Fe^{2+}
(Heme synthetase)
Erythrohepatic porphyria

HEME RING

Figure 4-3. Heme synthesis begins with succinyl coenzyme A and terminates with the insertion of iron (Fe) into protoporphyrin IX. Enzyme deficiencies in the heme-biosynthetic pathway are related to the various porphyrias (the name of the porphyria is placed by the enzyme that is deficient or dysfunctional). There is a buildup of the biosynthetic intermediates in the pathway prior to the enzyme deficiency, which results in an increase in these metabolites in the blood, feces, and urine. ALA = aminolevulinic acid.

(b) The common **laboratory profile** includes:

    (i) Slight elevations of bilirubin and alkaline phosphatase levels

    (ii) Increased urine ALA and porphobilinogen (PBG)

    (iii) Leukocytosis

(c) **Enzyme defects.** AIP is caused by **decreased levels of uroporphyrinogen I and III synthetase,** which results in increased production of ALA and PBG.

(2) **Hereditary coproporphyria** is a hereditary, autosomal dominant condition.

    (a) **Clinical symptoms.** Patients are either asymptomatic, or they are initially seen with **mild** neurologic, abdominal, or psychiatric symptoms. Patients commonly have **light-sensitive skin** because of increased levels of PBG.

      (b) The **laboratory profile** includes:

        (i) **Increased coproporphyrinogen III in feces**

        (ii) Intermittent **increases of coproporphyrinogen, ALA, and PBG in urine.**

      (c) **Enzyme defect.** Patients have a deficiency in **coproporphyrinogen decarboxylase activity.**

    (3) **Variegate porphyria** is a hereditary autosomal dominant condition that has a high incidence in the white population of South Africa.

      (a) **Clinical symptoms.** Symptoms are similar to AIP, with the additional symptom of **cutaneous lesions,** which are caused by highly photosensitive skin.

      (b) **Laboratory profile.** There are **increased levels of urinary ALA and PBG,** but there is also an increase in the levels of porphyrin precursors that occur further along the pathway.

      (c) **Enzyme defect.** Patients who have this disorder have a deficiency in **heme synthetase** (also known as **ferrochelatase deficiency**).

  c. **Chronic porphyrias** are more commonly associated with **solar photosensitivity of the skin** and include either genetic or acquired conditions.

    (1) **Congenital erythropoietic porphyria** is rare and is inherited as an autosomal recessive disorder.

      (a) **Clinical symptoms** of this disorder include:

        (i) Redness of the skin

        (ii) Hemolytic anemia

        (iii) Severe skin photosensitivity

        (iv) Splenomegaly

        (v) Often fatal early in life

      (b) **Laboratory profile.** Patients often excrete **red pigmented urine** because of **excessive excretion of coproporphyrin I and uroporphyrin I.**

      (c) **Enzyme defect.** Patients with this disorder show a deficiency in **uroporphyrinogen III cosynthetase.**

    (2) **Erythrohepatic protoporphyria** is an inherited disorder so named because the enzyme defects are localized in both the hepatic and erythropoietic cells.

      (a) **Clinical symptoms.** This porphyria is a disease of early adulthood that exhibits mild skin photosensitivity.

      (b) **Laboratory profile.** Patients who have this porphyria demonstrate an **increased level of RBC photoporphyrin and elevated levels of fecal coproporphyrinogen and photoporphyrin.**

      (c) The **enzyme defect** causing this disorder is deficient activity of **heme synthetase,** which leads to over-reactive ALA synthetase.

    (3) **Cutaneous hepatic porphyria (i.e., cutanea tarda)** is an **acquired** disorder.

      (a) **Clinical symptoms.** Patients are commonly first seen with **skin lesions** because of solar photosensitivity. Patients who have this porphyria have a medical history associated with liver disease, alcoholism, estrogen therapy, or ingestion of hexachlorobenzene.

(b) **Characteristic laboratory profile** results include an **elevated urine uroporphyrin,** with the Type I isomers being excreted in greater amounts than the Type III isomers.

(c) **Enzyme defect.** Patients diagnosed with this disorder have reduced activity of the enzyme **uroporphyrinogen III decarboxylase.**

(4) **Lead intoxication** is a commonly acquired porphyria that results from a block in several of the heme biosynthetic enzymes.

    (a) **Clinical symptoms** of lead poisoning include:

        (i) Abdominal pain

        (ii) Constipation

        (iii) Neuropathy

        (iv) Absence of skin photosensitivity, **ferrochelatase, and coproporphyrinogen oxidase**

    (b) The characteristic **laboratory profile** associated with lead toxicity includes:

        (i) **Elevated urinary ALA and coproporphyrin levels**

        (ii) **Increased RBC photoporphyrin**

        (iii) Hypochromic RBCs with **basophilic stippling** due to increased erythropoiesis

        (iv) **Toxic granulation in neutrophils**

    (c) **Enzyme defect.** Lead inhibits several enzymes of the biosynthetic pathway. The most severely affected **enzyme is ALA dehydrase.**

3. **Iron metabolism–associated disorders** most commonly occur as a result of an iron deficiency but can result from a block of the enzyme that inserts iron (i.e., ferrochelatase) into the heme ring (see Figure 4-3).

    a. Iron and its metabolism are vital to the body because a Hb molecule is nonfunctioning without iron, and two thirds or more of the total body iron is in the RBCs and their precursors.

    (1) Each milliliter of RBCs contains 1 mg of iron.

    (2) Storage iron is present in macrophages or normoblasts as **ferritin** (i.e., Fe^{3+} plus apoferritin) or **hemosiderin.**

    (3) The majority of iron used in Hb synthesis is from the iron released and **recycled** by Hb that is degraded in macrophages and transported to normoblasts by plasma **transferrin.**

    (4) Only 0.9–1.3 mg of iron per day is lost from the body.

    (5) The small amount of iron lost from the body is maintained by **dietary absorption,** which amounts to approximately **1 mg/d.**

        (a) In **men,** dietary iron averages approximately 15 mg/d, with only 6% intestinal absorption.

        (b) In **women,** dietary iron averages approximately 11 mg/d, with 12% intestinal absorption.

        (c) Dietary absorption is increased in an iron deficiency state, but only to a maximum of 20%.

        (d) Dietary iron is **digested in the ferric form** (i.e., Fe^{3+}) but is reduced to the **ferrous form** (i.e., Fe^{2+}) in the stomach by HCl and other reducing agents (e.g., food).

        (e) The **ferrous form is much more rapidly absorbed** by the mucosal cells of the duodenum and upper jejunum than is the ferric form.

(f) Once in the mucosal cell, the ferrous form is oxidized again back to the ferric form and coupled to the protein apoferritin, to form ferritin.

(g) Iron enters the circulation **bound to transferrin.**
   (i) The normal serum **iron concentration is 50–150 mg/dL.**
   (ii) **The normal TIBC of transferrin is 250–400 mg/dL.**
   (iii) Transferrin is normally only **30% saturated.**
   (iv) **Serum ferritin concentration is normally 15–200 ng/mL.**

(6) Normoblasts in the marrow have transferrin receptors and the capacity to extract iron from plasma transferrin.

(a) The **marrow** receives only 5% of the total cardiac output, but it **extracts 85% of the circulating iron.**

(b) Iron is also transferred to normoblasts via the **"nurse" macrophage.**

b. **Iron deficiency anemia (IDA)** is one of the most common forms of anemia in the United States.

(1) **IDA results** when iron **loss exceeds iron intake** for a long time, and the body's iron stores are depleted. Insufficient iron is available for normal heme production.

(a) Iron deficiency develops when there is an **increased need for iron,** such as in rapid growth in infancy, childhood, or during pregnancy. IDA is the most common cause of anemia in children who are between the ages of 6 and 24 months.

(b) Iron deficiency also develops when there is **excessive chronic loss of blood.**

(c) In the adult man, even with no dietary iron intake, body iron stores of 1000 mg would last for 3 or 4 years before iron depletion anemia would occur. **Most cases of IDA in adult men, therefore, are attributed to chronic blood loss.**

(2) The **development of IDA** is seen to occur in three stages.

(a) **Iron depletion stage** is the beginning of iron deficiency, when iron loss exceeds absorption. A negative iron balance develops, and iron is mobilized from iron stores. When this process begins, **storage iron decreases, plasma ferritin decreases,** gastrointestinal (GI) iron absorption increases to a limited extent, and the **amount of plasma transferrin (i.e., TIBC) increases.**

(b) **Iron deficient erythropoiesis stage** occurs when the tissue iron stores are depleted. **When transferrin saturation falls below 15%,** the percent of **marrow sideroblasts decreases,** and as a result of insufficient iron for heme synthesis, the **serum iron is decreased,** and **levels of RBC photoporphyrin increase.**

(c) By the **IDA stage,** a clinical anemia becomes detectable first as a normocytic/normochromic anemia, then gradually progressing to a microcytic/hypochromic anemia.

(3) Patients who have IDA are initially seen with the following **clinical symptoms:**

(**a**) Numbness and tingling of extremities

(**b**) Atrophy of the epithelium of the tongue with soreness

(**c**) Cracks or ulcers at the corners of the mouth

(**d**) Abnormal cravings for such things as dirt or ice (i.e., pica)

(**e**) Concave or spoon-shaped nails

(**4**) **Laboratory diagnosis** of IDA demonstrates characteristic findings in the blood and bone marrow.

    (**a**) Laboratory findings from a **peripheral blood** sample include the following:

        (**i**) Early stages of IDA may demonstrate normocytic/normochromic RBCs, but these eventually develop into **microcytic/hypochromic** RBCs with **marked anisocytosis and slight poikilocytosis.**

        (**ii**) **Reticulocytes are decreased,** except after iron therapy.

        (**iii**) **The MCV is low, and the RDW is increased.**

        (**iv**) The osmotic fragility is decreased.

        (**v**) In most cases, the **WBC count is normal,** but granulocytes may tend toward a maturation shift to the right (i.e., hypersegmentation).

        (**vi**) **Platelets are increased if the anemia is due to blood loss,** or platelets may be decreased in advanced, severe anemic stages.

        (**vii**) **Serum iron is decreased** (normal level is **50–150 mg/dL**).

        (**viii**) **TIBC is increased** (normal level is **250–400 mg/dL**).

        (**ix**) The **percent saturation of TIBC** [i.e., (serum iron ÷ TIBC) × 100] **falls below 15%** in IDA (normal is **20%–55%**).

        (**x**) **Serum ferritin** is in equilibrium with tissue ferritin and is a good reflection of storage iron. Ferritin values usually decline **below 12 ng/mL, which indicates low iron stores** (normal range is **15–200 ng/mL**).

        (**xi**) Level of RBC **intracellular photoporphyrin IX is increased** in RBCs when TIBC percent saturation falls below 15%.

    (**b**) **The marrow** of a patient who has IDA may have the following characteristics:

        (**i**) Normoblasts are smaller than normal, with frayed margins

        (**ii**) **Storage iron is absent** unless patient is receiving iron therapy

        (**iii**) **Sideroblasts are decreased to lower than 20%**

(**5**) **IDA must be differentially diagnosed** from other microcytic/hypochromic anemias such as **thalassemia, anemia of chronic disease, and sideroblastic anemia** (Table 4-2).

c. **Disorders of iron excess** result from the slow accumulation of excess quantities of tissue iron stores. This can result from **increased intestinal absorption,** administration from transfused blood (i.e., **transfusion hemosiderosis**), or **administration of iron-complex drugs or vitamins.**

(**1**) **General considerations**

Table 4-2. Differential Diagnosis of the Microcytic/Hypochromic Anemias Using Iron-Related Parameters

Disorder	Serum Iron	TIBC	% Sat	Ferritin	Bone Marrow Iron
Iron deficiency anemia	↓	↑	↓	↓	↓
Anemia of chronic disorders	↓	N to ↓	N to ↓	N to ↑	N to ↑
Sideroblastic anemia	↑	↓	↑	↑	↑
Thalassemia	N to ↑	N to ↓	N to ↑	N to ↑	N to ↑

N = normal; TIBC = total iron binding capacity; % Sat = percent transferrin iron saturation; ↑ = increased; ↓ = decreased.

    (a) Plasma iron increases to 200 mg/dL with 100% TIBC saturation.
    (b) Macrophages are no longer able to store the extra iron once the percent TIBC saturation increases higher than 50%.
    (c) Excess iron slowly damages organs over a period of years.
    (d) **Hemochromatosis** refers to the diseases and symptoms that arise from chronic iron overexposure.
    (e) Young **children are highly susceptible to acute iron poisoning** because of accidentally swallowing iron pills or vitamins. Iron poisoning in children can be fatal with as little as a 50-mg dose.
  (2) **Primary familial hemochromatosis** is a condition of iron excess that results from an abnormality in a gene on chromosome 6 that is closely linked with the human leukocyte antigen (HLA) locus.
    (a) Iron overload stems from an overall **increase in absorption by the intestinal mucosal cells.**
    (b) Patients chronically have an **increased serum iron level, increased transferrin saturation,** and iron-loading in macrophages and hepatocytes.
  (3) **Sideroblastic anemia** is a disorder of iron excess that is associated with defective synthesis of heme because of multiple enzyme defects, and a resulting iron overload in the mitochondria of normoblasts. This anemia is **now classified as a myelodysplastic syndrome.**
    (a) The patient's RBC morphology is hypochromic and often microcytic.
    (b) Patients are commonly seen with **increased serum iron levels, decreased TIBC, and greatly increased transferrin saturation.**
    (c) The marrow shows a greatly increased storage iron by an **increase in sideroblasts greater than 50%** and an increase in siderotic granules per cell, with granules surrounding the nucleus (i.e., **ring sideroblasts**).
    (d) Several variations of sideroblastic anemia have been noted:
        (i) **A hereditary,** X chromosome–linked type is found mostly in males and does not show up until adolescence.

      (ii) Acquired idiopathic sideroblastic anemia can occur in either sex and has its onset in late adulthood. Some of the RBCs may be megaloblastic, and 10% of patients who have this type of anemia develop acute leukemia.

      (iii) Pyridoxine-responsive (i.e., vitamin B_6) sideroblastic anemia can be treated with high amounts of vitamin B_6 to maintain normal Hb synthesis.

      (iv) Drug-induced sideroblastic anemia has been known to occur in patients chronically exposed to antituberculosis drugs (e.g., isoniazid); lead; chloramphenicol; or ethanol ingestion.

D. Globin chain disorders

  1. General considerations. Globin dysfunction can occur from genetic mutations giving rise to either of the following two anemia classifications:

    a. Hemoglobinopathies represent the majority of abnormal Hb disorders. These Hb disorders result from a **single amino-acid substitution** in one of the polypeptide chains (i.e., α, β, γ, δ).

    b. Thalassemias are caused by an abnormal long or short polypeptide resulting from gene coding termination errors, frame-shift mutations, crossover in phase, deletion of codons, or fused hybrid chains. These gene-coding abnormalities result in the **deficiency or absence** of one of the types of globin chains.

  2. Hemoglobinopathies

    a. Nomenclature

      (1) The abnormal Hb disorder is most commonly represented by its letter abbreviation. For example, sickle cell anemia is denoted as **Hb S,** methemoglobinemia is written as **Hb M.**

      (2) Hb variants can also be written to describe their amino acid substitution (**e.g., Hb S** = α_2, β_2 **6 val).**

    b. Sickle-cell disease (Hb SS) is a genetically **homozygous** condition that results in a serious chronic hemolytic anemia.

      (1) The anemia **shows up at childhood** and is often fatal by 30–40 years of age.

      (2) Hb S is found almost exclusively in the black population. Between 0.1% and 0.2% of American blacks are affected by this disorder.

      (3) Genetic alteration results in the **glutamic** amino acid in position 6 of the β-chain being **replaced by a valine amino acid.** This molecular alteration changes the Hb molecule's overall charge and electrophoretic mobility.

      (4) Hb S is freely soluble in its **fully oxygenated form.**

        (a) In its deoxygenated form, polymerization of the abnormal Hb molecules occurs, which leads to the formation of intracellular crystals that deform the RBC to the sickle shape.

        (b) With homozygous Hb SS disease, sickling occurs even at physiologic oxygen tensions.

      (5) The **rigidity** of the RBC in the sickle shape is responsible for the trapping and hemolysis of the RBCs. This **results in intravascular**

hemolysis, and the marrow becomes hyperplastic early in childhood, expanding the marrow space.

(6) Clinical complications accompanying Hb SS disease are serious, resulting in systemic organ damage.

  (a) Early in childhood, **bilateral painful swelling of the hands and feet** occur due to RBC sickling and capillary plugging (i.e., hand-foot syndrome).

  (b) Splenic complications occur because of splenic blood sequestration and pooling of blood, which causes rapid **splenomegaly and systemic hypovolemia.** Patients can develop functional asplenia, which leads to an **impaired immune system** and renders the patient more susceptible to infections.

  (c) Anoxic damage to the kidneys results from renovascular plugging. Patients cannot produce a concentrated urine; they commonly are seen with hematuria (i.e., RBCs in the urine).

  (d) Vaso-occlusive crises due to capillary occluding by sickle cells and loss of circulation to tissues intermittently affects patients with joint and abdominal pain.

  (e) Aplastic crises can occur in the marrow because of systemic intravascular hemolysis.

  (f) Leg ulcers are common because of capillary blocking and ischemic tissue.

(7) It is common for patients who have **homozygous Hb SS** to have the following **hematologic profile:**

  (a) Normocytic/normochromic anemia

  (b) Marked **polychromasia** on the blood smear

  (c) Normoblasts found on the blood smear

  (d) Numerous **target cells** and **Howell-Jolly bodies** because of asplenia

  (e) Sickled RBCs found on the blood smear

  (f) Decreased osmotic fragility test

  (g) Neutrophilia and **thrombocytosis**

(8) The marrow aspirate shows **normoblastic hyperplasia** and **increased iron storage.**

(9) Common **laboratory screening tests** for Hb S include the following:

  (a) Sickling of RBCs containing Hb S can be induced on a microscope slide with **sodium metabisulfite.**

   (i) Metabisulfite is a reducing substance that enhances deoxygenation and sickling.

   (ii) This test cannot differentiate homozygous Hb SS and heterozygous sickle cell trait (Hb AS).

  (b) Solubility (i.e., turbidity) tests screen for Hb S with **dithionite or toluene.**

   (i) The RBCs are first lysed, and Hb S is reduced by dithionite or toluene.

   (ii) Reduced Hb S is insoluble in concentrated inorganic buffers, and the polymers of Hb S produce turbidity. The amount of turbidity is proportional to the amount of Hb S in the RBCs.

(10) A **definitive diagnosis** of Hb SS can be made with a **hemoglobin electrophoresis** at alkaline pH. Table 4-3 shows the electrophoresis

Table 4-3. Differential Diagnosis of the Globin-Chain Disorders Based on Hemoglobin Electrophoresis Results at Alkaline and Acid pH

Globin-chain Disorder	Electrophoresis (pH 8.4–8.6)							Hemoglobin Electrophoresis (pH 6.0–6.2)				
	(−) o	(+) A_2/C/E	S/D/G	F	A	Bart's	(+) H	(+) C	S	o	A_2/A/D/G/E	(−) F
Normal adult	—	+/−	—	—	++++	—	—	—	—	—	++++	—
hemoglobinopathies:												
HgB-SS	—	+	+++	++	—	—	—	—	+++	—	+	++
HgB-AS	—	—	++	+	+++	—	—	—	++	—	+++	++
HgB-CC	—	+++	—	+	—	—	—	+++	—	—	—	+
HgB-AC	—	++	+++	+	+++	—	—	++	—	—	+++	+
HgB-DD	—	—	+++	+	—	—	—	—	—	—	++++	+
HgB-AD	—	—	++	+	+++	—	—	—	—	—	+++	+
HgB-EE	—	+++	—	+	—	—	—	—	—	—	++++	+
HgB-AE	—	++	—	+	+++	—	—	—	—	—	++++	+
HgB-SC	—	++	+++	+	—	—	—	++	++	—	—	+
HgB-SD	—	—	++++	—	—	—	—	—	++	—	++	—
Thalassemias												
β^{0}-Thal major	—	+	—	+++	—	—	—	—	—	—	—	—
β^{+}-Thal major (Mediterranean)	—	++	—	+++	+	—	—	—	—	—	—	—
β^{+}-Thal major (black)	—	—	—	++	++	—	—	—	—	—	—	—
β-Thal minor	—	+	—	+/−	+++	—	—	—	—	—	—	—
α-Thal major	—	—	—	—	+++	++*	++	—	—	—	—	—
α-Thal minor	—	—	—	—	+++	+*	—	—	—	—	—	—

o = origin or application of sample; +/− = slightly increased; + = 1%–25%; ++ = 26%–50%; +++ = 51%–75%; ++++ = 76%–100%; — = no data.
*Only shows up at birth.

results seen in homozygous Hb S. (**Note:** Abnormal hemoglobins **Hb D and Hb G produce the same electrophoresis mobility, but the sickle-cell screening tests are negative.**)

  c. **Hb AS** is a **heterozygous** β-chain defect and the most common hemoglobinopathy in the United States. The genetic trait is present in 9% of American blacks and normally has no clinical signs or symptoms.

    (1) With physiologic acidosis, hypoxia of high altitudes, respiratory tract infection, anesthesia, or congestive heart failure, sickling occurs, with the same symptoms as seen in the homozygous form.

    (2) **Hb AS protects persons from the lethal effects of falciparum malaria.**

    (3) The patient's RBC count and morphology are normal, except for a few target cells.

    (4) All **sickle cell tests are positive.**

    (5) Heterozygous Hb AS produces the Hb **electrophoresis results** at an alkaline pH (see Table 4-3).

  d. **Hemoglobin C disease (Hb CC)** is a genetically homozygous condition chiefly affecting blacks (0.02% in the United States) that presents as a moderate hemolytic anemia with splenomegaly, jaundice, and abdominal discomfort.

    (1) The **genetic alteration** results in a β-**chain** amino acid **substitution of the glutamate at position 6 with a lysine amino acid.**

    (2) Patients who have homozygous Hb CC are usually seen with the following **hematologic profile:**

      (a) The anemia is normocytic/normochromic with a **mixture of microcytes and spherocytes** on the blood smear.

      (b) A slight reticulocytosis is often noted.

      (c) **Numerous target cells (40%–90%)** are found on the blood smear.

      (d) The osmotic fragility test is biphasic.

      (e) Hexagonal or rod-shaped crystals (i.e., **Hb C crystals**) may be found in RBCs on the blood smear. These **crystals** result from cellular **dehydration** of older RBCs, which therefore increases their **rigidity, splenic trapping, and destruction.**

    (3) Homozygous Hb CC produces the Hb **electrophoresis results** as shown in Table 4-3.

  e. The milder **heterozygous form (i.e., Hb AC)**, found in 2%–3% of American blacks, is usually asymptomatic without anemia.

    (1) The most striking hematologic finding is a moderate number of **target cells** on the patient's blood smear.

    (2) Heterozygous Hb AC produces the Hb **electrophoresis results** as seen in Table 4-3.

  f. **Hb D disease and trait** is most common in persons of **Asian-Indian extraction.**

    (1) The **genetic alteration** in this disorder results in an amino acid substitution in the β-chain(s) at position 121 of the **glutamate with a glutamine amino acid.**

    (2) The heterozygous trait is asymptomatic with a normal blood profile.

(3) Hb D migrates on the electrophoretic gel with the Hb S fraction, but the sickle tests are negative. Hb D produces the Hb **electrophoresis results** as seen in Table 4-3.

g. **Hb E disease and trait is found mainly in individuals of Asian origin.**
   (1) Homozygous patients have a mild anemia with moderate microcytosis and target cells on their blood smear.
   (2) Hb E produces the Hb **electrophoresis results** shown in Table 4-3.

h. **Doubly heterozygous β-hemoglobinopathies** are disorders in which the individual inherits a different abnormal β-chain gene from each parent.
   (1) Hb SC disease has an incidence similar to the homozygous Hb SS disease that occurs in American blacks.
      (a) The severity of the disease is intermediate between sickle cell trait and sickle-cell disease.
      (b) Onset is in childhood, but physical difficulties do not occur until the teenage years.
      (c) Basically, the symptoms are the same as Hb SS, but **splenomegaly** is more common in patients with Hb SC.
      (d) Patients are commonly seen with the following **hematologic profile:**
         (i) Moderate-to-mild normocytic/normochromic anemia
         (ii) Moderate-to-severe anisocytosis and poikilocytosis
         (iii) Target cells can comprise up to 85% of the RBCs
         (iv) Sickle cells as well as Hb CC crystals on the blood smear
         (v) Positive sickle cell tests
      (e) Hb SC produces the Hb **electrophoresis** pattern shown in Table 4-3.
   (2) Hb SD disease simulates but is less severe than Hb SS anemia. This disorder cannot be distinguished between Hb SC or sickle cell trait.

i. **In some heterozygous hemoglobinopathies, the amino acid substitutions occur in the heme pocket, where they either increase the stability of the Hb M, or alter the affinity of the heme ring for oxygen.**
   (1) Some abnormal hemoglobins are associated with **cyanosis and Hb M.**
      (a) The reduction to the ferrous heme and binding of oxygen is prevented by an amino acid substitution near the heme ring.
      (b) With α-chain Hb M, cyanosis is present from birth. However, with β-chain Hb M, cyanosis does not occur until β-chain production reaches adult levels.
   (2) Some hemoglobinopathies result in **increased oxygen-affinity and polycythemia.**
      (a) Because of the high oxygen affinity, the tissue is hypoxic at any given oxygen tension. The result is increased EPO and hence, **polycythemia.**
      (b) Because the amino acid substitution is inside the molecule, the abnormality is indistinguishable from Hb A on Hb electrophoresis.
      (c) Example: Hemoglobin Chesapeake is an α-chain abnormality that results in a mild polycythemia.

    (3) Some hemoglobins are associated with **decreased oxygen affinity and cyanosis.** An example of such an abnormal Hb is **hemoglobin Kansas.**

  j. Unstable hemoglobins have an amino acid substitution at a place in the α or β chain that affects the formation of the bonds between chains. The majority of these hemoglobins are β-chain substitutions.

    (1) Hb precipitates out in the circulating RBC and attaches to the RBC membrane.

      (a) Heinz bodies are Hb intracellular precipitates.

      (b) Intracellular precipitates render the cells inflexible and **shorten RBC survival.**

    (2) The majority of Heinz bodies are removed from the RBCs by the spleen.

    (3) Jaundice and splenomegaly are common, and patients may have a darkly pigmented urine.

    (4) Following splenectomy, Heinz bodies are numerous in the circulating RBCs.

    (5) Unstable hemoglobins produce the following Hb **electrophoresis results** at an alkaline pH:

      (a) Approximately 25% of patients have a normal electrophoretic pattern

      (b) Hb A2; increased in β-chain variants

      (c) Hb F; increased to 10%–15%

    (6) Unstable hemoglobins can also be detected in the laboratory with the **heat instability test** and the **isopropanol precipitation test.**

3. Thalassemias

  a. Background

    (1) Thalassemias are **disorders of Hb synthesis** that occur mainly in persons of Mediterranean, African, and Asian ancestry.

    (2) The dysfunction is a **diminished rate of synthesis of certain globin chains,** but the chain formed in most cases is of normal amino acid sequence.

    (3) Total lack of α- or β-globin production is known as **thalassemia major.** Production at a decreased rate is known as **thalassemia minor.**

    (4) α-Thalassemia is associated with a decrease in the production of α-chains. β-Thalassemia is associated with a decrease in the production in β-chains.

  b. Globin-chain molecular defects and nomenclature includes the following:

    (1) β^0**-Thalassemia** denotes a condition in which β-chain synthesis is **absent.** The gene is not deleted, but the messenger ribonucleic acid (mRNA) is absent or nonfunctioning.

    (2) β^+**-Thalassemia** is a condition in which β-chain synthesis is only **reduced.** Such disorders result from defects in transcription and processing of mRNA.

    (3) $\delta\beta$**-Thalassemia** is caused by **gene deletions involving both the δ and β genes.**

    (4) $\gamma\delta\beta$**-Thalassemia** is caused by a **long deletion including the**

γ-genes and δ-genes that stops short of the β-gene, but also reduces the output of β-chains.

(5) **Lepore thalassemia** shows normal α-genes. **Abnormal $\delta\beta$-genes** caused by $\delta\beta$-**fusion of genes** results from gene crossover.

(6) α-**Thalassemias** are generally caused by gene deletions of various lengths and can also be α^o or α^+.

(7) **Hb constant spring** is caused by an abnormal termination codon in an α-gene. This results in an **elongated α-chain with 31 extra amino acids and** slowed or reduced α-globin synthesis.

c. **Homozygous β-thalassemia (thalassemia major)** results from either a decrease or an absence in β-chain production by **both gene alleles.**

(1) With a decrease in β-chain production, γ-chain production is high, which results in **increased Hb F.**

(2) There is an excess of α-chains due to a lack of matching β-chains.

    (a) **Unstable tetramers of α-chains (i.e., α_4) precipitate out of solution in the normoblast or RBC.**

    (b) These α-chain precipitates adhere to the inner membrane and **damage the cell,** which results in ineffective erythropoiesis and a severe **hemolytic anemia.**

(3) **Clinical symptoms** of β-thalassemia major include:

    (a) Jaundice and splenomegaly early in childhood

    (b) Prominent frontal bones (i.e., cheek, jaws)

    (c) Chronic marrow hyperplasia resulting in a thinned cortex of the long bones

    (d) Stunted growth and delayed puberty

    (e) **Hemochromatosis** from regular transfusions

    (f) Cardiac failure (i.e., major cause of death) due to myocardial siderosis by 30 years of age

(4) Patients who have homozygous β-thalassemia commonly present with the following **hematologic profile:**

    (a) **Unlike most hemolytic anemias, β-thalassemia is morphologically a microcytic/hypochromic anemia caused by a defect in either the rate of Hb synthesis or in the lack of synthesis.**

    (b) Peripheral blood smears show **extreme poikilocytosis and anisocytosis** in RBCs, as well as such morphologic abnormalities as target cells, ovalocytes, Howell-Jolly bodies, normoblasts, siderocytes, and Cabot's rings.

    (c) The **reticulocyte count** is less elevated than what would be expected for the degree of anemia because of the destruction of erythroid precursors in the marrow.

    (d) The **osmotic fragility test is decreased.**

    (e) **Serum iron is increased.**

    (f) The indirect bilirubin level is increased.

    (g) **The MCV is decreased, with an increased RDW.**

(5) Marrow aspirate reveals **normoblastic hyperplasia, increased storage iron, and sideroblasts.**

(6) Homozygous β-thalassemia can exist in three genetic forms, each producing a different **electrophoresis pattern** (see Table 4-3).

      (a) β^+**-Thalassemia** represents a partial decrease in β-chain production. Persons of **Mediterranean descent** with this form of thalassemia have severe clinical symptoms. They demonstrate the electrophoretic pattern as seen in Table 4-3.

      (b) β^+**-Thalassemia** is a less clinically severe disorder that occurs in persons of African descent. These patients show the electrophoretic pattern as seen in Table 4-3.

  d. **Heterozygous β-thalassemia** (i.e., thalassemia minor) results from the absence or decrease in β-chain production at **one gene allele.**

    (1) Patients may be seen with the following **clinical symptoms:**

      (a) The degree of anemia may vary from a severe microcytic/hypochromic anemia to normal clinical findings.

      (b) A moderate-to-severe anemia is more common in individuals of Mediterranean descent.

      (c) Patients who have more severe disease have a slight hemolytic jaundice and splenomegaly.

    (2) Patients who have heterozygous β**-thalassemia** are commonly seen with the following **hematologic profile:**

      (a) Characteristically, **the RBC count is increased, and the Hb and Hct are reduced.**

      (b) The RBC indices are commonly below normal, and the **RDW is increased.**

      (c) RBC morphology on the peripheral blood smear shows moderate poikilocytosis, **target cells,** and basophilic stippling.

      (d) **Osmotic fragility is decreased.**

      (e) **Serum iron levels are normal to high.**

    (3) Marrow often demonstrates the same characteristics as homozygous β-thalassemia.

    (4) Thalassemia minor produces the Hb **electrophoresis results** shown in Table 4-3.

    (5) $\delta\beta$**-Thalassemias** produce clinical symptoms similar to β-thalassemias.

      (a) Homozygotes have intermediate thalassemia symptoms, and their electrophoretic pattern shows an **absence of Hb A and Hb A2.**

      (b) Heterozygotes clinically have thalassemia minor symptoms and demonstrate **5%–20% Hb F and normal Hb A2** on their electrophoretic pattern.

    (6) **Hb Lepore syndromes** produce an abnormal Hb that has a **normal α-chain combined with a fused $\delta\beta$-chain.**

      (a) Because the $\delta\beta$-chain is synthesized at a slower rate, it results in a microcytic/hypochromic anemia and resembles a thalassemia.

      (b) **Hb Lepore migrates with the Hb S band** on electrophoresis gel at an alkaline pH.

  e. **Double heterozygotes for β-thalassemia and β-hemoglobinopathies** occur when an individual inherits a thalassemia gene from one parent and a hemoglobinopathy gene from the other parent.

    (1) Hb A levels are always less than levels of the variant Hb.

    (2) **Sickle cell thalassemia** (i.e., **Hb S β-thalassemia**) symptomatically differs from Hb SS in that patients have splenomegaly from childhood into adulthood.

  (a) This disorder is clinically similar to sickle-cell disease, except that the **MCV and MCH are lower, and Hb A2 is increased to greater levels** than that seen in Hb SS.

  (b) Patients are commonly seen with the following distinguishing **hematologic characteristics:**

     (i) **Marked microcytosis**

     (ii) Variable hypochromia

     (iii) Many target cells

     (iv) Rare sickle cells

     (v) Low MCV and MCH

     (vi) **Positive sickle cell tests**

  (c) **Hb S β^o–thalassemia** demonstrates the following electrophoresis pattern:

     (i) **Hb A: none**

     (ii) **Hb S: 75%–90%**

     (iii) **Hb F: 5%–20%**

     (iv) **Hb A2: greater than 4.5%**

  (d) **Hb S β^+–thalassemia** demonstrates the following electrophoresis pattern:

     (i) **Hb A: 15%–30%**

     (ii) **Hb S:** greater than 50%

     (iii) **Hb F:** 1%–20%

     (iv) **Hb A2:** increased greater than 4.5%

(3) **Hb C β–thalassemia** occurs mainly as a mild anemia in persons of African descent and as a severe anemia in a smaller percentage of persons of Mediterranean descent.

  (a) **Hb C β^o–thalassemia** demonstrates the following electrophoresis pattern:

     (i) **Hb C: 90%–95%**

     (ii) **Hb F: 5%–10%**

     (iii) **Hb A: none**

  (b) **Hb C β^+–thalassemia** demonstrates the following electrophoresis pattern:

     (i) **Hb A: 20%–30%**

     (ii) **Hb C: 70%–80%**

     (iii) **Hb F: normal**

     (iv) **Hb A2:** masked on electrophoresis by Hb C

(4) **Hb E β–thalassemia is a southeast Asian disease** resembling thalassemia major and demonstrates the following characteristic electrophoresis pattern:

  (a) **Hb E: 15%–95%**

  (b) **Hb F: 5%–85%**

  (c) **Hb A: none**

f. **α-Thalassemias** result from a partial or total decrease in the production of α-chains.

  (1) Although there are two β-globin genes per diploid genotype, **there are four α-globin genes per diploid genotype. These are normally designated as $\alpha\alpha/\alpha\alpha$.**

(a) **Mild** α-thalassemia (i.e., α^+-thalassemia) is a deletion of only one gene and is represented as -α/$\alpha\alpha$.

(b) **Severe** α-thalassemia (i.e., α°-thalassemia) is a deletion of two α-globin genes, and is represented as --/$\alpha\alpha$.

(2) **Hydrops fetalis with Hb Bart's** is the most severe form of α-thalassemia. Individuals who have this disorder have a diploid genotype of **--/--**, which represents the absence of all α-chains.

(a) The absence of all α-chains is **incompatible with life,** and infants who have this disorder are stillborn or die soon after birth.

(b) In the absence of α-chains, γ-chains and β-chains form **tetramers** known as **Hb Bart's and Hb H,** respectively. Both of these tetramer forms migrate faster than do Hb A on electrophoresis gel.

(c) This disorder demonstrates the following characteristic **electrophoretic pattern:**

(i) **Hb A, Hb F, and Hb A2: none**

(ii) **Hb Bart's: greater than 80%**

(3) **Hb H disease** (i.e., α-thalassemia major) is a thalassemia in which three of the four α-globin genes are absent (i.e., --/-α).

(a) Clinically, patients who have this disorder have a **chronic hemolytic anemia** that resembles an intermediate thalassemia.

(b) Patients are commonly seen with the following distinguishing **hematologic characteristics:**

(i) Decreased MCV and MCH

(ii) Hypochromia and target cells on the blood smear

(iii) Moderate anisocytosis and poikilocytosis on the smear

(iv) A reticulocyte count of 4%–5%

(v) **Moderate Heinz bodies,** which are Hb H precipitates

(c) This disorder demonstrates the characteristic **electrophoretic pattern** shown in Table 4-3.

(4) α-**Thalassemia minor** is clinically mild and resembles β-thalassemia minor. Genetically, patients are lacking two of the four α-globin genes (i.e., --/$\alpha\alpha$ or -α/-α).

(a) Patients have a **mild anemia, microcytosis, and normal serum iron.**

(b) This disorder demonstrates the following characteristic **electrophoretic pattern:**

(i) **Diagnosis is made by finding 5%–6% of Hb Bart's in cord blood.**

(ii) **Adults show no evidence of an Hb imbalance.**

(5) **Silent carrier of α-thalassemia** (i.e., heterozygous α^+-thalassemia) represents a disorder that has only one defective α-globin gene (i.e., -α/$\alpha\alpha$) and is not associated with any hematologic abnormalities.

(6) **Hemoglobin constant spring (Hb CS)** is **an α-chain variant with 31 extra amino acids.**

(a) α-Chains are functionally normal but synthesized more slowly, and therefore present a clinical picture of thalassemia.

(b) Hb CS **migrates slower than Hb A2** at an alkaline pH.

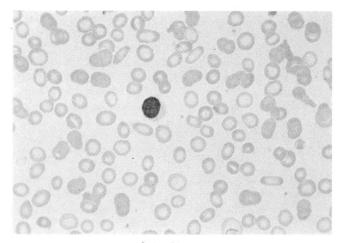

Color Plate 1

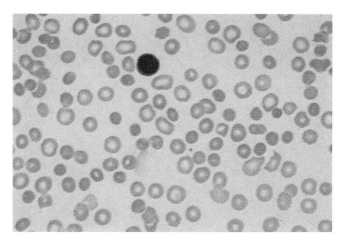

Color Plate 2

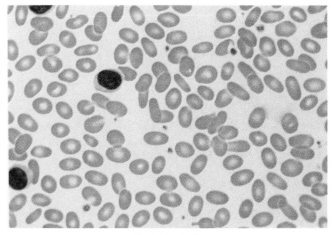

Color Plate 3

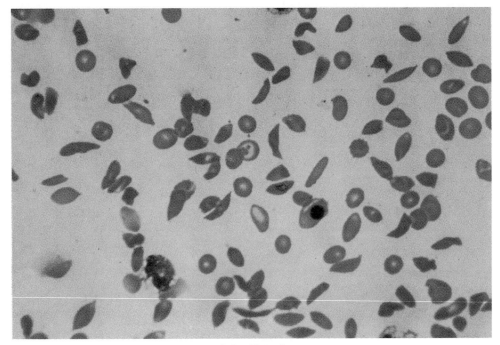

Color Plate 4

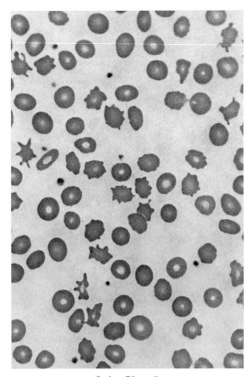

Color Plate 5

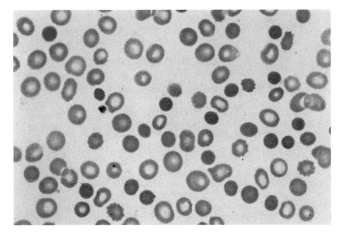

Color Plate 6

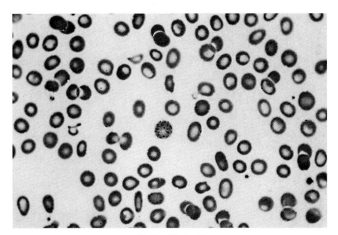

Color Plate 7

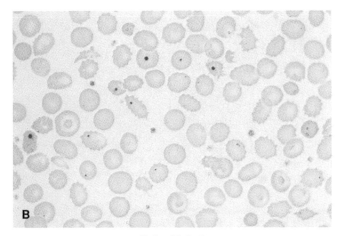

Color Plate 8

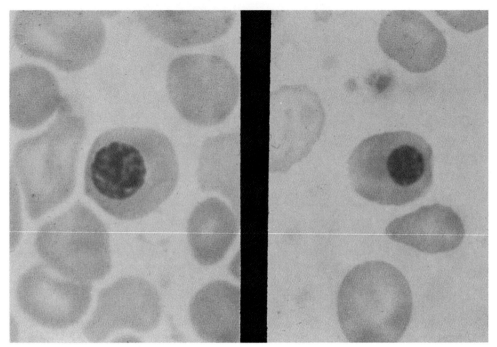

Color Plate 9

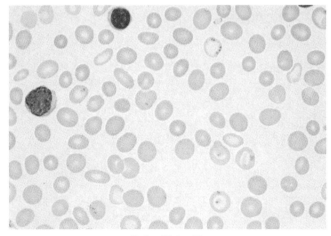

Color Plate 10

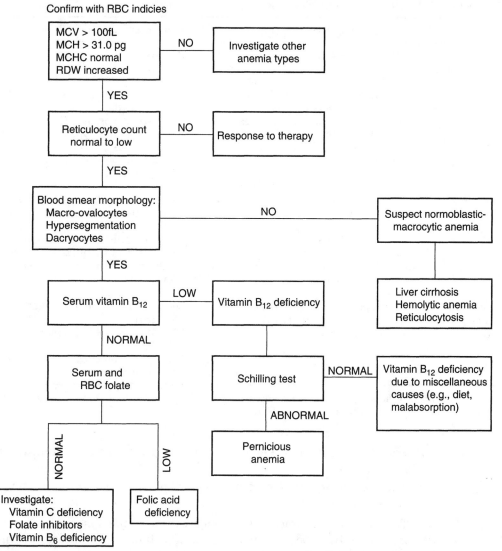

Confirm with RBC indicies

Figure 4-4. Algorithm for the differential diagnosis of the megaloblastic anemias from other macrocytic anemias. MCH = mean corpuscular hemoglobin; MCHC = mean corpuscular hemoglobin concentration; MCV = mean cell volume; RBC = red blood cell; RDW = red cell distribution width.

(c) This disorder demonstrates the following characteristic **electrophoretic pattern:**
(i) **Hb CS: 5%–6%**
(ii) **Hb A2: normal**
(iii) **Hb Bart's: trace**
(iv) **Hb A: major fraction**

E. **Deoxyribonucleic acid (DNA) disorders.** Megaloblastosis is almost always caused by deficiencies of vitamin B_{12} or folic acid.

1. **Megaloblastic anemia as a macrocytic condition.** Macrocytosis caused by megaloblastic anemia must be differentiated from macrocytosis with a normoblastic marrow (Figure 4-4).

Table 4-4. Laboratory Profiles of DNA Disorders

Disorder	Characteristics	Laboratory Profile
Megaloblastic anemia	Marrow has enlarged precursor cells Blood smear RBC morphology shows macrocytes mixed with microcytes, moderate anisocytosis and poikilocytosis, dacryocytes, basophilic stippling, Howell-Jolly bodies, Cabot's rings, and a few NRBCs	Pancytopenia Low RBC count Low hemoglobin Low hematocrit MCV > 100 fL Increased to normal MCH Leukopenia with hypersegmentation of neutrophils Mild thrombocytopenia Increased serum iron
Vitamin B_{12} deficiency	Same characteristics as megaloblastic anemia	Serum vitamin B_{12} assay indicates value < 100 ng/L (normal = 200–900 ng/L) Increased urinary methylmalonic acid Schilling test can indicate an intrinsic factor dysfunction or pernicious anemia
Folic acid deficiency	Leukopenia and thrombocytopenia are less common than with vitamin B_{12} deficiency	Serum folate < 3 μg/L (normal = 5–21 μg/L) RBC folate < 150 μg/L (normal = 150–600 μg/L) Urinary formimonoglutamic acid level is increased

DNA = deoxyribonucleic acid; MCH = mean corpuscular hemoglobin; MCV = mean corpuscular volume; NRBCs = nucleated red blood cells; RBC = red blood cell.

2. **Macrocytic anemia with a megaloblastic marrow** can result in **ineffective hematopoiesis.**

 a. **The laboratory profile** of a patient who has megaloblastic anemia is given in Table 4-4.

 b. The **marrow** is characterized by enlargement of precursor cells. Marrow is **hypercellular** because of increased EPO stimulation; however, erythropoiesis is ineffective (Figure 4-5).

3. **Vitamin B_{12} (i.e., cyanocobalamin)**

 a. **Metabolism** occurs in the small intestine. Dietary B_{12} is released from digestion of animal proteins in meats and is bound by gastric **intrinsic factor (IF).**

 b. **Normal serum vitamin B_{12} values** range from **200–900 ng/L.** If vitamin B_{12} intake is stopped, total body stores of 2–5 mg last for several years before a megaloblastic anemia results.

 c. **Vitamin B_{12} function** is related to DNA synthesis because vitamin B_{12} is a vital **cofactor in the conversion of methyl tetrahydrofolate (i.e., folic acid) to tetrahydrofolate.** This substrate is an important cofactor needed for the production of **thymidine,** which is a DNA base.

 d. **Common cause of vitamin B_{12} deficiency.** Inadequate dietary intake of vitamin B_{12} is extremely rare in the United States; it is usually seen in strict

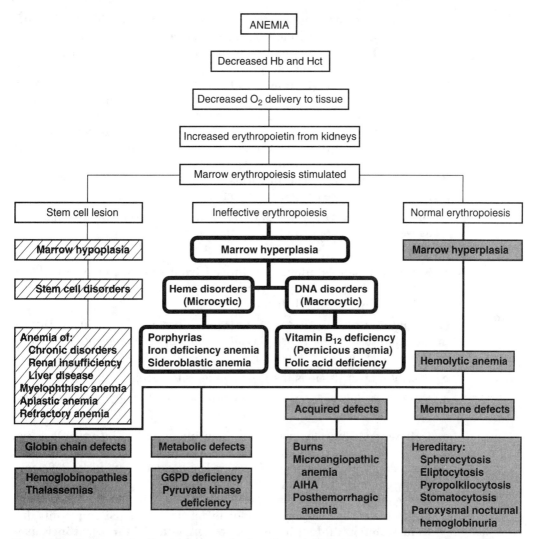

Figure 4-5. Summary algorithm of the anemias based on physiologic cause and bone marrow dynamics. AIHA = autoimmune hemolytic anemia; DNA = deoxyribonucleic acid; G6PD = glucose-6-phosphate dehydrogenase; Hb = hemoglobin; Hct = hematocrit.

vegetarians. The most common cause of vitamin B_{12} deficiency is **defective production of IF.**

   (1) Pernicious anemia (PA) is a "conditioned" nutritional deficiency of B_{12}, caused by failure of the gastric mucosa to secrete IF.

   (2) PA is an **inherited disorder,** most commonly occurring in persons older than 40 years (see Table 4-4). **Two types of autoantibodies** have been identified in PA patients:

      (a) An autoantibody that is **directed against the parietal cells** is found in 85%–95% of PA patients.

      (b) Autoantibodies can also develop that are directed against IF or the IF–vitamin B_{12} complex.

   (3) Other causes of PA include the following:

      (a) Gastrectomy (i.e., the surgical removal of part or all of the stomach) removes the source of IF and results in megaloblastic anemia if vitamin B_{12} supplements are not provided.

(b) **Defective absorption of vitamin B_{12}** into the intestinal mucosal cell can result in a secondary vitamin B_{12} deficiency, even if dietary intake is normal. **Lack of availability of vitamin B_{12}** in the small intestine can result from competition for dietary B_{12}.

(i) In some countries, infestation with the **fish tapeworm** *Diphyllobothrium latum* is common and results in vitamin B_{12} deficiency because the worm competes for the available dietary vitamin B_{12}.

(ii) **Bacterial infestation** in a blind loop of the intestine also uses ingested vitamin B_{12}.

e. **Diagnosis of vitamin B_{12} deficiency** is based upon clinical symptoms, as well as laboratory results (see Table 4-4).

4. Folic acid

a. **Sources.** Folate is primarily **acquired from the diet** in such foods as eggs, milk, leafy vegetables, yeast, liver, and fruits. A smaller percentage is formed by **intestinal flora.**

b. The **minimum daily dietary requirement** has been set at 50 mg. Dietary ingestion just barely meets the minimum daily requirement. The body's reserve lasts for only 3 months.

c. **Storage.** Liver tissue is the main storage site of folic acid.

d. **Normal serum reference values** are 5–21 μg/L, and 150–600 μg/L for RBC folate.

e. **Deficiency.** Clinically, symptoms from **inadequate dietary folate** can occur within weeks, as compared with years for a vitamin B_{12} deficiency. Leukopenia and thrombocytopenia are less common with folate deficiency than vitamin B_{12} deficiency, but the symptoms and the hematologic profile are generally the same (see Table 4-4). Unlike vitamin B_{12} deficiency, a megaloblastic anemia caused by folate deficiency is **most commonly due to insufficient dietary intake.** A woman's **demand for folate increases during pregnancy,** and pregnant women should receive folate supplements of approximately 500 mg/d.

f. **Causes of deficiency**

(1) **Liver disease associated with alcoholism** results in a dietary folate deficiency. A differential diagnosis is necessary to distinguish this condition from an **anemia of liver disease,** which has a normal folate but is macrocytic with a normoblastic marrow.

(2) **Defective absorption** of folate in the small intestine can result from malabsorbtion syndromes, such as nontropical sprue, intestinal blind-loop syndrome, and adult celiac disease.

(3) **Inadequate utilization** of folate in the body can be blocked with **chemotherapy drugs (e.g., methotrexate),** which are folic acid antagonists. In addition to inhibiting tumor growth, chemotherapeutic drugs also produce a megaloblastic anemia.

g. **Diagnosis of a folate deficiency** is based upon the common clinical symptoms, as well as laboratory results (see Table 4-4).

Table 4-5. Characteristics and Laboratory Profiles of RBC Membrane Disorders

Disorder	Characteristics	Laboratory Profile

Hemolysis	Normocytic/normochromic anemia
	Polychromasia on blood smear
	Normoblasts on blood smear if shift reticulocytosis is present
	Other RBC abnormalities
	Leukocytosis with maturation shift to left if hemolysis is acute
	Spherocytosis
		Increased serum bilirubin
		Decreased serum haptoglobin
		Bone marrow shows normoblastic hyperplasia
		Storage iron and sideroblasts increased
		Possible aplastic crisis
		  reticulocytopenia
		  erythroid hypoplasia
		Possible hemolytic anemia
		  reticulocytosis
		  erythroid hyperplasia

Hereditary spherocytosis	Spherocytic RBCs
	  intrinsically defective
	  smaller diameter
	  no central pallor
	Defect in spectrin
	Splenomegaly
		Osmotic fragility test increased
		MCHC increased

Hereditary elliptocytosis	Splenomegaly Few spherocytes	Osmotic fragility test decreased Abnormal autohemolysis test results
Hereditary pyropoikilocytosis	Microcytosis Marked poikilocytosis and RBC fragmentation Defective spectrin function	Abnormal RBC fragmentation at 45°C–46°C.
Paroxysmal nocturnal hemoglobinuria	Chronic normocytic/normochromic anemia Microcytic/hypochromic	Osmotic fragility test normal Increased autohemolysis

MCHC = mean corpuscular hemoglobin concentration; RBCs = red blood cells.

F. Survival disorders: hemolytic anemias

1. **Common laboratory characteristics of hemolysis.** Hemolysis occurs whenever there is **increased RBC destruction and shortened cell survival.** In general, all hemolytic anemias can be categorized into one of two groups (see Figure 4-5).

   a. **Intrinsic hemolytic anemias** are usually **hereditary** and occur from **defects in the RBC membrane, metabolism, or the Hb molecule.**

   b. **Extrinsic hemolytic anemias** represent the RBC survival disorders that are **acquired** and occur secondary to a primary condition or stimulus.

2. **Hemolysis caused by RBC membrane disorders.** The common clinical and laboratory characteristics of these disorders are given in Table 4-5.

   a. **Hereditary spherocytosis (HS)** is an autosomal dominant condition that exhibits a moderate-to-severe anemia.

      (1) **Cause. Splenomegaly** is the cause of the shortened RBC survival. The chronic hemolytic anemia is often corrected by splenectomy. HS is caused by a **defect in spectrin,** which is an RBC peripheral protein.

      (2) Laboratory tests useful in the diagnosis of HS include:

        (a) Blood smear with spherocytes

        (b) Osmotic fragility test

        (c) Autohemolysis test

  b. Hereditary eliptocytosis (HE) is an autosomal dominant condition that results in a defect of **spectrin** assembly during the formation of the RBC skeletal lattice.

    (1) Elliptocytes are abundant and often represent more than 25% of the RBC population.

    (2) Of all patients who have HE, 90% are nonanemic. The other 10% of patients have a mild-to-moderate hemolytic anemia.

  c. Hereditary pyropoikilocytosis (HPP) is an autosomal recessive, severe hemolytic anemia that **occurs rarely in blacks.** HPP is also thought to **involve defective spectrin function.**

  d. Hereditary stomatocytosis results in a mild-to-moderate hemolytic anemia.

    (1) Stomatocytes are RBCs that, on an air-dried blood film, have a slit-shaped central pallor rather than a circular central pallor.

    (2) Stomatocyte forms are not as flexible as the normal biconcave disk-shaped RBC, and they have a shortened survival time.

  e. Paroxysmal nocturnal hemoglobinuria (PNH) occurs more frequently in young adults as an **acquired intrinsic defect of the RBC membrane.** The defect renders the **RBCs hypersensitive to complement C3 binding,** and therefore, hemolysis.

    (1) PNH is characterized by **chronic intravascular hemolysis,** with or without hemoglobinuria.

    (2) Hemosiderinuria is also present. If excessive, it can lead to a serious iron loss.

    (3) Two or three different populations of RBCs with different degrees of complement sensitivity are present.

    (4) Platelets and neutrophils may also be hypersensitive to complement, and therefore **low in count.**

    (5) Laboratory tests useful in the diagnosis of PNH include the following:

      (a) The sucrose hemolysis test (i.e., sugar-water test) is based on the principle that sucrose provides a medium of low ionic strength and promotes the binding of complement to RBCs. **Patients who have PNH demonstrate a higher degree of hemolysis with this procedure.**

      (b) The acidified serum test (i.e., Ham test) is based on the principle that acidified serum activates complement by the alternate pathway. **Patients who have PNH demonstrate a higher degree of hemolysis with this procedure.**

3. Hemolysis caused by RBC metabolic disorders

  a. Glucose-6-phosphate dehydrogenase (G6PD) deficiencies are inherited as a sex-linked trait. Anemia caused by a G6PD deficiency is found in all races, but the highest incidence is among **African and Mediterranean cultures.**

(1) **Two genetic isoenzyme variations** of G6PD have been identified. These subtypes are **Type A and Type B, depending on their electrophoretic mobility.**

    (a) **Type A.** Approximately 10% of blacks who have Type A isoenzyme have an inherited deficiency that results in only 10%–15% G6PD enzyme activity. These individuals have **clinically mild conditions** but can be affected by oxidants to produce a hemolytic crisis.

    (b) **Type B.** Persons of Mediterranean descent who have a G6PD deficiency more commonly have a Type B deficiency. Patients who have a Type B deficiency have an enzyme activity of only 1%. These patients are **more susceptible to severe oxidant hemolysis** than are Type A individuals.

    (c) **Favism.** A subgroup of G6PD–deficient patients have severe life-threatening hemolysis that occurs within hours after eating **fava beans.**

(2) **Cause.** Nicotinamide-adenine dinucleotide phosphate reduction (NADPH) in the RBC is linked to **glutathione** (GSH) **reduction.** GSH is a vital reducer of oxidants, such as hydrogen peroxide. This metabolic pathway preserves vital enzymes and Hb. A deficiency of G6PD limits the regeneration of NADPH, and therefore GSH. Lack of GSH renders the RBC vulnerable to the oxidative degeneration of Hb.

    (a) G6PD is normally highest in young RBCs and decreases as the cell ages; therefore, the older RBCs are preferentially destroyed.

    (b) **Oxidized Hb denatures and precipitates intracellularly as Heinz bodies,** which adhere to the membrane and thus cause rigidity, a tendency to lyse, and splenic trapping.

    (c) A patient's susceptibility to hemolytic crisis can greatly increase with an illness or exposure to drugs that have oxidant properties.

    (d) Patients who have G6PD deficiency have a moderate-to-severe hemolytic anemia and a **high incidence of Heinz bodies** in their RBCs. **Laboratory tests** useful in the diagnosis of G6PD deficiency are given in Table 4-6.

b. Pyruvate kinase (PK) deficiency is a rare, autosomal recessive condition.

(1) **Cause.** The enzyme PK catalyzes the conversion of phosphophenol-pyruvate to pyruvate in the Embden-Meyerhof pathway, with the production of adenosine triphosphate (ATP). As a result of the decrease in ATP needed to maintain RBC membrane stability and flexibility, this deficiency results in a mild-to-moderate hemolytic anemia. The RBC loses its flexibility, and splenic trapping and removal of the RBC ensues. Patients who have PK deficiency may not have any observable RBC abnormalities until after splenectomy.

(2) **Laboratory tests** useful in the diagnosis of PK deficiency are given in Table 4-6.

4. Acquired extrinsic hemolysis

    a. Causes. Physical forces can destroy the shape of the normal RBC and result in fragmentation.

Table 4-6. Laboratory Tests Useful for Diagnosing Hemolysis Caused by Metabolic Disorders

Deficiency	Laboratory Test	Principle
G6PD deficiency	Methyl violet or crystal violet stains	Heinz bodies stain
	Dye reduction test	G6P, NADP, and brilliant cresyl blue dye mixture is incubated; if G6PD is present in hemolysate, NADP will be oxidized, and blue dye will change color
	Ascorbate cyanide test	Hemoglobin is oxidized to Hb M by ascorbate more rapidly in G6PD–deficient patients because they lack GSH
	Fluorescent spot test	A drop of G6P and NADP is placed on filter paper with patient's hemolysate; if G6PD is present, NADP is oxidized to NADPH, which fluoresces with UV light
	Quantitative assay of G6PD	Rate of reduction of NADP to NADPH can be measured spectrophotometrically at 340 nm
PK deficiency	Fluorescent spot test	RBCs with PK activity reduce any NADH to nonfluorescent NAD; if fluorescence persists, PK deficiency is indicated
	Quantitative assay for PK	Same principle as for G6PD; rate of decrease is measured at 340 nm

G6P = glucose-6-phosphate; G6PD = glucose-6-phosphate dehydrogenase; GSH = reduced glutathione; Hb M = hemoglobin M; NAD = nicotinamide adenine dinucleotide; NADH = reduced nicotinamide adenine dinucleotide; NADP = nicotinamide adenine dinucleotide phosphate; NADPH = reduced nicotinamide adenine dinucleotide phosphate; PK = pyruvate kinase; RBCs = red blood cells; UV = ultraviolet.

> **(1) Heat from extensive burns** results in a hemolytic anemia with RBC fragments.
> **(2) Cardiovascular disease and prostheses** can produce hemolysis due to mechanical damage of RBCs.

b. Microangiopathic hemolytic anemia with moderate RBC fragmentation can result as a secondary manifestation of the following conditions:

> **(1)** Chronic hypertension
> **(2)** Thrombotic thrombocytopenic purpura
> **(3)** Disseminated carcinoma
> **(4)** DIC

c. Immune hemolytic anemias result from immunoglobulin binding to the RBC membrane and splenic removal of the cells.

> **(1) Autoimmune hemolytic anemia (AIHA)** presents a hematologic picture of a hemolytic anemia **with a positive direct antiglobulin test** (i.e., Coombs' test).
>> **(a)** AIHA can be associated with **warm antibodies.** These immunoglobulins are usually **immunoglobulin G (IgG) autoantibodies**

directed against Rh antigens that demonstrate maximum RBC binding at 37°C.
- **(b)** AIHA associated with **cold antibodies** are most often **immunoglobulin M (IgM)** autoantibodies that react most strongly at or below 25°C.
  - **(i)** Cold hemagglutinin disease involves **complement-fixing autoantibodies against the I antigen.**
  - **(ii)** **Paroxysmal cold hemoglobinuria** is most often caused by a complement-fixing **IgG** autoantibody **directed against the P antigen.**
- **(2)** **Isoimmune hemolytic anemia** is caused by an immune response to a foreign antigen. An example is **hemolytic disease of the newborn (HDN),** which is caused by Rh or ABO incompatibility between mother and fetus.
- **(3)** **Drug-induced immune hemolytic anemias** are caused by the adsorption of drug-stimulated immune complexes to RBC membranes.
  - **(a)** The drug-induced antibody fixes complement that binds to the RBC membranes, which results in lysis.
  - **(b)** Drugs such as penicillin or cephalosporin can act as haptens, inducing an immune response when they attach to the RBC membrane.

5. Anemia of blood loss
- **a.** **Acute posthemorrhagic anemia,** caused by a sudden blood loss, first results in early hypovolemia without any signs of anemia.
  - **(1)** After approximately 24 hours, blood volume is returned to normal to maintain blood pressure. Fluid from tissues move into the circulation, increasing the plasma volume. When a systemic fluid shift occurs, anemia becomes evident.
  - **(2)** **Hematologic changes** seen with acute blood loss include the following:
    - **(a)** The earliest change is a **brief thrombocytopenia,** which soon returns to normal.
    - **(b)** A **moderate leukocytosis** with a shift to the left occurs for the first few days after hemorrhage.
    - **(c)** Hb and Hct do not decline until plasma volume is increased by inward movement of fluid.
    - **(d)** After 2–3 days, normocytic-normochromic anemia occurs with minimum anisocytosis and poikilocytosis.
    - **(e)** Increased erythropoietin release results in a **reticulocytosis** after 3–5 days and peaks at approximately 10 days after hemorrhage. With reticulocytosis, the anemia **may be macrocytic with polychromasia caused by shift reticulocytosis.**
- **b.** **Chronic posthemorrhagic anemia** is caused by slow, sustained blood loss (e.g., GI bleeding).
  - **(1)** The **reticulocyte count may be normal** or only slightly increased.
  - **(2)** The anemia that develops is one of iron deficiency and presents as a **microcytic-hypochromic anemia.**
  - **(3)** The **WBC count is normal or slightly decreased.**
  - **(4)** **Thrombocytosis** is common until iron deficiency is severe.

IV. LEUKOCYTE DISORDERS

A. Blood film white cell morphology and differential

1. **Staining the blood film**

   a. **Blood dyes** are of two general types: methylene blue and eosin. Cell structures are stained by either one or a combination of both dyes.

   (1) **Methylene blue** is known as a **basic stain.**

   (a) **WBC nuclei, cytoplasmic RNA, and platelets** are stained by basic stains.

   (b) Staining of cell structures with methylene blue is known as **basophilic staining.**

   (2) **Eosin** is known as an **acid stain. Hb** and other cytoplasmic cellular organelles are stained by eosin. Cell structures that take up acid stains are known as **acidophilic or eosinophilic.**

   b. **Wright's stain** is most commonly used for routine blood film staining. It contains both basic dyes and acid stains.

   (1) A good staining reaction is **pH dependent (i.e., 6.4–6.7). A properly stained blood smear** should demonstrate the following characteristics:

   (a) RBCs should be pink or a light red.

   (b) Color should be uniform.

   (c) Nuclei of WBCs should stain blue to dark purple.

   (d) Platelets should be clearly visible.

   (2) **Excessive basophilia** results from **overstaining** with the methylene blue portion of Wright's stain. The RBCs appear light blue. Basophilia can result from the following errors in staining technique:

   (a) Blood film **too thick**

   (b) **Prolonged staining** time

   (c) **Inadequate washing**

   (d) **Excessive alkalinity** of stain or buffer

   (3) **Excessive acidophilia** results from overstaining with the eosin component of Wright's stain. RBCs will stain bright red or orange, and the WBC nuclear material will appear pale blue. Acidophilia can result from the following errors in technique:

   (a) **Insufficient staining** time

   (b) **Prolonged washing** time

   (c) **Excessive acidity** of the stain or buffer

B. Phagocyte function and kinetics

1. **Leukocyte maturation** (Tables 4-7 and 4-8). The morphology of myeloid (i.e., granulocyte) maturation is important to know for differentiating and visually identifying cells of each maturation stage.

   a. **Myeloblasts** are the earliest recognizable stage of myeloid maturation.

   b. **Promyelocytes** are the second stage following one or more mitotic divisions of myeloblasts.

   c. The **myelocyte** stage of maturation begins with the appearance of a new type of granulocyte-specific granule. These granules (secondary granules) give the mature granulocyte its characteristic appearance and functional

Table 4-7. Morphology of Granulocyte Maturation

Stage	Cell Size	N-C Ratio	Nucleus Shape	Nucleus Chromatin	Nucleus Nucleoli	Cytoplasm Staining	Cytoplasm Granules	Normal Range in Peripheral Blood
Myeloblast	10–18 μm	4 : 1	Round and centralized	Smooth	2–5 obvious	Deeply basophilic	None	None
Promyelocyte	12–20 μm	2 : 1	Variable shape; centralized	Begins to condense	Still visible	Basophilic	Many azurophilic	None
Myelocyte	12–18 μm	1 : 1	Round or elongated, often eccentric	Slightly condensed	Faint	Mixture of basophilic and acidophilic staining	First appearance of secondary granules; could also be eosinophilic or basophilic granules	None
Metamyelocyte	12–15 μm	1 : 1	Indented, kidney-shaped	Slightly condensed	None	Beige or salmon staining	Many	None
Neutrophil band	12–13 μm	1 : 1–1 : 2	Uniform or elongated, U-shaped	Condensed	None	Beige or salmon staining	Faint	0%–6% or 0–700/mm^3
Segmented neutrophil	10–14 μm	1 : 2	2–4 lobes	Highly condensed	None	Beige or salmon staining	Faint	50%–75% or 2700–7000/mm^3
Eosinophil	12–15 μm	1 : 2	2–3 lobes	Condensed	None	Beige or salmon staining	Many large, round, orange granules	0%–4% or 0–450/mm^3
Basophil	12–15 μm	1 : 2	2–3 lobes	Condensed	None	Beige or salmon staining	Many large, round, purple granules	0%–2% or 0–200/mm^3

Table 4-8. Morphology of Monocyte Maturation

| Stage | Cell Size | N-C Ratio | Nucleus | | | Cytoplasm | | Normal Range in Peripheral Blood |
			Shape	Chromatin	Nucleoli	Staining	Granules	
Monoblast	12–20 μm	4:1	Round with folding and clefting	Smooth	1–2 obvious	Deeply basophilic	None	None
Promonocyte	15–20 μm	3:1	Oval, indented, or folded	Delicate	Faint	Basophilic with a frosted appearance	Few	None
Monocyte	14–20 μm	2:1–1:1	Variable	Slightly condensed	Obscure	Blue-gray with a frosted appearance; often vacuolated	Few	3%–7% or 120–800/mm^3

destiny. Therefore, the maturation of the myelocyte, which is based on granule type, **gives rise to neutrophils, eosinophils, or basophils.**

  (1) **Metamyelocytes** emerge after several mitotic divisions of the myelocytes.

  (2) The **band neutrophil** stage is reached after the round metamyelocyte nucleus flattens.

  (3) The final stage of **a segmented neutrophil** reaches full maturity once the band nucleus pinches off into segments.

2. **Function of granulocytes and monocytes**

  a. **Phagocytic function** involves the following general steps:

     (1) Increase in cell numbers at the infected site
     (2) Cell attachment to the foreign or dead material
     (3) **Engulfment of** foreign or dead material
     (4) **Dissolving of** foreign or dead material
     (5) **Disposition** of catabolic components

  b. **Granulocytes are the first line of defense against microbial organisms.**

     (1) **Neutrophil migration** is directed by **infections** or **inflamed tissue.**

        (a) Tissue injury results in the release of **vasoactive** and **chemotactic factors.**

           (i) **Vasoactive factors,** such as **prostaglandins** and **leukotrienes,** increase capillary permeability and induce local migration.

           (ii) **Chemotactic factors** direct the migration of neutrophils to a localized area of inflammation. Well-known chemotactic factors are activated complement C3b and C5a, lymphocyte secretions, and bacterial products, such as endotoxins or bradykinin.

        (b) Neutrophils have **receptors for the crystallizable fragment (Fc) portion of IgG and C3,** which bind to the coated microorganism and phagocytize.

        (c) **Degranulation.** Engulfed material is covered by internalized surface membrane, which forms a **phagosome.** Degranulation is the process by which activated lysosomal granules become attached to the phagosome and empty their hydrolytic enzymes into the phagosome, killing and dissolving their contents.

        (d) **Bacterial killing** occurs in the phagosome by processes that are either oxygen-dependent or oxygen-independent.

           (i) **Oxygen-dependent** bacterial killing in the phagosome results from the reduction of oxygen to a superoxide radical ($O^{\bullet}$) in the presence of an oxidase enzyme.

           (ii) Oxygen radicals bind with hydrogen to yield hydrogen peroxide (i.e., H_2O_2).

           (iii) Hydrogen peroxide, with the help of chloride and iodine ions and the enzyme **myeloperoxidase,** dissolve the bacterial membrane. The whole process is known as **peroxidation** (Figure 4-6).

           (iv) **Oxygen-independent killing** is accomplished by hydrogen ions, lysozymes, and bactericidal proteins.

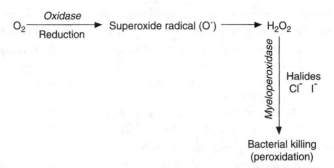

Figure 4-6. The process of peroxidation. Cl^- = chloride ions; H_2O_2 = hydrogen peroxide; I^- = iodine ion.

(v) Chronic granulomatous disease (CGD) is a fatal disorder seen in male children that results from a defect in the oxygen-dependent peroxidation pathway. The **nitroblue tetrazolium (NBT) test** can be used to test for leukocyte bactericidal effectiveness and to diagnose CGD.

(2) Eosinophils increase in circulating numbers in response to an immunologic stimuli mediated by T lymphocytes. Eosinophils decrease in number in the blood and migrate into tissue when the level of adrenocorticotropic hormone (ACTH) increases.

(a) Eosinophils **phagocytize foreign particles** and **antigen-antibody complexes,** but this is not their main function.

(b) Eosinophils may **modulate reactions** that occur when tissue mast cells and basophils degranulate.

(c) Eosinophils provide some **defense against helminthic parasites.**

(d) Eosinophils **have a role in allergic reactions** by lessening hypersensitivity reactions through the release of an **amine oxidase, which neutralizes histamine.**

(3) Basophils and mast cells (i.e., tissue-based basophils) are full of **granules that contain histamine, heparin, and peroxidase.**

(a) These cells synthesize and store histamine and **eosinophil chemotactic factor of anaphylaxis (ECF-A).**

(b) Basophils synthesize and release (when stimulated) substances known as **slow-reacting substance of anaphylaxis (SRS-A) and platelet activating factor (PAF).**

(c) Basophils are involved in **hypersensitivity reactions,** such as allergic asthma and delayed-onset allergy reactions.

(d) Immunoglobulin E (IgE) binds to basophil or mast cell membranes.

(i) When a specific antigen reacts with the membrane-bound IgE, degranulation occurs, with the release of mediators of hypersensitivity (e.g., histamine, SRS-A, PAF, heparin, ECF-A).

(ii) ECF-A leads to an accumulation of eosinophils at the site of inflammation, which acts to counteract and balance the mediators of inflammation.

(e) Basophils are also involved in **delayed hypersensitivity** reactions, such as contact allergies.

c. Monocytes and macrophages
  (1) The monocyte migrates into the tissue, where it is transformed into a macrophage (i.e., histiocyte).
  (2) Some macrophages are motile and respond to chemotactic factors and factors from activated lymphocytes. Other macrophages are tissue-based, such as **Kupffer's cells or alveolar macrophages.**
  (3) Monocytes become immobilized by **migration inhibiting factor** (MIF), which is released from activated lymphocytes.
  (4) Monocytes and macrophages become activated to phagocytize by complement, prostaglandins, or previously phagocytized material.
  (5) Functions. Monocytes and macrophages are highly versatile cells that perform many vital functions, including:
    (a) A defense against microorganisms such as mycobacterium, fungi, bacteria, protozoa, and viruses
    (b) A role in the **antigen-induced blast transformation of lymphocytes**
      (i) Monocytes secrete **interleukin-1 (IL-1),** which activates helper T cells.
      (ii) Monocytes physically **present and deliver the antigen to the specific membrane surface receptor sites.**
    (c) A major role in the **daily destruction of aged blood cells, denatured plasma proteins, and lipids**
    (d) Heme oxidase activity, which enables some tissue macrophages to break down RBC Hb and recycle it [see III C 3 a (3)].

3. **Granulopoiesis** is controlled by glycoproteins isolated from lymphocytes and monocytes. These glycoproteins are known as **interleukins (IL) and monokines,** respectively. Because most research in this area was done on bone marrow cultures, these growth stimulators are also known as **colony stimulating factors (CSF).**
  a. Multi-CSF (i.e., IL-3) production is stimulated by **endotoxin** released from infection.
    (1) Source. IL-3 is secreted by marrow fibroblasts, T lymphocytes, macrophages, and monocytes.
    (2) Function. IL-3 stimulates regeneration, maturation, and differentiation of multipotential and unipotential stem cells.
  b. Granulocyte/monocyte colony stimulating factor (GM-CSF) is important for myeloid maturation in the marrow.
    (1) Source. GM-CSF is secreted by T lymphocytes, marrow fibroblasts, marrow endothelial cells, and monocytes.
    (2) Function. GM-CSF stimulates neutrophil, eosinophil, and monocyte growth.
  c. Granulocyte colony stimulating factor (G-CSF) is a more specific granulocyte growth factor.
    (1) Source. G-CSF is secreted by monocytes, marrow fibroblasts, and endothelial cells.
    (2) Function. G-CSF stimulates the growth of neutrophils and enhances the functional response of neutrophils.

    d. Monocyte/macrophage colony stimulating factor (M-CSF), also known as CSF-1, is the primary monocytic growth factor.
      (1) Source. M-CSF is secreted by mature monocytes, marrow fibroblasts, and marrow endothelial cells.
      (2) Function. M-CSF stimulates macrophages and the release of G-CSF from monocytes. This monocytic growth factor also stimulates the release of tumor necrosis factor, interferon, and IL-1 from macrophages.

C. Quantitative and qualitative leukocyte abnormalities (Figure 4-7)
  1. Nonpathologic factors that affect WBC counts
    a. The age of the patient must be taken into account. At birth, the normal average WBC count is 18,000/mm^3.
    b. The patient's basal condition must be taken into account.
      (1) The WBC count is **lowest at complete physical and mental relaxation.**
      (2) Exercise increases the WBC count.
    c. Physiologic conditions other than disease can affect the WBC count. Convulsions, electric shock, and pregnancy can **lower** the WBC count.

  2. Quantitative abnormalities of leukocytes
    a. Granulocytopenia occurs with a **reduction of the absolute count to lower than 3000/mm^3. Neutropenia** results from the following **physiologic mechanisms:**
      (1) Decreased flow of neutrophils from marrow caused by decreased or ineffective production (see Figure 4-7)
      (2) Increased removal of neutrophils from the blood (i.e., decreased survival; see Figure 4-7)
      (3) Altered distribution between the circulating leukocyte pool (CLP) and the marginal leukocyte pool (MLP)
      (4) Combination of the aforementioned mechanisms
    b. Eosinopenia is hard to detect unless a manual count is performed. Eosinopenia can result from the following conditions:
      (1) Acute stress
      (2) ACTH and epinephrine secretion (e.g., Cushing's syndrome)
      (3) Acute inflammatory or infectious states (i.e., shift of WBCs into the MLP and migration into inflamed tissue)
    c. Granulocytosis refers to an absolute increase in the concentration of circulating leukocytes higher than normal for a certain age (i.e., **greater than 11,000/mm^3 in adults;** see Figure 4-7).
      (1) Physiologic neutrophilia
        (a) Granulocytosis results from the following **physiologic mechanisms:**
          (i) Increased rate of inflow of cells into the circulation from the marrow
          (ii) Shift in cells from the MLP into the CLP
          (iii) A decrease in the rate of outflow of cells from the blood

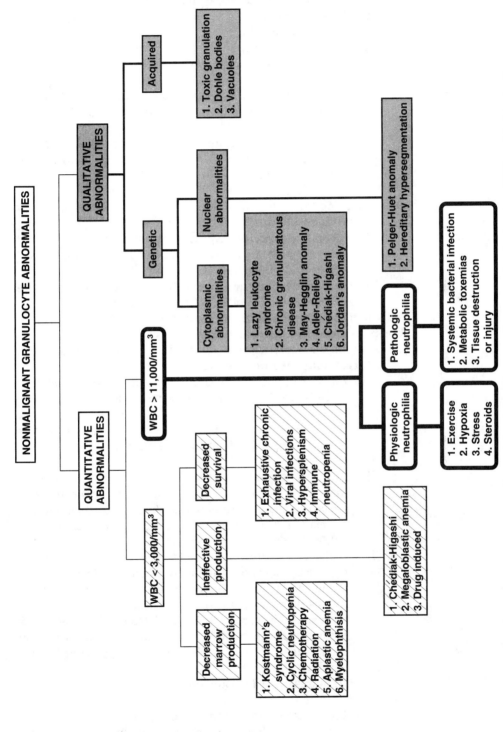

Figure 4-7. Algorithm demonstrating the differential diagnosis of the nonmalignant granulocytic disorders. WBC = white blood cell.

    (b) A **leukemoid reaction is a nonleukemic leukocytosis** with a WBC count greater than 30,000/mm^3.

        (i) This condition is characterized by the lack of myeloblasts in the peripheral blood.

        (ii) A maturation **shift to the left** occurs with increased band forms and few metamyelocytes or myelocytes in the peripheral blood.

        (iii) The **LAP level will be increased,** which is a distinguishing factor as compared with a leukemic granulocytosis (see V D 5 e (1) (c)).

        (iv) Leukemoid reactions are seen most **commonly in children who have infections** (e.g., pneumonia, meningitis, tuberculosis) and also in cases of severe hemolysis or metastatic cancer.

    (c) **Physiologic leukocytosis** is produced by factors that do not involve tissue damage.

        (i) Excessive exercise, hypoxia, or stress can cause a shift from the MLP into the CLP, which appears as an increased peripheral WBC count.

        (ii) **Increased outflow of cells from the marrow into the blood** increases both the CLP and the MLP.

(2) **Pathologic neutrophilia** results from disease, and is usually in response to tissue damage from a chronic infection.

    (a) Three physiologic phases of shifting WBC counts can be observed in **acute and chronic infections.**

        (i) **Phase I in early infection** results in the acute migration of cells from the MLP into tissue releasing chemotactic factor. Because the CLP and the MLP are in equilibrium, a **transient neutropenia** results. Myeloid growth factors are also released to stimulate the marrow to increase production.

        (ii) **Phase II is related to established chronic and severe infections** when the marrow supply slowly rises to the increased demand and increases the flow of cells into the circulation. This results in a **neutrophilia,** a shift to the left, and a decrease in eosinophils.

        (iii) **Phase III is related either to recovery from the infection or to marrow exhaustion** when the infection begins to subside, and the fever breaks. The total number of granulocytes decreases, and **the total number of monocytes increases** (i.e., secondary line of defense). If recovery does not occur, the marrow becomes depleted, and production cannot keep up with granulocyte loss. A **granulocytopenia results.**

    (b) **Miscellaneous disorders and conditions** associated with neutrophilia include the following:

        (i) **Toxic factors** that produce neutrophilia can be classified as either metabolic diseases (e.g., uremia, gout, diabetic acidosis) or as **drugs and chemicals** (e.g., lead, mercury, digitalis, epinephrine, ACTH).

(ii) **Tissue destruction or necrosis** involving a large amount of tissue can cause neutrophilia (e.g., myocardial infarction, burns, surgery, crush injuries, fractures).

(iii) **Hemorrhage,** if significant, can result in neutrophilia.

(iv) Acute massive **hemolysis** can increase the CLP.

(v) Hematologic disorders such as **myeloproliferative disorders** are associated with an absolute neutrophilia.

(3) **Eosinophilia** is clinically defined as an absolute eosinophil count higher than **400/mm³** in the peripheral blood. Disorders and conditions that demonstrate eosinophilia include the following:

(a) **Allergic diseases**

(b) **Skin disorders**

(c) **Parasitic infections** (e.g., trichinosis)

(d) **Infectious diseases** (e.g., scarlet fever with skin rash)

(e) **Pulmonary eosinophilias** (e.g., Löffler's syndrome)

(f) **Blood diseases** such as chronic myelogenous leukemia (CML) and other myeloproliferative disorders

(g) **Splenectomy**

(h) **Various drugs** (e.g., pilocarpine, digitalis)

(4) **Basophilia** is defined as an absolute basophil count higher than **40/mm³** in the peripheral blood. Basophilias have causes similar to eosinophilias.

(5) **Monocytosis** is defined as an absolute monocyte count higher than **800/mm³**. Monocytosis is commonly observed during the **recovery phase of infections and in various myeloproliferative diseases.**

3. Persons who have **qualitative leukocyte abnormalities** demonstrate a decreased resistance to infection, despite normal leukocyte counts.

a. **Lazy leukocyte syndrome** is a rare inherited condition seen in children. **Granulocytes do not respond to chemotactic factors;** therefore, they fail to accumulate at the inflamed tissue.

b. **CGD** is a qualitative disorder in which the granulocytes are capable of phagocytosis and degranulation [see IV B 2 b (1) (c)] but are **incapable of the subsequent bacterial killing process.**

(1) Lysozymes have lost their bactericidal properties due to a **decrease in the production of H_2O_2.**

(2) Granulocytes in this disorder, when stained with NBT, demonstrate a **weak staining** of **less than 10%** of the blood granulocytes.

(3) The disorder is clinically characterized by frequent infections, enlarged spleen and liver, lymphadenitis, and **granulomas** (i.e., aggregates of mononuclear cells) in many organs.

c. **Congenital and acquired qualitative disorders of neutrophils** can affect either the cytoplasm or the nucleus.

(1) Qualitative disorders affecting the **neutrophil cytoplasm** include the following:

(a) **Toxic granulation** appears as tiny, dark blue-to-purple cytoplasmic granules in the metamyelocyte, band, or segmented neutrophil stages.

(i) These granules are **peroxidase positive.**

(ii) They are most commonly **found in severe infections or other toxic conditions.**

(iii) Toxic granules are actually **azurophil granules** (i.e., secondary granules) that have retained their basophilic staining qualities because of lack of maturation or **skipped maturation divisions during accelerated granulopoiesis.**

(iv) **Cytoplasmic vacuoles** are also signs of toxic change.

(b) **Döhle's inclusion bodies** are small, oval inclusions in the peripheral cytoplasm of neutrophils that stain pale blue with Wright's stain.

(i) Döhle's bodies are **remnants of RNA and free ribosomes or** rough endoplasmic reticulum.

(ii) These cytoplasmic inclusions stain **positive** with the **periodic acid-Schiff (PAS)** cytochemical stain.

(iii) The appearance of Döhle's bodies is often associated with **scarlet fever,** and these inclusion bodies are occasionally seen in patients who have **burns; infectious diseases** (i.e., often with toxic granulation); **aplastic anemia;** and following **exposure to toxic chemicals.**

(c) **May-Hegglin anomaly** is a rare, autosomal dominant, qualitative leukocyte abnormality.

(i) The granulocytes of patients who have this disorder demonstrate pale blue inclusions that are larger and more prominent than the Döhle's bodies found with infections.

(ii) Compared with Döhle's bodies occurring secondary to chronic infection, the cytoplasmic inclusions in May-Hegglin anomaly are **PAS negative.**

(iii) Cytoplasmic inclusions result from structural RNA alterations.

(iv) Inclusions have been found in eosinophils, basophils, and monocytes, as well as neutrophils.

(v) Patients are seen to have a mild **thrombocytopenia, giant platelets,** and a slight bleeding tendency.

(d) **Alder-Reilly anomaly** is a genetic abnormality that results in **dense azurophilic granulation in all types of leukocytes.**

(i) Cytoplasmic granulation is not transient or related to an infectious disease, as it is with toxic granulation.

(ii) Granulation results from an abnormal deposition and storage of mucopolysaccharides.

(e) **Chédiak-Steinbrinck-Higashi anomaly** is an autosomal recessive disorder that results in qualitative abnormalities in all types of leukocytes.

(i) Large, coarse, irregular **lysosome granules are found in the cytoplasm of granulocytes and monocytes.**

(ii) Patients also demonstrate abnormal pigmentation, neuropathies, photophobia, and recurrent infections.

(iii) Leukocytes of both the blood and bone marrow are affected.

(f) **Jordan's anomaly** is a genetic qualitative disorder in which abundant **sudanophilic inclusions** (i.e., lipid) are found in the cytoplasm of granulocytes, lymphocytes, and plasma cells in the blood and marrow.

(2) Qualitative disorders affecting the **neutrophil nucleus** include the following:

(a) Pelger-Huët anomaly is an autosomal dominant condition in which there is a **failure of normal segmentation** of neutrophil nuclei.

  (i) Most nuclei are band-shaped, have two segments, or are peanut-shaped.

  (ii) The nuclear chromatin of these cells is coarse and clumped beyond the degree of clumping found in normal immature band forms.

(b) Hereditary hypersegmentation of neutrophils is a disorder in which the majority of the patient's neutrophils have four or more lobes. This disorder must be differentiated from the hypersegmentation of megaloblastic anemia.

d. Monocyte-macrophage qualitative abnormalities are rare, autosomal recessive **lipid-storage diseases.**

  (1) Common characteristics

  (a) There is a deficiency in one of the catabolic enzymes involved in the breakdown of **sphingolipids.**

  (b) Because macrophages play an important role in the catabolism of lipid-rich membranes, they can accumulate undegraded lipid products in their cytoplasm. This leads to the production of lipid-heavy and blocked **foamy macrophages,** which stimulate further macrophage production and result in an expansion of the monocyte-macrophage system.

  (2) Gaucher's disease is a genetic disorder that results in the **accumulation of glycosphingolipids** in the cytoplasm of monocytes and macrophages.

  (a) There is a **deficiency of β-glucosidase,** which is the enzyme that splits glucose from sphingolipids.

  (b) Macrophages and monocytes in this disease are PAS positive because of accumulated cytoplasmic carbohydrate (i.e., monocytes are normally weakly positive to negative for PAS).

  (c) Macrophage cytoplasm has a pale onion-skin appearance (i.e., Gaucher's cells).

  (3) Niemann-Pick disease is a similar disorder in which there is a deficiency in the enzyme that cleaves phosphoryl choline from sphingolipids. Macrophages and monocytes have a **"foam-cell"** appearance but are **PAS negative.**

D. Leukemias and cytochemical stains

  1. Common characteristics of leukemias

  a. Incidence. Leukemia is a relatively **common disorder** with approximately seven new cases per 100,000 population reported annually in the United States.

  b. Definition. Leukemia can be defined as a generalized abnormal neoplastic proliferation or accumulation of hemopoietic cells in the bone marrow, organs, and the peripheral blood.

c. **Clinical classifications**

(1) **Acute leukemias** are refractory to remission, usually fatal within 3 months, and demonstrate a bone marrow **packed with primitive cells (i.e., blasts)** of the cell type involved, with little differentiation.

(2) **Subacute leukemias** have a longer patient survival of 3–12 months, and usually have a clinical picture of an acute leukemia.

(3) **Chronic leukemias** are defined as having a survival of greater than 1 year if no remission occurs. Blasts are elevated in marrow and blood but are usually less than 5%. Maturation within a cell line still occurs.

d. **Cytologic classifications** are **myeloid or lymphoid.**

e. **Common laboratory results** include the following:

(1) **Anemia** (i.e., present in more than 90% of leukemia patients)

(2) **Leukocytosis**

(a) Almost 30% of leukemic patients demonstrate normal or decreased WBC counts (i.e., aleukemic leukemia).

(b) Approximately 20% of leukemic patients have WBC counts higher than 100,000/mm^3.

(c) The remainder of leukemic patients have elevated counts lower than 100,000/mm^3.

(3) **Thrombocytopenia** (present in 80% of leukemic patients)

(4) **Basophilia** in the peripheral blood and bone marrow

(5) **Immature precursor or blast cells** in the peripheral blood and marrow

(6) **NRBCs in the peripheral blood**

(7) **Decrease in the LAP level**

(8) Nonhematologic clues such as an elevation in **serum uric acid, lactate dehydrogenase, and vitamin B$_{12}$ levels or B$_{12}$-binding capacity** (i.e., due to increased amounts of **transcobalamin I** produced by neutrophils)

2. **Cytochemical stains** are useful diagnostic tools (Table 4-9). The cytochemical stains help **to differentiate the leukemic blasts** of acute myelogenous leukemia (AML) from leukemias of lymphoid origin. It is difficult to distinguish between leukemias with Wright's stain.

a. The **general principle** of most cytochemical stains is to incubate cells on a blood smear with a substrate that reacts with an intracellular marker (e.g., lipid, lysozyme, glycogen, enzyme). In enzymatic procedures, the reaction product is coupled with a diazonium salt (i.e., dye) to produce a visible reaction product.

b. **Sudan black B and peroxidase** (i.e., myeloperoxidase) cytochemical stains share a common staining pattern.

(1) **Sudan black B stains phospholipids and sterols** (i.e., lipids) in cytoplasmic lysosome and mitochondrial membranes.

(a) Azurophilic and specific neutrophil granules are stained.

(b) **Cytoplasmic granules stain faintly in myeloblast cells and strongly in mature neutrophils.** As the cell matures from the promyelocyte stage to the mature segmented neutrophil, each stage is generally more positive.

Table 4-9. Cytochemical Staining Reactions in Leukemias and Individual Cells

Cells	Sudan B Black	Chloracetate Esterase	α-Naphthyl Acetate Esterase	Periodic Acid Schiff	Acid Phosphatase	Acute Leukemias
Neutrophil	P	P	N	P	WP	AML
Myeloid Precursor	P 2+	P 2+	N (−)	WP +/−	WP +/−	AML
Monocyte	WP +/−	N +/−	P 3+	WP 1+	P 2+	AML-M4 and M5
Lymphocyte	N (−)	N (−)	WP[F] +/−[F]	WP[F] +/−[F]	P[F] +/−[F]	ALL
Normoblast	N (−)	N (−)	N (−)	N 2+[E]	WP[F] +/−[F]	AML-M6

ALL = acute lymphocytic leukemia; AML = acute myelogenous leukemia; AML-M4 = acute myelomonocytic leukemia; AML-M5 = acute monocytic leukemia; AML-M6 = erythroleukemia; [E] = positive in erythroleukemia; [F] = focal positivity; N = negative staining; P = strongly positive staining; WP = weakly positive staining; (−) = leukemia blasts stain negative; +/− = leukemia blasts stain weakly positive; 1+ = a few leukemic blasts stain positive; 2+ = leukemia blasts stain moderately positive; 3+ = leukemia blasts stain strongly positive.

        (c) Eosinophilic granules stain positive.

        (d) Monocytes are generally unstained or weakly positive with a few scattered positively stained cytoplasmic granules.

        (e) Lymphoblasts and lymphocytes are negative.

        (f) Leukemic myeloblasts demonstrate stronger positivity than normal blasts.

        (g) Auer bodies in leukemic myelogenous cells **stain positive.**

    (2) Peroxidase stains only azurophilic granules.

        (a) The stain reacts with the lysosomal enzyme in azurophilic granules to yield a black or brown reaction product.

        (b) Reactions with myeloperoxidase stain are generally the same as that for Sudan black B.

  c. Esterase cytochemical stains include either specific or nonspecific esterase procedures.

    (1) AS-D chloroacetate esterase stain (specific esterase) is more useful in separating monocyte precursors from granulocyte precursors than are the Sudan black B or peroxidase cytochemical stains.

        (a) Neutrophils and neutrophil precursors stain the most strongly positive of all cell lines.

        (b) Generally, **monocytes, lymphocytes, and their precursors stain negative.**

    (2) α-Naphthyl acetate esterase stain (nonspecific esterase) is also useful to differentiate neutrophil precursors from monocytes and their precursors in acute leukemias.

        (a) Monocytes stain strongly positive at all stages of maturity.

The addition of **sodium fluoride** to the incubation solution **inhibits the staining reaction in monocytes but not in granulocytes.**
- **(b)** Megakaryocytes and macrophages stain positive.
- **(c) Granulocytes at all stages of maturation stain negative or only weakly positive.**
- **(d)** Basophils, plasma cells, and T lymphocytes stain positive.

d. PAS is often useful for identifying some lymphocytic leukemias.
- **(1) Periodic acid (HIO$_4$)** is an oxidizing agent that converts hydroxy-groups on adjacent carbon atoms to aldehydes (e.g., carbohydrates).
  - **(a)** The resulting reaction product is red-colored at the site of hydroxy-group conversion.
  - **(b)** A positive reaction is seen in the presence of polysaccharides, mucopolysaccharides, glycoproteins, and other carbohydrates.
  - **(c)** A positive PAS reaction usually **indicates the presence of stored carbohydrates** in the cytoplasm of a cell.
- **(2) Neutrophils** are **positive at most stages of development,** but most strongly in the mature stage. **Myeloblasts are usually weakly positive or negative.**
- **(3)** Eosinophils are positive at all stages of development.
- **(4)** Monocytes are weakly positive in the form of fine granules.
- **(5) Lymphocytes may contain a few positive granules,** but in **lymphocytic leukemias** the malignant lymphocytes may have an **increased number of PAS-positive granules in a focal or blocklike positivity.**
- **(6)** NRBCs are negative, **but stain positive in the abnormal erythroid precursors of erythroleukemia.**
- **(7)** Megakaryocytes stain positive.

e. Acid phosphatase cytochemical staining is useful for confirming a diagnosis of **hairy-cell leukemia** and for differentiating a T-lymphocytic leukemia from a B-lymphocytic leukemia.
- **(1)** Acid phosphatase–containing cytoplasmic granules stain red.
- **(2) Monocytes stain strongly positive.**
- **(3)** Neutrophils and precursors stain positive but less intensely than do monocytes.
- **(4) T lymphocytes stain positive,** but B lymphocytes stain negative.
- **(5)** A variation of this staining procedure calls for the addition of **L-tartaric acid** into the staining reagent. This variation is known as the tartaric acid resistant acid phosphatase stain, or the **TRAP stain.**
  - **(a)** L-tartaric acid used in the staining solution **inhibits the isoenzymes of acid phosphatase,** and therefore results in a negative reaction in most cell types that normally stain positive.
  - **(b)** However, the acid phosphatase isoenzymes in the malignant lymphocytes of **hairy-cell leukemia are not inhibited by the addition of L-tartarate and will still stain positive.**

f. LAP staining is useful for distinguishing a leukemic neutrophilia from a nonleukemic neutrophilia seen with chronic inflammation and infection.

Box 4-4. Kaplow Count

Staining intensity		Number of cells		Score
0	X	45	=	0
1+	X	35	=	35
2+	X	15	=	30
3+	X	3	=	9
4+	X	2	=	8
			Kaplow count:	82

(1) This enzyme is found in neutrophils from the myelocyte stage to the mature segmented neutrophil stage.

(2) The enzyme is detected in its reaction with a naphthyl phosphate in the presence of a diazonium salt (e.g., fast blue or fast violet) at an alkaline pH of 9.5.

(3) After staining, a **Kaplow count is performed.** A total of 100 mature neutrophils are scored from 0 (negative) to 4 (strongly positive), based upon the intensity of the staining reaction. An example of how a count is scored is demonstrated in Box 4-4.

(4) The scores will range from a score of 0–400. Reference values are usually in the range of 20–200, although each hospital usually establishes its own normal range.

    (a) **Increased LAP** activity occurs in the following diseases or conditions:

        (i) Infections

        (ii) Polycythemia vera

        (iii) Hodgkin's disease

        (iv) Myelofibrosis with myeloid metaplasia

        (v) Pregnancy (i.e., last trimester)

    (b) **Decreased activity** occurs in the following diseases:

        (i) CML

        (ii) AML

        (iii) Paroxysmal nocturnal hemoglobinuria

        (iv) Aplastic anemia

        (v) Some viral infections (e.g., infectious mononucleosis)

E. Chronic and acute myeloproliferative disorders (Figure 4-8)

    1. Characteristics. Myeloproliferative disorders are a group of closely related diseases characterized by the **spontaneous proliferation** of erythroid, granulocyte, monocyte, or megakaryocyte precursors in the **marrow.** Some shared general characteristics include the following:

    a. The spleen, liver, and lymph nodes may be involved.

    b. All cell lines or only a single cell line may be involved.

    c. Myeloproliferative disorders are **clonal in origin, having arisen from a single pluripotential hemapoietic stem cell.**

    d. **Cytogenetic abnormalities** are common to most myeloproliferative disorders (Table 4-10).

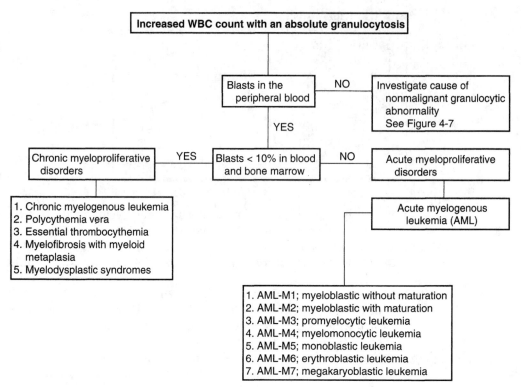

Figure 4-8. Algorithm demonstrating a comparison of acute and chronic myeloproliferative disorders. WBC = white blood cell.

2. **Chronic myeloproliferative disorders** include a group of leukemias that share a common stem cell lesion and are slow in their clinical course.
   a. **CML** occurs mainly in **middle-aged adults** with a **slow and unrevealing** onset of symptoms.

Table 4-10. Common Cytogenetic Abnormalities of Chronic and Acute Myeloproliferative Disorders as Compared to Their Common Monoclonal Immunofluorescent CD Markers

Myeloproliferative Disorder	Cytogenetic Abnormality	CD Marker
CML	Ph[1], t(9:22)	CD11b, CD33
AML-M2	t(8:21)	CD11b, CD33
AML-M3	t(15:17)	CD11b, CD33
AML-M4	16q	CD11b, CD14, CD33
AML-M5	t(9:11)	CD11b, CD14, CD33
MDS	−5, 5q−, −7, 7q−, trisomy 8, and 12 q	No data

AML = acute myelogenous leukemia (subdivided as M1–M7); AML-M4 = acute myelomonocytic leukemia; AML-M5 = acute monocytic leukemia; CD = cluster designation; CML = chronic myelogenous leukemia; MDS = myelodysplastic syndromes; Ph[1] = Philadelphia chromosome.

(1) **Clinical symptoms,** which are mainly caused by the body's increased load of myeloid cells and nutritional demands, include the following:

   (a) Anemia

   (b) Weight loss

   (c) Lack of energy

   (d) Spleen enlargement causing abdominal discomfort

   (e) Fever

   (f) Excessive bleeding or bruising (i.e., due to decreased platelet production)

(2) A patient who has CML typically is seen with the following blood and marrow **laboratory profile:**

   (a) A **WBC count usually higher than 50,000/mm^3 and possibly as high as 300,000/mm^3.**

      (i) CML has a characteristic differential count showing **complete maturation of granulocyte cells** from myeloblasts to segmented neutrophils and a **bimodal distribution,** with myelocytes and segmented neutrophils both exceeding other types in absolute numbers. **Myeloblasts are usually less than 10% in the blood and marrow.**

      (ii) **Basophilia** is almost always present.

      (iii) An absolute **eosinophilia and monocytosis** are also typical.

      (iv) **Normocytic/normochromic anemia** occurs in most cases due to decreased RBC production.

      (v) **Thrombocytosis** is seen in the early phases of the disease, and **thrombocytopenia** occurs in later phases.

      (vi) **NRBCs** on the blood smear are also commonly found.

   (b) **Bone marrow** is **hypercellular** because of granulocyte proliferation with all stages of maturation represented.

      (i) **Myeloid-erythroid ratios of 15:1 to 50:1** are common.

      (ii) Eosinophil and basophil precursors are often increased.

      (iii) **Blasts are increased, but usually less than 10%.**

   (c) **LAP is reduced or absent in more than 90% of CML patients.** In one third of CML patients who are in remission, the LAP level returns to normal.

   (d) **Cytogenetic abnormalities** found in CML are highly diagnostic.

      (i) Direct bone marrow preparations show that **90% of CML patients demonstrate the "Philadelphia" (Ph^1) chromosome.**

      (ii) The mutation results from a **translocation from the long arm of chromosome 22 to an arm of chromosome 9.**

      (iii) The 10% of CML patients who are **Ph^1 negative** have similar laboratory and clinical findings. However, this group is characterized by the following: a **larger proportion of children, not as good a response to therapy, and a shorter survival.**

   (e) Serum levels of vitamin B$_{12}$ and B$_{12}$-binding proteins are increased because of the increased total granulocyte pool.

   (f) Serum uric acid and muramidase are increased.

(3) **CML is treated** with chemotherapeutic agents such as **busulfan,**

which is an alkylating agent, or **hydroxyurea,** which is a folic acid antagonist.

- **(a)** Alkylating agents are thought to combine with guanine in DNA to inhibit rapidly growing cells.
- **(b)** Toxic effects of chemotherapy occur, such as bone marrow depression and bleeding.

(4) Remissions may last from several months to several years. The LAP level returns to normal, and the Ph^1 chromosome usually disappears.

- **(a)** When the patient comes out of remission, the disease changes into a more aggressive and **accelerated phase** characterized by a rising granulocyte count and spleen enlargement.
- **(b)** **When blasts exceed 30% of cells in the marrow or blood, it is known as the blastic phase of the disease, or blast crisis.**

b. Polycythemia vera (PV) is characterized by excessive proliferation of erythroid, granulocytic, and megakaryocytic elements of the marrow, and an increase in circulating RBC mass (see Figure 4-1).

(1) The **neoplasia** is classified as an **absolute primary polycythemia** and differentiated from secondary polycythemia by the hyperproliferation in all cell lines.

(2) A patient who has PV typically presents with the following blood and marrow **laboratory profile:**

- **(a)** The peripheral blood typically has an elevated **RBC count between 6.0 and 12.0 $\times$ 10^6/mm^3.**
  - **(i)** The Hb is elevated between **18 g/dL and 24 g/dL,** and the MCV, MCH, and MCHC are normal to low.
  - **(ii)** Blood smear RBC morphology shows some macrocytes, polychromatic cells, and normoblasts.
  - **(iii)** RBC production is increased, and RBC survival is normal, but RBC survival is reduced if the spleen is enlarged.
  - **(iv)** Oxygen Hb saturation is normal.
  - **(v)** Patients have a **leukocytosis of 10,000–30,000/mm^3,** and the presence of **immature myeloid and erythroid cells** on their peripheral blood smear.
  - **(vi)** **This disorder demonstrates an increased level of LAP.**
  - **(vii)** The serum vitamin B_{12} level and binding capacity are increased.
  - **(viii)** Patients who have PV have **decreased levels of serum and urine EPO.** This can be a diagnostic characteristic, because all **secondary polycythemias are the result of an increased level of EPO.**
- **(b)** Marrow aspirate demonstrates a **hypercellular marrow with all cell lines increased in absolute amounts. Iron storage is decreased or absent.**

(3) Treatment of PV is with one or a combination of the following methods:

- **(a) Phlebotomy**
- **(b) Chemotherapy**
- **(c) Radioisotope phosphorus 32**

    (4) A late **complication of PV** is **acute leukemia,** which is often caused by treatment with alkylating drugs and radiotherapy.

        (a) In 20%–40% of individuals who have PV, progressive **anemia, splenomegaly,** and **further leukocytosis occurs** with more circulating **immature granulocytes, normoblasts,** and **dacryocytes** apparent on blood smears.

        (b) Myelofibrosis in the marrow may increase.

        (c) Many cases of PV evolve into myelofibrosis with myeloid metaplasia (MMM).

  c. MMM is characterized by a **chronic, progressive panmyelosis with varying fibrosis of the marrow.**

    (1) Patients demonstrate a **massive splenomegaly caused by extramedullary hematopoiesis** (i.e., MMM).

    (2) A patient with MMM typically demonstrates the following blood and bone marrow **laboratory profile:**

        (a) The peripheral **blood** shows a moderate normocytic- normochromic **anemia** with some **basophilic stippling.**

           (i) RBC morphology shows moderate **anisocytosis** and **poikilocytosis** (e.g., fragmented forms); **dacryocytes; elliptocytes;** and **NRBCs.**

          (ii) Reticulocytosis is common.

         (iii) The **leukocyte count is normal or slightly increased,** and the differential shows a few **immature granulocytes.**

         (iv) The **LAP level is increased.**

          (v) Platelet counts can be normal or decreased, with the presence of abnormal platelets.

         (vi) The serum uric acid level is increased, but the serum vitamin B_{12} level is usually normal.

        (b) Marrow aspiration is usually "dry" because of the increase in reticulin fibers and patchy fibrosis.

    (3) The **usual course** of MMM is progressive anemia, enlargement of the spleen, and opportunistic infections.

  d. Essential thrombocythemia is a clonal malignancy most **closely related to PV.** It is characterized by a **predominance of megakaryocytic proliferation in the marrow.**

    (1) Clinically, patients are often seen with reoccurring, **spontaneous hemorrhages** (i.e., mostly GI in origin).

    (2) A patient who has thrombocythemia typically demonstrates the following blood and bone marrow **laboratory profile:**

        (a) The peripheral **blood** shows a **marked increase in platelets** (between 900,000/mm³ and 1,400,000/mm³), with abnormal giant forms and fragments of megakaryocytes.

          (i) Patients have a **leukocytosis.**

         (ii) The **LAP level is normal.**

         (iii) Many patients demonstrate a **hypochromic-microcytic anemia** due to chronic blood loss.

        (iv) Platelet function defects can be present, and platelets may show a decreased aggregation in response to epinephrine.

      (b) A hypercellular **marrow** demonstrates a **panmyelosis** with in-creased **megakaryocytes and increased reticulin** (i.e., may result in a "dry" aspiration).

    (3) Course. Thrombocythemia has a stable course for many years but may develop into other myeloproliferative disorders.

e. Myelodysplastic syndrome (MDS) is a family of marrow disorders found mainly in persons older than 50 years. MDS is **characterized by ineffective cellular production.**

    (1) MDS is believed to be caused by a defect in a member of the marrow stem cell pool, which results in increased proliferation and inadequate maturation or an imbalance in one or more cell lines.

    (2) This group of disorders has been termed **preleukemias** because most patients progress to have acute leukemias.

    (3) Between 40% and 90% of MDS patients have demonstrated chromosome abnormalities. Mutations have been commonly found on **chromosome 5, but also have been noted on chromosomes 7, 8, 12, and 20.**

    (4) MDS is classified into five subtypes, as defined by the French-American-British (FAB) Cooperative Pathology Group.

        (a) Refractory anemia (RA) has the following identifying characteristics:

            (i) Anemia with a decreased reticulocyte count

            (ii) Abnormal erythrocytes (e.g., ovalocytes)

            (iii) Blasts less than 1% in peripheral blood

            (iv) Approximately 10% of RA patients progress to AML

        (b) Refractory anemia with ring sideroblasts (RARS) has the following identifying characteristics:

            (i) Greater than 15% ring sideroblasts in the marrow (i.e., any nucleated erythroid precursor cell that contains stainable iron granules)

            (ii) Ring sideroblasts have a "necklace" of iron granules around the nucleus

            (iii) Approximately 10% of RARS patients progress to AML

        (c) Refractory anemia with excess blasts (RAEB) has the following identifying characteristics:

            (i) A cytopenia in two of the three cell lines

            (ii) Greater than 1% but less than 5% circulating blasts

            (iii) Between 5% and 20% blasts in the marrow

        (d) Chronic myelomonocytic leukemia (CMML) has the following identifying characteristics:

            (i) Chronic monocytosis greater than 1000/mm³

            (ii) Frequent **granulocytosis**

            (iii) Less than 5% circulating blasts

            (iv) Greater percent of promonocytes seen in marrow

        (e) RAEB in transformation (RAEBIT) has the following identifying characteristics:

            (i) Greater than 5% circulating blasts

            (ii) Between 20% and 30% blasts in the marrow

            (iii) Presence of **Auer bodies in blasts**

(iv) Approximately **60% of patients with RAEBIT transform into AML**

3. **Acute myeloproliferative leukemia (AML)** includes a group of leukemias that share a common stem cell lesion, are more refractory to treatment, and have a **rapid onset** in their clinical course.

   a. Patients diagnosed with AML share the following **common clinical symptoms and laboratory features:**

      (1) AML is a disease of **adulthood.**

      (2) Many cases are believed to be viral-induced or can be related to exposure to **radiation, chemicals,** or diseases with a long **preleukemic phase.**

      (3) Most patients have **very high WBC counts (e.g., 200,000/mm³).**

      (4) AML is **resistant to treatment** with chemotherapeutic agents.

      (5) The disease has a **rapid onset,** with symptoms often resembling an acute infection.

      (6) Ulcerations of mucous membranes are commonly seen.

      (7) Patients have a lack of energy.

      (8) Symptoms are due to the mass of leukemic cells blocking capillaries, crowding out normal bone marrow cells, and compromising the immune system, all resulting in anemia, hemorrhage, and infections.

      (9) In 1976, the **FAB group** published guidelines for the classification of AMLs based on the morphology of the cells involved. This classification system has come to be known as the **FAB classification** of AML and represents **seven subtypes (M1 to M7).**

   b. **AML-M1 and AML-M2** are known as **acute myeloblastic leukemias.**

      (1) **M1 is defined by a predominance of myeloblasts** in the marrow **with very little maturation beyond the blast stage.** Cytochemical staining reactions occur, as illustrated in Table 4-9.

      (2) **AML-M2** is different from M1 because of the finding of a significant number of **myeloid precursor cells in the marrow beyond the blast and promyelocyte stages (i.e., maturation is involved).**

         (a) **More than 50% of marrow cells are myeloblasts or promyelocytes.**

         (b) Patients who have M2 have a **common chromosome abnormality of t(8;21).**

      (3) **Maturation abnormalities** are often present with M1 or M2.

         (a) Hyposegmentation is seen in many of the neutrophils (i.e., **pseudo-Pelger Huët**).

         (b) **Myeloblasts** can show **bilobed or reniform** nuclear shapes.

         (c) Some blasts may present with **azurophilic granules.**

         (d) **Auer bodies** can be found in the cytoplasm of a few blasts.

            (i) These inclusions are linear or spindle-shaped, red-purple inclusions in the cytoplasm of blasts or promyelocytes.

            (ii) They are thought to be giant lysosomes, and they stain positive for Sudan black B, peroxidase, AS-D chloroacetate esterase, and acid phosphatase.

   c. **AML-M3** is known as **acute promyelocytic leukemia (APL).** Cytochemical staining reactions are summarized in Table 4-9.

(1) Promyelocytes instead of myeloblasts are the major abnormal cell found in the marrow and blood.

(2) These promyelocytes have an abundance of azurophilic granules.

(3) Auer bodies are found in most patients who have M3.

(4) Two variants of APL are found based on the staining intensity of promyelocyte granularity.

    (a) **Hypergranular promyelocytes** are the most common variety of M3.

        (i) Characteristically, promyelocytes may have **bundles of cytoplasmic Auer bodies and intensely staining azurophilic granules.**

        (ii) The **nucleus of these promyelocytes may vary in size and shape** (i.e., kidney-shaped or bilobed).

        (iii) Patients who have hypergranular M3 often have **bad bleeding problems. DIC** is easily initiated by procoagulant material released from granules of abnormal hypergranular promyelocytes.

        (iv) **The WBC count is not usually as greatly elevated as that seen with other AMLs.**

    (b) **Hypogranular promyelocytes (M3V)** may be easily confused with myeloblastic leukemia (i.e., M1 or M2) because promyelocytes are faintly granulated and may appear as myeloblasts.

        (i) **In approximately 60%** of patients who have M3V, a **t(15;17) chromosome translocation is demonstrated.**

        (ii) Patients who have this variant usually demonstrate **very high WBC counts** (up to 200,000/mm^3).

d. **AML-M4, acute myelomonocytic leukemia (AMML),** demonstrates a **predominance of both monocyte and granulocyte precursor cells** in the marrow and peripheral blood.

(1) This leukemia is defined as a malignancy in which more than 20% promonocytes and monocytes are found in marrow and peripheral blood, with the presence of more than 20% myeloblasts and abnormal granulocyte precursor cells.

(2) **Chromosome abnormalities are seen as a 16q mutation.**

e. **AML-M5 is a relative pure monocytic leukemia.**

(1) This leukemia is defined as a malignancy in which more than 20% promonocytes and monocytes, and less than 20% myeloblasts and granulocytic precursors are found in the marrow or peripheral blood.

(2) **Two subtypes of M5 are found.**

    (a) **Differentiated** monoblastic leukemia **(M5a)** has monocytes and promonocytes as the majority in the marrow and blood. The blood has a higher percentage of monocytes than the marrow, and the most common type of cell is the promonocyte.

    (b) **Poorly differentiated (M5b)** is characterized by a predominance of large blasts in the bone marrow and blood.

(3) **Chromosome abnormalities are seen in M5 as a t(9;11).**

(4) Promonocytes and leukemic monoblasts in AML-M5 demonstrate the following **morphologic characteristics:**

    (a) Delicate reticular chromatin

      (b) One to two nucleoli

      (c) Folded and indented nuclei

      (d) Moderate nucleus:cytoplasm (N:C) ratio (i.e., 1:1 to 2:1)

      (e) Phagocytosis of RBCs or cellular debris

      (f) Auer bodies

      (g) Abundance of basophilic-staining cytoplasm with pseudopodia and possibly rare azurophilic granules

   (5) AML-M5 may have **lymph node enlargement.**

   (6) Cytochemical staining reactions for M4 and M5 can be found in Table 4-9.

   (7) Patients who have monocytic leukemias characteristically have very **high levels of muramidase** in the serum or urine.

  f. AML-M6 or erythroleukemia was formerly known as Di Guglielmo syndrome.

   (1) This type of AML results from an **abnormal proliferation of both erythroid and granulocytic precursors, with a predominance of erythroid precursors in the marrow representing** 50% or greater of the marrow precursor cell population.

   (2) Myeloid-erythroid ratios decrease to between 1:2 and 1:4.

   (3) Erythremic myelosis is a variant of M6 that has a more rapid course and an arrest in the maturation of the erythrocytic precursors. Mainly, only the erythroblast stage of maturation is seen in the erythroid marrow.

   (4) Often, M6 terminates in AML-M1.

   (5) Erythroid precursors are abnormal in appearance, predominate in the marrow and blood, and demonstrate the following cellular **morphologic** characteristics:

      (a) Blasts irregular in outline, often with pseudopodia

      (b) Medium N:C ratio

      (c) Bizarre large nucleoli and nuclear shape

      (d) Numerous multinucleated giant forms

      (e) Cytoplasmic vacuolation

   (6) Myeloblasts are increased in the chronic form of erythroleukemia, and Auer bodies may be present.

   (7) Abnormal megakaryocytes are present, with giant forms and nuclear fragmentation. Atypical platelets may also be found in the blood.

   (8) The cytochemistry results of M6 show a **strong positivity to PAS.** Erythroid precursors are **normally PAS negative.**

   (9) Patients with AML-M6 have a poor prognosis.

  g. AML-M7 or acute megakaryoblastic leukemia (i.e., acute myelofibrosis) is the newest FAB classification of acute nonlymphocytic leukemias.

   (1) This leukemia demonstrates a **predominance of megakaryoblasts and megakaryocytes in the marrow, with an increase in reticulum fibrosis.**

   (2) M7 is the rarest subtype.

  h. Prognosis. As a group, AMLs generally have a terminal prognosis of approximately 3–6 months, and complete remission is achieved in 40%–60% of patients.

4. Rare forms of leukemia

    a. Acute stem cell leukemia is a leukemia in which the predominant hyperproliferating cells are blast forms that cannot be classified using cytochemical or immunologic techniques.

    b. Chloroma is a rare form of AML in which green-pigmented tumors of myeloblasts form in the tissues surrounding the bones.

    c. Myeloblastic sarcoma is a form of AML in which localized tumors of myeloblasts are found in tissues. This type differs from chloroma only in the absence of the green pigment found in the tumor.

    d. Eosinophilic leukemia can occur, although rarely, as a **variant of AML or CML.**

        (1) Types. There are acute and chronic forms.

        (2) Laboratory profile. Immature eosinophils infiltrate the tissues in the body. **Other immature myeloid precursor cells are usually involved, and their levels are increased in the blood and marrow.**

        (3) Differential diagnosis. This disorder must be distinguished from hypereosinophilic syndrome seen with parasitic infection.

        (4) Diagnosis. The identification of immature forms in the blood and an increase of eosinophils in the marrow of greater than 5% help diagnose eosinophilic leukemia.

    e. Basophilic leukemia can be a variant of CML in the accelerated phase. This variant is associated with an increase in blood histamine levels.

V. LYMPHOCYTE PHYSIOLOGY AND DISORDERS

  A. Lymphocyte development

    1. Development involves three major lymphoid compartments.

      a. The pool of **undifferentiated stem cells** is located in the **bursa-equivalent tissue of the bone marrow,** where proliferation and maturation occurs.

      b. Primary lymphoid tissues are the location of **antigen-independent** lymphopoiesis.

        (1) T-lymphocyte development occurs in the **thymus.**

        (2) B-lymphocyte development occurs in the **bone marrow.**

      c. Peripheral or secondary lymphoid development is antigen dependent. Secondary lymphoid tissues contain mixed T-cell and B-cell populations; these tissues are found in the spleen, lymph nodes, and gut-associated lymphoid tissue.

    2. B-lymphocyte development (see Chapter 6 II B)

    3. T-Lymphocyte development is centered in the thymus gland (see Figure 4-9; Chapter 6 II A).

  B. Lymphocyte structure

    1. From a morphologic basis, lymphocyte development consists of three recognized stages.

      a. Lymphoblasts are the youngest recognizable form of B lymphocytes or T lymphocytes based on staining characteristics.

        (1) Blast size is larger than a mature lymphocyte, averaging 16–24 mm.

Site of maturation

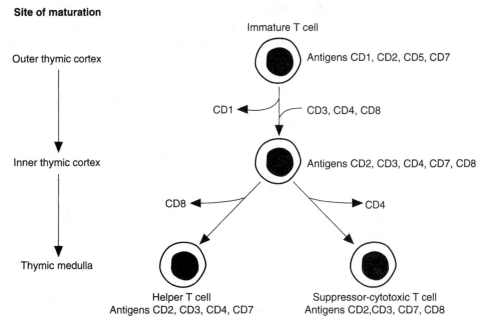

Immature T cell

Antigens CD1, CD2, CD5, CD7

Outer thymic cortex

CD1 ◄──── ── CD3, CD4, CD8

Inner thymic cortex   Antigens CD2, CD3, CD4, CD7, CD8

CD8 ◄────   ────► CD4

Thymic medulla

Helper T cell   Suppressor-cytotoxic T cell
Antigens CD2, CD3, CD4, CD7   Antigens CD2, CD3, CD7, CD8

Figure 4-9. Maturation of the T lymphocyte in the thymus. (Reprinted with permission from Besa EC: *Hematology.* Baltimore, Williams & Wilkins, 1992, pp 158.)

(**2**) Blasts have 1–2 easily recognizable large **nucleoli.**

(**3**) Chromatin in these blasts is finely divided into a smooth grainy texture.

(**4**) Lymphoblasts have the **highest N:C ratio** of any blast cell.

(**5**) Cytoplasm is scant and highly basophilic in staining.

b. The **prolymphocyte** is a middle stage in the development between the blast and mature lymphocyte.

(**1**) The size of this midstage cell is the same or slightly larger than the blast, averaging 18–28 μm.

(**2**) Nucleoli can still be easily recognized.

(**3**) The nuclear **chromatin** pattern is slightly **more condensed** than the blast stage.

(**4**) Prolymphocytes have a **high-to-moderate N:C ratio.**

(**5**) The cytoplasm is more abundant than the blast but still deeply basophilic.

c. **Mature lymphocytes** in the peripheral blood represent nondividing B lymphocytes or T lymphocytes between the primary and secondary development.

(**1**) **Size.** Small lymphocytes are just slightly larger than an RBC (i.e., 8–12 μm).

(**2**) **Organelles.** These cells have a sharply defined, round nucleus that contains heavy concentrations of **dense chromatin appearing blocked or "smudgy."** The nucleus stains deep blue to purple and is sometimes indented at one side. The cytoplasm stains a pale blue. Normally, lymphocytes do not demonstrate specific cytoplasmic granules.

(3) In a **small lymphocyte,** the nucleus occupies most of the cell area, and there may be just a thin perinuclear zone of cytoplasm.

(4) **Large lymphocytes** may be found in the peripheral blood, especially in children. These lymphocytes demonstrate the following **morphologic characteristics:**

  (a) 12–15 μm in diameter

  (b) Abundant cytoplasm

  (c) Nuclei less densely staining

  (d) Irregular borders and shape

  (e) May appear as a small monocyte

  (f) Few bluish purple cytoplasmic granules

(5) Lymphocytes average **25%–45%** of all circulating WBCs, with a total absolute count range of **1000–4800/mm³.**

(6) T and B lymphocytes cannot be distinguished from each other morphologically.

d. **Plasma cells originate from B lymphocytes.** They are cells designed for the **synthesis of immunoglobulin.**

(1) **Plasmablasts,** or **immunoblasts,** have a large blastlike nucleus with nucleoli, but have other plasma cell characteristics.

(2) Plasma cells are identified by their **eccentrically placed nucleus** and the following morphologic characteristics:

  (a) The nucleus is round, with a small indentation on the cytoplasm side.

  (b) Nuclear chromatin is distributed more regularly in a pattern. resembling the spokes of a wheel.

  (c) The **cytoplasm, except for one small area, stains deeply bluish green.**

  (d) The unstained portion of cytoplasm corresponds to the indented portion of the nucleus. A large Golgi apparatus exists here because of the large amount of protein synthesis.

2. **Lymphocytes demonstrate a heterogeneity of functional types.**

a. **B lymphocytes** function as **precursors for plasma cells.** They also **synthesize and release immunoglobulin,** which is easily detectable on their surface membranes.

(1) **Approximately 10%–15% of circulating blood lymphocytes are B cells.**

(2) **Diversity**

  (a) Individual B cells are limited to the one type of antibody they can synthesize and release.

  (b) **IgM or immunoglobulin D (IgD)** are found on most **circulating B cells.**

  (c) B lymphocytes with surface **IgM or IgG are found mainly in organized secondary lymphoid tissue.**

  (d) **Immunoglobulin A (IgA)- and IgE-bearing B cells are predominately at sites of external Ig secretion** (e.g., the GI and respiratory tracts, saliva).

(3) **B-lymphocyte surface receptors** include the following identifying markers:

> **(a) Fc receptors** (i.e., **CD7**) that recognize the Fc portion of immunoglobulins
> **(b) C3 receptors** (i.e., **CD21**) for complement fixation
> **(c) Specific receptor for the Epstein-Barr virus antigen**
> **(d) Mouse RBC receptor**

b. T lymphocytes are responsible for reactions of **cellular immunity and modulation of humoral immunity** (see Figure 4–9).

  (1) T cells interact with macrophages for the proper delivery of antigens to B lymphocytes.

  (2) T cell–mediated immunity is antigen directed; therefore, T cells must have surface receptors to recognize antigens.

    (a) T lymphocytes display a specific receptor for **sheep RBCs** (i.e., CD2), forming E-rosettes.

    (b) Fc receptors are present but not abundant.

    (c) T cell–specific antigens CD1 to CD8 are also abundant.

c. Null lymphocytes are lymphocytes that cannot be classified as either T or B types on the basis of surface properties. These cells constitute approximately **10% of the lymphocyte population.**

  (1) Null cells possibly represent undifferentiated stem cells, immature T or B cells, or those lymphocytes that have lost their recognizable surface receptors.

  (2) L cells are lymphocytes that do not proliferate in response to antigens but are capable of enhancing the responses of T lymphocytes in the presence of monocytes.

    (a) These lymphocytes bear **surface IgG and Fc receptors.**

    (b) L cells **do not develop into antibody-producing cells.**

  (3) Large granular lymphocytes (LGLs) mediate **antibody-dependent cytotoxicity.**

    (a) LGLs include **natural killer (NK)** and **killer (K)** cells.

    (b) NK cells mediate cytotoxic reactions without prior sensitization in defensive mechanisms against tumors and virally transformed cells.

C. Function and regulation of the immune response

  1. Monocyte-macrophages secrete **IL-1,** which activates the helper-inducer T lymphocytes. IL-1 also has pyogenic effects on the central nervous system (CNS) in raising body temperature.

  2. Helper-inducer T lymphocyte lymphokines, which are secreted in an immune reaction (see Chapter 6 II A), consist of the following substances:

    a. Once activated by IL-1, the helper-inducer T lymphocyte secretes **IL-2,** which stimulates other helper-inducer T lymphocytes to multiply.

    b. B-cell growth factor (BCGF) is released to stimulate B-cell proliferation.

    c. B-cell differentiation factor (BCDF) is released to halt replication of the immunospecific B cells and stimulates antibody production.

    d. Gamma-interferon is released to stimulate B-cell antibody production, activate killer T lymphocytes, and localize macrophages at the site of infection.

3. **B lymphocytes** (see Chapter 6 II B) produce and secrete an antigen-specific antibody.

D. **Lymphocyte pathophysiology**

1. **The normal circulating concentration of lymphocytes is 1500–4000/ mm³.**

   a. An absolute circulating lymphocyte count **below 1500/mm³ is considered clinically to be a lymphocytopenia.**

   b. The reduction in circulating lymphocytes affects mostly T cells, because they represent the greatest percentage of circulating lymphocytes.

2. **Nonmalignant disorders of lymphocytopenia** often include a **hypogammaglobulinemia** (Figure 4-10). A lymphocytopenia can be found in the following disorders or conditions:

   a. A **blockage of the lymphatic thoracic duct** results in a lymphocytopenia.

   b. **Radiation** overexposure is highly toxic to lymphopoiesis and results in a reduction of lymphocytes.

   c. **Acute stress** results in a reduction of lymphocytes in the circulating pool.

   d. **Therapy with corticoids** shifts distribution of lymphocytes from the blood into the extravascular spaces. Cell lysis and an inhibition of cell proliferation are minor drug-induced mechanisms of lymphopenia.

   e. **Chemotherapeutic alkylating drugs** interfere with lymphocyte proliferation.

   f. **Acquired immunodeficiency syndrome (AIDS)** is a virally induced lymphocytopenia.

      (1) The virus that causes AIDS has been named **human T-cell lymphotrophic virus-3 (HTLV-3), or human immunodeficiency virus (HIV).**

      (2) Patients who have AIDS have a **high risk of infections** because of a significant decrease in helper-inducer T lymphocytes.

         (a) The AIDS virus invades the helper-inducer T cells and renders them incapable of functioning.

         (b) The T lymphocyte helper-suppressor **(H-S) ratio is decreased below the normal range of 0.9%–2.9%.**

   g. **Primary immunodeficiency disorders** include several disorders caused by a developmental defect in either B or T lymphocytes.

      (1) **X-linked agammaglobulinemia (Bruton type)** is a **developmental defect of B cells** that primarily affects **male** infants.

         (a) B-cell zones of lymph nodes and spleen are depleted of B cells.

         (b) Blood lymphocyte counts are normal, but the **serum immunoglobulin concentrations are very low,** and patients suffer from recurrent infections.

      (2) **Hypogammaglobulinemia of infancy** is a decrease in immunoglobulins caused by delayed immune development in the first years of life.

         (a) Normally, following the gradual disappearance of maternal IgG, an infant's own IgG and IgM levels increase to approximately 75% of the adult level by 1 year of age.

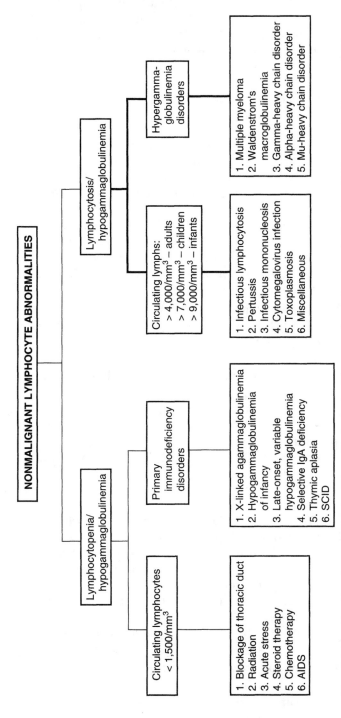

Figure 4-10. Algorithm demonstrating the differential diagnosis of the nonmalignant lymphocytic disorders. AIDS = acquired immune deficiency syndrome; IgA = immunoglobulin A; SCID = severe combined immunodeficiency.

(**b**) Infants who have this disorder have a **delayed onset of immuno-globulin synthesis** and are subject to recurrent infections.

(**c**) The disorder usually self-corrects by 2 years of age.

(**3**) **Late-onset variable primary hypogammaglobulinemia occurs in adults, usually by 30 years of age.**

(**a**) The pattern of immunoglobulin deficiency varies among individuals.

(**b**) There is a **defect in the differentiation of B lymphocytes into plasma cells.**

(**c**) Patients have an increased occurrence of infections and an increased incidence of autoimmune disorders.

(**4**) **Selective immunoglobulin deficiency** is an acquired decrease in one subtype of immunoglobulin. A lack of IgA is most common.

(**5**) **Thymic aplasia (DiGeorge syndrome) is a developmental defect of the thymus gland.**

(**a**) T-cell zones of the lymph nodes are depleted.

(**b**) Serum immunoglobulin levels are normal.

(**6**) **Severe combined immune deficiency** is a **defect in the common stem cell that leads to a deficiency of both T and B lymphocytes.**

3. **Lymphocytosis** is clinically defined as an absolute circulating increase in the lymphocyte count greater than **4000/mm³ in adults, 7000/mm³ in children, and 9000/mm³ in infants.** Disorders that demonstrate lymphocytosis include the following characteristics:

a. **Infectious lymphocytosis** occurs mainly **in children.**

(**1**) The disorder is believed to be **caused by** viruses (e.g., coxsackievirus A and B6, echoviruses, adenovirus).

(**2**) **Symptoms** include vomiting, fever, and abdominal discomfort.

(**3**) **Laboratory findings**

(**a**) A leukocytosis of 20,000–50,000/mm³ is one of the earliest findings.

(**b**) The blood differential shows **60%–95% normal lymphocytes.**

(**c**) Atypical lymphocytes **are not seen with this disorder.**

(**d**) **Eosinophilia** is common.

(**e**) The lymphocytosis usually lasts only 3–5 weeks and, in most cases, is acute and self-correcting. Rarely, some patients demonstrate a chronic course.

(**f**) Serologically, patients have a negative test for infectious mononucleosis (IM).

(**g**) **Bone marrow** of these patients is **normal.**

b. **Pertussis (i.e., whooping cough)** is a childhood inflammatory reaction of the respiratory system.

(**1**) **Cause.** The etiologic agent is the bacterium *Bordetella pertussis*.

(**2**) **Laboratory findings.** Patients demonstrate a significant **lymphocytosis** as high as 30,000/mm³. Lymphocytosis is highest in the first 3 weeks of the disease, then decreases after 4 weeks. Lymphocytosis is caused by the release of lymphocytosis-promoting factor (LPF) from *B. pertussis*. LPF induces an acute release of lymphocytes from lymph nodes and also inhibits the migration of lymphocytes from the circulation into the lymphatics.

(3) **Morphologic characteristics.** The lymphocytes in this disorder are small and mature.

c. **IM (see Chapter 6 XIII B)**

(1) **Serious complications** of IM may require hospitalization.

   (a) **AIHA** is reported in 1%–3% of patients, which is related to the development of an autoimmune **anti-i.**

   (b) Mild thrombocytopenia (i.e., approximately 5000–100,000/mm^3) is reported in 50% of patients who have IM.

   (c) **Liver involvement** can occur, which leads to mild jaundice and hepatitis.

   (d) **Splenomegaly** can also be a dangerous complication.

(2) Recognizing **hematologic features** of IM can result in a rapid diagnosis.

   (a) **Leukocytosis** between 12,000/mm^3 and 25,000/mm^3 persists for the first 3 weeks of infection, with a differential showing 60%–90% lymphocytes.

   (b) A **neutrophilia** occurs during the first week of infection, with a left shift, metamyelocytes, toxic granulation, and Döhle's bodies.

   (c) **Abundant atypical lymphocytes** are found on the peripheral blood smear. These are active or transformed lymphocytes involved in an immune reaction. **Atypical lymphocytes are not exclusive to IM** and are also found in the following disorders:

       (i) **Cytomegalovirus infections**
       (ii) **Toxoplasmosis**
       (iii) **Infectious hepatitis**
       (iv) **Viral pneumonia and mumps**

d. **Cytomegalovirus infection (CMV) demonstrates** clinical and laboratory symptoms that are in some ways identical to those of IM.

(1) **Patients receiving massive blood transfusions** are in a high-risk category for contracting CMV.

(2) **Presentation.** Patients have a **leukocytosis involving a lymphocytosis** in which **20% or more of lymphocytes may be reactive.**

(3) **Serologic tests.** Patients are negative for heterophil antibodies and Epstein-Barr virus (EBV) antibodies.

(4) **Diagnosis** is made by the **demonstration of CMV antibodies** by complement fixation or hemagglutination techniques.

e. **Toxoplasmosis** also produces clinical and laboratory symptoms similar to those of IM.

(1) **Presentation.** Patients have an absolute lymphocytosis and atypical lymphocytes on the peripheral blood smear.

(2) **Serologic tests** for EBV and heterophil antibodies are negative.

(3) **Diagnosis** is made by the demonstration of toxoplasmosis antibodies by the Sabin-Feldman dye test, fluorescent antibody, or hemagglutination techniques.

    f. Miscellaneous causes of lymphocytosis

      (1) Syphilis

      (2) Smallpox

      (3) Para-aminosalicylic acid hypersensitivity

      (4) Phenytoin (i.e., dilantin) and mesentoin hypersensitivity

4. Hypergammaglobulinemias are related disorders in which the levels of one or more serum immunoglobulins are increased above normal levels. Hypergammaglobulinemias may or may not be accompanied by an absolute lymphocytosis.

    a. Multiple myeloma (MM) is a monoclonal gammopathy (i.e., an abnormality of only one B-cell clone) in which only one type of gamma-globulin is increased.

      (1) MM involves a **neoplastic proliferation of plasma cells** primarily in the bone marrow. Plasma cell proliferation may be either **nodular or diffuse.**

      (2) Clinical symptoms of MM are found primarily in persons older than 40 years.

        (a) Bone pain is the most common symptom, and MM patients are often first seen with **bone fractures.**

        (b) Tumor growth in the marrow increases bone destruction, and **the serum calcium level is high.**

        (c) Patients have a high **susceptibility to infection.**

        (d) Renal insufficiency is also a common symptom of patients who have MM.

      (3) The **laboratory profile** of a patient who has MM includes the following results:

        (a) Normocytic/normochromic **anemia**

        (b) Normoblasts on the peripheral blood smear

        (c) Rouleau formation and increased erythrocyte sedimentation rate (ESR) (i.e., due to increase in serum globulins)

        (d) Possible **shift to the left with metamyelocytes**

        (e) Increased serum calcium level

        (f) Circulating plasma cells

        (g) An increase in one of the serum gamma-globulins as demonstrated by protein electrophoresis

      (4) Bone marrow examination **shows the presence of plasma cells varying from 1%– 90%.**

      (5) Serum **immunoglobulins are increased** in a variety of electrophoresis patterns among different patients. Serum protein electrophoresis usually shows a homogeneous band in the gamma or beta region of the electrophoretic tracing known as an **"M-spot."**

        (a) Most patients with MM are hypergammaglobulin producers, but in 25% of patients, only the light chains of the globulin are produced (i.e., **Bence Jones proteins**) by the abnormal plasma cells. A serum hypogammaglobulinemia is found in these patients, because light chains are cleared by the kidney into the urine.

        (b) Half of reported MM patients show an increase in IgG only.

        (c) A monoclonal increase in **IgA is found in approximately 20% of MM patients.**

(**d**) IgD is increased in approximately 1% of patients.

(**e**) IgE is rarely found to demonstrate a monoclonal increase.

(**f**) **Proteinuria with Bence Jones proteins can also be demon-strated in more than 50% of MM patients.**

(**6**) **Course.** MM usually has a chronic course, with the median survival approximately 3 years.

(**a**) In 5% of MM patients, AMML develops as a secondary manifestation of the malignancy.

(**b**) In some patients, large numbers of plasma cells may be found in the blood and bone marrow, and the disease is then classified as plasma cell leukemia.

b. Waldenström's macroglobulinemia (WM) is a hypergammaglobulinemia variant of chronic lymphocytic leukemia, in which there is a **greater degree of maturation of the B lymphocytes into plasma cells.**

(**1**) WM is characterized by a **generalized proliferation of B cells and plasma cells, and an increase of monoclonal IgM in the serum that amounts to at least 15% of the total serum protein.**

(**2**) **Clinical symptoms** of WM are primarily found in individuals older than 40 years. Symptoms are caused by the cellular proliferation and increased blood viscosity caused by the increased IgM. Patients who have WM are commonly seen with the following symptoms:

(**a**) **Neurologic abnormalities**

(**b**) **Renal insufficiency**

(**c**) **Heart failure**

(**d**) **Clotting abnormalities** (e.g., **DIC**)

(**3**) The **laboratory profile** includes the following results:

(**a**) **IgM in excess of 1.0 g/dL**

(**b**) Normocytic-normochromic **anemia** (i.e., occasionally hemolytic with a **positive direct Coombs' test**)

(**c**) **Thrombocytopenia** caused by IgM platelet clumping or pancytopenia caused by marrow infiltration

(**d**) **Lymphocytosis**

(**e**) **Marked rouleau and increased ESR**

(**f**) **Bence Jones proteinuria in 10% of patients**

(**4**) The **bone marrow** often cannot be aspirated easily. A biopsy demonstrates an **increase in small normal lymphocytes and plasma cells.**

c. Heavy-chain diseases are disorders related to the production and excretion of the immunoglobulin heavy chains without the light chains.

(**1**) **Gamma heavy-chain disease (γ-HCD) resembles a malignant lymphoma** rather than a myeloma.

(**a**) The patient has a blood picture of anemia, leukopenia, thrombocytopenia, atypical lymphocytes, and plasma cells.

(**b**) A broad serum protein "spike" is found in the beta-gamma region of the electrophoretic pattern, accompanied by serum hypogammaglobulinemia.

(**2**) **Alpha heavy-chain disease (α-HCD)** is more common than γ-HCD and occurs in a **younger age** group.

(**a**) **Common symptoms include intestinal involvement** with mal-

Table 4-11. Comparison and Differentiation of the Malignant Lymphoproliferative Disorders Based on Immunological Typing and Cytogenetic Abnormalities

Disorder	Cell Type	CD Marker	Cytogenetic Abnormality
Chronic lymphocytic leukemia	B cell; 95% T cell; 5%	CD5, CD19, CD20, CD22, CD24 CD2, CD3, CD8	+12; t(11:14)
HCL	B cell	sIg, CD5, CD19, CD20, CD22, CD25	
PLL	B cell	sIg, CD19, CD20, CD22, CD24	
Acute lympho-cytic leukemia			t(4:11)
CALLA	Early B; 70%	TdT, CD10, CD19, CD20	
Null cell	Pre-B	TdT, cIg	
T cell	Early T; 15%–20%	TdT, CD1, CD2	
Burkitt type	Late B	sIg, CD19, CD20, CD22, CD24	
Lymphoma			
NSCC	B cell	sIg, CD19, CD20, CD24	t(14:18)
Burkitt's	Late B cell	sIg, CD19, CD20, CD24	t(8 or 2, or 22:14)
SLL, DLCL	B cell	sIg, CD19, CD20, CD24	t(11:14)
TCL	Late T cell	CD2, CD3, CD4, CD5	t(7:14; or 11 or 9)

CALLA = common acute lymphocytic leukemia antigen; CD = cluster designation; cIg = cytoplasmic immunoglobulin; DLCL = diffuse large-cell lymphoma; HCL = hairy cell leukemia; NSCC = nodular small cleaved lymphoma; PLL = prolymphocytic leukemia; sIg = surface membrane immunoglobulin; SLL = small-cell lymphocytic lymphoma; t = chromosomal translocation; TdT = terminal deoxynucleotidyl transferase; + = trisomy.

absorption, diarrhea, and a massive lymphoplasmacytic infiltration in the intestinal mucosa.

  (b) The bone marrow and lymph nodes are not usually involved.

  (c) Protein electrophoresis is normal, but small amounts of alpha chain may be detected in serum and urine on immunoelectrophoresis.

  (3) Mu heavy-chain disease (μ-HCD) can be diagnosed only by a serum immunoelectrophoresis that demonstrates an increase in mu chains.

  5. Lymphoproliferative diseases

    a. These disorders represent a group of **clonal disorders** originating from cells of the lymphoreticular system (Table 4-11).

      (1) When neoplastic cells involve mainly the bone marrow and blood, the disorder is known as a **leukemia.**

      (2) When the disease is limited mainly to lymph nodes or organs, the disease is known as a **lymphoma.**

      (3) Occasionally, a lymphoma develops into a leukemia.

    b. Chronic lymphocytic leukemia (CLL) is a slowly progressing clonal malignancy of lymphocytes in an arrested stage of maturation.

      (1) The **clinical profile** of a patient who has CLL includes the following features:

   (a) CLL most commonly is seen in adults, with a **mean age of occurrence at 55 years.**
   (b) The disorder is twice as common in **men** as compared with
   women.
   (c) Onset is slow, unrevealing, and is commonly discovered inciden-
   tally or only in the late stages of the disease.
   (d) Patients are seen with **symptoms** such as weakness, fatigue,
   anorexia, weight loss, **enlarged lymph nodes,** and abdominal
   discomfort caused by liver and spleen enlargement.
(2) The **laboratory profile** of a patient who has CLL includes the following:
   (a) Patients have a **leukocytosis ranging from 10,000–150,000/
   mm^3 with 80%–90% lymphocytes** persistent over a period of
   weeks to months.
   (b) Smudge cells are commonly found on blood smears.
   (c) Lymphocytes in patients with CLL have a characteristic morphology.
      (i) The nuclear chromatin is coarsely condensed.
      (ii) Nucleoli may be demonstrable.
      (iii) Lymphocytes show **minimal size and shape variation.**
      (iv) The cytoplasm is small to moderate in amount.
   (d) Occasionally, **immature lymphocytes** (i.e., usually fewer than
   10%) may be found on the peripheral blood smear.
   (e) Patients who have CLL do not usually have **anemia or thrombocytopenia in early stages.** As lymphocyte proliferation replaces
   the marrow with leukemic cells, production of other cell lines
   may suffer, and the symptoms will appear.
   (f) **AIHA develops in 10%** of patients who have CLL. The patient's
   blood smear demonstrates spherocytes and reticulocytosis.
   (g) **Hypogammaglobulinemia** may also be present because of qualitative defects of the leukemic lymphocytes.
(3) A marrow aspirate commonly shows an **increase in morphologically
   mature lymphocytes.**
   (a) If AIHA is present, then a marrow picture of increased erythropoiesis is predominant.
   (b) In later stages of CLL, the lymphocytes overrun the marrow,
   replacing the other hemapoietic tissues.
(4) **Ninety-five percent of CLL patients immunologically type as
   having a B-cell leukemia.**
   (a) **Immunologic cell-marker** assays for lymphocytic membrane
   receptors, surface antigens, and enzymes are useful in differentiating between lymphocytic leukemias. **Cluster designation
   markers** for B lymphocytes include the following:
      (i) **CD5:** positive in B-lymphocyte CLLs and some lymphomas
      (ii) **CD22:** positive for late B cells and hairy-cell leukemia
      (iii) **CD24:** positive in all stages of B-lymphocyte development
         (i.e., Pan-B)
   (b) **Surface IgM** can be commonly detected but is weak.

(c) In most cases of B-cell leukemia, the ability of the lymphocytes to form spontaneous rosettes with mouse RBCs can be demonstrated (i.e., **M rosettes**).

(5) Five percent of CLL patients have a T-cell leukemia.

  (a) Leukemic T lymphocytes may have a **cleft-or clover-shaped nucleus** (i.e., Sézary cells).

  (b) **Skin involvement** and lymphocyte infiltration occur in 60% of T-cell CLL patients.

  (c) **Immunologic markers** for T-cell leukemia include the following:

  (i) **CD2: E-rosette** marker (i.e., sheep RBCs)

  (ii) **CD3:** positive for T-lymphocyte CLL, T-cell prolymphocytic leukemia, and infectious mononucleosis

  (iii) **CD8:** positive for T-lymphocyte CLL

(6) **Staging systems** have been devised to help categorize patients into prognostic groups.

  (a) **Criteria** for staging include lymphadenopathy, anemia, hepatosplenomegaly, and thrombocytopenia.

  (b) The absence of these symptoms indicates a good prognosis with a long survival (i.e., 20 years).

  (c) With these symptoms, the patient's survival can be up to 5 or 6 years with treatment.

(7) **Treatment of CLL** can include one or a combination of the following agents:

  (a) Chemotherapy with **alkylating drugs**

  (b) Glucocorticoid administration

  (c) Radiotherapy

(8) Treatment can relieve symptoms and improve life expectancy and blood counts. However, hypogammaglobulinemia is often not corrected with treatment, and patients can succumb to infection.

c. Several **clinical variations of CLL** can be found.

  (1) **Hairy-cell leukemia** (leukemic reticuloendotheliosis) is a rare form of CLL found **four times more in men than women.** The mean age of occurrence is 50 years.

  (a) The onset of the disease is slow and is characterized by proliferation of abnormal lymphocytes in the secondary lymphoid organs.

  (b) **Splenomegaly** is a common physical finding.

  (c) The **laboratory profile** of a patient who has hairy- cell leukemia includes the following:

  (i) **Pancytopenia, or a depression of two cell lines,** is common.

  (ii) The peripheral blood smear may have variable numbers of **"hairy-cell" lymphocytes.** These lymphocytes are medium-sized cells with a round, oval, notched, or dumbbell-shaped nucleus. The cytoplasm of these lymphocytes is moderate in amount, with numerous hairlike projections and frayed borders.

  (iii) Hairy-cell lymphocytes contain an acid phosphatase that is resistant to inhibition by L-tartarate, which results in a **positive TRAP stain.**

(iv) Lymphocytes in hairy-cell leukemia are **usually B cells** that demonstrate **strong surface membrane immuno-globulin (sIg)** and a positive reaction for **common B-cell markers, such as CD19; CD20; CD22; CD24;** and **CD25** (i.e., IL2 receptor), which is unique to patients who have hairy-cell leukemia.

(d) The median survival of patients who have hairy-cell leukemia is 5–6 years.

(2) **Lymphosarcoma cell leukemia** is a lymphocytic lymphoma that has transformed into a leukemic phase with the invasion of the marrow and blood of leukemic lymphocytes.

(a) The clinical course is **more aggressive than that in common B-cell CLL.**

(b) **Morphologic differences.** Leukemic lymphocytes are B cells, but they are morphologically different than those cells seen in regular B-cell CLL.

(i) The nuclear **chromatin is smoother,** and the **nucleus is oval or notched.**

(ii) **Distinct nucleoli** are easily seen in malignant lympho-cytes.

(iii) A **lower N:C ratio** is found in these lymphocytes when compared with the N:C ratio in regular B-cell CLL.

(iv) Lymphocytes demonstrate a **strong expression of sIg.**

(3) **Prolymphocytic leukemia (PLL)** is a variation of CLL in which there is a high number of morphologically immature larger lymphocytes, which appear as prolymphocytes.

(a) This variation is typically seen in **older men** (i.e., older than 50 years).

(b) The leukemia is characterized by a **high lymphocytosis up to 350,000/mm³.**

(c) Lymphocytes are the **B-cell type.**

(d) Prolymphocytes can be distinguished by their smooth nuclear chromatin and large nucleoli.

(e) Patients commonly have a **massive splenomegaly,** but their **lymph nodes are not enlarged.**

(f) The prognosis is usually subacute and more resistant to treat-ment than is common CLL. Patients have a mean survival of 1 year.

(g) Prolymphocytes of PLL commonly type positive with the **mem-brane markers** CD19, CD20, CD22, and CD24. They also strongly express sIg.

d. **Acute lymphocytic leukemia (ALL)** is a rapidly progressing clonal malignancy of early immature lymphocytes in an arrested stage of maturation.

(1) The **clinical profile** of a patient who has ALL includes the follow-ing features:

(a) ALL is mainly a **disease of childhood,** with a **peak incidence at 4 years.** The second peak of incidence (i.e., bimodal distribu-tion) is in young adults between **20 and 40 years.**

Table 4-12. Differentiation of Acute Lymphocytic Leukemia (ALL) Based on FAB Morphologic Classification and Immunologic Subtype

Characteristics	L1	L2	L3
Cell size	Homogeneous population of small blasts	Heterogeneous population of large blasts	Homogeneous population of large blasts
Nucleus	Homogeneous regular shape with slightly clumped chromatin; faint nucleoli	Variable shape with smooth chromatin; one or more large nucleoli	Regular shape with dense–fine homogeneous chromatin; one or more prominent nucleoli
Cytoplasm	High N:C ratio; slight-to-moderate basophilia	Moderate N:C ratio; moderate-to-deep basophilia	Moderate-to-low N:C ratio; deep basophilia with obvious vacuolation
Patient age	70% of childhood ALL	70% of adult ALL	Rare in children and adults
Immunologic markers	CALLA (CD10); TdT; CD19, CD20	TdT	sg; CD19, CD20, CD22, CD24

CALLA = common acute lymphocytic leukemia antigen; CD = cluster designation; FAB = French-American-British; N:C = nucleus:cytoplasm; sIg = surface membrane immunoglobulin; TdT = terminal deoxynucleotidyl transferase.

  (b) **Onset of leukemia is sudden,** with symptoms of anemia, bleeding, fever, and fatigue.
  (c) **The spleen, liver, and lymph nodes** are commonly **enlarged.**
 (2) The **laboratory profile** of a patient who has ALL includes the following results:
  (a) A **normocytic-normochromic anemia** is common.
  (b) Normoblasts are found on the peripheral blood smear.
  (c) The leukocyte count shows three patterns. The WBC count is occasionally very high (i.e., greater than 100,000/mm³); often is slightly elevated; but most often is normal or decreased.
  (d) The predominant cell type is the **lymphoblast or immature lymphocyte.**
  (e) The serum level of uric acid is often elevated.
  (f) A small percent of ALL patients are positive for the Ph¹ chromosome.
  (g) **Immunodeficiency or hypogammaglobulinemia is not as common as in CLL.**
 (3) A marrow aspirate commonly shows **diffuse infiltration of lymphoblasts.**
 (4) Acute lymphocytic leukemias are classified by the FAB group as **L1, L2, and L3** (Table 4-12).
  (a) Approximately **70% of children with ALL are Type L1,** and **27% are Type L2.** The remaining 3% are Type L3.
  (b) The **L2** type of ALL is the most common type of **adult ALL.**
  (c) **L3** represents the B-cell **Burkitt's lymphoma type of ALL,** with vacuolated lymphoblasts.

(5) The diagnosis of ALL cannot be made with complete certainty until **cytochemical staining** procedures have been performed to distinguish the lymphoblasts and lymphocytes from positively reacting cells of AML.

    (a) ALL blasts are **negative for Sudan black B, peroxidase, and naphthyl AS-D chloroacetate esterase.**

    (b) The **acid phosphatase reaction is positive in the 20%** of patients whose ALL is of the T-lymphocyte type.

    (c) **Terminal deoxynucleotidyl transferase (TdT)** is an **intracellular DNA polymerase** that is **present in T and B lymphoblasts.**

        (i) TdT is weakly positive in pre–B cells.

        (ii) TdT is strongly positive in **60%–85% of T-cell thymocytes.**

        (iii) Mature peripheral T cells and mature B cells are TdT negative.

        (iv) TdT is measured with an immunofluorescence assay that uses a specific antibody against TdT prepared in rabbits.

        (v) This assay is used in the diagnosis of ALL, lymphoblastic lymphoma, and the blast phase of CML. **Lymphoblasts in 90% of ALL patients are TdT positive,** but blasts in only 5% of nonlymphocytic leukemias (e.g., CML) stain positive for TdT.

(6) There are several **functional subclasses** of ALL based upon immunologic **membrane surface markers.**

    (a) **Common ALL antigen (CALLA),** which is also **CD10,** is the most common subtype.

        (i) Lymphocytes do not show surface features of B or T cells on blast membranes.

        (ii) This subtype is the **most common form of ALL in children** and morphologically, lymphocytes are of the FAB classification of **L1.**

    (b) **Null-cell ALL** is a proliferation of lymphocytes that type negative for **T-cell, B-cell, and CALLA surface antigens.**

        (i) This subtype includes a smaller proportion of children and **more adults.**

        (ii) Null-cell ALL is thought to be a **pre-B-cell leukemia.**

    (c) **T-cell ALL** accounts for **10%–20% of all patients who have ALL.**

        (i) This functional subtype occurs mainly in **boys.**

        (ii) Patients usually show a **high leukocyte count** pattern and have a **poor prognosis.**

        (iii) T-cell ALL is characterized by a high frequency of mediastinal tumor, skin, and CNS involvement.

        (iv) Malignant lymphoblasts demonstrate T-cell markers such as **CD2 (i.e., E rosettes); TdT; and CD1.**

    (d) **B-cell ALL** is the **rarest of subtypes,** and it corresponds to the **FAB classification Burkitt's Type L3.**

        (i) Patients who have Type L3 generally have a **poor prognosis.**

(ii) L3 can be diagnosed by demonstration of B-cell typical **surface Ig receptors.**

(iii) This disorder is thought to be a **memory-cell leukemia.**

(7) **Better prognosis is seen in female patients,** ALL patients who have **lower WBC counts,** and patients diagnosed with the FAB classification **L1 subtype.**

(8) **Treatment** is now able to produce complete remission in 95% of children and in 50%–70% of adults with ALL. Approximately 50% of children in remission show signs of being completely cured.

e. **Lymphomas** are a group of lymphoproliferative disorders in which there is **neoplastic proliferation** of an arrested stage of secondary lymphocyte maturation that usually begins in and **involves mainly the lymph nodes.** As the disease progresses, many other organs and tissues (e.g., spleen, liver, skin, marrow) can become invaded by malignant lymph. All lymphomas are categorized into either Hodgkin's lymphoma or non-Hodgkin's lymphoma.

(1) The general **laboratory profile** of a patient who has lymphoma includes the following results:

(a) The WBC count may vary, depending on the progression of the malignancy.

(i) Neutrophilia is seen only when lymph nodes are involved, but neutropenia persists when the bone marrow is involved.

(ii) Most frequent are WBC counts from 12,000–25,000/mm³, with **lymphophilia and monocytosis.**

(iii) Eosinophilia is found in 20% of patients who have lymphoma.

(iv) The platelet count depends upon the extent of marrow involvement.

(b) **Normochromic-normocytic severe anemia is seen in 50%** of patients.

(c) The **LAP level is elevated** in the active phases of the disease.

(d) **Reed-Sternberg cells,** which are the hallmark of Hodgkin's lymphoma, may be found in the lymph nodes and marrow of a patient who has this disease.

(i) These cells can be identified as giant binucleated or multinucleated cells with acidophilic nuclei.

(ii) This cell type is thought to originate from the monocyte-macrophage cell line.

(e) Bone marrow biopsy frequently reveals **granulocytic hyperplasia** with a shift to the left, slight monocytosis, and eosinophilia. Reed-Sternburg cells may be present, depending on the clinical subtype.

(2) The **Hodgkin's type** of lymphoma has an increased frequency of occurrence in persons between the ages of 15 and 30 years and after 50 years.

(a) The clinical subclassification and diagnosis of Hodgkin's lymphoma is made histologically from a **lymph node biopsy.**

(i) **Lymphocytic-predominant** Hodgkin's lymphoma is most frequent in **young men** and localizes to the cervical lymph nodes. Lymph-node biopsy reveals **numerous lymphocytes,** no fibrosis or necrosis, and few Reed-Sternberg cells.

(ii) **Nodular-sclerosis** Hodgkin's lymphoma is a common variety most often discovered as a mediastinal mass in **young women.** Lymph-node biopsy is **characterized by broad bands of collagen separating nodules of lymphoid tissue and the presence of lacunar cells, which are atypical histiocytes.** Few Reed-Sternberg cells are found.

(iii) The **mixed type** of Hodgkin's lymphoma is characterized on lymph-node biopsy by a **variety of all cell types** (e.g., lymphocytes, plasma cells, eosinophils, histiocytes, and numerous Reed-Sternberg cells). **Necrosis and fibrosis** may also be present.

(iv) **The lymphocyte depletion type** of Hodgkin's lymphoma is the rarest type. Lymph-node biopsy reveals **diffuse fibrosis** and a **lack of lymphoid growth.** This type is accompanied by **pancytopenia and lymphocytopenia,** because there is a more frequent involvement of bone marrow.

(b) **Clinical staging** of Hodgkin's lymphoma is based on the extent of lymph node and systemic involvement.

(i) **Stage I** of the disease is limited to lymph nodes in one or two anatomic regions on one side of the diaphragm.

(ii) **Stage II** of the disease involves more than two regions of lymph node involvement on one side of the diaphragm.

(iii) **Stage III** of the disease involves two or more regions of node involvement on both sides of the diaphragm.

(iv) **Stage IV** of the disease involves bone marrow and other organs, in addition to lymph nodes. Cell-mediated immunity is defective by this stage.

(c) **Treatment.** Without treatment, few patients survive as long as 10 years. With modern treatment methods, 85% of patients diagnosed in Stages I and II can be cured. The cure rate is 50% for patients diagnosed in Stages III or IV. Treatment consists of long-term chemotherapy and localized radiotherapy for infected lymph nodes.

(3) **Non-Hodgkin's lymphomas** are classified as a group of clonal proliferations of lymphocytes that have undergone malignant transformation at an arrested stage of their differentiation. Non-Hodgkin's lymphomas **involve mostly B lymphocytes and** are reported mostly in **middle-age and older patients.**

(a) The **Rappaport classification** of non-Hodgkin's lymphomas is based upon nodular and diffuse arrangement of malignant cells in a lymph-node biopsy, as well as on size characteristics of the predominating lymphocytes.

(b) Many subtypes of non-Hodgkin's lymphoma are closely related to a **defect in immune regulation.**

(c) Some subtypes of non-Hodgkin's lymphoma are believed to be **virally related.**

(i) **Burkitt's lymphoma, which is** associated with **EBV,** has a strong affinity for B cells; this affinity causes B-cell proliferation. When the cytolytic killer T lymphocytes' response is deficient, an unchecked B-cell proliferation can result in lymphoma.

(ii) Cutaneous T-cell lymphoma (i.e., mycosis fungoides) is an **HTLV-1**–promoted helper-inducer T-cell malignancy. This lymphoma is associated with a lymphocytosis of **Sézary cells.**

(d) Most patients who have non-Hodgkin's lymphomas have associated **chromosome abnormalities** (see Table 4-11).

(i) Nodular small cleaved-cell lymphoma is associated with a translocation between the genes of Ig heavy chains found on **chromosome 14** and an arm of **chromosome 18.**

(ii) Burkitt's lymphoma is associated with a translocation between chromosomes **8 and 2 or 22 and 14.**

(iii) Small lymphocytic lymphoma and **diffuse large-cell lymphoma** are associated with a translocation **between chromosomes 11 and 14.**

(iv) Cutaneous T-cell lymphoma is associated with a translocation between chromosomes **7 and 14 or 11 and 9.**

Study Questions

Directions: Each of the numbered items or incomplete statements in this section is followed by answers or by completions of the statement. Select the ONE lettered answer or completion that is BEST in each case.

1. Severe skin photosensitivity, excretion of excessive amounts of uroporphyrin I and coproporphyrin I, and fatality early in life are characteristics of which one of the following porphyrias?

a. acute intermittent porphyria
b. congenital erythropoietic porphyria
c. lead poisoning
d. coproporphyria

2. Pernicious anemia is a megaloblastic anemia with which one of the following causes?

a. a dietary deficiency in folate
b. liver disease or alcoholism
c. a conditioned deficiency of vitamin B_{12} due to autoimmune interference of intrinsic factor
d. a lack of availability of vitamin B_{12} due to intestinal bacterial infestation or infestation with *Diphyllobothrium latum*

3. An acute myelogenous leukemia (AML) patient demonstrated 40% blast cells on both peripheral and bone marrow Wright's-stained smears. For the pathologist to differentiate between AML-M4 and AML-M5 or between AML-M1 and AML-M5, what two cytochemical stains must be performed?

a. Sudan black B and peroxidase
b. chloroacetate esterase AS-D and alpha-naphthyl acetate esterase
c. chloroacetate esterase AS-D and leukocyte alkaline phosphatase (LAP)
d. periodic acid-Schiff (PAS) and LAP

4. A chronic lymphocyte leukemia (CLL) variant characterized by splenomegaly, a proliferation of abnormal lymphocytes in bone marrow and secondary lymphoid organs, and the findings of abnormal lymphocytes with hairlike projections that stain positive with acid phosphatase (even with L-tartrate inhibition) is most likely with which one of the following disorders?

a. Hodgkin's lymphoma
b. chloroma
c. lymphosarcoma cell leukemia
d. Hairy-cell leukemia

5. A monoclonal gammopathy caused by a proliferation of plasma cells would most likely be

a. acquired immunodeficiency syndrome (AIDS)
b. late-onset variable primary hypogammaglobulinemia
c. gamma heavy-chain disease
d. multiple myeloma (MM)

6. Acute myelogenous leukemia (AML) patients who have severe bleeding problems caused by procoagulant material released from the granules of abnormal cells would most likely have which type of AML?

a. AML-M1
b. AML-M2
c. AML-M3
d. AML-M4
e. AML-M5

7. The diagnosis of Hodgkin's lymphoma is made in part by which one of the following characteristics?

a. a certain number of Reed-Sternberg cells in the circulation
b. a lymph-node biopsy and the demonstration of Reed-Sternberg cells
c. lymphocyte surface membrane markers
d. circulating lymphoblasts

8. A rare autosomal dominant condition characterized by thrombocytopenia; giant platelets; and pale blue, periodic acid-Schiff (PAS)–negative, neutrophilic cytoplasmic ribonucleic acid (RNA) inclusions resembling Döhle's bodies is

a. Pelger-Huët anomaly
b. May-Hegglin anomaly
c. Alder-Reilly anomaly
d. Neimann-Pick disease

9. When interpreting a white blood cell (WBC) differential, a shift to the left indicates which one of the following actions?

a. a decrease in the hemoglobin (Hb) oxygen affinity
b. an increase in the percent of band neutrophils and other immature myeloid forms
c. an increase in the percent of lymphocytes that is higher than the percent of segmented neutrophils
d. an increase in the number of hypersegmented neutrophils

10. A mild form of anemia often occurs secondary to a serious chronic disorder because of which one of the following problems?

a. failure of the multipotential stem cell proliferation
b. the production of autoantibodies against erythroid precursor cells
c. a block in the endogenous iron recycling and storage, because the monocytes and macrophages have a reduced ability of moving iron to erythroid normoblasts
d. a high level of intravascular hemolysis occurring secondary to the chronic disorder

11. Under which one of the following conditions will an iron deficiency anemia demonstrate an increased reticulocyte count?

a. after treatment
b. at all times
c. before treatment
d. in the clinical iron-deficient erythropoiesis stage

12. A 25-year-old man was being evaluated for the cause of his chronic granulocytosis. His original white blood cell (WBC) count was 47,000/mm^3. His physician ordered a leukocyte alkaline phosphatase (LAP) test. The laboratory hematologist received the following results on the Kaplow count:

Grading scale: 4+ 3+ 2+ 1+ 0
Number of cells: 10 30 55 5 0

Based on his LAP results, which one of the following diseases can be eliminated for this patient?

a. leukemoid reaction
b. polycythemia vera (PV)
c. chronic myelogenous leukemia (CML)
d. myelofibrosis

Directions: Each of the numbered items or incomplete statements in this section is negatively phrased, as indicated by a capitalized word such as NOT, LEAST, or EXCEPT. Select the ONE lettered answer or completion that is BEST in each case.

13. All of the following statements about hereditary spherocytosis are correct EXCEPT

a. it is caused by a defect in spectrin
b. it is characterized by an abundance of red blood cells (RBCs) with an increase in membrane surface area
c. it characteristically has a population of RBCs that demonstrate an increased amount of autohemolysis after 48 hours with and without glucose
d. it is a normocytic/normochromic anemia

14. Granulocytes normally found in the peripheral blood include all of the following EXCEPT

a. basophils
b. lymphocytes
c. eosinophils
d. band neutrophils

15. Cold agglutinin disease is characterized by all of the following statements EXCEPT

a. it is an autoimmune hemolytic anemia (AIHA)
b. antibodies that are present react with maximum activity at or below 25°C
c. antibodies have specificity for the RBC Ii antigen system
d. a direct Coombs' test is negative

16. All of the following statements about β-thalassemia, which is a dysfunction of hemoglobin (Hb) synthesis, are correct EXCEPT

a. there is an increased production of β-globin chains
b. the patient is initially seen with clinical symptoms of jaundice, splenomegaly, prominent frontal bones, and stunted growth
c. the patient's blood smear demonstrates a picture of 3–4+ poikilocytosis, target cells, hypochromic/microcytic red blood cells (RBCs), and Howell-Jolly bodies
d. it is most common in persons of African and Mediterranean descent

17. Bone marrow hypoplasia may be caused by all of the following EXCEPT

a. antimitotic agents (e.g., chemotherapeutic drugs)
b. Fanconi's anemia
c. aplastic anemia
d. chronic hemorrhage

18. All of the following laboratory characteristics are common to both cytomegalovirus and toxoplasmosis infections EXCEPT

a. lymphocytosis
b. atypical lymphocytes
c. negative Monospot test
d. positive direct antiglobulin test

19. All of the following are myelodysplastic syndromes EXCEPT

a. refractory anemia (RA)
b. chronic myelomonocytic leukemia (CMML)
c. refractory anemia with excess blasts (RAEB)
d. erythroleukemia

20. Characteristics of non-Hodgkin's lymphomas include all of the following EXCEPT

a. they are mostly B-lymphocyte lymphomas
b. they are classified as a group of clonal proliferations of lymphocytes that have undergone malignant transformation at an arrested stage
c. they include Burkitt's lymphoma
d. they have a preleukemic history

Answers and Explanations

1. The answer is b [II C 2 c (1); Figure 4-3]. Congenital erythropoietic porphyria (CEP) is classified as a nonacute porphyria and is most commonly associated with solar photosensitivity of the skin.

2. The answer is c [II D 2 d (1)]. Pernicious anemia is a megaloblastic anemia that demonstrates low serum vitamin B_{12} levels. This type is not caused by a dietary deficiency but by an immune block of the binding of intrinsic factor to dietary vitamin B_{12} in the digestive tract.

3. The answer is b [IV D 2; Table 4-9]. Two cytochemical stains must be selected that will differentiate between myeloid and monocytoid cells. The leukemia AML-M4 demonstrates a mixture of myeloid and monocytoid cells and precursors. Pure monocytic leukemia (i.e., AML-M5) has very few myeloid cells. The leukemia AML-M1 is a predominantly myeloblastic leukemia. The chloroacetate esterase AS-D stains cells of the myeloid cell line, and the alpha-naphthyl acetate esterase stain is negative for myeloid cells but positive for monocytoid cells. The M1 leukemia is positive with AS-D esterase only; M4 demonstrates positivity with both; M5 is positive only with the alpha-naphthyl acetate esterase stain.

4. The answer is d [V D 5 c (1)]. Hairy-cell leukemia is a variant of chronic lymphocytic leukemia (CLL) that demonstrates lymphocytes that morphologically have a hairy appearance on a stained blood smear. The L-tartrate addition of the acid phosphatase cytochemical stain is used to aid in the diagnosis of this disorder. All other lymphocytes stain negative with the addition of L-tartrate, except the lymphocytes of hairy-cell leukemia. Hodgkin's lymphoma involves the lymph nodes and does not typically appear as a leukemia. Chloroma is a variation of acute myelogenous leukemia (AML) and does not involve lymphocytes. Lymphosarcoma cell leukemia is also a CLL variant; however, lymphocytes in this disorder do not stain positive with L-tartrate inhibition.

5. The answer is d [V D 4 a (1)]. Multiple myeloma (MM) is commonly known as a plasma cell dyscrasia, and it most commonly demonstrates a plasmacytosis in the blood and bone marrow.

6. The answer is c [IV E 3 d]. Patients who have acute myelogenous leukemia (AML) subtype M3 are at high risk for developing disseminated intravascular coagulation (DIC).

7. The answer is b [V D 5 e (1) (d)]. The finding of Reed-Sternberg cells in a lymph node biopsy is unique to patients who have Hodgkin's lymphoma.

8. The answer is b [IV C 3 c (1) (c)]. Pelger-Huët anomaly is hereditary hyposegmentation of neutrophils. Alder-Reilly anomaly is a genetic defect of leukocyte granularity. Neimann-Pick disease is a genetic disorder that affects sphingolipid degradation in monocytes and macrophages.

9. The answer is b [IV C 2 c]. The normal absolute concentration of band neutrophils is 0–700/ mm^3. During chronic infections or in any condition in which myelopoiesis in the marrow is increased, it is common to see an increase in the white blood cell (WBC) count with a granulocytosis. This granulocytosis includes an increase in immature forms such as bands and metamyelocytes.

10. The answer is c [III B 1]. The anemia of chronic disorders results partially from a defect in unipotential stem cell depression of colony-forming unit erythrocyte (CFU-E) and blast-forming unit erythrocyte (BFU-E) secondary to a chronic inflammatory disorder (e.g., infection, rheumatoid arthritis, neoplastic disease). This anemia can become microcytic because of a block in secondary iron storage and recycling of iron back to the marrow. The inflammatory response results in release of interleukin-1 (IL-1), which acts to block macrophage iron release. This anemia is classified as a production disorder, not a hemolytic disorder.

11. The answer is a [III C 3; Figure 4-3]. In iron deficiency anemia, there is a lack of available iron for heme-ring production; therefore, erythropoiesis occurs in the marrow. This results in microcytic red blood cells (RBCs) because of the ineffective erythropoiesis. There are fewer RBCs leaving the marrow per day, so the reticulocyte count remains normal to low as long as the body is deficient in iron. Once treatment begins, the patient receives the necessary iron. Bone marrow erythropoiesis responds with an accelerated rate of production to replace the needed RBCs. This results in an increased reticulocyte count for a period of 2–3 weeks.

12. The answer is c [IV E 2 a (2)(c)]. This patient's leukocyte alkaline phosphatase (LAP) level is 245 (normal is 20–200). Infections resulting in a leukemoid reaction, polycythemia vera, and myelofibrosis all demonstrate an increased LAP. Chronic myelogenous leukemia (CML) is associated with a decrease in the LAP level.

13. The answer is b [III E 2 a]. In patients who have hereditary spherocytosis, the mean cell volume (MCV) often is normal, but the mean corpuscular hemoglobin (MCH) concentration is increased, which reflects a decrease in cell-surface area of the spherocyte. The autohemolysis test can be useful in diagnosing hereditary spherocytosis.

14. The answer is b [IV B 1; Tables 4-7, 4-8]. Basophils, eosinophils, and neutrophils are granulocytes that can be found in normal blood. A lymphocyte is not a granulocyte.

15. The answer is d [III E 4 c (1) (b)]. Cold agglutinin disease is so named because the attached autoantibodies react most strongly to temperatures at or below 25°C. Because an antibody is attached to the red blood cell (RBC), the direct antiglobulin test would be positive.

16. The answer is a [III D 3 b–c]. Beta-thalassemia is attributed to a decrease or absence of β-chain production.

17. The answer is d [III B 6 i]. Antimitotic drugs, which are used as chemotherapeutic agents, are designed to halt mitotic cells. Aplastic anemia results from multipotential stem cell failure and marrow hypoplasia. Fanconi's anemia is the genetic predisposition to bone marrow failure, and it often results in pancytopenia and hypoplasia in infants and children. Chronic hemorrhage results in iron loss and erythroid hyperplasia.

18. The answer is d [V D 3 d,e]. Both cytomegalovirus and toxoplasmosis have similar symptomatic, clinical, and laboratory characteristics. Definite diagnosis must be obtained by the demonstration of specific antibodies. A positive direct antiglobulin test indicates that antibody is attached to the red blood cells (RBCs). These diseases are not accompanied, as a rule, by autoimmune complications.

19. The answer is d [IV E 2 e (4)]. There are five French-American-British (FAB) subclassifications of myelodysplastic syndromes: refractory anemia (RA), RA with ringed sideroblasts (RARS), RA with excess blasts (RAEB), chronic myelomonocytic leukemia, and RAEB in transformation (RAEBIT). Erythroleukemia is classified as an acute myeloblastic leukemia and is also referred to as AML-M6.

20. The answer is d [V D 5 e (3)]. Non-Hodgkin's lymphomas are a group of clonal proliferations of lymphocytes that have undergone malignant transformation at an arrested stage of their differentiation. They have no preleukemic history because they are not classified as leukemias. Leukemias originate in the bone marrow. Lymphomas originate in the lymph nodes.

5

Immunohematology

Jo Ann Tyndall Larsen

I. INTRODUCTION

A. Definitions

1. **Antigens** (Ag) are substances that are recognized as foreign by the body and, therefore, elicit immune responses. **Blood group antigens** exist on the surface of red blood cells (RBCs). Only a relatively small number of blood group antigens are considered clinically significant, but more than 600 have been described.

2. **Antibodies** (Ab) are immunoglobulins (Ig) that are developed in response to the presence of antigens.

   a. **Heteroantibodies (xenoantibodies)** are antibodies produced in response to antigens from another species.

   b. **Alloantibodies** are formed in response to antigens from individuals of the same species and are the type of antibodies involved in transfusion reactions.

   c. **Autoantibodies** are made in response to the body's own antigens.

B. Immunoglobulins are produced and secreted by activated B lymphocytes. All share the same basic structure of two heavy chains and two light chains held together by disulfide bonds. There are **five classes**—IgG, IgA, IgM, IgE, and IgD. Only IgG, IgM, and (rarely) IgA antibodies are produced against RBC antigens.

1. **IgA** antibodies against RBC antigens usually occur with IgG and IgM antibodies having the same specificity. They do not cross the placental barrier and do not fix complement. IgA antibodies can cause agglutination in saline.

2. **IgG** antibodies account for the majority of the clinically significant antibodies directed against blood group antigens. There are **four subclasses** of IgG: IgG1, IgG2, IgG3, and IgG4.

   a. Most IgG antibodies contain all four subclasses, but some are predominantly or exclusively composed of a single subclass.

   b. The subclasses display different biologic properties.

      (1) All bind to the crystallizable fragment (Fc) receptors on macrophages; all can cross the placental barrier; and all but IgG4 are able to bind complement through the classic pathway.

245

(2) IgG1 and IgG3 bind complement much more efficiently than does IgG2.

(3) IgG1 comprises 65%–70% of the total IgG found in serum.

3. **IgM** antibodies agglutinate very strongly in saline, so they are considered **complete** antibodies. IgM exists in serum as a **pentamer** and cannot cross the placental barrier. It strongly fixes complement through the classic pathway.

C. **Antigen-antibody reactions.** Antigen-antibody reactions important to immunohematology involve the **agglutination** of erythrocytes by antibodies.

1. **Hemagglutination** is agglutination of the RBCs. It occurs in **two stages.**

   a. **Sensitization** occurs when the antigen-binding sites of the antibodies become closely associated with the antigenic determinants of the RBC membrane. The antibodies and binding sites are held together loosely by noncovalent bonds.

   b. **Visible agglutination** occurs when several RBCs are physically joined together by the antigen-antibody union. This stage depends on many factors, such as the pH, temperature, and ionic strength of the suspension medium.

      (1) The use of **proteolytic enzymes** such as **papain** or **ficin** can enhance cell-to-cell contact.

      (2) RBCs sensitized by **incomplete antibodies** (antibodies that will not react in saline) agglutinate when antiserum against human IgG is added.

2. **The amount of available antigen and antibody** also affects hemagglutination.

   a. **Prozone** occurs when antibody molecules are in excess of available antigenic sites, resulting in false-negative reactions.

   b. **Equivalence**—optimal proportions of antigen and antibody present—allows hemagglutination to occur.

   c. **Antigen excess** also results in false-negative reactions.

D. **Complement** proteins play a number of biologic roles, but the most important role in immunohematology is their ability to lyse the cell membranes of antibody-coated RBCs. Because complement components are unstable and heat labile, it is important for serum specimens to be fresh for blood bank testing. The native precursor components are numbered from 1–9, with subcomponents of the proteins receiving the letters from a to e as they are cleaved. Complement is activated through two pathways: the **classic pathway** and the **alternate pathway.** Although these two pathways are independent, they converge at the C5 reaction, and the reactions from C5 to C9 are common to both pathways.

1. **The classic pathway** is activated by both IgG and IgM antibodies when the C1 component binds to the Fc portion of the antibody molecule. IgM and IgG3 antibodies are most efficient at complement activation.

2. **The alternate pathway** does not require specific antibody for activation, but is instead triggered by polysaccharides and lipopolysaccharides on the surfaces of certain target cells.

3. The reactions that take place from **C5 to C9** are termed the **membrane**

Table 5-1. Frequency (%) of ABO Phenotypes

Phenotype	Whites	Blacks	Native Americans	Asians
A	42	27	16	28
B	10	20	4	26
AB	4	4	<1	5
O	44	49	79	41

attack complex and result in lesions on the RBC surface. These lesions allow the rapid passage of ions, and the cell lyses from osmotic pressure changes.

II. BLOOD GROUP SYSTEMS

A. **The ABO blood group system** is the most important system in transfusion and transplantation therapy.

1. **Antigen inheritance.** ABO genes are inherited in a co-dominant manner following simple Mendelian genetics laws. Several other genetic loci interact with the ABO locus: H, Se, Le, I, and P. ABO group inheritance is controlled by the A, B, and H genes. These genes code not for the antigens themselves but for the production of **glycotransferases,** which are involved in the formation of their respective antigenic determinants.

   a. H gene: L-fucose

   b. A gene: N-acetylgalactosamine

   c. B gene: D-galactose

2. **Antigen development**

   a. **H antigens** are precursors for the A and B antigens. A, B, and H antigens may be found in other body secretions, including saliva, urine, tears, amniotic fluid, milk, bile, exudates, and digestive fluids. The presence of H substances in body secretions is controlled by the **Se gene.** Individuals who are homozygous (Se Se) or heterozygous (Se se) for this gene are called **secretors** (approximately 80% of the population).

      (1) **Group O secretors** have H antigen in their secretions.
      (2) **Group A secretors** have A and H antigens in their secretions.
      (3) **Group B secretors** have B and H antigens in their secretions.
      (4) **Group AB secretors** have A, B, and H antigens in their secretions.

   b. **Development.** A and B antigens begin to develop in the sixth week of fetal life but do not reach adult levels until 3 years of age. Antigen levels approximate 50% at birth.

   c. Because the O gene does not result in the conversion of H antigen to other antigens, the RBCs of group O individuals have the highest concentration of H antigen. Group AB individuals have the lowest concentration.

3. **Phenotypes.** ABO genes allow for five different phenotypes. Table 5-1 shows the frequency of the ABO phenotypes.

a. **A phenotype.** Group A individuals may be homozygous (**AA**) or heterozygous (**AO**). They have A antigens on their RBCs and anti-B antibodies in their serum or plasma. The two main subgroups, A_1 and A_2, can be differentiated by using the lectin anti-A_1 **reagent** made from *Dolichos biflorus* seeds.

   (1) This reagent agglutinates RBCs with the A_1 antigen but not cells with the A_2 antigen.

   (2) Approximately 80% of group A individuals are A_1; approximately 20% are A_2.

   (3) Anti-A_1 can be found in 1%–8% of group A_2 individuals.

   (4) Several other **subgroups of A** exist but are extremely rare. The most common, A_3, shows mixed field agglutination with anti-A or anti-AB reagents.

b. **B phenotype.** Group B individuals may be homozygous (**BB**) or heterozygous (**BO**). They have B antigens on their RBCs and have anti-A antibodies in their serum or plasma. A few weak **subgroups** of B exist but are less common than the rare A subgroups.

c. **AB phenotype.** Group AB individuals have both A and B antigens on their RBCs but lack both anti-A and anti-B antibodies in their serum or plasma.

d. **O phenotype.** Group O individuals are homozygous (**OO**) and have neither A nor B antigens on their RBCs. They have both anti-A and anti-B antibodies in their serum or plasma. Anti-AB antibodies are also found in the serum or plasma of Group O individuals.

e. **Bombay phenotype.** Although the H gene is necessary for the development of A and B antigens, some individuals lack the H gene and are homozygous for the **h gene,** which results in the absence of A, B, or H antigens. These individuals type initially as group O. However, with reverse typing, they react strongly not only to A_1 and B cells but also to O cells. Confirmatory testing is done using an anti-H reagent made from the *Ulex europaeus* plant. The Bombay phenotype is very rare; fewer than 200 cases have been documented worldwide.

4. **ABO antibodies** are mostly naturally occurring antibodies that develop shortly after birth following exposure to ABO-like antigens in the environment. They are mostly IgM and react best at room temperature or below. Immune ABO antibodies develop in response to exposure to ABO-incompatible RBCs or other sources of exposure to ABO antigens. The immune ABO antibodies are usually IgG and can cross the placental barrier.

5. **Testing**

   a. **Forward grouping** analyzes patient cells for the presence of ABO antigens. Testing is performed at room temperature by adding anti-A and anti-B reagents to the patient's RBCs. Cell suspensions used in blood banking procedures are usually 3%–5%. All group O donors should also be tested with anti-AB reagent. Agglutination is a positive reaction.

   b. **Reverse grouping** analyzes patient serum or plasma for the presence of anti-A or anti-B antibodies. In adults, anti-A or anti-B is present in the serum when the corresponding antigen is not present on the RBCs.

Because neonates have not developed these types of antibodies, they are not candidates for reverse ABO grouping. Testing is performed at room temperature by adding the patient's serum or plasma to suspensions of known A_1 and B RBCs. Agglutination is a positive reaction.

   c. **Discrepancies** may occur in ABO testing for a variety of reasons, including:

      (1) **Subgroups of A or B.** Individuals with subgroups of A or B forward type as group O but reverse type as group A or B. This discrepancy can be resolved by adsorbing and eluting anti-A or anti-B from the RBCs.

      (2) **Polyagglutination** can be caused by **Tn activation** or **acquired B phenomenon.** Tn activation occurs when a somatic mutation exposes a hidden RBC antigen. These discrepancies can be resolved by determining if the cells are Tn activated or have the acquired B antigen.

      (3) **Interfering substances in the serum or plasma.** False-positive agglutination can result from such substances as Wharton's jelly or increased serum proteins. The patient will forward type as AB. This discrepancy can be resolved by thoroughly washing the patient's RBCs and repeating the test.

      (4) **IgM alloantibodies.** Some IgM antibodies such as anti-Le^a, anti-P, anti-M, and anti-N can cause false-positive results. Reverse-grouping reagent cells may have the antigens against which the alloantibodies are formed. Patients may forward type as A or B but reverse type as O. This discrepancy can be resolved by identifying the alloantibody and retesting with reagent cells that lack the antigen.

      (5) **Strong autoantibodies.** Autoantibodies such as anti-I may cause a patient to forward type as A or B but reverse type as O. This discrepancy can be resolved by autoabsorbing the serum and using it to repeat the testing.

      (6) **Rouleaux** caused by increased serum proteins (e.g., myeloma proteins) can cause a patient to forward type as AB and reverse type as O. This discrepancy can be resolved by performing a saline replacement to repeat the testing.

      (7) **The age of the patient** can cause discrepancies in ABO typing. Neonates do not have ABO antibodies and cannot be reverse typed, which makes it impossible to confirm the forward typing. Elderly patients may have weakened levels of ABO antibodies.

      (8) **Disease.** Certain diseases associated with hypogammaglobulinemia or agammaglobulinemia can result in patients reverse typing as AB.

 B. **The Rh blood group system** is one of the most complex systems, because nearly 50 different Rh antigens have been identified.

   1. **Nomenclature.** Three different nomenclature systems have been developed to identify the Rh antigens and to describe phenotypes. **Table 5-2** compares the nomenclature and frequency of the most common Rh phenotypes.

      a. **Fisher-Race.** Rh antigens are inherited as three closely linked sets of alleles with little or no crossing over between loci. The five major Rh antigens are defined as **D, C, E, c, and e.**

Table 5-2. Most Common Rh Phenotypes and Their Frequencies

Phenotype Nomenclature			Frequency (%)	
Fisher-Race	**Wiener**	**Rosenfield**	**Whites**	**Blacks**
CDe	Rh_1	Rh: 1,2,−3,−4,5	42	17
cde	rh	Rh: −1,−2,−3,4,5	37	26
cDE	Rh_o	Rh: 1,−2,3,4,−5	14	11
cDe	Rh_o	Rh: 1,−2,−3,4,5	4	44

    b. Wiener. Rh antigens are inherited as products of single genes at single loci. The five major Rh antigens are defined as **Rh_o, rh′, rh″, hr′, and hr″,** which correspond to D, C, E, c, and e, respectively.

    c. Rosenfield. Rh antigens are assigned numbers to correspond to antigens already designated by other nomenclature. Newer antigens are numbered based on the order of their discovery. The five major Rh antigens are defined as **Rh1, Rh2, Rh3, Rh4, and Rh5,** which correspond to D, C, E, c, and e, respectively.

2. **D antigen** is the most clinically significant of all non-ABO antigens. It is so highly immunogenic that a single exposure to D-positive blood results in the formation of anti-D antibodies in more than 50% of D-negative individuals.

    a. The D antigen is the only Rh antigen that undergoes **routine testing,** except in the case of investigation of unexpected antibodies.

    b. The D antigen is comprised of several component antigens that are inherited as a group. **Incomplete D antigens** result when some of the component parts are missing. Individuals with these incomplete D antigens are called **D mosaics.**

    c. D^u is a weakened form of the D antigen. D-negative donors and obstetric patients must be tested for D^u. D^u-positive individuals are classified as D positive in blood donor testing. D^u-positive recipients should always receive D-negative blood. A D-negative, D^u-positive infant born to a mother with anti-D in her serum can suffer from severe **hemolytic disease of the newborn (HDN) [see X].** D^u can be inherited three ways:

        (1) As an **incomplete antigen** (D mosaic)
        (2) Due to **position effect,** which results in steric hindrance
        (3) As a result of genetic coding for **weakened D expression**

3. The genes for **C and c antigens** are co-dominant. These antigens are less immunogenic than D antigens. Other alleles can be inherited in place of C or c at the C locus, and although they typically occur with low frequency, the antibodies stimulated by these antigens may sometimes be clinically significant. However, the **c-like antigen (Rh26)** is seen often and is found on almost all c-positive RBCs.

4. **E and e antigen** expression is co-dominant. E antigens are almost as

immunogenic as D antigens, although e antigens are the least immunogenic of the five major Rh antigens.

5. **G antigens** are produced by the same Rh gene complexes that produce C and D antigens. Most C-positive and D-positive RBCs are also G-positive.

6. **Compound antigens** occur when two Rh genes are on the same chromosome. The five compound antigens of the Rh system are:

   a. f (ce)

   b. rh_i (Ce)

   c. cE

   d. CE

   e. V (ce^s)

7. **D-deletion genes** lack alleles at the Ee locus or the Ee and Cc loci and are associated with unusually strong D antigens.

8. **Rh$_{null}$** RBCs lack all Rh antigens including **Rh29.** Rh29 is present on all RBCs except Rh$_{null}$ individuals and is the highest incidence antigen in the Rh system. The lack of RBC antigens results in the characteristic **stomatocytes** seen in Rh$_{null}$ individuals, who also suffer from a compensated hemolytic anemia.

9. **LW antigens** are rarely clinically significant, but must be considered when a D-positive person appears to have developed an anti-D antibody. Anti-LW reacts more strongly with D-positive than D-negative cells. Of the three alleles, the most common is **Lw^a. LW^b** is encountered much less frequently, and the third allele, **LW,** is silent.

10. **Rh-system antibodies** are usually RBC–stimulated, either through transfusion or during pregnancy. Most are **IgG1** or **IgG3,** and appear between 6 weeks and 6 months after exposure to the Rh antigen.

    a. They **do not agglutinate in saline** unless there is a major IgM component.

    b. They **react best at 37°C** and can be demonstrated by testing in high-protein media or by the **indirect antiglobulin test.**

    c. Reaction is **enhanced** by the use of **enzyme-treated** RBCs.

    d. They do not usually bind **complement.**

    e. Rh antibodies **often occur together,** for example, anti-D and anti-G, or anti-Ce and anti-C.

    f. They **cross the placenta** and **can cause HDN.**

11. **Rh-antigen–detection reagents.** There are several types of reagents used to detect Rh antigens.

    a. **High-protein IgG anti-D reagents** are the most commonly used and require the use of an anti-D control.

    b. **IgM anti-D reagents** are used in immediate-spin saline testing and are not suitable for D^u testing.

    c. **Chemically modified IgG anti-D reagents** may be used in direct saline agglutination testing.

    d. Monoclonal anti-D reagents are combinations of monoclonal IgM and IgG, which can detect Rh antigens both at immediate spin and in the antiglobulin test phase.

    e. Reagents are also available to test for C, c, E, and e antigens.

12. **Testing** is optimal at **37°C.** If the RBCs are coated with immunglobulin, the immunoglobulins may first be heat eluted, and the cells are then tested with saline reagents.

    a. False-positive reactions may be caused by:

        (1) Positive direct antiglobulin test (DAT). The most common cause of Rh-typing discrepancies is a positive DAT. This type of discrepancy can be resolved by using low-protein reagents.

        (2) Rouleaux [see II A 5 c (6)]

        (3) Cold autoagglutinins. False-positive reactions may occur because of the presence of cold autoagglutinins. The patient sample should be warmed to 37°C and immediately retested. The autoantibody should be investigated and identified.

    b. False-negative reactions may be caused by:

        (1) Incorrect cell suspension. False-negative reactions can occur if the patient RBC suspension is too concentrated.

        (2) Improper procedure. Failure to follow the manufacturer's directions can result in false-negative results.

C. The Lewis blood group system

1. **Antigens** in the Lewis blood group system do not develop as integral parts of the RBC membrane, but are **adsorbed** by the RBCs from the surrounding plasma.

    a. Expression. The amount of antigen present is variable and is partially dependent on the individual's ABO phenotype and age, because Lewis antigens develop gradually. Lewis **antigen expression is affected by H, Se, and Le genes.** Lewis antigen expression may decrease dramatically during pregnancy.

    b. The **most common phenotypes** are:

        (1) Le (a+b−)

        (2) Le (a−b+)

        (3) Le (a+b+)

        (4) Le (a−b−)

    c. Most **neonates** type as Le (a−b−) regardless of which Lewis genes they have inherited.

2. **Lewis antibodies**

    a. Anti-Le^a antibodies are usually **IgM** but may also be **IgG,** in total or in part.

        (1) Most **of these antibodies react best at room temperature** but may react at 37°C.

        (2) Although most Le^a antibodies are considered clinically insignificant, they can **bind complement** and are therefore **capable of triggering in vitro hemolysis.** Although Le^a antibodies are not associated with HDN, the antibodies that react at 37°C or that cause in vitro hemolysis may be associated with **hemolytic transfusion reactions (HTR).**

(3) Anti-Le^a activity is **enhanced by enzyme treatment.**

    b. Anti-Le^b antibodies are usually **IgM** and react best at **room temperature.** They **bind complement poorly.** Anti-Le^b activity is **enhanced by enzyme treatment.** Le^b antibodies are not associated with HDN and rarely cause HTR.

    c. Lewis antibodies **may appear transiently during pregnancy** in Le (a−b−) women but disappear after delivery.

    d. Lewis antigens **neutralize** Lewis antibodies. Because both anti-Le^a and anti-Le^b react with most cells on routine RBC panels, **Lewis substance** can be used to neutralize the antibodies and allow the detection of any other antibodies present.

D. The MNS blood group system

    1. Antigens

        a. The MNS antigens are determined by the MN and Ss loci; **MN** is associated with **glycophorin A; Ss** is associated with **glycophorin B.**

        b. There are five principal antigens in the MNS system: **M, N, S, s,** and **U.** RBCs with the S or s antigen also have the U antigen.

        c. MNS antigens are important markers in **paternity studies.**

    2. Antibodies

        a. Anti-M antibodies are relatively common. They are usually **naturally occurring** and may be **both IgM and IgG.** Anti-M antibodies **do not bind complement** and react optimally at **room temperature or below.** They are only **rarely associated with HDN or HTR.**

        b. Anti-N antibodies are rare. They are **weak, naturally occurring IgM** antibodies that react best at **room temperature or below.** They are **not usually associated with HDN or HTR.**

        c. Anti-S, anti-s, and anti-U antibodies are **rare.** These IgG antibodies usually develop following RBC stimulation, and all have been associated with **severe HDN and HTR.** Although S, s, and U antibodies are usually **reactive in the antiglobulin phase** of testing, some saline reactive antibodies have been reported.

    3. Testing

        a. In addition to human, rabbit, and monoclonal serum-typing reagents, lectin reagents are also used to test for M and N antigens. Examples include *Vicia graminia* and several *Bauhinia* species for anti-N, and several *Iberis* species for anti-M.

        b. Many M, N, and S antibodies demonstrate a **dosage effect;** that is, they react more strongly with homozygous than heterozygous cells.

        c. M and N antigens are **destroyed by enzyme treatment,** whereas S, s, and U usually are not.

E. The P blood group system

    1. Antigens. P blood group antigens are structurally related to ABO antigens and exist as glycoproteins and glycolipids. There are **five phenotypes:**

a. P_1 is one of the two most common phenotypes. Approximately 75% of the population possess the P_1 phenotype. P_1 individuals have both P and P_1 antigens. The **P antigen** is well developed at birth; the **P_1 antigen** is poorly developed at birth. P expression in adults is widely variable.

b. P_2 is the other most common phenotype. Individuals with this phenotype have only P antigen on their RBCs.

c. P_1^k phenotype is very rare. Individuals with this phenotype have both P_1 and P^k antigens on their RBCs.

d. P_2^k phenotype is also very rare. Individuals with this phenotype have both the P_2 and P^k antigens on their RBCs.

e. The **p** phenotype is extremely rare. The RBCs of individuals with this phenotype are negative for P, P_1, and P^k antigens.

2. **Antibodies**

   a. **Anti-P_1 antibodies** are **naturally-occurring, cold-reacting, IgM** antibodies often seen in individuals with the P_2 phenotype. They **rarely react at higher than room temperature,** but they do **bind complement.** Anti-P_1 antibodies **do not cause HDN** and are **rarely associated with HTR.**

   b. **Anti-P antibodies** are produced by individuals with P_1^k or P_2^k phenotypes and **can trigger severe HTR. Autoanti-P** (the **Donath-Landsteiner antibody**) is a **cold-reacting** antibody associated with **paroxysmal cold hemoglobinuria (PCH).**

   c. **Anti-PP, P^k,** and **anti-p antibodies** occur only rarely.

F. **The I blood group system**

   1. **Antigens.** The I blood group antigens are structurally related to the ABO antigens and are found on RBC membranes as well as in plasma, milk, and amniotic fluid. Both **I and i antigens** are found on all RBCs. I antigens are poorly developed at birth. As the I antigenic strength increases, i antigen strength decreases. Most adults have strong I antigen expression and weak i antigen expression.

   2. **Antibodies**

      a. **Anti-I antibodies** are **naturally occurring, cold-reacting IgM** antibodies. They fail to react with cord RBCs. Some anti-I antibodies react in a broader temperature range and can cause **cold-agglutinin disease (CAD).** CAD may be idiopathic or may be associated with diseases such as *Mycoplasma pneumoniae* infections. Anti-I antibodies are **not associated with HDN.**

      b. **Anti-i antibodies** are rare. Like anti-I, they are **cold-reacting** antibodies. They may be seen in cases of **infectious mononucleosis** and may cause an **associated hemolytic anemia** that disappears as the infection resolves.

   3. **Testing** for anti-I or anti-i antibodies is done at 4°C using group O RBCs or cord RBCs.

G. **The Duffy blood group system.** The Duffy system **(FY)** has four alleles that are responsible for the major antigens and resulting phenotypes: **Fy^a, Fy^b, Fy,** and **Fy^x.**

1. **Antigens.** Fy^a and Fy^b antigens are produced by co-dominant alleles. Fy^x is a weakened form of Fy^b, and the Fy allele produces no gene product. There are four **phenotypes:**

   a. Fy (a+b−)

   b. Fy (a−b+)

   c. Fy (a+b+)

   d. Fy (a−b−) (There is a high incidence of this phenotype among blacks. The RBCs of individuals with this phenotype are resistant to infection by ***Plasmodium vivax.***)

2. **Antibodies.** The most common FY antibodies are Fy^a and Fy^b,. which are both commonly encountered in blood banks. Other Duffy antibodies are very rare. Anti-Fy^a and anti-Fy^b antibodies are usually **IgG,** often **bind complement,** and generally **react only at the antiglobulin phase** of testing. Both are destroyed by proteolytic enzyme treatment and heating to 56°C. Anti-Fy^a antibodies are seen more frequently than Fy^b antibodies, and both occur more commonly in combination with other RBC antibodies than alone. Although **both can cause delayed HTR,** only Fy^a has occasionally been implicated in HDN.

H. **The Kell blood group system (see Cases 13 and 16)**

1. **Antigens.** The Kell (K) system is comprised of 21 high- and low-incidence antigens, the **most significant** of which are **K** and **k.** The **K$_o$** or **K$_{null}$** phenotype lack all Kell antigens. An antigen associated with the Kell system, **Kx,** is located on the X chromosome. RBCs that lack the Kx antigen also have greatly weakened expression of the other Kell system antigens. These RBCs are morphologically acanthocytes, have decreased survival, and are less permeable to water. This syndrome, known as **MacLeod syndrome,** is also characterized by splenomegaly, reticulocytosis, and occasional association with **chronic granulomatous disease (CGD).** Kell antigens are **destroyed or inactivated by sulfhydryl reagents.**

2. **Antibodies.** The two most important antibodies of the Kell system are **anti-K** and **anti-k (Cellano).**

   a. The K antigen is second only to the D antigen in immunogenicity, and the resulting antibody is relatively common in transfusion practice. Finding K-negative donor units is rarely a problem, however, because more than 90% of the population is K-negative.

   b. **Anti-K antibodies** are usually **IgG** antibodies that **react best at 37°C** and **may occasionally bind complement.** They can **cause both HDN and HTR.**

   c. **Anti-k antibodies** are rare but can cause both HDN and HTR.

   d. Antibodies to K$_o$ (K$_{null}$) antigens are called **anti-Ku or anti-KEL5** antibodies and are considered clinically significant. K$_o$ patients should be transfused with K$_o$ cells. In testing, K$_o$ cells can be made by treating normal RBCs with 2-aminoethylisothiouronium **(AET)** bromide or dithiothreitol (DTT) plus cysteine-activated papain **(ZZAP).**

I. The Kidd blood group system

1. Antigens

a. There are two major antigens in the Kidd (JK) system, **Jk^a** and **Jk^b**, which allows for four **phenotypes:**

    (1) Jk (a+b−)
    (2) Jk (a+b+)
    (3) Jk (a−b+)
    (4) Jk (a−b−)

b. A third antigen, **JK3,** is present on both Jk^a- and Jk^b-positive RBCs. Both Jk^a and Jk^b may exhibit dosage effect; reactivity may be enhanced by **enzyme treatment.**

2. Antibodies.

Although Jk^a and Jk^b antigens are **poorly immunogenic,** the resulting antibodies **can cause severe HTR,** and both are especially noted for causing delayed reactions. Both can occasionally **cause mild HDN.** Most Jk^a and Jk^b antibodies are **IgG1 or IgG3** and **bind complement** very efficiently. Both **react best at 37°C** in the **antiglobulin phase** of testing, but saline-reactive antibodies may be seen. Jk^a and Jk^b antibodies can be difficult to detect, and enhancement techniques such as enzymes, low ionic strength saline (LISS), or polyethylene glycol (PEG) can help identify them.

J. The Lutheran blood group system

1. Antigens

a. The two most common antigens in the Lutheran (Lu) system are Lu^a and Lu^b, which allows for four **phenotypes:**

    (1) Lu (a+b−); rare
    (2) Lu (a+b+); rare
    (3) Lu (a−b+); common
    (4) Lu (a−b−); extremely rare

b. The genes encoding for the Lu antigens are linked to the Se (secretor) genes.

2. Antibodies.

Both the anti-Lu^a and the anti-Lu^b antibodies are **rarely seen. Lu^a antibodies react best at 37°C** and give a **mixed field agglutination** reaction. **Lu^b antibodies react best at 37°C** in the antiglobulin phase of testing. Lu^b antibodies can cause mild HTR, but cause mild HDN only rarely. Lu^a antibodies are often naturally occurring, whereas Lu^b antibodies usually develop after RBC stimulation by transfusion or pregnancy.

K. Other blood group systems

1. The Cartwright (Yt) system

has two antigens, Yt^a and Yt^b. The majority of individuals are Yt (a+). **Antibodies are rare.** If they develop, they are **IgG** antibodies that **react best in the antiglobulin phase** of testing and are **not clinically significant.**

2. The Colton (Co) system

has three antigens, **Co^a, Co^b, and Co^{ab}. Antibodies** to Co^a and Co^b are **rare** but **can cause HTR.** Neither cause HDN.

3. The Diego (Di) system

has two antigens, **Di^a and Di^b. Antibodies** to both antigens are **rare,** although they have been reported as causes of rare cases of HDN. The **Di^a** antigen is useful as a **racial marker,** because it is seen

almost exclusively in individuals of Mongolian extraction, such as North, Central, and South American Indians, Japanese, and Chinese.

4. **The Dombrock (Do) system** has two antigens, **Do^a** and **Do^b. Antibodies are rare. Anti-Do^a** antibodies **can cause HTR,** but neither cause HDN.

5. **The Scianna (SC) system** has three antigens, **SC1, SC2,** and **SC3. Antibodies** to SC1 and SC2 are **rare IgG** antibodies that can be clinically significant.

6. **The Xg system** has only one antigen, Xg^a, and two resulting phenotypes: Xg (a+) and Xg (a−). The Xg^a antigen is **X linked** and is **more common in women.** The antigen is **destroyed by enzyme treatment.** Xg^a antibodies are usually **IgG** antibodies that **bind complement** but do not cause HDN or HTR.

7. **The Cromer system** is composed of eight high-incidence antigens (Cr^a, Tc^a, Tc^{ab}, Dr^a, Es^a, WES^b, UMC, and IFC) and three low-incidence antigens (Tc^b, Tc^c, and WES^a). These antigens are located on the decay-accelerating factor on the RBC membrane. Patients with paroxysmal nocturnal hemoglobinuria have weakly expressed or absent Cromer-related antigens.

L. **Miscellaneous blood group antigens.** Several other RBC antigens have been identified but have not been classified as part of any blood group system.

1. **Bg antigens.** There are three Bg antigens: **Bg^a, Bg^b,** and **Bg^c.** Bg antigens are related to human leukocyte antigens (HLA) on RBCs. Antibodies to Bg antigens are not clinically significant.

2. **Sd^a antigens** are **high-incidence** antigens found in several tissues and body fluids. Antibodies to these antigens are not clinically significant. Mixed-field agglutination is characteristically seen with Sd^a antibodies.

3. **High-titer low-avidity (HTLA) antigens** occur with high frequency, but the resulting antibodies are very weak and have little or no clinical significance. They **do not cause HDN or HTR.** There are several HTLA antigens:
   a. **Chido (Ch^a) and Rodgers (Rg^a)** genes are **linked to HLA** genes, and the **antigens are associated with the C4d** component of complement. Both antigens are denatured by proteolytic enzymes.
   b. **Cost-Sterling (Cs^a) and York (Yk^a) antigens**
   c. **Knops (Kn^a) and McCoy (McC^a) antigens**

4. **Independent high-frequency antigens** rarely produce antibodies.
   a. **Gregory (Gy^a) and Holley (Hy^a)** antibodies are **IgG** antibodies that can cause accelerated red cell destruction. They do not cause HDN.
   b. **The Gerbich** collection of antigens includes five antigens. Antibodies are extremely rare but may cause HDN or accelerated RBC destruction.
   c. **Vel antigens.** Antibodies to Vel antigens may cause HTR but not HDN. They are usually IgG and can bind complement.

5. **Independent low-frequency antigens** very rarely cause antibody forma-

Table 5-3. Frequency of Common Blood Group Antigens

Antigen	Frequency (%)	
	Whites	**Blacks**
Le^a	22	23
Le^b	72	55
M	78	70
N	22	30
S	55	31
s	45	3
P	21	6
P$_1$	79	94
Fy^a	66	10
Fy^b	83	23
K	9	2
k	99	98
Jk^a	77	91
Jk^b	72	43

tion. Such antibodies are not clinically significant. **Table 5-3** outlines the frequency of the most common blood group antigens.

III. DONOR SELECTION AND BLOOD COLLECTION

A. **Blood collection for homologous donors** begins with **donor selection.** The careful screening of donors ensures that the donation will not harm the donor and the donated blood will not harm the recipient. Certain guidelines established by the **Food and Drug Administration (FDA)** and the **American Association of Blood Banks (AABB)** are followed to help establish the safest possible blood supply. Following is a brief description of these guidelines:

1. **Age.** In general, donors should be between 17 and 65 years of age.

2. **General appearance.** The donor should appear to be in good health.

3. **Weight.** Donors should weigh at least 110 pounds to donate a full 450-mL unit. Donors weighing less than 110 pounds should have proportionately less blood drawn.

4. **Temperature** measured orally should not exceed 37.5°C (99.5°F).

5. **Pulse** should be between 50 and 100 beats per minute.

6. **Blood pressure.** Systolic pressure should be no higher than 180 mm Hg; diastolic pressure should be no higher than 100 mm Hg.

7. **Hemoglobin and hematocrit.** Blood for hemoglobin and hematocrit determination may be collected by earlobe puncture, venipuncture, or fingerstick.

   a. By **earlobe puncture,** the hemoglobin and hematocrit measurements for men should be no lower than 14.0 g/dL and 42%, respectively; for women, these measurements should be no lower than 13.0 g/dL and 39%, respectively.

   b. By **venipuncture or fingerstick,** the hemoglobin and hematocrit measurements for men should be no lower than 13.5 g/dL and 41%; for women, these measurements should be no lower than 12.5 g/dL and 38%.

8. **Time between donations.** At least 8 weeks should lapse between donations.

9. **Temporary deferrals.** Certain conditions are cause for temporary deferrals and include:

   a. Being pregnant or in the 6-week postpartum period

   b. Having had a blood transfusion in the past 12 months

   c. Undergoing tattooing or ear piercing in the past 12 months

   d. Having had close contact in the last 12 months with a person with viral hepatitis

   e. Having had malaria in the past 3 years

   f. Having received one of the following **vaccinations:**
      (1) Smallpox, measles, mumps, yellow fever, or oral poliomyelitis vaccine in the past 2 weeks
      (2) Rubella in the past 4 weeks
      (3) Rabies in the past 12 months
      (4) Hepatitis B immunoglobulin in the past 12 months

   g. Taking one of the following **medications:**
      (1) Isotretinoin in the past 30 days
      (2) Antimalarial drugs in the past 3 years
      (3) Aspirin within the last 3 days (if the donor is to be the sole source of platelets)

10. **Permanent deferrals** are caused by the following conditions:

   a. History of hepatitis B or hepatitis C infection

   b. Active pulmonary tuberculosis

   c. Cirrhosis of the liver

   d. History of coronary heart disease

   e. Acquired immunodeficiency syndrome

   f. Male homosexual contact since 1979

   g. Past or present history of intravenous drug abuse

   h. Hemophilia A or B

      i. Immigration from Haiti since 1977

      j. Sexual contact with anyone in a high-risk group

      k. History of lymphoma or leukemia

      l. Taking human growth hormone or injectable insulin

  11. Other questions concerning a donor's **medical history** may reveal underlying medical problems that could be cause for deferral. Any case in question should be referred to the donor center's medical director. Most **prescription** and **over-the-counter medications** are not cause for deferral, although any questions should be referred to the medical director.

B. Apheresis donors. The same selection criteria that apply to whole blood homologous donors apply to apheresis donors. Additionally:

  1. Plasmapheresis donors must have a serum total protein of at least 6.0 g/dL. A serum protein electrophoresis should be performed in these individuals every 4 months. There should also be at least 48 hours between donations.

  2. Plateletpheresis donors should have a platelet count of at least 150×10^9/L. Aspirin ingestion within 3 days of donation is cause for temporary deferral. There should be at least 8 weeks between donations.

  3. Leukapheresis donors must have an absolute granulocyte count of at least 4×10^9/L.

  4. Therapeutic apheresis may be performed for certain conditions, such as Goodpasture's syndrome, thrombotic thrombocytopenic purpura, myeloid leukemia with hyperleukocytosis, and acute complications of sickle-cell disease.

C. Criteria for autologous donors are not as well defined or regulated as are those for homologous donors. Some general guidelines for autologous donor suitability have been established by the AABB, but the facility medical director should make final decisions. In general, donors should have a hemoglobin of at least 11.0 g/dL and should not have signs or symptoms of active infection. Blood should not be donated within 72 hours of scheduled surgery or transfusion.

D. Donor reactions. Although rare, some blood donors experience donation-related reactions, ranging from mild to severe.

  1. Symptoms include:

    a. Pallor

    b. Sweating

    c. Dizziness

    d. Nausea and vomiting

    e. Twitching and muscle spasms

    f. Loss of consciousness

  2. True convulsions are extremely rare.

  3. Phlebotomy should be discontinued immediately, and the donor should be treated symptomatically.

E. Anticoagulants and preservatives. Several anticoagulants are currently approved by the FDA for storage of blood and blood components. FDA approval for anticoagulants and additive solutions requires that 70% of transfused RBCs must be present and viable 24 hours after transfusion.

1. The **purposes** of anticoagulants and preservative solutions are:

   a. Preventing physical changes to maintain the viability and function of the blood constituents

   b. Preventing bacterial contamination

   c. Minimizing cell lysis

2. **Citrate-phosphate-dextrose (CPD)** can be used to store blood for 21 days when stored between 1°C and 6°C. The **citrate** functions as an anticoagulant by binding calcium. The **phosphate** helps to increase adenosine triphosphate (ATP) production, and the **dextrose** provides energy for the RBCs.

3. The **adenine** in citrate-phosphate-dextrose-adenine (**CPDA-1**) provides a substrate for ATP production. The shelf life of blood collected in CPDA-1 is 35 days.

4. Although not used for routine blood collection, **heparin** may be used as an anticoagulant. Because heparin has no preservative qualities, blood collected in heparin must be transfused within 24–48 hours, preferably within 24 hours.

5. Stored RBCs may be **rejuvenated** up to 2–3 days after their expiration date by the addition of a solution containing pyruvate, inosine, glucose, and phosphate. They may be either washed and transfused within 24 hours or glycerolized and frozen.

IV. DONOR PROCESSING

A. **Homologous donor processing.** The FDA and AABB require that certain tests be performed on all blood units collected for homologous transfusion. All reagents used for donor blood processing must be FDA approved, and accurate and thorough record keeping is critical.

1. **ABO and Rh typing.** Forward and reverse ABO typing must be performed on each donor unit. The Rh type must be determined using anti-D and an appropriate reagent control. All units that are initially anti-D negative must have a D^u test performed. If the D^u test is positive, the unit is labeled Rh positive. If the D^u test and the Rh control are negative, the unit is labeled Rh negative.

2. **Antibody screen.** Although the AABB requires that screens for unexpected antibodies be performed only on donors with a history of transfusion or pregnancy, most blood centers perform antibody screens on all donors. The method used must be able to demonstrate clinically significant antibodies.

3. **Serologic tests for syphilis.** The FDA requires that a serologic test for syphilis be performed on all donor units.

4. **Hepatitis.** All donor units must be tested for **hepatitis B surface antigen** (HBsAg), **hepatitis B core antigen** (HBcAg), and **hepatitis C.** Units that are repeatedly reactive for any of these markers must be discarded, and the donors must be permanently deferred. Tests for **alanine aminotransferase (ALT)** must also be performed on each unit as an indicator of possible liver

Box 5-1. Testing Required for Homologous Donor Processing

ABO and Rh typing
Antibody screen
Serologic tests for syphilis
Hepatitis B surface antigen
Hepatitis B core antigen
Hepatitis C
Alanine aminotransferase (ALT)
HIV-1
HIV-2
HTLV-III

disease. Units with ALT values 1.5 times higher than an established cutoff value must be discarded, and the donors must be temporarily deferred. Donors with ALT values equal to or greater than 2 times the cutoff value should be permanently deferred.

5. **Human immunodeficiency virus (HIV) and human T-lymphotropic virus (HTLV).** All donor units must be tested for HIV-1, HIV-2, and HTLV-III antibodies. Any units reactive by screening methods for any of these markers must be discarded, and the donor must be permanently deferred.

6. **Cytomegalovirus (CMV).** Testing for CMV is not required but is often performed on donor units. The transfusion of CMV-negative units may be clinically indicated for low-birth-weight neonates, as well as organ or bone marrow transplantation patients, and other immunocompromised or immunodeficient patients. Box 5-1 summarizes the testing required for homologous donors.

B. **Autologous donor processing.** Requirements for processing autologous donor units differ somewhat from those for homologous units.
   1. **Testing.** In addition to ABO and Rh typing, testing for HBsAg, syphilis, and HIV-1 are required for processing autologous donor units. Most donor facilities perform all tests normally required for homologous units to allow unused autologous units to be used for other transfusion purposes.

   2. **Labeling.** Donor units dedicated for autologous use must be clearly labeled "for autologous use only," and a biohazard label must be attached to any unit repeatedly reactive for any of the previously mentioned tests for infectious diseases.

   3. **Storage.** In addition to being stored between 1°C and 6°C, autologous units must be stored separately from homologous units.

V. **BLOOD COMPONENTS AND COMPONENT THERAPY.** A wide variety of blood components can be prepared from routinely drawn units of whole

Table 5-4. Blood Component Therapy

Component	Indication for Use
Whole blood	Rapid blood loss Neonatal exchange transfusion
Packed RBCs	Symptomatic anemia
Deglycerolized RBCs	Avoid febrile or allergic transfusion reactions
Washed RBCs	Avoid febrile or allergic transfusion reactions
Leukocyte-poor RBCs	WBC antibodies
FFP	DIC Vitamin K deficiency Massive transfusions
Platelets	Thrombocytopenia DIC ITP
Plasma	Volume expander
Cryoprecipitate	Hemophilia A Factor XIII deficiency Hypofibrinogenemia
Granulocytes	Neutropenia Sepsis

DIC = disseminated intravascular coagulation; FFP = fresh frozen plasma; ITP = immune thrombocytopenia purpura; RBCs = red blood cells; WBC = white blood cell.

blood for many different therapeutic applications. Table 5-4 summarizes blood components and the clinical indications for their use.

A. Whole blood

    1. Preparation. Normally, approximately 450 mL of blood are collected into a bag containing 63 mL of anticoagulant, usually CPD or CPDA-1.

    2. The shelf life of whole blood collected in CPD is 21 days when stored between 1°C and 6°C. The shelf life is extended to 35 days when the blood is collected in CPDA-1 anticoagulant. A unit of blood must be transfused within 24 hours if the seal on the bag is broken to remove plasma. If the blood is not transfused in that time period, it must be disposed of.

    3. Therapeutic uses. Each unit of whole blood should increase the hematocrit from 3%–5%, or the hemoglobin from 1–1.5 g/dL. There are few clinical indications for whole blood transfusions, although they may be appropriate for patients with rapid blood loss when increased volume as well as increased RBC mass are needed. Whole blood may also be used in exchange transfusions, especially in neonates.

B. Packed RBCs

    1. Preparation. Each unit of packed RBCs contains approximately 250 mL.

Packed cells are prepared by removing approximately 200–250 mL of plasma from a unit of whole blood. The cells may be prepared in an open system by allowing the cells to sediment, then removing the plasma. A closed system may also be used in which multiple bags are attached to the unit, and the plasma is expressed into one of the satellite bags. The hematocrit of RBCs separated by these methods should not exceed 70%–80%.

2. **Shelf life.** Cells separated in an open system must be transfused within 24 hours. If the cells are separated in a closed system, they have the same expiration date as the original unit of whole blood. RBCs separated in a closed system with an additive bag can have a second preservative solution added that will extend the shelf life to 42 days. They should be stored between 1°C and 6°C.

3. **Therapeutic uses.** The increase in hemoglobin and hematocrit in response to one unit of packed RBCs is the same as for whole blood. Packed RBCs are used to increase the RBC mass in patients who have symptomatic anemia.

C. **Deglycerolized frozen RBCs**
   1. **Preparation.** RBCs to be frozen are collected in CPD, CPDA-1, or other additive systems and normally should be frozen within 6 hours. The cells are warmed and mixed with high molar concentrations of glycerol, then frozen at −65°C. Frozen units must be stored for up to 10 years. The cells must be **deglycerolized** before they can be transfused. **Deglycerolization** begins with thawing the cells at 37°C, then washing multiple times in a gradient concentration of saline, beginning with hypertonic concentrations and ending with an isotonic saline solution containing glucose. One unit of deglycerolized RBCs contains approximately 180 mL of cells.

   2. **Shelf life.** Deglycerolized RBCs are stored between 1°C and 6°C and must be transfused within 2 hours of deglycerolization.

   3. **Therapeutic uses.** The increase in hemoglobin and hematocrit in response to one unit is the same as for whole blood or packed cells. Freezing cells allows for long-term storage of rare donor units or autologous units. Transfusing deglycerolized RBCs also minimizes febrile or allergic reactions.

D. **Washed RBCs**
   1. **Preparation.** Plasma is removed from whole blood after centrifugation, and the remaining RBCs are washed three times with 0.9% saline.

   2. **Shelf life.** Washed RBCs have a shelf life of 24 hours after the original unit is opened, and they should be stored between 1°C and 6°C.

   3. **Therapeutic uses.** One unit of washed RBCs increases the hemoglobin and hematocrit by the same amount as do unwashed cells. Washing RBCs removes most of the leukocytes and plasma from a unit of blood, which greatly reduces the risk of febrile or allergic reactions in susceptible patients.

E. **Leukocyte-poor RBCs**
   1. **Preparation.** Leukocyte-poor RBC preparations have at least 70% of the original white blood cells (WBCs) removed, and at least 70% of the original RBCs are left. There are several different methods of obtaining leukocyte-poor RBCs, including centrifugation, filtration, and washing.

   2. **Shelf life.** If a closed preparation system is used, the shelf life is the same

as the original unit of blood. The shelf life is reduced to 24 hours if an open system is used. Leukocyte-poor RBCs should be stored between 1°C and 6°C.

3. **Therapeutic uses.** In addition to increasing RBC mass, leukocyte-poor RBCs also minimize febrile transfusion reactions in patients who have leukocyte antibodies.

F. **Fresh frozen plasma (FFP)**

1. **Preparation.** Plasma is separated from whole blood and frozen within 6 hours of collection. Plasma can be removed from whole blood using a double bag collection system to preserve a closed system. The plasma is immediately frozen at or below −18°C.

2. **Shelf life.** After freezing, the plasma should be stored at or below −18°C. FFP has a shelf life of 1 year after collection of the original unit of blood. It should be thawed at 37°C and transfused within 24 hours of thawing. Thawed FFP should be stored between 1°C and 6°C if it is not transfused immediately.

3. **Therapeutic uses.** Because FFP contains all of the coagulation factors, it can be used to treat patients who have liver failure, vitamin K deficiency, and disseminated intravascular coagulation (DIC), or patients who have received massive transfusions.

G. **Platelets**

1. **Preparation.** Platelet-rich plasma is separated at room temperature by centrifugation from RBCs within 6 hours of collection of whole blood. The platelet-rich plasma is then centrifuged, and the resulting platelet-poor plasma supernatant is removed, which leaves approximately 50 mL of plasma with the platelet concentrate.

2. **Shelf life.** Platelets are stored at room temperature with continuous gentle agitation and have a shelf life of 3–5 days, depending on the type of bag used. If several units of platelets are pooled, the shelf life is reduced to 4 hours following pooling.

3. **Therapeutic uses.** Platelet concentrate is used to treat patients who have thrombocytopenia, dysfunctional platelets, DIC, and idiopathic thrombocytopenia purpura (ITP), or patients who have received massive transfusions. Each unit of platelet concentrate should increase the platelet count by $5 \times 10^9/L$ to $10 \times 10^9/L$.

H. **Plasma derivatives**

1. **Preparation.** Plasma other than that prepared as FFP may be separated from whole blood at any time during the unit's shelf life up to 5 days after the expiration date. The plasma may be pooled, purified, or fractionated into **albumin** or **plasma protein fraction.**

2. **Shelf life.** Plasma derivatives have a shelf life of 5 years when stored between 1°C and 6°C.

3. **Therapeutic uses.** Plasma derivatives such as albumin are used primarily as volume expanders.

I. **Cryoprecipitate**

1. **Preparation.** Cryoprecipitate is the insoluble fraction of plasma. Each unit

contains 80–120 units of **factor VIII** and approximately 150–250 mg of **fibrinogen,** as well as significant amounts of **factor XIII** and **fibronectin.** Each unit of cryoprecipitate contains approximately 15 mL. It is prepared from FFP that has been partially thawed between 1°C and 6°C, centrifuged, and has had the supernatant removed. The remaining cryoprecipitate is immediately frozen at or below −18°C.

2. **Shelf life.** After freezing, the optimal storage temperature is at or below −30°C, and the shelf life is up to 12 months following the collection of the original unit.

3. **Therapeutic uses.** Cryoprecipitate is used in the treatment of hemophilia A, factor XIII deficiency, and hypofibrinogenemia.

J. **Granulocytes**

1. **Preparation.** Granulocyte preparations may be prepared by leukapheresis or from a freshly drawn donor unit.

2. **The shelf life** of granulocyte preparations is 24 hours after separation when stored at room temperature. However, granulocytes should be transfused as soon as possible because their half-life is only 6 hours.

3. **Therapeutic uses.** Granulocytes have been given to severely neutropenic patients or patients who have overwhelming sepsis. Success has been limited.

K. **Irradiation of blood products.** The immunologically active lymphocytes present in most blood components can create special problems for immunocompromised patients. **Graft-versus-host disease (GVHD)** is an especially serious complication for these patients. Irradiating blood products can help reduce the risk of GVHD and other related complications.

1. **Indications for use.** Irradiated blood products may be indicated for:

   a. Patients receiving chemotherapy or radiotherapy

   b. Organ transplantation recipients who have been immunosuppressed

   c. Low-birth-weight neonates

   d. Patients with genetically deficient immune systems

2. **Irradiation**

   a. Blood components should be irradiated immediately before transfusion.

   b. Doses of 1500–5000 rad are usually used.

   c. Irradiation does not affect the shelf life of the blood component.

VI. ANTIGLOBULIN TESTING

A. **Reagents.** Patient RBCs are tested to detect the presence of in vivo and in vitro antibodies using **antihuman globulin (AHG)** reagents. These reagents may be **monoclonal** or **polyclonal** and may be monospecific or polyspecific.

1. **Monospecific reagents** are made against a specific immunoglobulin class or complement component. **Anti-IgG is most commonly used** because most clinically significant antibodies are IgG. These IgG reagents are directed specifically against the heavy chain component of the immunoglobulin molecule. Some monospecific reagents are specific for the C3b and C3d components of complement.

2. **Polyspecific reagents** are made against a combination of immunoglobulin

Table 5-5. Agglutination Reactions

Grade	Appearance
4+	One large aggregate of RBCs against a clear background
3+	Several large aggregates against a clear background
2+	Many small-to-medium aggregates against a clear background
1+	Many small aggregates against a cloudy background
±	Many very small, easily broken aggregates against a cloudy background
(+)*	No agglutination visible macroscopically; agglutination visible microscopically
mf*	Mixed field reaction; tiny aggregates against a background of free RBCs
0*	Negative; no agglutination visible macroscopically or microscopically
H	Hemolysis

RBCs = red blood cells.
*Negative or weakly positive reactions are read microscopically.

classes and complement components, but always contain **anti-IgG** and **anti-C3d.**

B. **Direct antiglobulin testing (DAT)**

1. **Application.** DAT is used to demonstrate the in vivo coating of RBCs with antibody or complement. It may be used to investigate the following disorders:

   a. HDN (see X)

   b. Autoimmune and drug-induced hemolytic anemias

   c. HTR

2. **Testing.** Patient RBCs are saline washed and mixed with AHG reagents at room temperature, then centrifuged, resuspended, and examined for agglutination. Table 5-5 describes a typical system for grading agglutination reactions.

   a. Negative results are confirmed by the addition of **Coombs' control cells,** which should yield a positive reaction after centrifugation.

   b. Coombs' control cells are coated with IgG or C3d, depending on the specificity of the AHG reagent used. If the patient's RBCs have been properly washed, the IgG or C3d on the control cells reacts with any antibody or complement bound to the surface of the patient's RBCs.

   c. Patient RBCs should be collected in ethylenediamine tetraacetic acid (EDTA), acid-citrate-dextrose, or CPD anticoagulants.

3. **False-positive reactions** can be caused by:

   a. Dirty glassware

   b. Septicemia

   c. Overcentrifugation

    4. False-negative reactions can be caused by:

      a. Inadequately washed RBCs (most common cause)

      b. Undercentrifugation

      c. Delayed testing after specimen collection

C. Indirect antiglobulin testing (IAT)

  1. Application. The IAT is used to demonstrate the presence of antibody or complement in patient serum, which results in the in vitro coating of RBCs by the antibody or complement component. **Uses of IAT include:**

    a. Detecting and identifying antibodies

    b. Compatibility testing

    c. Investigating HDN (see X)

    d. Investigating HTR

    e. Investigating autoimmune hemolytic anemias (AIHA)

  2. Testing. Patient serum is incubated at 37°C with RBCs (e.g., donor cells, antibody screening cells). After incubation, the cells are washed with saline to remove unbound antibody, and the AHG reagent is added. The AHG reagent reacts with the RBCs that have been sensitized by any antibodies present. Negative results are confirmed by the addition of Coombs' control cells, which should yield a positive result after centrifugation. Reactions may be enhanced by the use of one of the following reagents to the incubation phase of testing:

    a. Bovine serum albumin at 22% or 30%, which increases the test's sensitivity

    b. LISS solutions, which also increase sensitivity and shorten incubation times

    c. Other reagents to increase sensitivity, such as **polybrene** and **PEG**

  3. False-positive reactions may be caused by:

    a. Polyagglutination resulting from in vivo coated RBCs (+DAT)

    b. Overcentrifugation

    c. Dirty glassware

  4. False-negative reactions may be caused by:

    a. Inadequately washed RBCs (most common cause)

    b. Undercentrifugation

    c. Delayed testing after specimen collection

    d. Incorrect cell-serum ratio

VII. UNEXPECTED ANTIBODIES

A. Detection. Clinically significant unexpected antibodies against blood group antigens occur in less than 3% of the population. Antibodies occur more frequently in women than in men because of the possibility of sensitization during pregnancy. Multiple antibodies are more commonly seen in patients older than

Table 5-6.   Characteristics of Clinically Significant Antibodies

Antibody	Class*	Phase†	HDN	HTR	Binds Complement
D	IgG	AHG	Yes	Yes	No
C	IgG	AHG	Yes	Yes	No
E	IgG	AHG	Yes	Yes	No
e	IgG	AHG	Yes	Yes	No
Le^a	IgM	RT	No	Yes	Yes
Le^b	IgM	RT	No	No	Yes
M	IgG, IgM	≤37°C	Rare	Yes	No
N	IgG, IgM	≤37°C	Rare	Rare	No
S	IgG, IgM	AHG	Yes	Yes	No
s	IgG	AHG	Yes	Yes	No
P$_1$	IgM	4°C	No	Rare	Yes
Fy^a	IgG	AHG	Yes	Yes	Yes
Fy^b	IgG	AHG	Yes	Yes	Yes
K	IgG	AHG	Yes	Yes	Yes
k	IgG	AHG	Yes	Yes	Yes
Jk^a	IgG	AHG	Yes	Yes	Yes
Jk^b	IgG	AHG	Yes	Yes	Yes
Lu^a	IgM, IgG	RT	Rare	No	Yes
Lu^b	IgM, IgG	AHG	Rare	Rare	Yes

AHG = antihuman globulin; HDN = hemolytic disease of the newborn; HTR = hemolytic transfusion reactions; RT = room temperature.
*Class = immunoglobulin class to which majority of antibodies belong.
†Phase = phase at which most of the antibodies react optimally.

60 years who have undergone transfusion multiple times. Table 5-6 summarizes the characteristics of clinically significant antibodies.

1. **Screening cells** are Group O cells that have known antigens present. Commercially available sets of screening cells contain D, C, E, c, e, M, N, S, s, Le^a, Le^b, P, K, k, Fy^a, Fy^b, Jk^a, and Jk^b antigens. **Testing** is performed in three consecutive phases using patient serum screening cells:

   a. **Immediate spin** in saline at room temperature

   b. **37°C incubation** with enhancement medium (e.g., albumin, LISS, polybrene)

    c. **AHG phase** after incubated cells are washed with saline

2. An **autocontrol** (using patient cells and patient serum) is also performed. A negative result effectively rules out the presence of an autoantibody.

3. **Results. IgM antibodies** usually **react on immediate spin** and include **M, N, Le^a, Le^b, and P$_1$. IgG antibodies** such as **Kell, Rh, Kidd, and Duffy** usually **react in the AHG phase.**

B. **Antibody identification. Antibody panels** are used to identify an unexpected antibody detected by antibody screening. These panels usually contain 10–15 vials of Group O cells, each of which yields a different antigen reaction pattern. **Cord cells** are useful in identifying cold antibodies because they strongly express the i antigen and weakly express the I antigen.

1. **Testing.** The patient's serum is mixed with the panel cells and tested, along with an autocontrol, in the three consecutive phases:

    a. **Immediate spin** in saline at room temperature

    b. **37°C incubation** with enhancement medium (e.g., albumin, LISS, polybrene)

    c. **AHG phase** after the incubated cells are washed with saline

2. **Techniques to enhance antigen-antibody reactions** may be used. These include:

    a. **Enzyme treatment** with **ficin, papain, trypsin,** or **bromelin to enhance the reactions** of some antibodies (e.g., Rh and Kidd) or **denature** others (e.g., M, N, S, and Duffy) [Table 5-7]

    b. **Increasing the amount of serum** to increase the number of available antibody molecules

    c. **Lengthening incubation time**

    d. **Concentrating** the antibody by adsorption and elution

3. **Other techniques** may be used to eliminate clinically insignificant reactions and make identification of significant antibodies easier. These include:

    a. **Enzyme treatment** as described previously

    b. **AET, DTT,** and **ZZAP,** which inactivate some antigens (especially Kell)

    c. **Thiol reagents,** which denature IgM immunoglobulins

    d. **Saline, LISS, albumin**

    e. **Increased or decreased incubation temperatures**

    f. **Saline replacement** to remove abnormal proteins

    g. **Adsorption and elution** to remove unwanted antibodies, such as cold or warm autoantibodies, or to help resolve multiple antibodies

4. **Titrations** may be used to detect the antibody present in the highest concentration in patients with multiple antibodies.

5. **Results.** The manufacturer's sheet supplied with each antibody panel (Figure 5-1) indicates the presence or absence of specific antigens in each vial of panel cells. Results should be consistent with the characteristics of the identified antibody, such as optimal reaction temperatures.

    a. **Patient reactions** are recorded and compared to those in the panel,

Table 5-7. Effect of Proteolytic
Enzymes on Antigen–Antibody
Reactivity

Antigen–Antibody	Reactivity
ABO	Enhanced
Rh	Enhanced
Le^a	Enhanced
Le^b	Enhanced
M	Destroyed
N	Destroyed
S	Destroyed
P_1	Enhanced
I	Enhanced
i	Enhanced
Fy^a	Denatured
Fy^b	Denatured
Jk^a	Enhanced
Jk^b	Enhanced
K	No effect
k	No effect
Lu^a	Destroyed
Lu^b	Destroyed
Xg^a	Destroyed

and antigens whose reactions do not match the patient's reactions are eliminated until the antibody or antibodies are identified.

   b. **Hemolysis** should also be noted because some antibodies, especially those in the ABO, P, Le, Jk, and Vel systems, can cause hemolysis.

C. **Troubleshooting** (Table 5-8)

   1. If the autocontrol and all panel cells agglutinate at room temperature but react less strongly at 37°C and in the antiglobulin phase, then the presence of one of the following should be suspected:

   a. **Cold-reacting antibody** such as anti-I

   b. **Rouleaux**

Cell	D	C	E	c	e	M	N	S	s	Le^a	Le^b	P_1	K	k	Fy^a	Fy^b	Jk^a	Jk^b	IS	37	IAT	enzyme
1	0	+	0	+	+	+	0	0	+	0	+	0	0	+	0	+	0	+	0	0	0	
2	+	+	0	0	+	+	+	+	+	0	+	+	0	+	+	0	0	+	0	0	2+	
3	+	+	0	+		+	0	+	+	+	0	+	+	0	+	+	+	0	0	0	2+	
4	+	+	0	0	+	+	0	+	0	0	+	+	0	+	0	+	+	+	0	0	0	
5	0	0	0	+	+	+	0	+	+	0	+	0	0	+	+	+	+	+	0	0	2+	
6	0	0	0	+	+	0	+	+	0	0	+	+	+	+	+	+	+	0	0	0	2+	
7	+	0	0	+	+	0	+	+	+	0	+	+	0	+	0	0	+	+	0	0	0	
8	+	0	+	+	0	0	+	0	+	+	0	+	0	+	0	+	0	+	0	0	0	
9	+	0	+	+	+	+	0	+	0	+	0	+	0	+	+	+	+	+	0	0	2+	
10	0	0	0	+	+	+	+	+	+	0	0	+	0	+	+	0	+	0	0	0	2+	
																	auto		0	0	0	

Figure 5-1. Antibody panel in which a single alloantibody, Fy^a, has been identified. Enzyme testing was not necessary.

2. If the autocontrol and all panel cells agglutinate only in the antiglobulin phase, then the problem may be a **warm autoantibody**.

3. If the autocontrol is negative, and all panel cells agglutinate, then there may be:

   a. **Multiple antibodies**

   b. **Antibody** against a **high-frequency antigen** found on all the panel cells

4. If the autocontrol is positive in the antiglobulin phase, and the panel cells

Table 5-8. Troubleshooting Antibody Panels

	Room Temperature	37°C	AHG	Possible Problem
Autocontrol	3+	1+	1+	Cold autoantibody, rouleaux
Panel cells	3+	1+	1+	
Autocontrol	0	0	+	Warm autoantibody
Panel cells	0	0	+	
Autocontrol	0	0	0	Multiple antibodies, antibody to high-frequency antigen in panel
Panel cells	+	+	+	
Autocontrol	0	0	+	Warm autoimmune hemolytic anemia
Panel cells	var	var	var	

AHG = antihuman globulin; var = variable.

are negative or give variable positive reactions, then the problem may be a **warm AIHA.**

VIII. COMPATIBILITY TESTING

  A. Patient specimens. Pre-transfusion testing begins with a properly collected and identified patient specimen.

    1. Patient identification. Proper identification of the patient is imperative; the patient must have a wristband with identification information. The tube should be labeled at bedside immediately after the sample is drawn. In addition to patient information, the label should also include the date and time of collection and the name of the person who collected the sample. A sample should never be collected into a previously labeled tube.

    2. Collection. Serum is the preferred specimen for compatibility testing. Hemolysis should be avoided. Blood should not be drawn from an intravenous site unless absolutely necessary. In such a case, the infusion should be stopped, the line should be flushed with normal saline, and the first 5–10 mL of blood should be discarded before the specimen is collected.

    3. Age of specimen. The freshest sample possible should be used for compatibility testing. If the patient has previously undergone transfusion or if the transfusion history is unknown, the sample should be no older than 72 hours. Pregnant patients should also be tested with samples not more than 72 hours old.

    4. Sample storage. The AABB requires that patient samples must be stored between 1°C and 6°C for at least 7 days following transfusion.

  B. Compatibility testing for homologous transfusion. The selection of donor units compatible for homologous transfusion includes:

    1. ABO and Rh on donor units

    2. ABO and Rh on recipient, including both forward and reverse ABO grouping [Rh is determined using anti-D reagents, and D^u testing may be performed on D-negative patients (although this is generally considered unnecessary, except in the case of obstetric patients)]

    3. Antibody screening of recipient

    4. Antibody identification, if necessary [If an unexpected antibody is identified, it should be determined if the antibody is clinically significant (Table 5-9). If so, all donor units should be tested for that antibody, and only those units lacking the antigen should be used.]

    5. Autocontrol to detect the presence of autoantibodies

    6. Crossmatch

      a. The **major crossmatch** tests **donor cells against the recipient's serum** and primarily functions to determine the ABO compatibility of the donor cells.

      b. The **minor crossmatch using recipient's cells and donor serum** is no longer required as part of the crossmatch procedure.

      c. The crossmatch is tested in **three phases:**

        (1) Immediate spin in saline at room temperature

Table 5-9. Clinically Significant Antibodies

Frequently Significant	Sometimes Significant
ABO	Le^a
Rh	Lu^a
Fy^a	Lu^b
Fy^b	M
K	N
k	P$_1$
Jk^a	
Jk^b	
S	
s	

(2) Incubation at 37°C with enhancement medium

(3) Antiglobulin phase after washing incubated cells with saline

C. **Compatibility testing for autologous transfusion** includes:

1. **ABO and Rh** on autologous units

2. **ABO and Rh** on recipient

3. **Antibody screening and major crossmatch** (not required, although an immediate-spin major crossmatch is often performed)

D. **Compatibility testing for neonatal transfusion** includes:

1. **ABO and Rh** on the infant

2. **Antibody screen** on the infant or the mother

   a. If the antibody screen is negative, a crossmatch is not necessary.

   b. If the donor cells are not group O, the infant must be tested for anti-A and anti-B antibodies. If either is present, ABO-compatible RBCs should be used. A crossmatch is not necessary.

E. **Troubleshooting incompatible crossmatches** (Table 5-10)

1. **Negative antibody screen, negative autocontrol, and positive major crossmatch** may be caused by:

   a. Incorrect ABO grouping of donor or recipient

   b. Donor unit with a positive DAT

   c. Donor with an alloantibody to a low-incidence antigen

2. **Positive antibody screen, negative autocontrol, and positive major crossmatch** may be caused by a recipient alloantibody to an antigen(s) on donor cells.

3. **Positive antibody screen, positive autocontrol, and positive major crossmatch** may be caused by:

Table 5-10. Troubleshooting Incompatible Crossmatches

Antibody Screen	Autocontrol	Major Crossmatch	Possible Problem
Negative	Negative	Positive	ABO/Rh typing error Donor unit with positive DAT Low-incidence antibody in donor unit
Positive	Negative	Positive	Donor alloantibody
Positive	Positive	Positive	Patient alloantibody Rouleaux

DAT = direct antiglobulin test.

    a. Recipient autoantibody

    b. Recipient alloantibody to recently transfused RBCs

    c. Rouleaux

        (1) Positive reactions are seen at 37°C.

        (2) Washing before the addition of AHG reagent should remove the excess protein that is causing the rouleaux formation.

        (3) The AHG phase should be negative.

F. Selection of donor units according to ABO and Rh

    1. The ABO group of the recipient (Table 5-11) is the most important consideration for selecting donor units for transfusion. Whenever possible, the donor units should be the same ABO group as the recipient. If this is not possible, the donor units must be ABO compatible with the recipient's serum and must be given as packed RBCs.

    2. The Rh type of the recipient is the second most important consideration.

        a. Rh-positive recipients may receive either Rh positive or Rh negative units.

        b. Rh-negative recipients should only receive Rh negative RBCs to avoid being sensitized to the D antigen. Rh-negative recipients may receive Rh positive RBCs if it has been demonstrated that anti-D is not present in the recipient.

Table 5-11. Selection of Whole Blood Donor Units and Packed Red Blood Cells (RBCs) In Order of Preference

Recipient ABO	Whole Blood	Packed RBCs			
		1st Choice	2nd Choice	3rd Choice	4th Choice
O	O	O	—	—	—
A	A	A	O	—	—
B	B	B	O	—	—
AB	AB	AB	A	B	O

3. Group O-negative RBCs are the component of choice for **neonatal transfusions.** Group-specific blood may be given if the mother and infant are the same ABO type. The donor RBCs must be compatible with the mother's serum.

4. **Emergency situations** may call for the release of uncrossmatched blood. In such cases, O-negative or group-specific blood should be given, and compatibility testing should be performed as soon as possible.

IX. **TRANSFUSION REACTIONS** include any adverse signs or symptoms associated with a transfusion and may be **acute** or **delayed.**

A. **Acute reactions** may have **immunologic** or **nonimmunologic** causes.

1. **Acute HTR** are **rare immunologic** reactions that may be life-threatening and are **usually caused by ABO incompatibilities.** The associated **hemolysis is intravascular.** The most common signs of an acute hemolytic reaction are **fever, chills, and hemoglobinuria.** Dyspnea and hypotension leading to shock are seen in severe reactions. The most severe cases may result in DIC and renal failure.

2. **Nonhemolytic febrile transfusion reactions** are **mild immunologic** reactions that are caused by **HLA class I antigens on transfused WBCs or platelets.** They are the **most common** type of transfusion reaction (1 in every 200 transfusions). Fever and chills are the most common symptoms. The use of leukocyte filters when transfusing blood can help reduce the frequency of these reactions (see Case 12).

3. **Allergic reactions** are the **second most common** type of transfusion reactions. These **acute immunologic** reactions are typically associated with **urticaria** and are thought to occur in response to reactions between recipient antibodies and soluble proteins in the donor units. **Antihistamines** given before the transfusion can reduce the risk of an allergic reaction. **Anaphylactic reactions are very severe allergic reactions.** Although rare, they **can be life-threatening.** They are usually caused by **antibodies to IgA.**

4. **Transfusion-related acute lung injury** is a rare but life-threatening transfusion reaction caused by HLA antibodies. Symptoms are the same as those seen in adult respiratory distress syndrome and include acute respiratory distress, hypoxemia, pulmonary edema, fever, and hypotension.

5. **Acute nonimmunologic reactions** may be caused by:

a. Bacterial contamination of the blood product

b. Circulatory overload caused by too rapid transfusion

c. Blood that has been hemolyzed by improper storage or mechanical stress (e.g., heart-lung machine)

B. **Delayed reactions** may also have immunologic or nonimmunologic causes.

1. **Delayed HTR** are characterized by the accelerated destruction of transfused RBCs and are most commonly **associated with a secondary (amnestic) response** to an RBC antigen. Delayed reactions may not be recognized for days, weeks, or even months after a transfusion, until a rapid decline in the recipient's hematocrit is noticed. Patients may experience fever and mild

jaundice. The associated **hemolysis is generally extravascular. IgG antibodies** to Rh, MNS, Kell, Kidd, and Duffy antigens are often implicated.

2. Transfusion-associated **GVHD** (TA-GVHD) reactions may be either **acute or chronic.** An **extremely high mortality rate** is associated with TA-GVHD. These reactions occur when immunologically competent lymphocytes are transfused into an immunoincompetent host. Bone marrow transplantation recipients may also develop TA-GVHD, but these patients typically have a chronic, milder disease with a much lower mortality rate. The transfusion of irradiated units can prevent TA-GVHD in immunocompromised patients.

3. **Post-transfusion purpura** is a rare transfusion reaction usually seen in older female patients who have been sensitized to platelet antigens, either by previous transfusion or pregnancy. These reactions are characterized by mild-to-severe immune thrombocytopenia, with clinical bleeding in severe cases.

4. **Other nonimmunologic transfusion reactions** include:
   a. **Citrate toxicity** from anticoagulant
   b. **Hypothermia** from transfusing cold blood
   c. **Hyperkalemia** from the increased potassium levels in banked blood
   d. **Transfusion-induced hemosiderosis** (iron overload) in patients who have undergone chronic transfusion

C. **Investigating transfusion reactions** requires strict adherence to the following steps:
   1. All patient records and blood product containers must be checked for proper identification. **Clerical error** is the most common cause of HTR.
   2. **A post-transfusion sample** from the patient is centrifuged, and the serum or plasma is examined for **icterus or hemolysis** and compared against the pretransfusion sample.
   3. A **DAT** is performed on a **post-transfusion EDTA specimen.** A DAT is performed on the pre-transfusion specimen if the post-transfusion specimen has a positive DAT. An antigen-antibody incompatibility is assumed if the post-transfusion specimen DAT is positive, and the pre-transfusion DAT is negative.
   4. **Other tests** to further investigate the cause of the incompatibility may be performed, including:
      a. **ABO and Rh** on the recipient's pre- and post-transfusion specimens and on the donor units
      b. **Repeat compatibility testing** with pre- and post-transfusion specimens
      c. **Serum bilirubin** on samples drawn 5–7 hours after transfusion
      d. **Gram's stain** on recipient's plasma and **culture** of donor unit bag
      e. **Haptoglobin** on pre- and post-transfusion specimens
      f. **Urine hemoglobin**
      g. **Coagulation studies**

X. HEMOLYTIC DISEASE OF THE NEWBORN (HDN) is sometimes

referred to as **erythroblastosis fetalis.** It occurs when the mother is alloimmunized to antigen(s) found on the RBCs of the fetus, which results in the destruction of the fetal RBCs by the mother's IgG antibodies. This hemolysis causes anemia in the fetus and anemia and hyperbilirubinemia in the newborn (see Case 14). **ABO and Rh** antibodies are most frequently implicated in HDN, although other alloantibodies (e.g., M, N, S, Kell, Duffy, Kidd, Lutheran) can also cause HDN. ABO-HDN is the most common form of the disease and is a milder disease than that caused by Rh antibodies. Anti-D, anti-CD, and anti-CE are associated with the most severe forms of the disease. Anti-c, anti-E, and anti-k (Cellano) are associated with moderate forms.

A. **Pathophysiology.** If a woman's first child has a RBC antigen(s) foreign to the mother, sensitization occurs during delivery, when the normal fetomaternal bleed allows some of the infant's RBCs to enter the mother's circulation. If subsequent fetuses have the same antigen(s) as the first, the mother's IgG antibodies against that antigen cross the placental barrier and enter the fetal circulation. This secondary antibody response results in the hemolysis of the fetus's RBCs, and the released hemoglobin is converted to **bilirubin.**

1. **Before delivery,** the glucuronyl transferase in the mother's liver converts the bilirubin to excretable conjugated bilirubin.

2. **After delivery,** however, the infant's liver cannot convert unconjugated bilirubin to conjugated bilirubin because newborns are deficient in glucuronyl transferase. This unconjugated bilirubin accumulates in the infant's tissues, causing jaundice and brain damage **(kernicterus).**

B. **Laboratory evaluation of disease.** In addition to being caused by different types of antibodies, there are other differences between ABO-HDN and Rh-HDN that are identified by several laboratory tests. The **hyperbilirubinemia** and the **degree of anemia** are the primary indicators of the severity of the disease, which can range from mild to severe.

1. **ABO-HDN** is characterized by a weakly positive or negative DAT. Anemia is absent or very mild, but spherocytes and reticulocytes are increased. Jaundice, if present, is usually mild and does not appear for 24–48 hours after delivery. ABO-HDN is seen most often in group A_1 or B infants who have group O mothers.

2. **Rh-HDN.** In contrast to ABO-HDN, Rh-HDN is characterized by a positive DAT. Anemia is present, and reticulocytes are increased. Jaundice appears within the first 24 hours, and bilirubin levels are greatly increased.

C. **Prenatal testing to asses risk of HDN.** If a prenatal antibody screen detects an antibody in the mother, it should be identified. The class of immunoglobulin involved is important because IgG antibodies cross the placenta, but IgM antibodies do not. In the case of antibodies that have both an IgG and an IgM component, DTT can be used to eliminate the agglutinating capability of the IgM portion, which allows the IgG component to be titered.

D. **Fetomaternal bleeds,** and thus the risk of sensitization, can be assessed by:

1. A qualitative test, such as the **rosetting test,** distinguishes Rh-positive fetal RBCs from Rh-negative maternal RBCs. Anti-D is added to maternal RBCs. Any Rh-positive cells present will attach to the anti-D. D-positive test cells are then added and form rosettes with any anti-D coated fetal cells present.

2. A quantitative test, such as the **Kleihauer-Betke stain,** distinguishes hemoglobin F–containing fetal RBCs from those adult cells that contain hemoglobin A. An alcohol-fixed blood smear is treated with an acid buffer to elute the hemoglobin A. The cells are then counterstained. Hemoglobin F–containing cells stain, and the hemoglobin A–containing cells appear as ghost cells.

E. Treatment of HDN can include:

1. Intrauterine transfusion to correct anemia in the fetus

2. Early delivery, usually at or after 34 weeks' gestation, and when fetal lung maturity has been determined

3. Transfusion to correct anemia in the newborn in mild cases

4. Exchange transfusion in severe cases:

a. To decrease bilirubin levels

b. To correct anemia

c. To remove the infant's sensitized RBCs

d. To decrease the concentration of incompatible antibodies

5. Donor blood cell characteristics

a. Must be group-specific or must be negative for the antigen against which the mother's antibodies are directed

b. Should be group O or the same ABO group as the mother and infant, if both are the same

c. Must not have any unexpected antibodies

d. Must be less than 7 days old

e. Should be negative for CMV

f. Should be negative for hemoglobin S

F. Prevention of HDN

1. The only type of HDN now preventable is that caused by anti-D. The administration of **Rh immune globulin (RhIG)** within 72 hours after delivery of the first D-positive infant from a D-negative mother prevents the sensitization of the mother to subsequent D-positive fetuses. D-negative or D^u-negative patients can be given RhIG at approximately 28 weeks' gestation. RhIG is made of purified, concentrated anti-D gamma globulin.

2. Criteria for administering RhIG

a. Mother must be D-negative; D-negative, D^u positive patients are not usually given RhIG

b. Mother must have no detectable anti-D in her serum

c. Infant must be D-positive

d. The DAT on the cord blood must be negative

e. The amount of RhIG to be given is calculated by performing a Kleihauer-Betke test and using the following formula:

Table 5-12. Autoimmune Hemolytic Anemias (AIHA)

AIHA Type	Reaction Temperature (°C)	DAT IgG	C3d	Reactive Eluate	Antibody in Serum
Warm	37	+	+	yes	yes
Cold	<37	0	+	no	yes
Mixed	≤37	+	+	yes	yes
PCH	≤37	0	+	no	yes
Drug-induced					
Adsorption	37	+	0	yes	yes
Immune complex	37	0	+	no	yes
Membrane modification	37	+	+	no	no
Drug-induced	37	+	0	yes	yes

DAT = direct antiglobulin test; PCH = paroxysmal cold hemoglobinuria.

$$\frac{\text{Number of fetal cells}}{1000 \text{ Adult cells}} \times 5000 = \frac{\text{mL fetal whole blood}}{30} = \text{Number of vials to give}$$

One vial of RhIG should be given if no fetal cells are detected.

XI. **AUTOIMMUNE HEMOLYTIC ANEMIAS (AIHA).** Autoantibodies may be responsible for **decreased RBC survival** and **may interfere with pre-transfusion testing.** There are several categories of AIHA (Table 5-12).

A. **Warm AIHAs** account for the **majority** of cases of AIHA. **Antibodies** involved are **usually IgG and react best at 37°C.** The **DAT is almost always positive.** If the antibody screen is positive, **adsorption and elution studies** may be necessary to determine if the antibodies present are autoantibodies, alloantibodies, or both.

B. **Cold AIHAs** are the **second most common** type of AIHA. These are usually **IgM antibodies** and may be **harmless or cause disease,** such as **cold agglutinin disease. PCH** is often associated with transient infections. The antibody involved is auto-anti-P (the **Donath-Landsteiner antibody**). Pathologic autoantibodies bind to RBCs at temperatures between 30°C and 32°C. Hemolysis occurs when the temperature increases to 37°C. Such antibodies are referred to as **biphasic.** The **DAT is positive** because of the presence of **C3d** on the RBCs. Cold-reacting antibodies may interfere with pre-transfusion testing, and adsorption studies may be helpful in determining if alloantibodies are present.

C. **Mixed-type AIHAs** cause **severe hemolysis.** These AIHAs have **features of** both **warm and cold** AIHAs. The **DAT is positive** because of the presence of both **IgG** and **C3d** on the RBCs. Adsorption studies may be necessary in pre-transfusion testing.

D. **Drug-induced immune hemolytic anemias** will give a **positive DAT.** Table

Table 5-13. Drugs Capable of Causing
Autoimmune Hemolytic Anemias (AIHA)

Mechanism of AIHA	Drug
Drug adsorption	Penicillin Cephalothin Quinidine
Immune complex	Rifampin Phenacetin Quinine
Membrane modification	Cephalothin
Autoantibody	Methyldopa Levodopa Mefenamic acid

5-13 lists some drugs known to cause AIHAs. Four different **mechanisms** of drug-induced hemolysis have been identified:

1. **Drug adsorption.** The involved **antibodies are IgG** and are directed against drugs such as **penicillin** that are adsorbed onto the surface of the RBCs. Eluates react only with drug-sensitized RBCs.

2. **Immune complex type.** Antibodies to drugs such as **quinine** and **quinidine** form immune complexes with the drugs and **activate complement.** C3d is usually found on the RBCs. Eluates are nonreactive.

3. **Membrane modification.** Drugs such as **cephalothin** modify the RBC membrane and allow the nonspecific adsorption of protein. Eluates are nonreactive.

4. **Drug-induced hemolytic anemias.** The **DAT is usually positive** because of the presence of **IgG** on the RBCs and becomes positive within 3–6 months after starting therapy with procainamide, levodopa, methyldopa, or mefenamic acid. A positive DAT may persist for up to 2 years after the particular drug has been discontinued. Eluates in this type of AIHA are reactive with normal RBCs.

XII. TRANSFUSION-TRANSMITTED DISEASES. Many different infectious diseases can be transmitted through transfused blood and blood products. Although the careful testing of donor units has significantly decreased the incidence of such diseases, the risk of acquiring them through transfusion still exists. These diseases include:

A. **Hepatitis**

1. **Hepatitis A** infection through blood transfusion is extremely rare.

2. The incidence of **hepatitis B** infection through blood transfusion has been greatly reduced by mandatory testing of all donor units for HBsAg.

3. **Hepatitis C** infection was the cause of 90% of all cases of non-A, non-B post-transfusion hepatitis. Recently developed testing methods have reduced

the risk of transfusion-transmitted infection. All donor units must be tested for hepatitis C.

    4. Hepatitis D infection is seen only in conjunction with hepatitis B infections.

B. HIV. HIV-1 and HIV-2 are known to cause disease in humans, although HIV-2 infection is currently extremely rare in the United States. Testing for HIV-1 and HIV-2 is required on all donor units. Improved testing techniques have greatly reduced the risk of transfusion-transmitted HIV infections.

C. HTLV-I and HTLV-II antibodies have been identified in some intravenous drug users. All donor units are tested for both viruses, and transfusion-related transmission is rare.

D. CMV transmission is of concern in low-birth-weight neonates and immunocompromised patients. Because the virus is transmitted by leukocytes, the transfusion of leukocyte-depleted donor units is helpful in reducing the risk of infection.

E. Malaria. Risk of transfusion-transmitted malarial infections is extremely rare. There are no screening tests, but persons with a history of disease are temporarily excluded from blood donation.

F. Babesiosis. Risk of transfusion-transmitted infection by *Babesia microti* infection is extremely rare. There are no screening tests.

G. Syphilis is rarely transmitted through blood transfusion, because the period that viable spirochetes can be found in the blood is very brief. The FDA requires syphilis testing on all donor units.

XIII. THE MAJOR HISTOCOMPATIBILITY COMPLEX (MHC) AND HUMAN LEUKOCYTE ANTIGENS (HLA)

A. The MHC is a set of closely linked genes found in all vertebrates that are capable of mounting an immune response. The cell-surface antigens that are encoded for by these genes play a major role in both immunity and disease. There are three classes of MHC proteins (see XIII B 1–3):

    1. Class I MHC proteins

    2. Class II MHC proteins

    3. Class III MHC proteins

B. HLA. The MHC in humans is called the HLA complex. The antigens in this system are identified as **HLA-A, -B, -C, -DP, -DQ, or -DR,** all of which can be classified as class I, II, or III.

    1. Class I HLA antigens are **HLA-A, HLA-B, and HLA-C** proteins. They are found on all tissue cells in the body as well as on platelets. They are present only in very small amounts on RBCs. These RBC HLA antigens are the **Bg antigens,** which include HLA-B7, HLA-B17, and HLA-A28.

    2. Class II HLA antigens are **HLA-DP, HLA-DQ, and HLA-DR.** These antigens are capable of inducing a humoral immune response. They are expressed only on B lymphocytes and antigen-presenting cells such as monocytes, macrophages, dendritic cells, Langerhans cells, and Kupffer's cells. All cells that express class II MHC proteins also express class I proteins.

    3. Class III HLA antigens include the complement precursors C2 and C4, as well as the Chido and Rodgers RBC antigens.

Table 5-14. Selected Human Leukocyte Antigens (HLA) and Associated Diseases

HLA Antigen	Associated Disease
HLA-B7	Multiple sclerosis
HLA-B8	Myasthenia gravis Systemic lupus erythematosus Graves' disease Addison's disease
HLA-B27	Ankylosing spondylitis Juvenile rheumatoid arthritis Reiter's syndrome
HLA-DR2	Goodpasture's syndrome Narcolepsy
HLA-DR3	Juvenile diabetes mellitus
HLA-DR4	Rheumatoid arthritis Juvenile diabetes mellitus

C. **HLA and disease.** Many diseases, including a significant number of autoimmune diseases, have been associated with specific class II HLA antigens. Determining an individual's HLA type can help predict the risk of certain diseases. Table 5-14 lists some diseases and the HLA antigens associated with an increased risk of developing these diseases.

D. **Organ transplantation.** The cellular and humoral immune responses that can result in organ-graft rejection are caused by HLA antigens. Testing of both donor and recipient for HLA compatibility greatly reduces the risk of rejection. **HLA-A, HLA-B, and HLA-DR** antigens are the most important antigens in compatibility testing for solid organ transplants.

E. **Bone marrow transplantation** can result in severe GVHD and graft rejection. Donor marrow that matches the recipient's **HLA-A, HLA-B, HLA-C, and HLA-DR** antigens is less likely to stimulate rejection.

F. **Paternity testing. HLA-A** and **HLA-B typing** in combination with **RBC antigen testing** can exclude an individual as a father in 95% of cases. There are two types of exclusions.

    1. **Direct or first-order exclusion** is established when a child inherits a trait that neither the alleged mother nor the alleged father has.

    2. **Indirect or second-order exclusion** is established when:

       a. The alleged father is homozygous for an antigen that the child does not have.

       b. The child is homozygous for an antigen that the mother has but the alleged father does not have.

       c. The child does not have two antithetical antigens that the alleged father has.

Study Questions

Directions: Each of the numbered items or incomplete statements in this section is followed by answers or completions of the statement. Select the ONE lettered answer or completion that is BEST in each case.

1. Blood group antibodies belong to which one of the following immunoglobulin classes?

a. IgM, IgG, IgA, IgE, IgD
b. IgM, IgG, IgE
c. IgM, IgG, IgA
d. IgM, IgG

2. Which one of the following classes of immunoglobulins is capable of crossing the placental barrier?

a. IgA
b. IgG
c. IgM
d. IgD

3. Which one of the following is the "membrane attack complex" in the classic pathway of complement activation?

a. C1
b. C3
c. C4b, C2a
d. C5, C6, C7, C8, C9

4. Which one of the following characteristics apply to individuals who have A antigens on their red blood cells (RBCs)?

a. they have anti-A in their serum
b. they have anti-B in their serum
c. they have anti-A and anti-B in their serum
d. they have neither anti-A or anti-B in their serum

5. Extracts from the seeds of *Dolichos biflorus* agglutinate the red blood cells (RBCs) of which one of the following groups?

a. H
b. A_1
c. A_2
d. B

6. Mixed-field agglutination in ABO typing would most likely be caused by

a. Bombay phenotype
b. A_3 red blood cells (RBCs)
c. positive indirect antiglobulin test
d. cold autoantibody

7. Antibodies in the Rh system are generally

a. the result of transfusion or pregnancy
b. inhibited by enzymes
c. IgM antibodies
d. complement binding

8. Rh antibodies react best at which one of the following temperatures?

a. 22°C
b. 18°C
c. 4°C
d. 37°C

9. D^u red blood cells (RBCs) have which one of the following characteristics?

a. they react in the saline phase with anti-D
b. they are classified as D positive in blood donor testing
c. they react with anti-D^u
d. they are classified as D negative in blood donor testing

10. In vitro hemolysis may be associated with which one of the following antibodies?

a. anti-Le^a
b. anti-s
c. anti-k
d. anti-M

11. Which one of the following blood group phenotypes is associated with resistance to *Plasmodium* infections?

a. Fy (a+b−)
b. Fy (a−b+)
c. Fy (a+b+)
d. Fy (a−b−)

12. Which one of the following characteristics best describes anti-Lu^b antibodies?

a. they are often naturally occurring antibodies
b. they can cause hemolytic transfusion reactions (HTR)
c. they react best at room temperature
d. they are not able to bind complement

13. Which one of the following antigens is seen almost exclusively in persons of Mongolian extraction?

a. k (Cellano)
b. Do^b (Dombrock)
c. Di^a (Diego)
d. Ch^a (Chido)

14. The Kell antigen is best described as

a. absent from the red blood cells (RBCs) of neonates
b. strongly immunogenic
c. destroyed by enzymes
d. very common in the random population

15. Proteolytic enzyme treatment of red blood cells (RBCs) usually destroys which one of the following antigens?

a. Jk^a
b. E
c. Fy^a
d. Le^a

16. Anti-Jk^a antibodies have which one of the following characteristics?

a. they can cause severe, delayed hemolytic transfusion reactions (HTR)
b. they are usually IgM
c. they react best at room temperature
d. they are strongly immunogenic

17. Which one of the following is grounds for permanent rejection of a blood donor?

a. receiving a tattoo 5 months before donation
b. recent close contact with a patient with hepatitis B
c. having two units of blood transfused 4 months previously
d. having a confirmed positive test for HBsAg 10 years ago

18. After a unit of whole blood stored between 1°C and 6°C has been entered, what is the maximum allowable storage time?

a. 4 hours
b. 6 hours
c. 24 hours
d. 72 hours

19. The shelf life of a unit of blood collected in citrate-phosphate-dextrose-adenine (CPDA-1) is

a. 21 days
b. 35 days
c. 42 days
d. 45 days

20. The optimum storage temperature for whole blood is

a. 1°C to 6°C
b. 12°C to 15°C
c. −20°C to −25°C
d. −75°C to −80°C

Answers and Explanations

1. The answer is c [I B]. The majority of antibodies against blood group antigens are of the IgG class of immunoglobulins. Most of the rest are IgM. Only a few rare blood group antibodies are IgA. There are no IgD or IgE blood group antibodies.

2. The answer is b [I B]. IgG is the only class of immunoglobulin capable of crossing the placental barrier.

3. The answer is d [I D 3]. Although the classic and the alternate pathways are activated through different mechanisms, they converge at C5. Components C5 through C9 form the membrane attack complex. Cell lysis occurs when C8 and C9 attach to the cell membrane.

4. The answer is b [II A 3 a]. Anti-B antibodies are found in the serum of individuals who have A antigens on their red blood cells (RBCs). Individuals with B antigens on their RBCs have anti-A antibodies in their serum.

5. The answer is b [II A 3 a]. Reagents made from *Dolichos biflorus* seeds can be used to differentiate group A_1 from A_2. The extract agglutinates A_1 red blood cells (RBCs) but not A_2 RBCs.

6. The answer is b [II A 3 a]. A_3 is the most common of the A subgroups after A_1 and A_2. Mixed-field agglutination is often seen when A_3 red blood cells (RBCs) react with anti-A or anti-AB reagents. The A_3 subgroup should be considered when mixed-field agglutination is seen in ABO forward typing.

7. The answer is a [II B 10]. Most antibodies against Rh system antigens are IgG antibodies that develop as a result of a previous transfusion or by sensitization during pregnancy.

8. The answer is d [II B 10 b]. Rh antibodies are mostly IgG antibodies that react optimally at 37°C.

9. The answer is b [II B 2 d]. D^u is a weakened form of the D antigen that can elicit an antibody response in D-negative patients. D^u-positive donors and obstetric patients should always be considered to be D positive.

10. The answer is a [II C 2 a]. Anti-Le^a antibodies bind complement strongly, and as a result they are capable of triggering in vitro hemolysis. Anti-s, anti-k, and anti-M antibodies do not trigger in vitro hemolysis.

11. The answer is d [II G 1 d]. There is a high incidence of the Fy (a−b−) phenotype among people of African descent. Red blood cells (RBCs) having this phenotype are unusually resistant to infection by *Plasmodium vivax*.

12. The answer is b [II J 2]. Although Lu^a antibodies are rare, naturally occurring antibodies, Lu^b antibodies may be seen following transfusions or pregnancy and can cause mild hemolytic transfusion reactions (HTR). Both antibodies are capable of binding complement.

13. The answer is c [II K 3]. The Di^a antigen is rarely seen in white or black populations, but is a high-incidence antigen in people of Mongolian extraction (e.g., North, Central, and South American Indians; Chinese; and Japanese).

14. The answer is b [II H 2]. The Kell antigen is second only to the D antigen in immunogenicity. Fewer than 10% of the population is positive for the Kell antigen.

15. The answer is c [II G 2]. Fy^a and Fy^b antigens are both denatured by treatment with proteolytic enzymes such as ficin and papain. Jk^a, E, and Le^a antibodies are all enhanced by enzyme treatment.

16. The answer is a [II I 1, 2]. Both Jk^a and Jk^b antigens are poorly immunogenic, but antibodies

286

against them can cause severe hemolytic transfusion reactions (HTR). They are typically IgG antibodies that react best at 37°C.

17. The answer is d [III A 10 a]. A history of active hepatitis B infection will permanently disqualify a blood donor. The other situations are all cause for temporary deferrals.

18. The answer is c [V A 2]. Once the seal on a unit of blood has been broken and the unit is entered, the unit must be transfused within 24 hours. If it is not transfused within 24 hours, it must be disposed of.

19. The answer is b [V A 2]. Blood collected in the anticoagulant citrate-phosphate-dextrose (CPD) has a shelf life of 21 days. CPDA-1 (CPD with adenine added) extends the storage time to 35 days.

20. The answer is a [V A 2]. Whole blood collected for transfusion should be stored between 1°C and 6°C.

6

Immunology and Serology

Jo Ann Tyndall Larsen

I. INTRODUCTION

A. Antigens and haptens. An **antigen** is a substance that stimulates antibody formation and has the ability to bind to an antibody. A **hapten** is a low-molecular-weight, nonantigenic substance that, when combined with an antigen, changes the antigenic specificity of that antigen.

B. An **antibody** is a glycoprotein substance (immunoglobulin) that is produced by B lymphocytes in response to an antigen.

    1. Antibodies may be **monoclonal** or **polyclonal. Monoclonal antibodies** are derived from a single B-cell clone and are produced as a single class of immunoglobulin with specificity unique to the antigenic stimulus.

    2. Polyclonal antibodies are produced as different classes of immunoglobulins by many B-cell clones in response to an antigen.

    3. Antibodies produced in response to antigens from another species are called **heteroantibodies** or **xenoantibodies.**

    4. Alloantibodies are formed in response to antigens from individuals of the same species.

    5. Autoantibodies are produced by the body's immune system against "self" antigens. They function by facilitating phagocytosis and microbial killing and by neutralizing toxic substances. They also combine with antigens on cell surfaces, which results in either intravascular or extravascular destruction of the target cells.

C. Antigen-antibody reactions

    1. An **epitope** is the part of an antigen that reacts specifically with an antibody or T-cell receptor (Figure 6-1).

    2. Agglutination is the clumping of particulate antigens by antibodies specific for the antigens.

    3. Affinity is the tendency that an epitope has for combining with the antigen-binding site on an antibody molecule.

    4. Avidity is the strength of the bond between the antigen and the antibody.

289

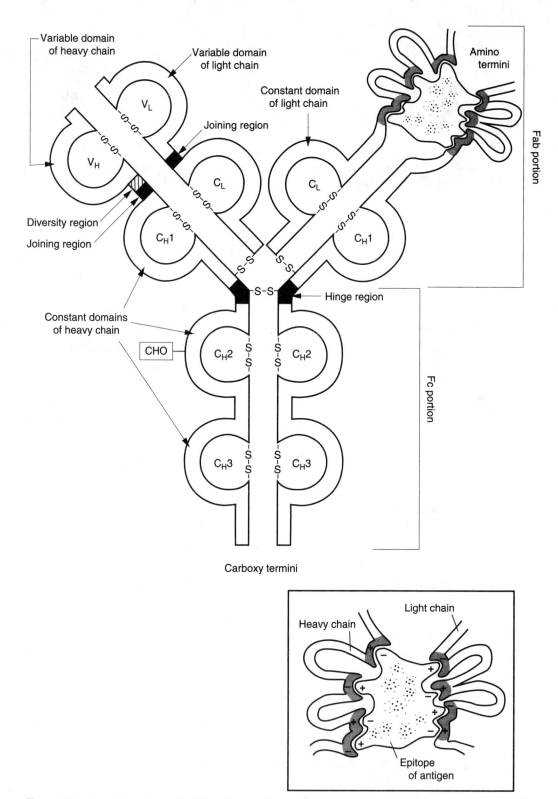

Figure 6-1. Basic immunoglobulin (Ig) molecule. Four polypeptide chains are linked covalently by disulfide bonds (S-S). The loops correspond to domains within each chain. *V* = variable domain; *C* = constant domain; *L* = light chain; *H* = heavy chain; *CHO* = carbohydrate side chain. The *inset* shows the hypervariable complementarity-determining regions as *shaded* areas. Similar hypervariable regions are found in the alpha and beta chains of the T-cell receptor for antigen. (Reprinted with permission from Hyde RM: *Immunology*, 3rd ed. Baltimore, Williams & Wilkins, 1995, p 40.)

Table 6-1. Characteristics of Immunoglobulins (Ig)

Immunoglobulin Class	Subclasses	Form	Crosses Placenta	Fixes Complement	Serum Levels (mg/dL)
IgA	2	Monomer, dimer	No	No	77–400
IgD	0	Monomer	No	No	3–5
IgE	0	Monomer	No	No	17–450
IgG	4	Monomer	Yes	Yes*	591–1965
IgM	0	Pentamer	No	Yes	50–311

*IgG4 does not fix complement.

    5. Sensitivity is the smallest amount of antigen or antibody that can be detected.

    6. Specificity is the ability of an antibody to bind to an antigen with complementary determinants and not to an antigen with dissimilar determinants.

  D. Immunoglobulins are glycoprotein substances secreted by antigen-stimulated B cells. All classes of immunoglobulins share the same basic structure: two **heavy chains** and two **light chains** joined by varying numbers of disulfide bonds (see Figure 6-1). Heavy chains determine the isotype, or class, of immunoglobulin. There are five immunoglobulin classes: **IgA, IgD, IgE, IgG, and IgM** (Table 6-1). Each molecule of immunoglobulin has either two **kappa** light chains or two **lambda** light chains.

    1. IgA exists as a monomer in serum and as a dimer in body secretions. It is the predominant immunoglobulin in secretions such as tears, saliva, sweat, breast milk, and respiratory tract, genital, and intestinal secretions. IgA binds antigens and prevents their adherence to mucous membranes to keep them from invading the body. It also confers immunity from mother to infant through breast milk. The normal range for serum IgA is 77–400 mg/dL.

    2. IgD exists as a monomer, and its function is unknown. Normal serum values of IgD are 3–5 mg/dL.

    3. IgE exists in serum as a monomer. It binds to crystallizable fragment (Fc) receptors on mast cells and basophils and is elevated during parasitic infections and Type I allergic reactions. Normal serum values for IgE are 17–450 mg/dL.

    4. IgG is the predominant immunoglobulin in the adult. There are four subclasses of IgG: IgG1, IgG2, IgG3, and IgG4. IgG binds complement, has roles in opsonization and antibody-dependent cellular cytotoxicity (ADCC), and neutralizes toxins. It is also the only immunoglobulin that crosses the placental barrier, thus transferring immunity from mother to infant. IgG precipitates and agglutinates in vitro. Normal serum values for IgG are 591–1965 mg/dL.

    5. IgM is the largest of the immunoglobulins, existing as a pentamer (Figure

6-2). It binds complement, neutralizes toxins, and agglutinates antigens in vitro. IgM is the first immunoglobulin to be produced after exposure to an antigen. Normal serum values are 50–311 mg/dL.

E. **Complement.** The complement system is a group of proteins synthesized in mononuclear phagocytes, hepatocytes, fibroblasts, and some endothelial cells. The native precursor components are numbered from 1–9, with subcomponents of the proteins receiving the letters a to e as they are cleaved.

1. **Function.** Complement proteins are involved in the disruption of microbial cell walls, inflammation mediation, regulation of phagocytic activity, and the metabolism of immune complexes. Complement can be activated through either the **classic pathway** or the **alternate pathway.**

   a. **The classic pathway** requires IgG or IgM for activation. **Table 6-2** describes the classic pathway of complement activation.

   b. **The alternate pathway** does not require specific antibody for activation, but is instead triggered by polysaccharides and lipopolysaccharides on the surfaces of certain target cells.

2. **Membrane attack complex.** Although these two pathways are separate and function independently, they converge at the C5 reaction, and the reactions from C5 to C9 are common to both pathways. These last components compose the common pathway and are also called the **membrane attack complex.** The C567 complex acts on C8 and C9. As C8 and C9 are inserted into the cell membrane, the resulting lesions allow the rapid passage of ions, and the cell lyses from osmotic pressure changes.

II. **CELLS AND TISSUES OF THE IMMUNE SYSTEM.** There are several cell types and body tissues that work together in the immune system. Many surface antigens or **surface markers** have been identified that help to characterize these cells according to their function. These markers are referred to as **clusters of differentiation (CD).** An international nomenclature system has been developed to standardize the CD numbers. Table 6-3 lists examples of CD markers.

A. **T Lymphocytes**

1. **T lymphocytes** are derived from cells in the bone marrow. This subset of lymphocytes migrates to the **thymus,** where they mature and acquire and express certain surface antigens. T lymphocytes are responsible for **cell-mediated immune responses.** They exist in several subpopulations with specific functions.

   a. **T helper cells (T_H)** are **CD4** positive and produce the lymphokines **interleukin-2 (IL-2), interleukin-3 (IL-3), granulocyte-monocyte colony-stimulating factor (GM-CSF),** and **gamma interferon (IFN-γ).** They aid in B-cell differentiation, and they stimulate other T-cell populations.

   b. **T suppressor cells (T_s)** are **CD8** positive and produce factors that inhibit the action of other T cells.

   c. Most **cytotoxic T cells (T_c)** are **CD8** positive. They secrete **lymphotoxins** and release **perforins,** which destroy cells recognized as foreign.

   d. **Delayed-type hypersensitivity T cells (T_{DTH})** are **CD4** positive. They

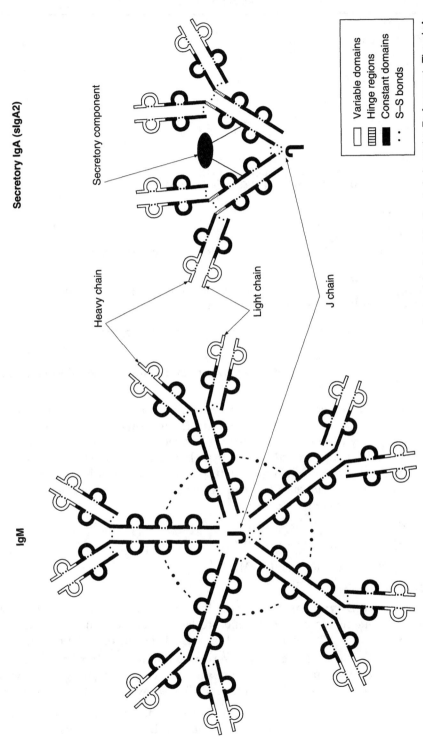

Figure 6-2. Structural models of IgM and secretory IgA (sIgA). IgM has a pentameric structure linked by the J chain at the Fc fragment. The sIgA molecule has a dimeric structure, plus joining (J) chain, plus secretory component. Shown is the dominant IgA2 subclass. (Reprinted with permission from Hyde RM: *Immunology*, 3rd ed. Baltimore, Williams & Wilkins, 1995, p 47.)

Table 6-2. Classic Pathway of Complement Activation

Activation of C1
  C1 is activated by IgG or IgM

Activation of C4
  C4 is activated by C1s

Activation of C2
  C1s interacts with C4 to cleave C2
  C2 combines with C4 to form C42 complex (C3 convertase)

Activation of C3
  C3 is activated by C42, resulting in C3a and C3b
  C3b combines with C42 to form C423 (C5 convertase)

Membrane attack complex
Activation of C5, C6, and C7
  C5 convertase splits C5 into C5a and C5b
  C5b binds to C6 and C7, forming C567 complex on the cell membrane

Activation of C8 and C9
  C8 and C9 are acted on by C567 and insert themselves into the cell membrane
  Resulting channels allow water to enter the cell
  Lysis occurs

---

secrete **macrophage chemotaxin** and **macrophage migration inhibition factor (MIF)**.

2. If a T lymphocyte has surface receptors for a specific antigen, contact with that antigen stimulates **blastic transformation.** The resulting large lymphocyte then subdivides to produce two expanded populations of T cells: small lymphocytes and medium lymphocytes, both of which have the same antigenic specificity. Several **mitogenic substances** have been found to stimulate T cells and thus can be used in laboratory evaluation of T-cell function, including:

   a. Concanavalin A (ConA)

   b. Phytohemagglutinin A (PHA)

   c. Pokeweed mitogen (PWM)

B. **B Lymphocytes**

   1. **Mature B lymphocytes** secrete immunoglobulin. These cells develop in the bone marrow in adults and are later localized also in the spleen and lymph nodes. There are several identifiable stages of B-cell maturation.

      a. Both T and B **stem cells** have **terminal deoxynucleotidyl transferase (TdT).** Stem B cells also have **immune response (Ir) gene products,** which are **major histocompatibility complex (MHC)** proteins.

      b. **The pre–B cell** is characterized by immunoglobulin gene rearrangement and the appearance of heavy chains in the cell's cytoplasm.

      c. In the **immature B cell,** light chain genes are rearranged, and the light chains appear in the cell's cytoplasm. Coupled with the heavy chains, the light chains form IgM, which is confined to the cell surface **(sIgM).**

Table 6-3.   Clusters of Differentiation (CD)

CD	Leukocytes
CD2	T lymphocytes
CD4	T lymphocytes
CD8	T lymphocytes
CD10	Pre–B lymphocytes, common ALL
CD12	Monocytes, granulocytes, platelets
CD15	Granulocytes
CD19	B lymphocytes
CD24	B lymphocytes, granulocytes
CD27	T lymphocytes, plasma cells
CD33	Myeloid leukemia
CD34	Hematopoietic stem cells
CD39	B lymphocytes, macrophages
CD41a	Glycoprotein IIb/IIIa
CD45	Leukocytes
CD47	Leukocytes, platelets
CD68	Macrophages
CD69	Activated Lymphocytes
CDw70	Reed-Sternberg cells
CD77	Activated B cells

ALL = acute lymphocytic leukemia.

   d. The mature B cell expresses both surface IgM and surface IgD, as well as MHC proteins. TdT is no longer present. Receptors for the Fc portion of the heavy chain of IgG are present, as well as complement receptors.

   e. Plasma cells develop in response to antigen stimulus in several stages:

     (1) Antigen-antibody complexes aggregate on the mature B-cell surface (capping), and the antigen is internalized.

     (2) Interleukins from T cells stimulate the B-cell growth cycle.

     (3) The new plasma cell synthesizes and secretes immunoglobulin.

     (4) Class switching allows the plasma cells to produce only one class of immunoglobulin.

 2. In addition to antigens and T-cell products, B cells also respond to a variety of other mitogens, including:

    a. Lipopolysaccharides found on the cell surface of gram-negative bacteria

    b. Protein A found on the surface of *Staphylococcus aureus*

    c. PHA

    d. PWM

    e. Phorbol myristate

    f. Anti-IgM antibody

C. Non-T, non-B lymphocytes have neither T-cell nor B-cell markers and have been classified as **killer cells (K), natural killer cells (NK),** and **lymphokine-activated killer cells (LAK).** It is unclear as to whether they represent separate populations or are the same cells with different functions.

    1. K cells express surface immunoglobulin receptors and lyse target cells by **ADCC.**

    2. NK cells play a role in tumor host defense because they have the ability to recognize and destroy tumor cells.

    3. LAK cells use IL-2 to help lyse tumor cells.

D. Phagocytes play a major role in the immune system.

    1. Polymorphonuclear leukocytes (PMNs) include **eosinophils, basophils, and neutrophils.**

        a. Eosinophil granules contain antimicrobial agents.

        b. Basophil granules contain **histamine** and **heparin,** which play a role in **anaphylactic reactions.**

        c. The two major populations of neutrophil granules are primary and secondary granules.

            (1) Primary granules contain **myeloperoxidase (MPO)** and **lysozyme,** which are important bactericidal agents.

            (2) Secondary granules also contain lysozyme. Neutrophils have **chemotactic receptors,** which allow them to respond to chemotaxins produced at sites of inflammation.

                (a) Chemotaxins commonly involved in this process include the **C5a** component of complement, **formyl peptides** found in bacteria, and **arachidonic acid metabolites** released from damaged cell membranes.

                (b) The ingestion of bacteria and other foreign particles by these cells is enhanced if the particles are coated with immunoglobulin or the C3b component of complement (**opsonization**).

    2. Monocytes and macrophages

        a. Function. As circulating monocytes respond to chemotaxins, they leave the circulation and enter the tissues, where they are converted to macrophages. These cells are important in **antigen processing** and **antigen presentation.**

        b. Surface receptors. Macrophages have several different surface receptors, including the **integrin Mac 1-CR3,** which binds the C3b component of complement; **Fc receptors,** which bind immunoglobulin; **CR1,** which binds C3b and C4b; and **Class II MHC receptors.**

    c. Secreted products. Macrophages secrete products that assist in the Ir.

        (1) Interleukin 1 (IL-1) stimulates T-cell growth.

        (2) Interleukin 6 (IL-6) stimulates B cells.

        (3) Tumor necrosis factor (TNF$_a$) has antitumor and antibacterial activity and stimulates production of IL-1 and interferon.

        (4) Endothelial leukocyte adhesion molecule (ELAM-1) plays a role in diapedesis (migration of cells into tissues from the circulation).

E. Other cells involved in antigen presentation are:

    1. Dendritic cells

    2. Langerhans cells

    3. B lymphocytes

F. Lymphoid tissues are found throughout the entire body.

    1. Distribution

        a. Spleen

        b. Thymus

        c. Thoracic duct

        d. Lymph nodes

        e. Bone marrow

        f. Peyer's patches

        g. Tonsils

        h. Appendix

    2. Concentration. Although both T and B lymphocytes can be found in all lymphoid tissues, the highest concentration of T cells is found in the thymus. The highest concentration of B cells is found in the bone marrow.

III. IMMUNITY may be **natural** or **acquired.**

A. Natural immunity is present at birth and provides protection against disease and aids in recovery from disease. However, it also provides the basis for organ rejection after transplantation. Factors involved in natural immunity include:

    1. Physical barriers, such as skin and mucous membranes

    2. Genetically controlled **susceptibility and nonsusceptibility** to certain diseases

    3. Inflammation, which involves a vascular response and a cellular response by phagocytic cells

    4. Acute-phase plasma proteins, such as C-reactive protein, haptoglobin, and fibrinogen, which are produced in response to injury and aid in wound healing

B. Acquired or specific immunity results when immunologic memory and antibody specific to a foreign antigen develop in response to the antigen. Acquired immunity may be **active** (through immunization or disease) or **passive** (through transplacental transfer). This type of immunity involves both cell-mediated and humoral immune responses.

IV. IMMUNE RESPONSE (IR). The Ir may be roughly divided into two components, **cell-mediated** and **humoral.** Although most Ir contain elements of both, certain antigens elicit a strong humoral response with little cell-mediated involvement, and other antigens elicit primarily a cell-mediated response.

   A. Humoral immunity involves **immunoglobulin** (antibody) production by B lymphocytes. **Complement** can also be considered a humoral component because it can be activated by immunoglobulin. The humoral response occurs in three phases:

   1. **Antigen elimination.** This phase is accomplished by phagocytosis. Most injected antigen is removed within minutes, but complete removal may take months or years.

   2. **The primary response.** After exposure to an antigen, there is a latent period of approximately 5–15 days before antibody appears in the serum. The antibody titer increases, plateaus, then decreases. **IgM** is the first immunoglobulin to appear. Although a small amount of IgG is made later, the majority of immunoglobulin produced during a primary response is IgM.

   3. **The secondary response.** A second or any subsequent exposure to the same antigen elicits a secondary response. This time, there is a rapid antibody response, usually within 2–4 days after antigen exposure. **IgG** is the predominant immunoglobulin. The circulating antibody titer is much higher and lasts longer than that seen in the primary response.

   B. Cell-mediated immunity is especially important in viral and fungal infections and in infections caused by acid-fast bacilli (e.g., tuberculosis, Hansen's disease).

   1. **Macrophages, T_c, and NK cells** play a role in cell-mediated immunity (see II A 1 c, C 2, D 2).

   2. **ADCC.** Cells with cytolytic activity and Fc receptors, especially NK cells, are able to directly lyse antibody-coated (usually IgG) target cells.

   3. **Cytokines** are protein messengers produced by cells. Many play a role in cell-mediated immunity.

      a. **Lymphokines** are produced primarily by activated T lymphocytes and include:

         (1) IL-2
         (2) IL-3
         (3) IL-4
         (4) GM-CSF
         (5) B-cell growth factor 2
         (6) Macrophage activating factor
         (7) MIF
         (8) IFN-γ

      b. **Monokines** are produced by monocytes and include:

         (1) IL-1
         (2) TNF_α

V. HYPERSENSITIVITY is an enhanced immune reaction to an antigen. These immune reactions are classified into four different types, depending on their patho-

Table 6-4. Hypersensitivity Reactions

Type	Mechanism	Example
I	Immediate-type	Urticaria Hay fever Bronchial asthma
II	Cytotoxic	HTR HDN ITP Some drug allergies
III	Immune complex	Immune glomerulonephritis Serum sickness Arthus reaction
IV	Delayed-type	Tuberculin skin test Contact dermatitis

ITP = immune thrombocytopenic purpura; HDN = hemolytic disease of the newborn; HTP = hemolytic transfusion reactions.

physiology (Table 6-4). Types I, II, and III are humoral (i.e., antibody mediated), and type IV hypersensitivity reactions are cell-mediated.

A. **Type I** reactions are **immediate-type hypersensitivities** that can range from **mild food allergies** to **anaphylactic shock.** Antigens complex with IgE and attach to basophils or tissue mast cells, which results in the release of **histamines** and the synthesis of **leukotrienes** C4, D4, and E4. Although Type I reactions can be systemic, most are localized. Examples include:

1. **Urticaria** (hives)

2. **Hay fever**

3. **Bronchial asthma**

4. **Food allergies**

B. **Type II** reactions are **cytotoxic responses.** In these reactions, complement-fixing IgG or IgM antibodies are directed against cellular or tissue antigens such as those found on the surface of white blood cells (WBCs) and platelets. Examples include:

1. **Hemolytic transfusion reactions (HTR)**

2. **Hemolytic disease of the newborn (HDN)**

3. **Immune thrombocytopenia**

4. **Certain drug allergies**

C. **Type III** reactions are **immune complex reactions.** IgG and IgM antibodies form soluble immune complexes with antigens. These complexes may be deposited in extravascular tissues, which results in infiltration by neutrophils and local tissue damage. Complement is also activated and contributes to the inflammatory response. Examples include:

1. **Immune glomerulonephritis**

2. **Serum sickness**

3. Arthus reaction

D. Type IV reactions are **delayed-type hypersensitivity reactions.** CD4-positive T lymphocytes react with the foreign antigen and release lymphokines, some of which are chemoattractants that attract PMNs, monocytes, and macrophages. These cells release substances such as proteases, collagenases, cathepsins, and TNF_α, which mediate inflammation. Examples include:

1. Tuberculin skin test

2. Contact dermatitis

VI. AUTOIMMUNITY is an expression of the Ir that occurs when the body's self-tolerance system fails. The body's immune cells are no longer able to recognize "self" and thus mount an Ir against its own antigens. This can result in a variety of apparently unrelated diseases known as **autoimmune diseases.** However, all autoimmune diseases involve immune complexes. The autoimmune response is strongly influenced by MHC antigens and can involve either Class I or Class II MHC proteins. Many autoimmune diseases are associated with specific Class II human leukocyte antigens (HLA), and determining an individual's HLA type can help predict the risk of certain diseases.

A. Mechanisms. Autoantibodies form in response to many different immunogenic stimuli. The autoimmune response may be triggered by:

1. Sequestered antigens, which do not normally circulate in the blood and, as a result, fail to establish immunogenic tolerance

2. Foreign antigens, which may cross-react with self-antigens

3. Altered antigens, which become denatured or mutated because of physical, chemical, or biologic changes

4. Mutation of immunocompetent cells, which may become responsive to self-antigens

5. Dysfunction of T cells, which may lose their ability to regulate the Ir

B. Autoimmune diseases may be **organ-specific** or **systemic** (Table 6-5).

1. Organ-specific autoimmune diseases. Virtually any organ system can be affected by autoimmune diseases. Examples include:

a. Hematologic disorders

(1) Paroxysmal cold hemoglobinuria

(2) Warm autoimmune hemolytic anemias (AIHAs)

(3) Immune thrombocytopenia purpura (ITP)

b. Endocrine disorders

(1) Graves' disease

(2) Hashimoto's thyroiditis

(3) Insulin-dependent diabetes mellitus

c. Neuromuscular disorders

(1) Myasthenia gravis

(2) Multiple sclerosis

d. Renal disorders

(1) Goodpasture's syndrome

(2) Tubulo-interstitial nephritis

Table 6-5. Antibodies Associated with Autoimmune Diseases

Disease	Associated Antibodies
SLE	Anti-DNA Antinuclear Anti-ribosome Anti-DNP
Primary biliary cirrhosis	Anti-mitochondrial
Myasthenia gravis	Anti-acetylcholine receptor binding Anti-acetylcholine receptor blocking
Pernicious anemia	Anti-intrinsic factor Anti-parietal cell
Multiple sclerosis	Anti-myelin
Scleroderma	Anti-centriole Anti-Scl
Sjögren's syndrome	Anti-SS-A Anti-SS-B
Graves' disease	Anti-thyroglobulin
Polymyositis	Anti-Jo-1 Anti-Ku Anti-Mi-1 Anti-PM-1
Goodpasture's syndrome	Anti-glomerular basement membrane
ITP	Anti-platelet
Insulin-dependent diabetes	Anti-islet cell

DNP = deoxyribonucleoprotein; ITP = idiopathic thrombocytopenic purpura; SLE = systemic lupus erythematosus.

e. Gastrointestinal disorders
  (1) Pernicious anemia
  (2) Primary biliary cirrhosis
2. Systemic diseases are characterized by widespread involvement. Autoantibodies are not confined to any one specific organ. Examples include:
  a. Rheumatoid arthritis (RA)
    (1) General considerations. RA is characterized by the presence of abnormal circulating IgM autoantibodies known collectively as rheumatoid factor (RF). These antibodies react specifically with the Fc portion of IgG molecules. RF may also be seen in patients with chronic hepatitis, systemic lupus erythematosus (SLE), syphilis, hypogammaglobulinemia, or hypergammaglobulinemia.
    (2) Testing. There are a variety of tests for RF, including:
      (a) Latex fixation

(b) Latex agglutination (commonly used test; considered positive for RF if the titer is at least 20)
(c) Sheep red cell agglutination
(d) Quantitation of IgM RF

b. **Polymyositis**

(1) Description. Polymyositis is characterized by inflammation and degeneration of skeletal muscle.

(2) Autoantibodies. Antinuclear antibodies (ANA), RF, and anti-Jo-1 antibodies are present.

c. **SLE**

(1) Description. SLE is a systemic rheumatic disorder that is characterized by the presence of circulating immune complexes.

(a) Epidemiology. It is most commonly seen in women and persons of African descent.

(b) Symptoms. More than half of SLE patients develop a characteristic rash or other skin abnormalities during the course of the disease. Other common symptoms include myocarditis, lymphadenopathy, glomerulonephritis, and serositis.

(c) Causes. SLE may be **idiopathic** or **drug-induced.** Drugs such as **procainamide, phenytoin, methyldopa, penicillin,** and **sulfonamides** may cause a lupus-like syndrome. ANA are present and may persist for months after the drug has been discontinued.

(2) Pathophysiology. Antibodies to native or altered self-antigens are produced and form circulating immune complexes with the antigens. Typically, the antigens involved are nuclear antigens, especially deoxyribonucleic acid (DNA). These complexes are deposited in various organs and cause inflammation, which eventually results in tissue injury.

(3) ANA are autoantibodies that react with the body's nuclear proteins, DNA, or histones. In general, they are neither organ-specific nor species-specific, and they can cross-react with nuclear material from humans or animals. Although ANAs can be demonstrated in disease-free, healthy individuals, they are most often associated with various systemic rheumatoid diseases. The ANAs formed in SLE are usually IgG but may be IgM or IgA. Several different antibodies to DNA and DNA components may be seen in SLE.

(a) Anti-ds (double-stranded)-DNA antibodies
(b) Anti-ss (single-stranded)-DNA antibodies
(c) Anti-ribonucleic acid (RNA) antibodies
(d) Anti-extractable nuclear antigen antibodies
  (i) Smith (Sm) antigens
  (ii) Microsomal antigens (MA)
(e) Anti-histone antibodies
(f) Anti-deoxyribonucleoprotein (DNP) antibodies **[LE factor; see VI B 2 c (4) (b)]**

(4) Diagnosis (Table 6-6)

(a) ANA testing

(i) The fluorescent antinuclear antibody test (FANA)

Table 6-6. Antinuclear Antibody Interpretation

Staining Pattern	Associated Antibodies	Associated Diseases
Homogeneous	nDNA, dsDNA, ssDNA DNP, histones	RA SLE Sjögren's syndrome
Preipheral	nDNA, dsDNA, DNP	Sjögren's syndrome SLE
Speckled	RNP, Sm	Scleroderma RA Sjögren's syndrome SLE Dermatomyositis
Nucleolar	Nucleolar RNA	Scleroderma Sjögren's syndrome SLE
Anti-centromere	Centromeric chromatin	Scleroderma

DNP = deoxyribonucleoprotein; dsDNA = double-stranded DNA; nDNA = native DNA; RA = rheumatoid arthritis; RNP = ribonucleoprotein; SLE = systemic lupus erythematosus; Sm = Smith; ssDNA = single-stranded DNA.

is an indirect immunofluorescence technique used for ANA screening. Mouse or rat liver cells are commonly used as substrate cells. ANAs bind to the substrate cells' nuclei. Fluorescein-conjugated antihuman globulin is added and binds to any antibodies present.

(ii) **ANA testing by immunohistochemistry** is also commonly used. Human epithelial cells are used as substrate cells. Horseradish peroxidase (HRP)–conjugated antihuman globulin binds to any ANA that has bound to the nuclei of the cells.

(iii) **Interpretation.** Positive results can be categorized by several different staining patterns: **homogeneous, peripheral, speckled, nucleolar, and anti-centromere.**

(b) **The LE cell test** demonstrates a phenomenon often seen in SLE patients as well as patients who have other diseases (e.g., **RA, scleroderma, polydermatomyositis**). The LE factor is detected in more than 95% of patients with SLE, and it is responsible for the LE cell phenomenon. In the presence of the LE factor, disrupted homogenous nuclei of lymphocytes and neutrophils are phagocytized by neutrophils. True LE cells must be distinguished from **rosette formation** (several neutrophils attempting to engulf one nucleus) and **tart cells** (monocytes phagocytizing whole cells or nonhomogenous nuclei).

VII. IMMUNODEFICIENCIES. Deficiencies of the immune system include disorders of phagocytic cells, B lymphocytes, a combination of T and B lymphocytes, and the complement system.

A. **Phagocytic cell deficiencies**

 1. Phagocytic cell deficiencies result in a decreased ability to phagocytize and kill bacteria.

 a. **Chronic granulomatous disease (CGD)** is a genetic disease characterized by ineffective killing of bacteria by neutrophils.

 (1) **Cause.** CGD is caused by a defect in **cytochrome b,** which results in **decreased hydrogen peroxide production.** Hydrogen peroxide is necessary for producing the **toxic superoxides** that are critical in bacterial killing.

 (2) **Diagnosis.** The **nitroblue tetrazolium (NBT) reductase test** is used to detect impaired neutrophil phagocytosis. The neutrophils of CGD patients fail to reduce the NBT dye.

 (3) **Symptoms.** Patients with CGD suffer from recurrent infections caused by catalase-positive bacteria and yeast and fungi.

 (4) **Treatment** includes the use of GM-CSF or G-CSF and IFN-γ.

 b. **MPO deficiency** is inherited as an autosomal recessive trait and is one of the most common inherited disorders. The **MPO** in the primary granules of neutrophils is **decreased or absent,** and although **phagocytosis takes place normally,** bacterial killing is inefficient. **Fungal killing** is more seriously impaired than bacterial killing. Although otherwise healthy patients with MPO deficiency do not have an increased frequency of infection, diabetic patients who have this disorder may have an increase in *Candida sp* infections.

 c. **Glucose-6-phosphate dehydrogenase (G6PD) deficiency** is another inherited disorder in which the aerobic system of neutrophils is impaired. This deficiency results in a substantial **decrease in the amount of hydrogen peroxide produced** during phagocytosis, and thus decreased bacterial killing efficiency. Patients with G6PD deficiency experience recurrent bacterial infections.

 d. **CR3 (iC3b receptor) deficiency** is a rare, autosomal recessive trait characterized by a **decrease or absence of specific complement component receptors** on neutrophils, monocytes, and lymphocytes. These receptors are responsible for **adherence-related functions.** Abnormalities result in **defective margination and diapedesis of neutrophils, impaired chemotaxis, and ineffective phagocytosis.** T lymphocytes adhere poorly to target cells. Clinically, there is an increased frequency of bacterial infections, a decreased inflammatory response, and neutrophilia.

 e. **Specific granule deficiency** is inherited as an autosomal recessive trait. **Neutrophils fail to develop specific granules** during myelopoiesis, and as a result, patients who have this disorder experience severe, recurrent bacterial infections.

 f. **Chédiak-Higashi syndrome** is an inherited disorder that is characterized by the **abnormal fusion of primary granules** in neutrophils. During phagocytosis, degranulation is impaired, and **little or no MPO is released into the phagosome.** Patients who have Chédiak-Higashi syndrome have recurrent bacterial infections and are also characterized by albinism and extreme photosensitivity.

    g. Lazy leukocyte syndromes include:

      (1) Job syndrome, also known as **hyperimmunoglobulin E,** is characterized by poor chemotaxis and recurrent skin infections and abscesses.

      (2) Tuftsin deficiency. Tuftsin is a **chemotaxin** that also improves phagocyte motility, engulfment, and oxidative metabolism. Affected persons experience recurrent bacterial infections.

      (3) Actin dysfunction. A deficiency of the **cytoskeletal protein actin** can result in **decreased cell motility and chemotaxis.** Patients experience recurrent bacterial infections.

B. B-lymphocyte immunodeficiencies may be **inherited** or **acquired** and account for more than half of all immunodeficiencies. **Affectedness varies widely,** depending on the class of immunoglobulin that is deficient. A deficiency of a minor immunoglobulin, such as IgD, causes little if any increase in the incidence of bacterial infections. However, because 75%–85% of total immunoglobulin is IgG, an individual deficient in IgG would be significantly affected.

    1. Bruton's agammaglobulinemia is a **sex-linked** disorder that primarily affects men. It is usually recognized early in life when **antibodies fail to develop.** Pre–B cells may be found in the bone marrow, but they do not mature. Few mature B cells are found in the peripheral blood. **Gamma globulin levels are markedly decreased.** This disorder may be treated with gamma globulin preparations.

    2. Common variable hypogammaglobulinemia is an **acquired** disorder in which **one or two immunoglobulin classes are deficient.** Total immunoglobulin levels may be normal, because a decrease in one immunoglobulin is often compensated by an increase in the production of another. **Selective IgA deficiency is one of the most common** of these deficiencies. Typically, only those patients whose disease includes IgG deficiency suffer from increased bacterial infections.

    3. Neonatal hypogammaglobulinemia is caused by the normal immaturity of the neonate's immune system. It corrects itself between the ages of 6 and 12 months as the infant's immune system matures.

C. T-lymphocyte immunodeficiencies without an accompanying loss of B-cell function are rare, composing only 7% of all immunodeficiencies. These disorders may be acquired or inherited.

    1. DiGeorge syndrome results when the **thymus gland develops abnormally** during embryogenesis. Abnormalities of other endoderm-derived tissues are also seen. **T lymphocytes are usually decreased,** but may be normal. Most patients have a **high CD4-CD8 ratio.** Although antibody responses may be normal, cell-mediated immune responses are impaired.

    2. Nezelof syndrome is an **autosomal recessive** disorder. Patients are **athymic** and are especially susceptible to viral and fungal infections, which can be fatal in these patients.

D. Combined B- and T-lymphocyte immunodeficiencies are the most serious of the immunodeficiencies, because both cell-mediated and humoral immune responses are affected.

    1. Bare-lymphocyte syndromes are characterized by defects in Class I MHC antigen expression, Class II MHC antigen expression, or a combination of both. CD4-positive T lymphocytes are decreased in number, and B- and T-cell activation is reduced.

2. **Severe combined immunodeficiency disease** may be inherited as autosomal recessive or X-linked traits. All are characterized by markedly decreased numbers of both T and B lymphocytes.

3. **Acquired immunodeficiency syndrome (AIDS)** is caused by the **human immunodeficiency virus 1 (HIV-1) or the human immunodeficiency virus 2 (HIV-2).** The **CD4-positive T lymphocytes are the primary target cells.** Approximately 5% of B lymphocytes are also infected.

   a. **Transmission** of the HIV virus is primarily through sexual contact with infected persons and parenteral routes (e.g., transfusion of infected blood and blood products). Other body fluids may also transmit the virus.

   b. There are **three stages of clinical manifestation** of HIV infection.

      (1) **The primary stage** may last from many months to years. Infected persons may experience an initial flulike illness, and then remain asymptomatic or exhibit only chronic lymphadenopathy for many years.

      (2) **The intermediate stage** is also known as **AIDS-related complex (ARC).** There are physical symptoms but no opportunistic infections.

      (3) **The final stage, AIDS,** is usually seen within 2–10 years after initial infection with the HIV virus. Opportunistic infections are common and include *Pneumocystis carinii* pneumonia, candidiasis, and histoplasmosis.

   c. **Effects on the immune system** primarily involve CD4-positive T lymphocytes.

      (1) The CD4-CD8 ratio is reduced from normal (2:1 to 0.5:1).
      (2) CD4-positive T-cell counts are decreased.
      (3) CD4-positive T-cell function is impaired.
      (4) B-cell activation is abnormal.
      (5) Macrophage function is impaired.
      (6) NK cell function is impaired.

   d. **Laboratory detection of HIV infection.** A number of tests have been developed to detect the presence of HIV antigens, antibodies, DNA, and RNA.

      (1) **Tests for antigens.** The presence of HIV antigen indicates active infection.

         (a) **The HIV isolation technique** can detect antigens before antibodies develop and can be used to monitor antiviral treatment. The patient's monocytes are stimulated and grown in culture. The culture supernatant can be tested for the presence of antigens.

         (b) A **modified enzyme-linked immunosorbent assay (ELISA)** can be performed on plasma, serum, cerebrospinal fluid (CSF), and culture fluids to detect the presence of HIV antigens.

         (c) **Immunofluorescence assay (IFA)** can be used to detect HIV antigens.

(2) **Tests for antibodies.** The presence of HIV antibodies indicates **prior exposure** to the HIV antigen. Antibody development follows a predictable course following exposure. The **p24 core protein** is the major structural protein of the HIV-1 virus. **IgM antibody against the p24 core protein** usually develops within 6–8 weeks after infection. Within weeks, IgG antibodies against p24 appear, as do antibodies against envelope gene products (i.e., gp160, gp120, gp41) and polymerase gene products (i.e., p31, p51, p66).

    (a) **The ELISA** is the most commonly performed screening test for HIV antibodies. Both false-positive and false-negative results may occur. Repeatedly reactive results necessitate confirmatory testing.

    (b) **Western blot assays** are the most commonly used confirmatory test for HIV antibodies. Protein from disrupted virus is separated onto polyacrylamide gels by electrophoresis. False-positive reactions may occur.

    (c) **Other tests** for HIV antibodies include:

        (i) **IFA**

        (ii) **Radioimmunoassay (RIA)**

        (iii) **Radioimmunoprecipitation assay**

        (iv) **Slide agglutination tests**

(3) **Tests for DNA and RNA**

    (a) **In situ hybridization and filter hybridization** can be used to detect viral RNA. Cells from peripheral blood and lymph nodes can be used.

    (b) **Southern blot hybridization** can be used to detect viral DNA in infected cells.

    (c) **Polymerase chain reaction (PCR) techniques** can be used to amplify both RNA and DNA, which provides extremely sensitive systems for RNA and DNA detection.

VIII. TECHNIQUES IN IMMUNOLOGY AND SEROLOGY

A. Agglutination assays demonstrate the presence of antigen-antibody reactions by the visible aggregation of antigen-antibody complexes. These tests are simple to perform and are often the most sensitive test method.

1. **Flocculation tests.** Antibody is detected when soluble antigen interacts with antibody and a precipitate is formed. Antigen is bound to reagent particles; visible agglutination results when the particles bind to antibody.

2. **Latex agglutination.** Antibody is bound to latex beads; visible agglutination occurs when antigen binds to the latex-bound antibody.

3. **Direct bacterial agglutination.** Antibodies bind to the surface antigens of bacteria in suspension, which results in visible agglutination.

4. **Hemagglutination** tests are used to detect antibodies to red blood cell (RBC) antigens. In **passive or indirect hemagglutination tests,** soluble antigens are adsorbed onto the surface of RBCs. These antigens then bind to any corresponding antibody present, and the RBCs agglutinate.

5. **Agglutination inhibition assays** are very sensitive and can detect small amounts of antigen. In **hemagglutination inhibition (HAI) assays,** anti-

A. Nonidentity reaction

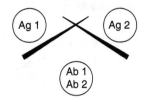

B. Partial identity reaction

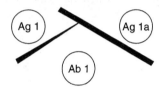

C. Identity reaction

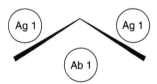

Figure 6-3. Reaction patterns of double immunodiffusion (Ouchterlony test). **A,** Nonidentity reaction: Non–cross-reacting antigens. **B,** Partial identity reaction: Antigenic determinants are partially shared. **C,** Identity reaction: Antigenic determinants are shared. (Reprinted with permission from Stites DP, Terr AI: *Basic and Clinical Immunology,* 7th ed. Norwalk, Conn, Appleton & Lange, 1991, p 219.)

gen and antibody are bound to RBCs. If antibody is present in the test sample, agglutination does not occur because there is already antibody bound to the antigen. Agglutination is a negative result. In other assays, antigen and antibody are bound to latex particles.

B. **Precipitation assays.** When both are present in proper proportions, antigens and antibodies interact and form visible precipitates. The largest amount of precipitation is seen when antigens and antibodies are present in optimal proportions; this is known as the **equivalence zone.** False-negative reactions can occur when either antigen or antibody is present in excess.

1. **Double immunodiffusion (Ouchterlony method).** Antigens and antibodies are allowed to diffuse in a semisolid medium such as agar or agarose. When the antigens and antibodies meet, a precipitate forms. Three basic reaction patterns (Figure 6-3) can result from this interaction.

   a. **Identity.** A single smooth arc of precipitation forms between the antigens and antibodies, which indicates that the antibodies are precipitating identical antigen specificities.

      b. Nonidentity. Two separate lines of precipitation cross each other, which indicates that the antigens and antibodies are unrelated and do not precipitate together.

      c. Partial identity. The two precipitating lines meet, forming a spur. This indicates that the antigens share some common epitopes, but that one of the antigens has a unique epitope.

  2. Radial immunodiffusion (RID) is a single diffusion method that can be used to quantitate immunoglobulins and other serum proteins. Samples are introduced into wells cut in agarose containing antiserum and allowed to diffuse, usually overnight. The diameters of the resulting precipitation rings correspond to the amount of antigen present (Figure 6-4).

  3. Electroimmunodiffusion combines the speed of electrophoresis with the sensitivity of immunodiffusion.

      a. Countercurrent immunoelectrophoresis (CIE). This technique is essentially a double diffusion technique in which voltage is applied to move the antigens and antibodies together. A precipitin band forms when a zone of equivalence is reached.

      b. Rocket electrophoresis. This technique applies an electrical charge to a RID assay, which results in a rocket-shaped line of precipitation. The height of the rocket is proportional to the antigen concentration.

C. Electrophoresis

  1. Immunoelectrophoresis (IEP) is often used to diagnose monoclonal gammopathies. After the serum or urine specimen is electrophoresed in a gel medium, a trough is cut in the agar parallel to the line of separated proteins. Monoclonal or polyclonal antisera are loaded into the trough, and the gels are incubated to allow the antigens and antibodies to diffuse toward each other. Precipitation lines become visible when a zone of equivalence is reached. Typically, control serum is run above the trough, and the patient sample is run below the trough for easy comparison.

  2. Immunofixation electrophoresis (IFE). After serum, urine, or CSF samples are electrophoresed in an agarose gel, cellulose acetate impregnated with antiserum is placed on the gel. The antiserum from the cellulose acetate diffuses into the gel, and antigen-antibody precipitates form. The cellulose acetate is stained to visualize the precipitation bands. IFE and IEP are often used together to work up monoclonal gammopathies.

D. Labeling immunoassays can be qualitative or quantitative and can occur in the soluble or solid phase. Radioactive, enzyme, chemiluminescent, or fluorescent labels can be used.

  1. RIA is a rapid and sensitive method that can be used to detect small amounts of antigen or antibody. However, exposure to radioisotopes can damage DNA and lead to radiation sickness, an increased incidence of neoplasms, or death. These potential hazards are a disadvantage to the RIA method.

  2. Radioallergosorbent test (RAST) is an RIA method specifically designed to measure antigen-specific IgE.

  3. Radioimmunosorbent test (RIST) is a competitive binding technique used to quantitate IgE.

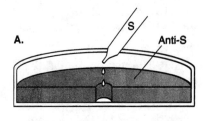

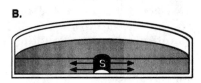

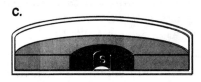

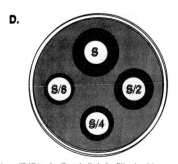

Figure 6-4. Radial immunodiffusion (RID). **A,** Petri dish is filled with semisolid agar solution containing antibody to antigen S. After agar hardens, the center well is filled with a precisely measured amount of material containing antigen S. **B,** Antigen S is allowed to diffuse radially from the center well for 24–48 hours. **C,** Where antigen S meets corresponding antibody to S in the agar, precipitation results. After reaction proceeds to completion or at a timed interval, a sharp border or ring is formed. **D,** By serial dilution of a known standard quantity, rings of progressively decreasing size are formed. The amount of antigen S in unknown specimens can be calculated and compared with a standard. (Reprinted with permission from Stites DP, Terr AI: *Basic and Clinical Immunology,* 7th ed. Norwalk, Conn, Appleton & Lange, 1991, p 221.)

4. **ELISA** is similar in principle to RIA and has the same sensitivity, but uses an enzyme label instead of a radioactive label. **HRP** and **alkaline phosphatase (ALP)** are the most commonly used enzymes. ELISAs can be used to detect extremely small amounts of antigen or antibody.

5. **Immunofluorescence assays (IFA)** are often used to identify antigens in tissue sections or air-dried smears of peripheral blood, bone marrow aspirates, touch preparations, or fine needle aspirate samples.

   a. **Labeling. Fluorescein isothiocyanate** is the most commonly used fluorescent label. **Labeling may be direct** (using a labeled antibody) **or**

indirect (using a labeled secondary antibody). After staining, the slides are washed and dried and immediately examined using a fluorescence microscope. Fluorescence quenches quickly when exposed to light, which is the major disadvantage of immunofluorescence methods.

b. **Immunocytochemical techniques** are modifications of the direct and indirect immunofluorescence methods; **enzyme labels** such as HRP and ALP are used instead of fluorescent labels. These reaction products do not fade, so slides may be stored to provide permanent records.

E. **Nephelometry (turbidimetry)** photometrically measures the turbidity of solutions created by particles in suspension. It is accurate, rapid, and precise and is often used to **quantitate immunoglobulins, complement components, and immune complexes.** This method can also be used to **measure antigen concentration.** The light source in nephelometry instruments produces a wavelength of **840 nm.**

F. **Neutralization tests.** Neutralizing antibodies can destroy the infectivity of viruses, which provides the basis for assays that can determine the amount of viral antibody present. These techniques are often used to detect antibodies against herpes simplex virus Types 1 and 2 (HSV-1 and HSV-2) and echovirus.

G. **Cellular assays.** A wide variety of techniques exists for assessing the function of the cells of the immune system.

1. **Functional assays.** These tests are rarely performed except in large medical centers and reference laboratories. Some tests are even considered obsolete. Functional assays include the following.

   a. **ADCC assays** use bacteria-infected tumor cells to assess the killing ability of NK cells.

   b. **The Boyden chamber** uses chemotactic substances to assess the chemotactic response of neutrophils.

   c. **Cell-mediated monocytolysis** uses tumor cells to assess the killing functions of monocytes.

   d. **Latex bead ingestion** assesses phagocytic activity.

   e. **Lymphocyte transformation tests** assess the ability of lymphocytes to respond to mitogens or specific antigens.

   f. **Lympholysis tests** assess the ability of T_c to lyse labeled target cells.

   g. **Microcytotoxicity studies** are used to detect HLA antigens and antibodies.

   h. **Migration inhibition** techniques determine the ability of lymphocytes to produce chemotactic factors in response to granulocytes and monocytes.

   i. **Mixed-lymphocyte cultures** are used to assess the human leukocyte antigen D (HLA-D) compatibility of donor and recipient lymphocytes.

   j. **NBT reductase tests** are used to assess the intracellular killing ability of neutrophils.

   k. **Phagocytosis assays** mix bacteria with neutrophils to assess the cells' phagocytic ability.

2. **Flow cytometry** can be used to identify subpopulations of cells such as

reticulocytes, granulocytes, T-cell subsets, B lymphocytes, and others. Fluorescent dyes, such as **fluorescein, acridine orange, and phycoerythrin,** are bound specifically to the cell marker of interest. Cells in suspension pass singly through a laminar-flow saline sheath. As the stained cells pass through a laser beam (usually argon or krypton), the dye is activated, and the cell fluoresces. The fluorescence is detected and collected by sensors placed at 90° relative to the source beam, and the information is processed by a computer.

IX. SYPHILIS SEROLOGY

A. **Human syphilis** is caused by the spirochete *Treponema pallidum.* Antibodies against treponemal antigens and nontreponemal cardiolipin antigens (Wassermann antigens) develop and elicit a cell-mediated and humoral Ir, which results in the formation of immune complexes.

B. **Disease.** Sexual contact with infected persons is the most common form of transmission of human syphilis. Transmission through blood or blood-product transfusion can occur but is rare now because of effective pre-transfusion testing. In addition, syphilis can be passed from an infected pregnant woman to her fetus. There are **four clinical stages** of disease.

1. **Primary (early) syphilis.** Inflammatory lesions (chancres) appear 2–8 weeks after infection and last for 1–5 weeks. Serum tests for syphilis are positive in 90% of patients after 3 weeks. The antibodies that develop are predominantly IgM.

2. **Secondary syphilis** usually occurs 6–8 weeks after chancres first appear. This stage is characterized by a generalized rash, and secondary lesions may develop in the eyes, joints, or central nervous system (CNS). These lesions are highly contagious, but heal spontaneously within 2–6 weeks. Serologic tests are positive in secondary syphilis. Antibodies are mostly IgG.

3. **The latent stage** of syphilis is contagious and is generally considered to begin after the second year of infection. There are no clinical symptoms, although serologic tests are still positive. After 4 years, syphilis is not usually contagious; however, the disease may still be transmitted from mother to fetus.

4. **Tertiary syphilis** is characterized by granulomatous lesions known as **gummata.** These lesions may develop in skin, mucous membranes, joints, muscles, and bones, causing little or no clinical problems. Approximately 80% of patients experience CNS involvement, which can result in paralysis or dementia. Approximately 10% of patients develop cardiovascular problems, which can result in aortic aneurysm.

C. **Congenital syphilis.** Syphilis can be transmitted to a fetus after the 18th week of gestation. Treatment of the infected mother before the 18th week will prevent infection; treatment after the 18th week will cure it.

D. **Treatment.** Syphilis is easily and effectively treated. Penicillin is the drug of choice, although tetracycline or erythromycin can also be used. Treatment may or may not result in serologic tests becoming nonreactive, depending on the stage of the disease at the time of treatment.

1. **Primary stage.** A seropositive patient in the primary stage of disease usually becomes nonreactive approximately 6 months after treatment.

2. **Secondary stage.** If treatment occurs during the secondary stage, the patient usually becomes nonreactive within 12–18 months after treatment. Patients treated 10 years or more after infection may always remain seropositive.

E. **Tests for syphilis** are based on the detection of **nontreponemal antibodies** or **treponemal antibodies.**

1. **Nontreponemal antibody detection. Reagin antibodies** are formed after exposure to *Treponema pallidum* and react with lipoidal antigens used in screening tests for syphilis. The most commonly performed reagin tests are:

a. **The Venereal Disease Research Laboratory (VDRL) slide test.** The VDRL is a qualitative agglutination test using heat-inactivated patient serum. CSF can also be used. The test can be modified and used as a quantitative test.

b. **The rapid plasma reagin (RPR) test.** The RPR is an agglutination test. In addition to lipoidal antigens and cholesterol, the antigen reagent contains charcoal to facilitate macroscopic interpretation of results. Unheated serum is the specimen of choice, although plasma may be used.

c. **Results.** VDRL and RPR test reactions are graded as **nonreactive (NR), weakly reactive (WR), or reactive (R).** False-positive and false-negative reactions may occur.

(1) **False-positive** reactions may be caused by:
   (a) SLE
   (b) RA
   (c) Infectious mononucleosis
   (d) Pregnancy
   (e) Old age
(2) **False-negative** reactions may be caused by:
   (a) Technical errors
   (b) Low antibody titers
   (c) Prozone phenomenon

2. **Treponemal antibody detection.** The serum of patients who have syphilis also contains an antibody distinct from the antireagin antibody. Tests for these antibodies are used as confirmatory tests when reactive results are obtained using screening methods. These tests are also used to determine antibody titers. The most commonly used treponemal tests are:

a. **The fluorescent treponemal antibody absorption test (FTA-ABS).** The FTA-ABS test detects treponemal antibodies by using a killed suspension of *T. pallidum* as an antigen and a fluorescein-conjugated antihuman globulin reagent.

b. **The microhemagglutination assay for** *T. pallidum* **(MHA-TP)** uses RBCs coated with treponemal antigens to detect antibodies.

X. **ACUTE PHASE PROTEINS** are a group of plasma proteins whose levels increase significantly and independently during the acute phase of an inflammatory process. They are primarily produced in the liver by the parenchymal cells.

A. **Alpha$_1$-antitrypsin** is a serine protease inhibitor that inhibits the action of specific proteases that cause lung damage and pulmonary inflammation. Heterozygous deficiencies result in increased risk of liver disease, glomerulonephritis, and connective tissue diseases. Homozygous deficiencies result in premature emphysema and liver disease.

B. Alpha$_2$-macroglobulin is a protease inhibitor that plays a role in the coagulation, fibrinolytic, and complement components of hemostasis.

C. Ceruloplasmin is a major copper-transport protein. An absence or deficiency of ceruloplasmin is associated with Wilson's disease.

D. C-Reactive Protein (CRP) is normally present in trace amounts in serum, but may increase to 1000 times normal in many inflammatory processes. It is the first of the acute reactive proteins to appear following tissue injury or inflammation. CRP levels can be used to assess disease severity and monitor therapy. Elevated levels are seen in rheumatic diseases such as RA, bacterial and viral infections, burn injuries, malignancies, tuberculosis, and renal transplantation. Levels also rise rapidly following myocardial infarction and correspond with elevated CK-MB levels. The latex agglutination test is the most commonly used method for CRP testing.

E. Fibrinogen plays an active role in wound healing after tissue injury. It is primarily responsible for an elevated erythrocyte sedimentation rate (ESR).

F. Haptoglobin is a plasma protein that binds to free hemoglobin. Decreased levels may be caused by intravascular hemolysis or decreased synthesis secondary to liver disease. Haptoglobin levels increase twofold to fourfold following tissue injury.

XI. HEPATITIS is an inflammation of the liver and usually refers to the diseases caused by a group of viruses identified as hepatitis A, B, C, D, and E.

A. Hepatitis A (infectious hepatitis) is caused by the hepatitis A virus (HAV).

  1. Transmission. HAV is transmitted most commonly through the fecal-oral route and is frequently seen in epidemics in areas with poor sanitation. Raw shellfish from contaminated water can also transmit the disease.

  2. Disease course. HAV infections are almost always acute and self-limiting. There is no carrier state. Symptoms, if present, are vague and relatively nonspecific; patients may complain of fatigue, malaise, and anorexia. Jaundice may be present, although most patients are anicteric. Many cases are subclinical, especially those in children.

  3. Laboratory diagnosis. Liver function test results, especially alanine aminotransferase (ALT), are elevated. Total bilirubin levels may be elevated. Antibodies to HAV can be detected by enzyme immunoassay (EIA) and RIA methods. IgM anti-HAV antibodies develop during the acute phase of the disease and persist for 3–12 months after onset of the disease. As IgM titers decrease, levels of IgG anti-HAV antibodies increase and persist throughout life. These IgG antibodies confer lifelong immunity.

  4. Prevention. Household and sexual contacts of infected persons should receive immune globulin injections within 2 weeks of exposure. A recently developed vaccine against HAV is now available.

B. Hepatitis B virus (HBV) was formerly known as the Australia or hepatitis-

Box 6-1. Order of Appearance of
Hepatitis B Markers

> Hepatitis B surface antigen (HBsAg)
> Hepatitis Be antigen (HBeAg)
> Hepatitis B core antibody (HBcAb)
> Hepatitis Be antibody (HBeAb)
> Hepatitis B surface antibody (HBsAb)

associated antigen. Box 6-1 summarizes the order of appearance of HBV markers.

1. **Transmission.** HBV is transmitted parenterally or through sexual contact with infected persons. Common parenteral routes include intravenous drug use, transfusion of contaminated blood or blood products, and cutaneous or mucous membrane exposure (e.g., needlestick injuries; splashes in the eyes, nose, or mouth).

2. **Disease course.** The average incubation period is 2–3 months. HBV infections may be acute, chronic, or fulminant, or the patient may be a chronic asymptomatic carrier. Symptoms are similar to those seen in HAV infections. Jaundice may or may not be present. Approximately 95% of all cases of hepatitis B are acute. Acute HBV infections can be complicated by circulating HBV antigen-antibody complexes, which can cause polyarteritis, arthritis, glomerulonephritis, pancreatitis, or cryoglobulinemia. Chronic hepatitis B can progress to cirrhosis, which may later progress to hepatocellular carcinoma.

3. **Laboratory diagnosis.** Elevated ALT levels peak approximately the same time symptoms appear. Serologic tests not only identify HBV as the cause of the disease, but can also be used to pinpoint the stage of the disease.

   a. **Hepatitis B surface antigens (HBsAg)** appear 1 week to 2 months after exposure, and approximately 2 weeks to 2 months before the onset of symptoms. HBsAg disappears during the convalescent phase of acute disease and is an indicator of acute infection or chronic infection with unresolved antigenemia.

   b. **Hepatitis B surface antibodies (HBsAb)** appear as the antigens disappear. The presence of these antibodies indicates recovery and lifelong immunity.

   c. **Hepatitis B core antibodies (HBcAb)** appear shortly after the surface antigens appear. At this time, the ALT levels begin to rise. HBcAb persist throughout life and are a marker for previous infection.

   d. **Hepatitis Be antigen** appears before the onset of clinical disease, after the appearance of the surface antigens, and disappears within approximately 2 weeks. The presence of the Be antigen indicates active viral replication, and HBV is most infectious when the Be antigen is detectable.

   e. **Antibodies to Hepatitis Be antigen** appear shortly after the antigen disappears. Their presence in patients with acute hepatitis B suggests that the infection is resolving. In most cases of chronic hepatitis B infection, the presence of hepatitis Be antibodies indicates that the infection is resolving or that there is no complicating liver disease. Hepatitis Be antibodies may be seen in chronic asymptomatic carriers.

4. **Prevention.** Avoidance of high-risk behavior (e.g., intravenous drug abuse and sexual contact with infected persons) is a major factor in preventing HBV infection. A vaccine against HBV has been available since 1982. In a health care setting, HBV vaccination and the use of universal precautions can greatly reduce the risk of occupationally acquired HBV. The HBV vaccine also protects against HDV infection, because HDV infection only occurs with HBV infection.

C. **Hepatitis C** virus (HCV) has recently been identified as the causative agent in the majority of cases of what was previously known as non-A, non-B hepatitis (see Case Study 17).

1. **Transmission.** Like HBV, HCV is transmitted most commonly by parenteral routes or through sexual contact with infected persons. The majority of post-transfusion non-A, non-B hepatitis cases are caused by HCV.

2. **Disease course.** The average incubation period is 7–8 weeks. HCV infections may be acute or chronic. Symptoms are similar to those seen in HAV and HBV infections. Approximately 50% of HCV-infected patients are chronic carriers. Approximately 20% of these patients develop cirrhosis, and approximately 20% of those patients eventually develop hepatocellular carcinoma. HCV is also associated with immune-complex glomerulonephritis.

3. **Laboratory diagnosis.** Elevated ALT levels are associated with HCV infection. EIA and RIA assays have been developed to detect antibodies to the HCV antigens, but a high number of false-positive results are seen with these methods. Identifying infected persons is also difficult because antibody tests are positive in only 70%–85% of patients with post-transfusion HCV and in only 50% of patients with disease from other causes. Additionally, it can take up to 12 months for an infected person to seroconvert and test positive for HCV antibodies. Serum or liver tissue can be analyzed for HCV RNA by PCR, but this method largely remains a research tool.

4. **Prevention.** As with HBV, avoiding high-risk behavior (e.g., intravenous drug abuse and sexual contact with infected persons) is important in preventing HCV infections. No vaccine for HCV currently exists.

D. **Hepatitis D** is associated exclusively with HBV infections, either as a co-infection or as a superinfection. It is seen most commonly in intravenous drug users and hemophiliacs. No vaccine is available. The only means of preventing hepatitis D infection is to prevent HBV infection.

E. **Hepatitis E** causes sporadic and epidemic hepatitis in developing countries such as India, Pakistan, Africa, and Mexico. The disease clinically resembles HAV infections and is transmitted through the fecal-oral route. There is no chronic infection, and the Hepatitis E virus is not associated with hepatocellular carcinoma.

XII. **STREPTOCOCCAL SEROLOGY.** *Streptococcus pyogenes* is a gram-positive coccus responsible for a number of human infections, some of which can have serious sequelae. The M protein is the major virulence factor for *S. pyogenes;* more than 60 M serotypes have been identified.

A. **Bacterial toxins.** Two hemolysins are produced by virtually all strains of *S. pyogenes.*

    1. **Streptolysin O (SLO)** is an oxygen-labile enzyme that causes hemolysis by binding to cholesterol in the RBC membrane. It is antigenic, and the presence of antibodies to SLO is an indicator of recent streptococcal infection.

    2. **Streptolysin S** is a nonantigenic, oxygen-stable enzyme. It causes hemolysis by disrupting the selective permeability of the RBC membrane.

B. **Infections and sequelae**

    1. **Skin infections** caused by *S. pyogenes* include:

       a. Cellulitis

       b. Impetigo

       c. Erysipelas

    2. **Upper respiratory tract infections** caused by *S. pyogenes* are characterized by fever, sore throat, and pharyngeal edema.

    3. **Scarlet fever** is caused by a strain of *S. pyogenes* that produces an erythrogenic toxin, which results in a characteristic rash. Fever and sore throat are also present.

    4. **Rheumatic fever (RF)** is a complication seen following upper respiratory tract infections. All M serotypes that cause pharyngitis have been implicated in RF. RF results in damage to heart valves, and patients with rheumatic heart disease have an increased risk of developing endocarditis and other cardiac problems in later years.

    5. **Post-streptococcal glomerulonephritis** may occur after pharyngitis or skin infections. Only a few M serotypes cause this type of glomerulonephritis. Patients have an increased risk of developing renal failure later.

    6. **The mechanisms** by which these sequelae occur are not fully understood. Antibodies to streptococcal cell membranes cross-react with myosin in cardiac muscle cells, which results in cell damage. Antigen-antibody complexes form at the glomerular basement membrane and attract inflammatory cells that cause renal tissue damage.

C. **Laboratory diagnosis.** During an infection with *S. pyogenes*, the SLO produced elicits an Ir, and specific antibodies are formed. These antibodies neutralize the hemolytic activity of the SLO; this neutralization provides the basis for the most commonly used test in the detection of streptococcal infections.

    1. **Antistreptolysin O (ASO) titer.** The ASO titer begins to increase approximately 7 days after infection and peaks after 4–6 weeks.

       a. **Principle.** SLO is added to serial dilutions of patient serum, along with group O RBCs as indicator cells. If the patient serum contains antibodies against SLO, the antibodies will complex with the corresponding antigens. These complexes block the hemolytic activity of the antigen, and no hemolysis occurs. The ASO titer is reported as the reciprocal of the highest dilution that shows no hemolysis and is expressed in Todd units.

       b. **Normal values.** ASO values vary widely among healthy individuals, making it difficult to establish normal values. Most healthy adults have ASO titers of less than 166 Todd units, with the usual titer decreasing after 50 years of age. Although an elevated titer is generally regarded as evidence of recent streptococcal infection, a 30% rise in titer above a previous level is of greater significance than a single titer. The titer can remain elevated for weeks or months following acute disease. Approximately 80%–85% of patients with RF have increased ASO titers.

2. **Anti-DNAse B (AD-B).** Streptococci produce the enzyme deoxyribonuclease B (DNAse B). The anti-DN-B test is a neutralization test that can demonstrate recent streptococcal infection. Anti-DN-B neutralizes the activity of DNAse B. Anti-DN-B levels are increased in the 15%–20% of RF patients who do not have elevated ASO titers.

3. **Other tests.** Several rapid tests are now available to detect streptococcal antigens. The advantage is their speed over other test methods. However, a significant number of false-negative results occur.

XIII. EPSTEIN-BARR VIRUS (EBV) SEROLOGY

A. **Description.** EBV is the causative agent of **Burkitt's lymphoma, nasopharyngeal carcinoma,** and most commonly, **infectious mononucleosis (IM).** The virus is ubiquitous; 80%–90% of healthy adults have EBV antibodies. EBV infects B lymphocytes.

B. **Infectious mononucleosis (IM)** is an acute, self-limiting disease typically seen in young adults. The disease is characterized by fever, sore throat, cervical lymphadenopathy, splenomegaly, and mild hepatitis. The WBC count is elevated, and reactive lymphocytes are seen in the peripheral blood. There is a relative and absolute lymphocytosis. The average incubation period is approximately 2–8 weeks (see Case Study 18).

C. **Antigens and antibodies**
1. **Viral capsid antigen (VCA)** is found in the cytoplasm of EBV-infected lymphocytes. IgM antibodies against VCA are detectable early in the infections but disappear within 2–4 months. IgG antibodies against VCA develop within 1 week after infection and can persist for life.

2. **Early antigen-diffuse (EA-D) and early antigen-restricted (EA-R) antigens** are found in the cytoplasm of infected B lymphocytes. EA-D is also found in the nucleus. IgG antibodies to EA-D can be indicators of active disease. IgG antibodies to EA-R are sometimes seen in young children who have active IM infection, but not in infected young adults.

3. **Epstein-Barr nuclear antigen (EBNA)** is found in the nuclei of all infected cells. IgG antibodies to EBNA develop slowly but can remain detectable throughout life.

4. **Heterophile antibodies** are stimulated by one antigen and will react with unrelated antigens from different mammalian species. The heterophile antibodies of IM are IgM antibodies and are seen in 50%–70% of patients with IM. They persist for 4–8 weeks after infection.

D. **Testing**
1. **The Monospot test** is based on the principle that horse RBCs are agglutinated by the heterophile antibodies of IM. Horse RBCs contain both Forssman and IM antigens; patient serum must be differentially absorbed to

distinguish the antibodies. The patient serum is absorbed with guinea pig kidney, which will absorb only heterophile antibodies of the Forssman type, and beef erythrocyte stroma, which will absorb only the heterophile antibodies of IM. The Monospot test is positive if the horse RBCs are agglutinated by the patient serum absorbed with guinea pig kidney, and not agglutinated by the patient serum absorbed with beef erythrocyte stroma.

2. **The Davidsohn differential test** can distinguish heterophile sheep cell agglutinins in human serum caused by IM, serum sickness, and Forssman antigen.

3. **The Paul-Bunnell test** can detect only the presence or absence of heterophile antibodies. It cannot determine the specificity of the antibodies.

XIV. RUBELLA SEROLOGY

A. The rubella virus is the causative agent of **acquired rubella,** which is also known as **German measles or 3-day measles.** It is highly contagious, although its incidence has decreased dramatically because of vaccination. Rubella is characterized by rash, fever, and lymphadenopathy. Both IgG and IgM antibodies develop during acute infection. IgM antibodies disappear within a few weeks, but IgG antibodies persist and confer lifelong immunity.

B. **Congenital rubella syndrome** is caused by infection during pregnancy and can result in a wide spectrum of birth defects. In utero infection can also result in fetal death. The fetus is most likely to develop anomalies if the mother becomes infected during the first month of pregnancy.

C. **Testing.** Because IgM antibodies disappear quickly after infection, their presence is indicative of a current or very recent infection. However, because IgG antibodies appear early in the course of the disease and persist, their presence does not necessarily indicate current or recent infection. Because IgM does not cross the placental barrier, demonstration of IgM rubella antibodies in a neonate is diagnostic of congenital rubella syndrome. Pregnant women are often tested for rubella early in their pregnancy. Several methods of detecting rubella antibodies are commonly used:

1. **HAI** is the most widely used test for the detection and quantitation of rubella antibodies. It does not distinguish between IgG and IgM antibodies and is therefore most useful as an indicator of immune status. A titer of at least 8 is considered to be indicative of prior infection.

2. **Other tests include:**

   a. **Passive latex agglutination,** which is faster and more convenient than the HAI

   b. **Quantitative methods,** such as EIA and IFA

XV. FEBRILE DISEASE SEROLOGY

A. **Febrile diseases** are a group of microbial infections characterized by fever and the production of antibodies known as **febrile agglutinins.** These diseases include:

1. **Brucellosis,** which is caused by the bacteria *Brucella abortus*

2. **Paratyphoid fever,** which is caused by *Salmonella paratyphi*

3. **Rocky Mountain spotted fever,** which is caused by rickettsiae

4. Tularemia, which is caused by *Francisella tularensis*

5. Q fever, which is caused by rickettsiae

B. Tests for febrile diseases include:

1. **Widal's test,** which can detect antibodies in **typhoid fever, tularemia, and brucellosis**

2. **The Weil-Felix test,** which is an agglutination test based on the cross-reactivity of rickettsial antibodies with antibodies to the somatic "O" antigens of the OX-19 and OX-2 strains of *Proteus vulgaris* and the OX-K strain of *Proteus mirabilis*

   a. The Weil-Felix test is useful for identifying several rickettsial diseases, such as murine typhus and Q fever.

   b. Titers of 160 are usually considered significant.

Study Questions

Directions: Each of the numbered items or incomplete statements in this section is followed by answers or by completions of the statement. Select the ONE lettered answer or completion that is BEST in each case.

1. Which one of the following types of cells secretes antibodies?

a. killer cells (K)
b. bone marrow stem cells
c. mast cells
d. B cells

2. The immunoglobulin class typically found in saliva, tears, and other body secretions is

a. IgG
b. IgA
c. IgM
d. IgD

3. In adults, the predominant immunoglobulin is

a. IgA
b. IgG
c. IgM
d. IgD

4. Which one of the following is the C3 activation unit in the classic pathway of complement activation?

a. C1
b. C3
c. C42
d. C5-C9

5. An immune response (Ir) that leads to the production of antibody is

a. humoral and mediated primarily by B lymphocytes
b. humoral and mediated primarily by T lymphocytes
c. cellular and mediated primarily by B lymphocytes
d. cellular and mediated primarily by T lymphocytes

6. The first immunoglobulin produced after exposure to an antigen is

a. IgA
b. IgG
c. IgM
d. IgE

7. Which one of the following immunoglobulins is produced in the greatest amount during the secondary antibody response?

a. IgA
b. IgM
c. IgG
d. IgE

8. Cell-mediated immunity involves which one of the following groups of cells?

a. macrophages, natural killer (NK) cells, plasma cells
b. macrophages, plasma cells, cytotoxic T cells (T_c)
c. plasma cells, T_c, NK cells
d. macrophages, T_c, NK cells

9. Which one of the following substances is an important monokine?

a. tumor necrosis factor (TNF_α)
b. interleukin-2 (IL-2)
c. B-cell growth factor 2
d. macrophage migration inhibitory factor (MIF)

10. Bronchial asthma is an example of

a. type I hypersensitivity
b. type II hypersensitivity
c. type III hypersensitivity
d. type IV hypersensitivity

11. The LE factor in the blood of patients with systemic lupus erythematosus (SLE) and other autoimmune diseases is

a. anti-deoxyribonucleoprotein antibody (anti-DNP)
b. anti-Jo-1 antibody
c. anti-Ku antibody
d. anti-Mi-1 antibody

12. Substrate cells that are commonly used to screen for double stranded (ds)-DNA antibodies using immunohistochemical techniques are

a. human laryngeal tumor cells (HEp-2)
b. mouse kidney cells
c. *Crithidia lucilia*
d. mouse liver cells

13. A latex agglutination test for rheumatoid factor (RF) is considered positive for RF if the titer is at least:

a. 20
b. 40
c. 80
d. 160

14. Anti-parietal cell antibodies are often seen in patients with which one of the following conditions?

a. Goodpasture's syndrome
b. insulin-dependent diabetes mellitus
c. systemic lupus erythematosus (SLE)
d. pernicious anemia

15. A confirmatory test commonly used to detect the presence of human immunodeficiency virus (HIV) antibodies is

a. radioimmunoassay (RIA)
b. Western blot
c. immunofluorescence
d. enzyme-linked immunosorbent assay (ELISA)

16. The first detectable antibodies to appear in human immunodeficiency virus (HIV) infection are antibodies against

a. p24
b. gp41
c. p51
d. gp120

17. A defect in neutrophil chemotaxis associated with a genetic defect in primary granules is:

a. Chédiak-Higashi syndrome
b. chronic granulomatous disease (CGD)
c. myeloperoxidase (MPO) deficiency
d. Pelger-Huët anomaly

18. The CD4-CD8 ratio typically seen in AIDS patients is

a. 4:1
b. 2:1
c. 1:2
d. 0.5:1

19. A single immunodiffusion technique that is often used to quantitate immunoglobulins and other serum proteins is

a. the Ouchterlony method
b. counter immunoelectrophoresis
c. radial immunodiffusion (RID)
d. enzyme-linked immunosorbent assay (ELISA)

20. Lipoidal antigen reagents composed of cardiolipin, lecithin, cholesterol, and charcoal are used in which one of the following tests?

a. rapid plasma reagin (RPR)
b. Venereal Disease Research Laboratory (VDRL)
c. Wassermann test
d. microhemagglutination-*Treponema pallidum* (MHA-TP)

21. The acute phase protein that demonstrates the most dramatic rise during acute inflammation is

a. fibrinogen
b. C-reactive protein (CRP)
c. alpha$_2$-macroglobulin
d. haptoglobin

22. In patients with hepatitis B, specific serologic markers appear in which one of the following orders after infection?

a. HBcAg, HbeAg, HBcAb, HBsAb, HBsAg
b. HBcAg, HBsAb, HBeAg, HBsAg, HBcAb
c. HBeAg, HBcAg, HBsAg, HBsAb, HBcAb
d. HBsAg, HBeAg, HBcAb, HBeAb, HBsAb

23. Vaccination against hepatitis B protects against

a. only hepatitis B infection
b. hepatitis A and B infection
c. hepatitis B and C infection
d. hepatitis B and D infection

24. Twenty percent of individuals chronically infected with which one of the following viruses will later develop hepatocellular carcinoma?

a. hepatitis A
b. hepatitis B
c. hepatitis C
d. hepatitis D

25. In the antistreptolysin O (ASO) test, if the patient's serum contains sufficient antistreptolysin antibody to neutralize the antigen, which of the following events occurs?

a. hemolysis
b. no hemolysis
c. agglutination
d. a clot forms

26. After an infectious mononucleosis (IM) infection, heterophile antibodies usually remain elevated for approximately what length of time?

a. 1–2 weeks
b. 3–4 weeks
c. 4–8 weeks
d. 12–24 weeks

27. The greatest risk of birth defects caused by maternal rubella infection occurs during

a. the first month of gestation
b. the second trimester
c. the third or fourth month of gestation
d. the third trimester

28. Which one of the following is considered to be a significant titer in a Weil-Felix test?

a. 20
b. 30
c. 80
d. 160

Directions: Each of the numbered items or incomplete statements in this section is negatively phrased, as indicated by a capitalized word such as NOT, LEAST, or EXCEPT. Select the ONE lettered answer or completion that is BEST in each case.

29. Complement does NOT play a major role in the

a. mediation of inflammation
b. regulation of phagocytic activity
c. production of cytokines
d. metabolism of immune complexes

30. A positive test for rheumatoid factor (RF) may be seen in patients with all of the following conditions EXCEPT

a. systemic lupus erythematosus (SLE)
b. chronic hepatitis
c. syphilis
d. infectious mononcleosis (IM)

Answers and Explanations

1. The answer is d [I A]. Antibodies are produced when mature B cells are stimulated by antigens. They may be monoclonal or polyclonal.

2. The answer is b [I D 1]. Immunoglobulin A (IgA) exists as a dimer in body secretions. In addition to saliva and tears, it is also found in breast milk, sweat, and intestinal secretions. The monomeric form of IgA and the other classes of immunoglobulins are found in the serum.

3. The answer is b [I D 4]. Immunoglobulin G (IgG) is the predominant immunoglobulin in the adult.

4. The answer is c [Figure 6-1]. In the classic pathway, C1 is the recognition unit; C42 is the C3 activation unit; and C5-C9 is the membrane attack complex.

5. The answer is a [IV A]. Immune responses (Ir) may be humoral or cell-mediated. Although overlaps occur, the humoral response is primarily mediated by B lymphocytes and results in the production of antibody. Cell-mediated responses primarily involve T lymphocytes.

6. The answer is c [IV A 2]. Within days after exposure to an antigen, immunoglobulin M (IgM) is detectable in the serum. This is referred to as the primary response.

7. The answer is c [IV A 3]. Any exposure to a specific antigen following a primary exposure results in the rapid production of immunoglobulin, the vast majority of which is IgG.

8. The answer is d [IV B 1]. Macrophages, cytotoxic T cells (T_c), and natural killer (NK) cells are important in cell-mediated immunity. Plasma cells are mature B cells that have been stimulated to produce antibody; they are not involved in cell-mediated immunity.

9. The answer is a [IV B 3 b (1)]. Monokines are cytokines produced by monocytes. Tumor necrosis factor (TNF_α) is an example. Interleukin-2 (IL-2), B-cell growth factor 2, and macrophage inhibiting factor (MIF) are lymphokines, which are produced by lymphocytes.

10. The answer is a [V I 3]. Most Type I hypersensitivity reactions are localized reactions. Histamines and leukotrienes are released when antigens complex with IgE and attach to the surface of basophils or tissue mast cells. Examples of Type I reactions include bronchial asthma and hay fever.

11. The answer is a [VI B 2 c (3)(f)]. Anti-deoxyribonucleoprotein (DNP) is an IgG antibody known as the LE factor. It is present in more than 95% of patients who have systemic lupus erythematosus (SLE) but can also be seen in patients who have rheumatoid arthritis (RA) and scleroderma.

12. The answer is a [VI B 2 c (4) (a) (ii)]. Human laryngeal tumor cells (HEp-2) are often used as substrate cells in immunohistochemical tests for antinuclear antibodies (ANA) such as double-stranded (ds)-DNA. Mouse kidney and liver cells and *Crithidia lucilia* are commonly used substrates for fluorescent antinuclear antibody (FANA) techniques.

13. The answer is a [VI B 2 a (2) (b)]. The latex agglutination test is one of several tests used to detect the presence of rheumatoid factor (RF), which is present in clinically significant amounts when the titer reaches at least 20.

14. The answer is d [Table 5-5]. The parietal cells produce intrinsic factor, which is necessary for the normal production of red blood cells (RBCs). Antibodies against these cells block the production of intrinsic factor, and pernicious anemia can result.

15. The answer is b [VII D 3 d (2) (b)]. An enzyme-linked immunosorbent assay (ELISA) procedure is the screening test most commonly used to detect human immunodeficiency virus (HIV) antibodies. Positive results from ELISA tests are usually confirmed by the Western blot technique.

16. The answer is a [VII D 3 d (2)]. Within 6–8 weeks after infection with the human immunodeficiency virus (HIV)-1, IgM antibodies against the p24 core protein are detectable.

17. The answer is a [VII A 1 f]. Chédiak-Higashi syndrome is characterized by the abnormal fusion of primary granules in neutrophils, which results in impaired bacterial killing.

18. The answer is d [VII D 3 c (1)]. The normal CD4-CD8 ratio in healthy individuals is 2:1. In persons with acquired immune deficiency syndrome (AIDS), the CD4-positive T cells are greatly reduced in number, and the CD4-CD8 ratio changes to approximately 0.5:1.

19. The answer is c [VIII B 2]. The radial immunodiffusion (RID) technique is a single diffusion method that is often used to quantitate serum immunoglobulins. The Ouchterlony method is a double diffusion technique. Counter immunoelectrophoresis does not use immunodiffusion. The enzyme-linked immunosorbent assay (ELISA) is a labeled immunoassay that does not use diffusion.

20. The answer is a [IX E 1 b]. Lipoidal antigens are used as reagents in nontreponemal tests for syphilis, such as the Venereal Disease Research Laboratory (VDRL) test and the rapid plasma reagin (RPR) test. The RPR test antigens also contain charcoal to facilitate macroscopic interpretation of the test results.

21. The answer is b [X D]. Of all of the acute phase proteins, the level of C-reactive protein (CRP) has the greatest increase during inflammation. Levels may increase up to 1000 times normal.

22. The answer is d [XI B 3]. Hepatitis B surface antigens (HbsAg) appear before the onset of clinical disease. Shortly after their appearance, Be antigens and core antibodies appear. Be antibodies appear after the Be antigens disappear. Surface antibodies develop as the surface antigens disappear.

23. The answer is d [XI B 4]. Because hepatitis D infections occur only as co-infections or superinfections with hepatitis B, vaccine against hepatitis B also prevents hepatitis D infections.

24. The answer is c [XI C 2]. Approximately 20% of patients who have hepatitis C infection develop chronic infections. Of those chronically infected individuals, approximately 20% of them will eventually develop hepatocellular carcinoma.

25. The answer is b [XII C 1 a]. If streptolysin antibodies are present, they will complex with the streptolysin O (SLO) added to the patient's serum. These complexes block the hemolytic activity of the antigen, and no hemolysis will occur.

26. The answer is c [XIII C 4]. IgM heterophile antibodies develop in 50%–80% of persons who have infectious mononucleosis (IM) and are detectable for 4–8 weeks following infection.

27. The answer is a [XIV B]. The greatest risk to the fetus from maternal rubella infection occurs during the first month of gestation. The later the stage of pregnancy at the time of infection, the lesser the risk to the fetus.

28. The answer is d [XV B 2]. Rickettsial diseases detected by the Weil-Felix test typically demonstrate significant titers of 160.

29. The answer is c [I E 1]. The complement components play major roles in both the cell-mediated immune response (Ir) and the humoral response. They are not involved in cytokine production.

30. The answer is d [VI B 2 a (1)]. The presence of rheumatoid factor (RF) is characteristic of rheumatoid arthritis (RA), but it may also be detected in patients with systemic lupus erythematosus (SLE), hepatitis, and syphilis. RF is not associated with infectious mononucleosis (IM).

7

Current Issues in Laboratory Management

Hal S. Larsen
Mary Ann Harrison

I. QUALITY ASSURANCE

A. Introduction

1. **Quality assurance (QA) is a comprehensive set of policies, procedures, and practices** that are followed to ensure that a laboratory's results are reliable. QA evaluates the quality of the services provided. QA provides a way to prevent problems as well as deal with problems that occur. It differs from quality control (QC) in that QC is included as part of a QA program. QC ensures that a particular test method is working properly and that results of that test are reliable.

2. **QA includes record keeping, maintenance and calibration of equipment, proficiency testing, quality control, and training of personnel.** QA is a commitment to quality. Physician and patient relations are a part of this plan.

B. Quality assurance plan

1. **All policies and procedures are in writing** and available.

2. **Staff performance** is routinely evaluated.

3. **Continuing education** is used and documented.

4. **A safety program** is in place for both staff and patients.

   a. **Occupational Safety and Health Administration (OSHA) standards** are met.

   b. Hazardous materials are identified and labeled.

   c. Material Safety Data Sheets (MSDS) are available for each hazardous material.

   d. Employee safety training is documented.

   e. Records of any accidents (e.g., needle stick) are kept and reported to appropriate authorities.

   f. Hazardous waste is properly disposed.

327

    g. Universal precautions are strictly followed.

    h. Safety equipment (e.g., fire extinguishers, fire blankets, safety showers, goggles) is available to staff, and training in the use of this equipment is performed and documented.

    i. Electrical checks of all equipment are routinely performed.

5. Specimen collection and handling as well as correct patient preparation follows written guidelines and is documented.

6. A quality control (QC) program is in place. This ensures that the instruments, reagents, and personnel are functioning properly. A QC program comprises several areas:

    a. A **written QC program** is required that specifies:

        (1) Frequency of performing controls

        (2) Number of controls to be used

        (3) Type of controls

        (4) Acceptable limits for control results

        (5) Corrective action required if controls are out of range

    b. **QC plots** of control results are used to detect shifts (a sudden upward or downward change of four or more consecutive values) and trends (the tendency of results to gradually increase or decrease over a period of time).

    c. **Equipment maintenance** is performed and documented.

    d. **Temperatures** of incubators, certain instruments, and the room are noted and documented.

7. Checklists are used to ensure that scheduled activities and duties are performed.

8. The laboratory must participate in and document results of proficiency testing (PT). This allows comparison of results from a number of laboratories. Specimens from PT sponsors are to be treated exactly like patient specimens.

9. The laboratory must be accredited by an appropriate agency. This gives official approval and states that the laboratory follows all of the guidelines set forth by the accrediting agency. Inspectors representing the accrediting agency view records, documents, and visit the laboratory.

II. LABORATORY REGULATIONS

A. Clinical Laboratory Improvement Amendments of 1988 (CLIA 88)

    1. Background. CLIA 88 is **intended to establish regulations for all laboratories,** regardless of size or location, where clinical testing is performed for the purpose of diagnosis, treatment, or monitoring of patients' health. The law was **published in the February 28, 1992** issue of the *Federal Register.* The law **became effective** for all laboratories **on September 1, 1992.**

        a. Modifications to the law, which were published in the January 19, 1993 issue of the *Federal Register,* list the complexity of tests.

        b. Additional modifications, which were published in the *Federal Register* on April 24, 1995, define alternative routes for personnel qualifications.

    2. Laboratory accreditation

        a. All laboratories must have a CLIA certificate to perform testing and receive federal reimbursement.

b. Certification is based on the **level of test complexity.**

    (1) Waived testing constitutes approximately 0.5% of all testing. The analyte or test must be performed on the test system mentioned in the following list and only on the facility's own patients.

        (a) Urinalysis reagent testing (e.g., dipstick strip, reagent tablet)

        (b) Fecal occult blood

        (c) Home use ovulation

        (d) Urine pregnancy

        (e) Erythrocyte sedimentation rate (ESR) [manual]

        (f) Hemoglobin (Hb)

            (i) Copper sulfate method

            (ii) HemoCue instrument

        (g) Blood glucose

            (i) Home use instrumentation

            (ii) HemoCue B-glucose analyzer

            (iii) Cholestech LDX system

        (h) Spun microhematocrit

        (i) Chemtrak cholesterol accumeter

        (j) Ovulation kits

        (k) _Helicobacter pylori_ (serum Pyloritek test kit)

        (l) Streptococcus Gp. A (Quidel Quickvue In-Line One-Step Strep A test)

        (m) Total cholesterol (Cholestech LDX system)

        (n) High-density lipoprotein cholesterol (Cholestech LDX system)

        (o) Triglycerides (Cholestech LDX system)

    (2) Provider-performed microscopy (PPM) constitutes approximately 0.5% of testing and includes:

        (a) Wet mount

        (b) Potassium hydroxide (KOH) preparation

        (c) Urine sediment

        (d) Pinworm slides

        (e) Fern test

        (f) Vaginal smears

        (g) Nasal smear examinations for granulocytes

        (h) Fecal leukocyte examinations

        (i) Semen analysis

            (i) Qualitative examination

            (ii) Presence or absence

            (iii) Motility

    (3) Moderately complex testing constitutes approximately 74% of all testing and includes:

        (a) Hematology

        (b) Chemistry

        (c) Serology

        (d) Coagulation

        (e) Therapeutic drug monitoring

        (f) Blood gases

        (g) Urine colony counts

        (h) Blood type and Rh factor

        (i) Limited immunology

        (j) Manual differential (limited identification; normal cells only)

        (k) Gram's stain

            (i) Urethral for gas chromatography (GC)

            (ii) Cervical for GC

        (l) Throat culture screen only

            (i) Hemolysis

            (ii) Bacitracin

            (iii) Strep select agar

       (m) Microscopic urinalysis (non-PPM)

       (n) Rapid kits

     (4) **Highly complex testing** constitutes approximately 24% of all testing and includes:

       (a) Microbiology

       (b) Immunohematology

       (c) Bacteriology

       (d) Cytology

       (e) Histopathology

       (f) Mycology

       (g) Manual hematology counts

       (h) Manual differential

            (i) Identification of abnormal cells

            (ii) Complete identification

       (i) Nonautomated chemistry tests

  c. **The certificate fee and biennial inspection fee,** which are based on the size of the laboratory and number of tests performed annually, must be paid.

  d. **Accreditation by a private organization** is an alternative option for certification.

     (1) The Health Care Financing Administration (HCFA) may deem a laboratory to meet all of the CLIA requirements if the laboratory is accredited by a private, nonprofit organization that is certified as having **deemed status.** This means that the certifying agency must:

       (a) Provide reasonable assurance to HCFA that it requires the laboratories it accredits to meet all of the requirements equivalent to the CLIA requirements in the law

       (b) Inspect its laboratories per condition level requirements of the law

     (2) Approved **state laboratory programs** are responsible for accreditation of laboratories in their state, if this is a requirement of the department of health of that state.

3. **Personnel requirements must be met** by laboratories performing moderately or highly complex testing. These positions can be held by the same person or by different persons who meet the qualifications.

  a. **Moderately complex laboratories** must have the following personnel:

     (1) **Laboratory director**

     (2) **Technical consultant**

     (3) **Clinical consultant**

     (4) **Testing personnel**

       (a) Each person performing moderately complex testing must:

          (i) Follow laboratory procedures

          (ii) Maintain records

          (iii) Adhere to policies

          (iv) Identify problems

          (v) Document corrective actions

      (b) Testing personnel must have **documented training** in all areas of testing performed.

  b. Highly complex laboratories are required to have the same personnel as a moderately complex laboratory, but must also have:

    (1) General supervisor

    (2) Technical supervisor

    (3) All personnel must meet the qualifications published in the April 24, 1995 issue of the *Federal Register*.

4. Quality control (QC) must be performed on all moderately and highly complex testing.

  a. General QC procedures are performed on:

    (1) All **specialties and subspecialties** as specified in Sections 493.1201 through 493.1285 of the February 28, 1992 issue of the *Federal Register*

    (2) Procedures not found in the *Federal Register,* which must be conducted according to the manufacturer's protocol that has been approved by the Food and Drug Administration

  b. The laboratory **must establish and follow written QC procedures** for monitoring and evaluating the test process to assure accuracy and reliability of results.

  c. There must be documentation of all **calibration procedures.**

  d. A minimum of **two levels of control materials** are run on each day of testing.

  e. All QC records must be retained for **2 years.**

  f. QC must be tested in a manner that provides results within the laboratory's stated performance requirements.

  g. The laboratory **must have instruments, reagents, and supplies** sufficient for the type and volume of tests performed.

  h. There must be defined **criteria for proper storage of reagents and specimens.**

  i. A **procedure for remedial actions** must be established when QC fails.

  j. All reagents, solutions, medias, QC materials, and standards **must be labeled.**

  k. Different **lot numbers are not to be interchanged** unless specified by the manufacturer.

5. Proficiency testing (PT) is mandatory for all moderately and highly complex tests listed on the **Compiled List of Clinical Laboratory Systems, Assays, and Examinations Categorized by Complexity,** published on July 26, 1993, in the *Federal Register*.

  a. There are **more than 20 HCFA-approved PT** programs available.

  b. Laboratories receive between **three and five challenges** for each analyte that requires PT.

    c. Challenges are received **three times a year.** The same personnel who routinely perform the test procedures must perform the PT.

    d. Laboratories are required to score **80%** on all analytes to be considered in compliance.

    e. Blood bank specimens require a score of **100%.**

6. A procedures manual must be written to include all testing methods used in the laboratory. It must be available and followed by all testing personnel.

    a. The **manual must include:**

      (1) The **principle and methodology** of each test

      (2) Criteria for **specimen collection, processing, and rejection**

      (3) Instructions for **microscopic examination procedures**

      (4) Test procedures
        (a) Step-by-step instructions
        (b) Result interpretation

      (5) Preparation of materials
        (a) Required solutions (e.g., reagents, controls, calibrators, stains, slides) and their location
        (b) Step-by-step preparation of all materials needed
        (c) Storage after preparation
        (d) Labeling and dating instructions
        (e) Safety precautions needed
        (f) Solutions used in preparation (e.g., deionized water, diluent)

      (6) Calibration procedures
        (a) Step-by-step instructions
        (b) Verifications of calibration results
        (c) Concentration and number of calibrators used
        (d) Calibration schedule

      (7) Control procedures
        (a) Materials used, name, lot number, level, frequency used
        (b) Preparation of materials
        (c) Instructions for testing controls
        (d) Control limits
        (e) Description of how and where control results are recorded
        (f) Corrective actions taken when controls are not within limits

      (8) Actions taken when results deviate from expected values:
        (a) Recalibration
        (b) Troubleshooting
        (c) Repeats
        (d) Dilutions

      (9) Limitations
        (a) Interfering substances
        (b) Common sources of error

    (10) Result reporting
        (a) Reference ranges
          (i) Range for different specimens (e.g., serum, plasma, urine)
          (ii) Demographic variables (e.g., age, sex)
        (b) Panic values
          (i) Life-threatening results

                     (ii) Results needing special attention (critical results)
         (11) References
                  (a) Manufacturer's product literature (e.g., inserts, manuals)
                  (b) Literature (e.g., textbooks, professional magazines)
         (12) Specimen retention
                  (a) How long specimen is kept
                  (b) Where specimen is stored
         (13) System for reporting patient results
                  (a) Unacceptable results
                  (b) How results are reported to physician
                  (c) Protocol for panic and critical values
         (14) Course of action for problems
         (15) Specimen referral
                  (a) To whom or where specimen is referred
                  (b) How the specimen is sent
                  (c) How results are received

     b. The manual must be approved. To obtain approval, the manual must be:
                  (a) Signed by the laboratory director
                  (b) Reviewed by all personnel using the procedure
                  (c) Reviewed and updated by the supervisor or director

     c. The manual must be rewritten when new procedures are implemented.

     d. The manual must be retained for future reference.

   7. A quality assurance (QA) plan must be established and followed **to monitor and evaluate the quality of tests.**

     a. The program **must be an ongoing process.**

     b. It must **evaluate** all facets of **the testing process.**

     c. The program must **extend to the interactions of other health care professionals** in the ordering of tests.

     d. It must **allow for actions to be taken** to correct errors or problems.

     e. The program **must monitor and evaluate:**
         (1) Specimen requirements
         (2) Collection
         (3) Handling and processing
         (4) Corrective actions taken in QC and PT
         (5) Result reporting
         (6) Employee competence

     f. All QA activities must be **documented and evaluated** monthly.

   8. Inspections are conducted every 2 years by the Department of Health and Human Services (HHS) or its designee.

     a. Laboratory **inspectors have the right** to:
         (1) Interview all employees
         (2) Access all areas of a facility
         (3) Observe all testing
         (4) Review all information and data records
         (5) Determine that the laboratory is operated in a safe manner

(6) Determine that the laboratory is performing tests only within their complexity category

(7) Evaluate any complaints from the public

b. The **inspector may also:**

(1) Conduct unannounced inspections at any time during hours of operation

(2) Ask personnel to perform testing on test samples that the inspector supplies

(3) Re-inspect a laboratory at any time to evaluate accurate and reliable results

9. Sanctions may be imposed on laboratories that are found to be out of compliance with one or more of the conditions for Medicare coverage.

a. Suspension, limitations, or revocation of a certificate can be imposed.

b. A **civil suit** can be brought against a laboratory to forbid testing.

c. Imprisonment or fines can be levied against persons convicted of violations.

d. HHS publishes annually a list of laboratories that have been sanctioned.

B. Occupational Safety and Health Administration (OSHA) regulations for **Occupational Exposure to Bloodborne Pathogens** (OSHA Instruction CPL 2-2.44A) require laboratories to establish workplace safety practices to prevent accidental exposure to etiologic agents in blood.

1. The final rules were published in the ***Federal Register*** on **December 2, 1991.**

2. Regulations became effective on March 6, 1992.

3. The regulations limit occupational exposure to blood and other potentially infectious materials that can transmit bloodborne pathogens and **include but are not limited to:**

a. Hepatitis B virus (HBV)

b. Human immunodeficiency virus (HIV)

4. The basis for all preventive measures is the practice of **universal precautions.** This is described in a report published in *Morbidity and Mortality Weekly Report* on June 24, 1988. These are recommendations from the **Centers for Disease Control and Prevention (CDC).**

a. Laboratory personnel **must treat all human blood and other potentially infectious body fluids** as if they were infected with HIV, HBV, and other bloodborne pathogens.

b. This includes **materials** that are **contaminated with blood.**

5. A written exposure control plan must be in place that describes the procedures established to minimize employee exposure to bloodborne pathogens.

a. There must be **identification of job classification,** tasks, and procedures in which there is the **potential of exposure.**

(1) A determination must be made of the job types in which exposure could occur.

(2) All tasks must be included in the job description.

b. An explanation of **personal protective equipment (PPE)** available and in use must be included.

(1) Appropriate protective equipment **must be supplied to employees** at no cost to them.

(2) **Equipment is considered appropriate** only if it does not permit blood or other potentially infectious materials (PIMs) to pass through to an employee's clothes, skin, mouth, or other mucous membranes.

(3) **Types of PPE** are gloves, gowns, laboratory coats, face shields or masks, and eye protection.

(4) All **employers are responsible** for providing, maintaining, laundering, disposing of, replacing, and assuring the proper use of all PPE.

c. **Engineering controls** must be in place to minimize exposure.

(1) These are devices that **isolate or remove the pathogen hazard** from the workplace.

(2) These devices must be **made available** to all employees.

(3) **Examples** of engineering controls include:

(a) Sharps containers and biosafety bags

(b) Splash guards and self-sheathing needles

(c) Biosafety cabinets and fume hoods

(d) Mechanical pipetting devices

(e) Handwashing facilities, eyewash stations, and showers

d. **Work practices** must be developed to reduce or eliminate employee exposure to blood or PIMs during the execution of their work tasks.

(1) **Employees must fully understand** these procedures.

(2) The procedures **must be implemented,** when appropriate.

(3) **Work practice procedures include,** but are not limited to:

(a) Handwashing

(b) No recapping of contaminated needles

(c) No food or drink allowed in the laboratory

(d) No mouth pipetting

(e) Warning labels affixed where needed, and biohazard symbols placed appropriately

(f) A dress code that ensures safety

e. **Housekeeping procedures** are necessary for maintaining a clean and sanitary work site, which is a responsibility of employers.

(1) All equipment and **work surfaces** must be decontaminated.

(2) **Sharps containers** must be puncture resistant.

(3) Containers for **biohazard materials** must be constructed to contain all contents and prevent leakage during handling, storage, transport, and shipping.

(4) **Procedure for disposal** of biohazard materials will be based on federal, state, and local regulations.

(5) All housekeeping personnel will handle contaminated materials with the use of PPE.

f. An **HBV vaccination program** must be established.

(1) HBV vaccine and vaccination series **must be made available** to all employees who are identified as being exposed to PIMs.

(2) The vaccination series will be **offered within 10 days** of the employee being assigned to an area of possible exposure.

(3) The vaccination series must be offered at **no cost to the employee.**

(4) The program **must be established using the protocol** outlined in the *Federal Register*.

(5) The program must include **procedures for evaluation** of the circumstances of an exposure incident to prevent further incidents.

(6) Exemptions to the HBV vaccination program are:

(a) Employees who have already completed the HBV series

(b) Employees whose antibody tests reveal an immunity

(c) Employees for whom vaccination is contraindicated for medical reasons

(7) Employees who decline the HBV series **must sign** the **declination statement** published in Addendum A of the *Federal Register*.

(8) All records are part of the employee's permanent file and **are confidential information**.

g. **Post-exposure and follow-up evaluations** are available at no cost to any employee who sustains an exposure.

h. The **communication of hazards to employees** is required by OSHA regulations.

(1) All employees must receive **free biosafety training** during working hours.

(2) Training sessions must be presented in a way that can be clearly understood.

(3) These sessions must be **designed for the particular situation** and institution involved.

(4) Generic information and signing of a statement **will not satisfy** the requirements.

(5) Instructors must be knowledgeable and must:

(a) Demonstrate use and location of all safety devices

(b) Document all training

(c) Ensure that employees understand how to cope with hazards they may come in contact with during their employment

i. A **record-keeping** policy must be in place.

(1) All documentation of **training and exposure incidents** must be a part of each employee's permanent record.

(2) All files are **confidential information**.

(3) Medical records are transferred when an employee leaves.

(4) All records are kept on file for the duration of employment plus **30 years**.

C. **OSHA regulations** for **Occupational Exposures to Hazardous Chemicals in Laboratories** were published on January 31, 1990, in the *Federal Register* (vol 55, no. 21, pp 3300–3335) and are codified as 29 CFR 1910.1450.

1. **The laboratory** must develop a systematic approach **to significant risk determination**.

a. The standard **defines "employee"** as an individual employed in a laboratory workplace who **may be exposed to hazardous chemicals** in the course of his or her assignments.

b. The **standard defines "toxic or hazardous chemicals"** as any substance that has the capacity to produce personal injury or illness to man through ingestion, inhalation, or absorption through any body surface.

    c. The significant risk findings **must be based** on the following factors:

        (1) Epidemiologic information relating to disease and mortality rates

        (2) Evidence that shows **significant risk for specific substances** that are used in the laboratory

        (3) General recognition that safe work practices are necessary to prevent adverse health effects

        (4) Reported information about adverse health effects resulting from exposures to substances commonly used in the laboratory

        (5) Relevant **policy considerations**

2. Exposure monitoring of employees is required only when there is reason to believe that permissible exposure limits (PEL) or action levels for a substance are routinely exceeded.

3. The standard has a provision for a written chemical hygiene plan (CHP) to be formulated and implemented by the employer.

    a. Under the law, **employees have the right to know** any operations in their work area where hazardous chemicals are present.

    b. The location and availability of the **written hazard communication program** and **material safety data sheet (MSDS)** are required.

    c. A designated **chemical hygiene officer (CHO)** oversees the development, implementation, and administration of the CHP. The **duties of the CHO** include:

        (1) Developing a **standard operating procedure** that is relevant to the safety and health of persons who work with hazardous chemicals (This need not be developed for each chemical. A generic approach that groups chemicals by their physical and chemical properties is acceptable.)

        (2) Setting criteria that will be used by the laboratory to **determine the need** for and the implementation of **measures to control and reduce employee exposures** (The criteria should address engineering controls and PPE.)

        (3) Describing the laboratory's **employee information and training program**

        (4) Explaining the laboratory's program to provide OSHA-required **medical examinations and consultations**

        (5) Designating **specific operations** that cannot be performed without prior approval

        (6) Making provisions for **providing additional protection** for work with particularly hazardous materials, including:

            (a) Selected **carcinogens**

            (b) Reproductive toxins

            (c) Substances with a **high acute toxicity**

        (7) Labeling all chemicals to reflect the degree of hazard involved in their use

D. OSHA's final rule for **Occupational Exposure to Formaldehyde** was published on May 27, 1992.

    1. The risk of exposure in the laboratory is great without proper engineering controls and good work practices.

2. **A policy to maintain the permissible exposure limit (PEL)** must be in place.
   a. **PEL** at or below 0.75 parts per million (ppm)
   b. **Short-term exposure limit** of 2.0 ppm per 15 minutes of exposure
   c. **Action level** is 0.5 ppm
3. **The formaldehyde exposure control plan** must include:
   a. **Monitoring** of employees prone to exposure
   b. **Limitation of access to regulated areas** to authorized persons who have been trained to recognize the hazards
   c. Establishment of identified and located **engineering controls and work practices**
   d. Provision of the necessary **PPE and clothing** at no cost to the employee
   e. A **quick-drench shower and eyewash facility** located within the immediate work area
   f. **Visual inspections for spills** as a housekeeping procedure and cleaning up spills using formaldehyde-resistant clothing
   g. Performance by a licensed physician of all **medical surveillance procedures** without cost to the employee
   h. **Training of employees** at the time of employment, annually, and whenever a new exposure to formaldehyde is introduced into the work area
   i. **Environmental monitoring record keeping** for 30 years
E. **Guidelines from OSHA** for **Preventing the Transmission of *Mycobacterium tuberculosis* in Health Care Facilities** were published October 28, 1994, in the *Federal Register*.
   1. **Each laboratory** is responsible for having a policy on **prevention of *M. tuberculosis* transmission,** based on their own personnel's exposure to tuberculosis.
   2. **This policy must include** but is not limited to the following:
      a. **Control measures** must include the use of administrative measures to reduce the risk of exposure to persons who have infectious tuberculosis by **developing risk assessments.**
      b. **Engineering controls** include preventing the spread and reducing the concentrations of infectious droplets, as well as using **personal respiratory tract protective equipment** in areas where there is a risk of exposure. The most efficient of these is the **high-efficiency particulate air (HEPA) filter.**
      c. **Risk assessments** must be performed to identify and manage personnel who have tuberculosis. Management includes early treatment and isolation.
      d. A **tuberculosis screening program for employees** must be developed and must include the use of skin tests and follow-up treatment of all employees who have positive test results.
      e. All **employees must be trained and educated** in the use of PPE, hygiene, and handling of patients who have tuberculosis.

    f. The **evaluation of tuberculosis infection control programs** must include the effectiveness of the program and the outcome of exposures.

3. Three levels for preventing the transmission of tuberculosis include the following:

    a. The **first level** is to develop and implement policies for **rapid identification.** If a person is seen by a health care worker, who, from a history and examination, suspects tuberculosis, there should be a way to alert all other health care workers of the possibility. Each facility must determine their own policy for rapid identification.

    b. The **second level** is the use of PPE and respiratory tract protection (e.g., HEPA filter) to protect health care workers from the disease. This includes education and training programs for all employees, as well as the prompt evaluation of possible exposures to tuberculosis, including purified protein derivative skin tests and radiographs, if necessary.

    c. The **third level** is the coordination of activities with the local public health department. This includes the reporting of all cases, as well as continuation and completion of therapy.

STUDY QUESTIONS

Directions: Each of the numbered items or incomplete statements in this section is followed by answers or by completions of the statement. Select the ONE lettered answer or completion that is BEST in each case.

1. The purpose of a quality assurance (QA) program is to

a. ensure that a laboratory's results are reliable
b. ensure that a particular analyzer is working properly
c. ensure that only certified technologists are hired
d. ensure that instrumentation is updated

2. Which one of the following statements accurately describes proficiency testing (PT)?

a. it allows the laboratory to compare results of the same specimen to other laboratories' results
b. it ensures that a laboratory's quality assurance (QA) program is working
c. it ensures that proper specimen collection procedures are being used
d. it replaces the need for daily temperature checks of laboratory equipment

3. Which one of the following statements most accurately describes the practice of universal precautions?

a. all patient test results are considered invalid until the quality control (QC) data is verified for accuracy
b. all blood and body fluids are considered infectious
c. all electrical connections are considered hazardous
d. all laboratory reagents are considered hazardous

Directions: Each of the numbered items or incomplete statements in this section is negatively phrased, as indicated by a capitalized word such as NOT, LEAST, or EXCEPT. Select the ONE lettered answer or completion that is BEST in each case.

4. Which one of the following would NOT be part of a quality assurance (QA) program?

a. the use of universal precautions
b. a written procedure manual
c. a record of employee pay scales
d. enrollment in a proficiency testing program

5. Laboratory safety programs include all of the following EXCEPT

a. identification and labeling of hazardous materials
b. proper waste disposal
c. electrical checks
d. daily inspection of employees

6. The Clinical Laboratory Improvement Amendments of 1988 (CLIA 88) establishes regulations in all of the following areas EXCEPT

a. complexity of tests performed
b. personnel requirements
c. proficiency testing
d. pay and salary levels

Answers and Explanations

1. The answer is a [I A, B]. Although personnel and instrumentation are included in a quality assurance (QA) program, the entire program serves to ensure that results are reliable.

2. The answer is a [I B 8; II A 5]. Proficiency testing (PT) allows for comparison of results between laboratories using the same methodology. The PT sponsor determines if results are within range and acceptable.

3. The answer is b [II B 4]. Occupational Safety and Health Administration (OSHA) and Centers for Disease Control (CDC) requirements dictate that all blood and body fluids are to be considered capable of transmitting an infectious agent. There are a number of standard precautions that are taken when working with these specimens. The precautions are called "universal" precautions because they are practiced with all specimens, not only with those known to be infected.

4. The answer is c [II]. Inadequate pay may very well affect the performance of employees; however, recording pay scales is not part of a quality assurance (QA) program.

5. The answer is d [I B 4 a–i]. A safety program consists of policies and procedures that make the workplace safe for the employees and any visitors. There are at least nine components of a safety program: Occupational Safety and Health Administration (OSHA) standards, identification and labeling of hazardous materials, available material safety data sheets (MSDS), training, record keeping, waste disposal, universal precautions, safety equipment, and electrical checks.

6. The answer is d [II A]. The Clinical Laboratory Improvement Amendments of 1988 (CLIA 88) establishes requirements for laboratory operations. Personnel issues such as pay are not a part of CLIA 88.

8

Clinical Microbiology

Hal S. Larsen

I. BACTERIAL CELL STRUCTURE

A. The cell membrane serves as an osmotic barrier and may be a site of antibiotic action. An intact membrane is essential for bacterial viability.

B. The cell wall

1. The most prominent layer of the **gram-positive cell wall** is the rigid peptidoglycan layer, which is the site of action of the penicillins and cephalosporins.

2. More complex than the gram-positive cell wall, the **gram-negative cell wall** contains a thinner peptidoglycan layer but also an outer lipopolysaccharide (LPS) layer. LPS is an endotoxin that is an important virulence factor. An endotoxin causes shock, sepsis, fever, disseminated intravascular coagulation (DIC), and leukopenia.

C. A polysaccharide capsule covers many bacteria and serves to prevent or inhibit phagocytosis. For many organisms (e.g., *Streptococcus pneumoniae*), the capsule is the chief determinant of virulence.

D. Pili, also called fimbriae, are short, hairlike structures that serve to attach bacteria to target cells. For many bacteria (e.g., *Neisseria gonorrhoeae*), interference with attachment prevents infection. The exchange of deoxyribonucleic acid (DNA) between bacteria during conjugation occurs through the pili.

E. Flagella determine motility and can be used in classification.

F. Spores are a means of survival that make disease control very difficult. The two spore-forming genera of importance are *Bacillus* and *Clostridium*.

II. STAINS

A. Gram's stain

1. **Crystal violet** is the primary stain. **Iodine** binds the crystal violet within the cell (mordant). **Decolorizer** washes out any unbound dye. **Safranin O** is a counterstain.

   a. **Gram-positive** cells retain the crystal violet and stain purple.

      b. Gram-negative cells are decolorized, stained with safranin O, and stain red.

    2. Clinical use. Gram's stain is especially useful for examining smears of clinical specimens. Initial treatment, and often a presumptive identification, can be made from Gram's stain results. White and red blood cells (WBCs and RBCs), as well as cellular debris, stain pink. This can serve as an internal control.

B. Acridine orange stain is an orange fluorescent stain used to detect bacteria in body fluids in which numbers of bacteria may be few (e.g., blood and spinal fluid). It is very sensitive and can detect small numbers of bacteria that are living or dead. The procedure consists of flooding a methanol-fixed smear with acridine orange for 2 minutes, washing, and then observing with a fluorescence microscope.

C. Methylene blue stain is especially helpful for demonstrating metachromatic granules and characteristic morphology of *Corynebacterium diphtheriae* from Loeffler coagulated serum medium. The procedure consists of flooding a fixed smear with methylene blue, followed by washing.

D. Acid-fast stain is used to detect organisms that do not stain well with other conventional stains (e.g., *Mycobacterium* spp., *Nocardia*, *Actinomyces*). These organisms have a high lipid content in their cell walls. Once stained, they are very resistant to decolorization by acid alcohol. The most commonly used method is the **Kinyoun modification method.** The primary stain is **carbolfuchsin,** which contains a surface-active detergent to facilitate penetration of the stain without heating. After washing, methylene blue is used as a counterstain. Acid-fast organisms appear red against a blue background.

E. Auramine-rhodamine stain is a fluorescent stain that detects mycolic acids and so can be used for acid-fast organisms. The smear is stained with auramine-rhodamine, decolorized with acid alcohol, and then flooded with potassium permanganate. It is observed with a fluorescence microscope. The cells appear yellow against a dark background.

F. Calcofluor white stain binds specifically to chitin, which is found in fungal cell walls. It is used to detect yeast cells and hyphae in skin scrapings and other specimens. The fungal elements appear green or blue-white.

III. NORMAL FLORA describes the microorganisms that are frequently found on or in the bodies of healthy persons.

  A. General characteristics

    1. Local conditions select for those organisms that are suited for growth in a particular area.

    2. **Resident flora** colonize an area for months or years.

    3. **Transient flora** are present at a site temporarily.

    4. Organisms that live at the expense of the host are **parasites.**

    5. Organisms that benefit the host are **symbionts.**

    6. **Commensals** have a neutral effect on the host.

    7. A **carrier** harbors the organism without manifesting symptoms but is capable of transmitting infection (carrier state).

8. **Opportunists** are organisms that do not normally cause infection but do so if the condition of the host changes (i.e., immunosuppression).

B. **Normal flora of the skin**

1. The skin contains a wide variety of microorganisms that are not eliminated by washing or superficial antisepsis.

    a. *Propionibacterium acnes* colonizes the sebaceous glands.

    b. *Micrococcus, Staphylococcus* **spp.**, and diphtheroids are common.

2. Intact skin is an effective barrier to microbial invasion.

C. **Normal flora of the mouth.** The mouth contains large numbers of bacteria, most commonly **Streptococcus** spp. (especially viridans species), coagulase-negative *Staphylococcus, Peptostreptococcus,* and other **anaerobes.**

D. **Normal flora of the respiratory tract**

1. The respiratory tract beyond the oropharynx is normally sterile.

2. The ciliary action of epithelial cells and mucus movement remove invading organisms.

3. The nose and nasopharynx contain *Staphylococcus aureus, S. epidermidis,* and *Streptococcus* **spp.** The following may be present transiently during community outbreaks of infection: *Streptococcus pneumoniae, Haemophilus influenzae, and N. meningitidis.*

4. The normal flora in the oropharynx mirrors that of the mouth.

E. **Normal flora of the gastrointestinal tract**

1. Most microorganisms are destroyed in the stomach. The survivors multiply in the colon.

2. More than 90% of the microbial population is comprised of anaerobes.

3. Alteration of the normal flora by antibiotics may allow a superinfection by *Clostridium difficile* (necrotizing enterocolitis), *Candida albicans,* or *S. aureus.*

4. The most commonly found organisms in the gastrointestinal tract are: *Bacteroides* spp., *Clostridium* spp., *Eubacterium* spp., **anaerobic streptococci,** *Enterococcus,* and Enterobacteriaceae.

F. **Normal flora of the genitourinary tract**

1. The outermost segment of the **urethra** is colonized by skin organisms.

2. The **vagina** is colonized with *Lactobacillus,* **anaerobic gram-negative rod-shaped bacteria, and gram-positive cocci.**

IV. COLLECTION AND HANDLING OF CLINICAL SPECIMENS

A. **Collection.** A properly collected specimen is absolutely crucial to quality diagnostic information and patient care.

1. **Safety**

    a. **Universal precautions** are followed throughout the collection and handling process. Persons collecting or handling specimens should wear gloves and a laboratory coat. Eye protection should also be worn if splashing is a possibility.

    b. Accidents or injuries must be reported immediately.

2. **General guidelines**

   a. The specimen should be from the infection site and not contaminated by the surrounding area (e.g., culture within a wound and not the surface or the surrounding skin).

   b. Whenever possible, the specimen should be collected before antimicrobials are administered.

   c. Appropriate collection devices and containers should be used and must be sterile. Aseptic technique is required.

   d. The specimen container should be labeled with the patient's identification and the date and time of collection.

3. **Collection from various body sites**

   a. **Throat.** The tongue should be depressed before swabbing between the tonsillar pillars and behind the uvula. The cheek, tongue, and teeth should not be touched.

   b. **Nasopharynx.** A flexible wire nasopharyngeal swab should be gently inserted through the nose into the posterior nasopharynx, rotated, then removed.

   c. **Sputum.** Whenever possible, the patient should gargle with water (not mouthwash) immediately before sampling. Early morning specimens are best. Specimens from a deep cough should be collected into a sterile specimen cup.

   d. **Stool** should be collected in a clean, wide-mouthed container with a tight-fitting lid. If the specimen cannot be plated within 1 hour of collection, it should be mixed with a transport medium (e.g., buffered glycerol saline, Cary-Blair transport medium). The change in pH and temperature over time is detrimental to *Shigella* spp.

   e. **Urine.** Midstream clean-catch is the most common collection method. Proper cleansing of the urethral area is important, especially in women. The first few milliliters, which flush out the ureter, are discarded. The specimen is collected into a sterile specimen cup. The specimen is transported immediately to the laboratory or refrigerated, because contaminants grow readily at room temperature.

   f. **Blood.** Two to three cultures should be collected at random times during a 24-hour period. Collecting more than three sets of cultures in a 24-hour period does not significantly increase the probability of detecting bacteremia. Skin is disinfected with 70% alcohol, followed by iodine. The disinfectant is allowed to dry. The puncture site should not be palpated after disinfection. Ideally, 20–30 mL of blood per culture is collected from an adult (1–5 mL from infants and small children). Iodine should be cleaned from the puncture site with alcohol.

   g. **Cerebrospinal fluid** should be collected aseptically by a physician. This specimen should be processed immediately and not exposed to heat or refrigeration.

   h. **Abscesses and synovial, pericardial, and chest fluid** should be collected by a physician with a needle and syringe. The use of swabs may inhibit growth of anaerobes. Care should be taken not to inject an air bubble into the syringe.

i. Genital tract

(1) **Men.** Exudate may be expressed from the urethral orifice, or a small-diameter swab may be inserted 3–4 cm into the urethra. The specimen should be plated immediately on the appropriate media and not allowed to dry or be exposed to cold temperatures. A Gram's stain smear should be prepared.

(2) **Women.** Cervical specimens are obtained by a physician with the aid of a speculum. Lubricants, which may be lethal to *Neisseria gonorrhoeae*, should not be used on the speculum. The cervical mucus plug is removed, and a sterile swab is inserted into the cervix, rotated, and allowed to remain for a few seconds. The specimen is plated immediately to the appropriate media.

B. Handling

1. **Transport** all specimens to the laboratory promptly. Anaerobic specimens must be in an anaerobic transport system. If transport cannot occur immediately, most specimens can be held at 2°C–8°C. Exceptions to this include specimens that likely contain temperature-sensitive organisms (e.g., *Neisseria*), blood culture bottles, and cerebrospinal fluid (CSF). Generally, swabs are the least desirable collection and transport method. However, organisms can be successfully cultured if the swab is handled and transported properly (i.e., not allowed to dry out). Swabs are inappropriate for culturing anaerobes.

2. **Processing**

   a. **Media selection.** Specific reactions of the various clinical isolates on various media are contained within the individual organism groups. Some general principles apply to the use of primary media. In most cases, the concern is that the primary media will grow and isolate all or a majority of the possible organisms from a clinical specimen. In those cases in which certain organisms are excluded, the decision is based on time, cost, and probability of isolation information. In many cases, the choice of some primary media is an individual laboratory choice. Of primary importance is for the microbiologist to understand the range and purpose of each primary isolation medium, as well as the various reactions of the organisms.

      (1) **Substitutions** may be made with acceptable results (e.g., MacConkey agar in place of eosin-methylene blue agar).

      (2) Most isolation protocols call for **blood agar.**

      (3) **Chocolate agar** is used for fastidious isolates.

      (4) **Specialized media** [e.g., mannitol salt agar, bismuth sulfite agar, *Campylobacter* agar, thiosulfate-citrate-bile salts-sucrose (TCBS) agar] are used when specific organisms are suspected.

   b. **Specimen rejection criteria.** Rejection criteria should be part of the written policy of every clinical laboratory. They should be clearly listed and made available to anyone who might submit specimens for culture. Processing and culture of inappropriate specimens leads to increased costs and misinformation. In each case, the person submitting the request should be contacted and informed. In some cases, the difficulty of collection makes culturing necessary, although the results are not optimal. The following situations or specimen types should be rejected (this is not intended to be a comprehensive list):

(1) 24-hour urine or sputum collections

(2) Specimens received in nonsterile or contaminated containers (including those in which the specimen has leaked out)

(3) Specimens contaminated with barium or other foreign substances

(4) Culturing of Foley catheter tips

(5) Saliva instead of sputum

(6) Unrefrigerated urine specimens 2 hours or more post-collection

(7) Anaerobic culturing of midstream urine, upper respiratory tract, superficial skin, or feces specimens (certain *Clostridium* species may be appropriately cultured from feces)

V. Micrococcaceae

A. General characteristics

1. Members of the family Micrococcaceae are gram-positive cocci, aerobic or facultative anaerobes, and catalase positive (except *Stomatococcus*).

2. Most are members of the indigenous flora and are commonly isolated from a wide variety of diseases.

3. *Staphylococcus* (Table 8-1; Figure 8-1)

   a. The staphylococci are catalase-positive, nonmotile, facultative anaerobes that are normal inhabitants of the skin and mucous membranes. These organisms commonly cause human infections.

   b. Species are initially differentiated by the **coagulase test.** The most important coagulase-positive species is *S. aureus*. Some animal species produce coagulase but are rarely isolated from human samples.

   c. Staphylococci that do not produce coagulase are called "coagulase-negative staphylococci." The most prominent species are *S. epidermidis* and *S. saprophyticus*.

4. *Micrococcus* (see Table 8-1 and Figure 8-1). Micrococci are opportunistic pathogens found only in immunocompromised persons. *Micrococcus* is of

Table 8-1. Differentiation of the Micrococcaceae

Characteristic	Staphylococcus	Micrococcus	Stomatococcus
Catalase	+	+	−
Growth on 6.5% NaCl agar	+	+	−
Modified oxidase test	−	+	−
Resistance to bacitracin (0.04 μM) disk	+	−	−
Resistance to furazolidone (100 μg) disk	−	+	−

+ = positive; − = negative.

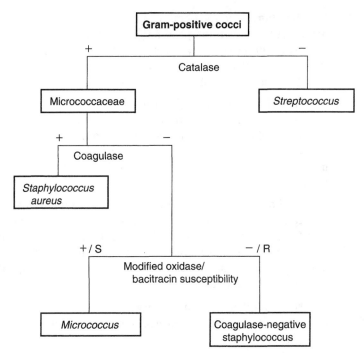

Figure 8-1. Identification of Micrococcaceae species.

low pathogenic significance but may be isolated as a contaminant or as part of the normal flora.

5. ***Stomatococcus*** (see Table 8-1 and Figure 8-1). This genus is part of the normal oral flora and is rarely isolated from infection. The colonies adhere strongly to the agar surface.

6. **Differential tests** include the following.

   a. **Modified oxidase test.** Modified oxidase reagent (6% tetramethylphenylene diamine hydrochloride in dimethyl sulfoxide) is added to a small amount of growth smeared onto a filter paper. Micrococci turn dark blue within 2 minutes.

   b. **Bacitracin susceptibility.** Isolate is streaked onto a sheep blood Mueller-Hinton medium. A 0.04-U bacitracin disk is placed onto the streaked area, and the plate is incubated overnight and observed for a zone of inhibition.

   c. **Furazolidone susceptibility** is tested exactly as for bacitracin susceptibility, except a disk containing 100-μg furazolidone is used.

B. ***Staphylococcus aureus***

   1. **Infections**

      a. **Skin and wound infections** caused by *S. aureus* are suppurative and pyogenic. Some common skin infections are boils, carbuncles, furuncles, and folliculitis.

      b. **Food poisoning.** *S. aureus* produces enterotoxins that are associated with food poisoning. The source of contamination is usually an infected food handler. Infection occurs when an individual ingests food contaminated with enterotoxin-producing strains. The heat-stable toxins are preformed in the food. Symptoms appear rapidly (2–6 hours after ingestion) and resolve within 8–10 hours. Symptoms may include nausea, vomiting, headache, abdominal pain, and severe cramping.

c. **Scalded skin syndrome (Ritter's disease)** is an extensive exfoliative dermatitis that occurs primarily in newborns and is caused by staphylococcal exfoliative or epidermolytic toxin. It can also occur in adults, most frequently among those who have chronic renal failure or are immunocompromised. The mortality rate is low in children but high in adults.

d. **Toxic shock syndrome (TSS)** is a multisystem disease characterized by high fever, rash, hypotension, shock, desquamation of the hands and feet, and possible death. It is caused by a toxin-producing strain of *S. aureus*. There is an association between use of tampons and TSS, although the disease may occur in both sexes if a toxin-producing strain of *S. aureus* has caused infection.

e. **Other staphylococcal infections**
   (1) Staphylococcal **pneumonia** secondary to influenza can occur. The mortality rate is high.
   (2) **Osteomyelitis** can occur secondary to **bacteremia.**

2. **Laboratory identification of *Staphylococcus aureus***
   a. **Microscopic examination** of stained smears from clinical specimens can be especially helpful. Numerous gram-positive cocci with polymorphonuclear cells are usually seen.

   b. *S. aureus* grows readily on common laboratory **media.** On sheep blood agar, colonies appear as round, smooth and white or pigmented (yellow-orange). They are usually β-hemolytic.

   c. *S. aureus* is most often identified by the **coagulase test.** Isolates may show cell-bound (clumping factor) or free (extracellular) coagulase. Cell-bound coagulase is identified by mixing the suspected organism with a drop of rabbit plasma on a glass slide. If clumping occurs, the isolate demonstrates cell-bound coagulase and is identified as *S. aureus.* Isolates that do not clump are tested for free coagulase by the tube method, in which the organism is mixed with 0.5 mL of rabbit plasma and incubated at 37°C for 4 hours.

   d. **Selective media** that can be used to isolate *S. aureus* from heavily contaminated specimens or when it is the only isolate of concern are **mannitol salt agar (MSA)** and **phenylethyl alcohol (PEA) blood agar.**
      (1) MSA provides mannitol as a fermentable carbohydrate source as well as 6.5% sodium chloride (NaCl). Generally, only *Staphylococcus* species grow because of the high salt content. *S. aureus* ferments the mannitol to produce acid, which turns the pink agar yellow. The colonies are identified by a yellow halo. This test is presumptive because some strains of *S. epidermidis* can also ferment mannitol.

(2) PEA agar inhibits the growth of gram-negative organisms, whereas the gram-positive bacteria, including *Staphylococcus species*, grow well.

  e. **Rapid methods** use plasma-coated latex particles. The plasma detects clumping factor and causes agglutination of the particles. Other methods use protein A–coated *S. aureus* as a nonspecific carrier of antibodies against specific antigens.

C. **Coagulase-negative staphylococci**

  1. **General characteristics.** The coagulase-negative staphylococci are found as normal flora in humans and animals. The incidence of infection by these organisms has increased. They are often hospital-acquired (nosocomial). Predisposing factors include catheterization, prosthetic device implants, and immunosuppressive therapy. The most common species isolated from clinical infections are *S. epidermidis* and *S. saprophyticus*. *S. saprophyticus* has been associated with urinary tract infections in young, sexually active women. Other species of coagulase-negative staphylococci are not isolated frequently. Three species that can cause a wide range of infections, but do so only occasionally, are *S. haemolyticus*, *S. lugdunensis*, and *S. schleiferi*. The latter two produce clumping factor and may yield a positive slide coagulase test.

  2. **Laboratory identification of coagulase-negative staphylococci**

    a. On sheep blood agar, colonies are usually round, smooth, and white without hemolysis.

    b. The most common isolates are *S. epidermidis* and *S. saprophyticus*.

    c. Urine isolates that are coagulase negative are further tested to presumptively identify *S. saprophyticus*. This is done by testing for novobiocin susceptibility using a 5-mg novobiocin disk. *S. saprophyticus* is resistant to novobiocin, whereas other coagulase-negative staphylococci are susceptible.

    d. Species identification of the coagulase-negative staphylococci requires a large number of characteristics. Various commercial identification systems exist and may be used if appropriate.

D. **Antibiotic susceptibility**

  1. Penicillin resistance is so high, especially in *S. aureus* isolates (85%–90%), that other antibiotics must often be used. There is variability in the susceptibility patterns.

  2. A common resistance mechanism is a production of β-lactamase.

  3. Various β-lactamase resistant penicillins have been developed. Methicillin is the most frequently used.

  4. Methicillin-resistant strains have increased in number. Vancomycin has been used as an alternative treatment of methicillin-resistant strains. However, vancomycin resistance is increasing.

VI. *STREPTOCOCCUS, ENTEROCOCCUS,* AND RELATED GENERA

A. **General characteristics**

1. The organisms included in this group are **catalase-negative, gram-positive cocci** (old cells may stain gram negative or gram variable) that are arranged in **pairs** or **chains** and are **facultative anaerobes.** Growth requirements may be complex, and the use of blood or enriched medium is necessary for isolation. Their role in human disease ranges from well-established and common, to rare but increasing.

2. **Hemolysis patterns on sheep blood agar** are helpful in identification.

B. *Streptococcus*

1. *Streptococcus pneumoniae*

   a. *S. pneumoniae* is often part of the **normal flora** of the respiratory tract.

   b. The key **virulence factor** is an antiphagocytic **capsule.** There are approximately 80 antigenic types.

   c. *S. pneumoniae* is an important human pathogen, causing **pneumonia, sinusitis, otitis media, bacteremia,** and **meningitis.** It is frequently isolated as a pathogen and as a member of the normal respiratory flora. Direct smears often reveal leukocytes and numerous **gram-positive cocci in pairs.** The ends of the cells are slightly pointed, giving them an oval or lancet shape.

   d. Complex media, such as brain-heart infusion agar, trypticase soy agar with 5% sheep blood, or chocolate agar are necessary for good growth. Isolates **may require increased CO_2** for growth during primary isolation. Colonies are **alpha-hemolytic.** Young cultures produce a round, glistening, wet mucoid, dome-shaped appearance.

   e. **Laboratory identification.** *S. pneumoniae* is **susceptible to optochin** (ethylhydrocuprein hydrochloride). The **bile solubility** test is also used for identification. An alpha-hemolytic streptococcus that is optochin susceptible or bile soluble can be identified as *S. pneumoniae.* Other alpha-hemolytic streptococci are negative for both tests.

2. *Streptococcus pyogenes*

   a. The cell wall contains the Lancefield group A carbohydrate. This organism is also referred to as **group A streptococcus** or **beta-hemolytic group A streptococcus.**

   b. **Virulence factors**

      (1) The most well-defined virulence factor is **M protein.** There are more than 80 different serotypes. Resistance to infection is related to the presence of type-specific antibodies to the M protein. The M protein molecule causes the streptococcal cell to resist phagocytosis. It enables the bacterial cell to adhere to mucosal cells.

      (2) **Streptolysin O** causes hemolysis of RBCs. Its role in virulence is unknown. Antibodies to streptolysin O indicate a recent infection **(antistreptolysin O titer).**

      (3) **Hyaluronidase** (spreading factor) may favor the spread of the organism through the tissues.

      (4) All strains form at least one deoxyribonuclease (DNAse). The most common is **DNAse B.** These enzymes are antigenic, and antibodies to DNAse can be detected following infection.

Table 8-2. *Streptococcus* Hemolysis Patterns

Type	Characteristic
Alpha (α)	**Greenish discoloration** in medium surrounding colony due to partial lysis of red blood cells
Alpha-prime (α')	Small ring of no hemolysis around the colony, which is surrounded by a wider zone of complete hemolysis (also called "wide zone" hemolysis)
Beta (β)	**Clearing** of red blood cells surrounding the colony due to complete lysis
Nonhemolytic	**No change**

      (5) Some strains of *S. pyogenes* cause a red spreading rash referred to as scarlet fever. This condition is caused by erythrogenic **toxin.**

  c. Infections

      (1) Pharyngitis is one of the most common *S. pyogenes* infections. "Strep throat" is most frequently seen in children between the ages of 5 and 15 years. Diagnosis relies on a throat culture or a positive quick "strep" test, in which group A antigens are detected from a throat swab in a matter of minutes. A throat culture is recommended if the antigen-detecting test is negative.

      (2) Skin infections include **impetigo, necrotizing fasciitis,** and **pyoderma.**

      (3) Scarlet fever is a red rash that appears on the upper chest and spreads to the trunk and extremities following infection with *S. pyogenes.*

      (4) Rheumatic fever and glomerulonephritis may result from infection at other sites. Damage appears to result from cross-reactivity of the streptococcal antigens with host tissue antigens.

      (5) Streptococcal TSS is similar to that caused by *Staphylococcus.*

  d. Laboratory identification (Table 8-2). Colonies of *S. pyogenes* on blood agar are small, transparent, and smooth, and they show beta hemolysis. Gram's stain reveals gram-positive cocci with some short chains.

  3. *Streptococcus agalactiae*

    a. The cell wall contains the Lancefield group B carbohydrate. This organism is also referred to as **group B streptococcus.** It may be found as normal flora in the genitourinary tract.

    b. Virulence factors

      (1) The capsule is the most important virulence factor.

      (2) Other factors (e.g., DNAse, hyaluronidase) have not been shown to be factors in infection.

    c. Infections

      (1) Neonatal sepsis (usually manifest as **pneumonia** or **meningitis**) occurs soon after birth. The most important factor in infection is the presence of group B streptococcus in the vagina of the mother.

(2) **Postpartum fever and sepsis** may occur after birth and may manifest as endometritis or a wound infection.

d. **Laboratory identification** (Table 8-3). Group B streptococci grow on blood agar as grayish white mucoid colonies surrounded by a small zone of beta hemolysis. They are gram-positive cocci that form short chains in clinical specimens and long chains in culture.

4. **Groups C and G**

a. There are three hemolytic species in group C that are occasionally isolated from clinical specimens: ***S. equi, S. zooepidemicus,* and *S. equisimilis.*** The major species found in group G is ***S. canis.*** It occasionally causes infection, and is part of the normal skin flora. Minute colony types of group G are part of the ***S. milleri*** group, with ***S. anginosus*** being the most prominent species.

b. These groups produce a variety of infections similar to those caused by groups A and B. Group C can cause pharyngitis.

c. **Laboratory identification.** Groups C and G can be identified by extensive biochemical tests. However, serologic tests to identify the group carbohydrate in the cell wall of the isolate (e.g., agglutination) are best.

5. **Group D** (see Table 8-3)

a. The group D streptococci include ***S. bovis*** and ***S. equinus.*** They may be found as normal intestinal flora.

b. The group D streptococci may produce bacterial **endocarditis, urinary tract infection,** and other diseases, such as **abscesses** and wound infections. An association has been made between bacteremia due to *S. bovis* and the presence of gastrointestinal tumors. Isolation of *S. bovis* from a blood culture may be the first indication that the patient has an occult tumor.

c. Hemolysis is usually absent, or alpha hemolysis is present. A key reaction of group D is a **positive bile esculin** test with **no growth in 6.5% NaCl broth.** Group D can be separated from *Enterococcus* by the L-pyrrolidonyl-β-naphthylamide **(PYR)** test because it is negative and *Enterococcus* is positive. Serotyping should be done to identify an isolate such as *S. bovis*, because it cannot be distinguished from some of the viridans group by biochemical tests alone.

6. ***Enterococcus*** (see Table 8-3)

a. This genus is found in the intestinal tract. The species found in this genus include ***E. faecalis,*** which is the most common isolate, ***E. faecium, E. avium,*** and ***E. durans.*** These enterococcal species share a number of characteristics with the group D streptococci, including the group D antigen. They show resistance to several of the commonly used antibiotics, so differentiation with *Streptococcus* and susceptibility testing is important.

b. The **infections** caused are similar to that of the group D streptococci. The most common is a **urinary tract infection.**

Table 8-3. Identification of *Streptococcus* and Related Organisms

	S. pyogenes	*S. agalactiae*	*Enterococcus*	Group D	*S. pneumoniae*	Viridans streptococci	Aerococcus	Pediococcus	Leuconostoc
Hemolysis	β	β	α, β, non	α, non	α	α, non	α	α	α
Susceptibility to:									
Vancomycin	S	S	S	S	S	S	S	R	R
Bacitracin	S	R	R	R	S	R	—	—	—
SXT	R	R	R	V	S	S	—	—	—
Optochin	R	R	R	R	S	R	—	—	—
Hippurate hydrolysis	—	+	—	—	—	—	+	+	—
PYR hydrolysis	+	—	+	—	—	—	+	—	—
CAMP test	—	+	—	—	—	—	—	—	—
Bile esculin hydrolysis	—	—	+	+	—	—	V	+	—
Growth in 6.5% NaCl	—	—	+	—	—	—	+	+	—

PYR = L-pyrrolidonyl-β-naphthylamide; R = resistant; S = susceptible; SXT = sulfamethoxazole trimethoprim; V = variable; — = negative; + = positive; — = tests not done (vancomycin is the key characteristic).

    c. It is not difficult to differentiate between *Enterococcus* and group D isolates. In addition to being **positive for bile esculin,** *Enterococcus* species grow in 6.5% NaCl broth and are **PYR positive.**

7. Viridans streptococci

    a. The viridans group includes those alpha-hemolytic streptococci that lack Lancefield group antigens and do not meet the criteria for *S. pneumoniae.* They are part of the normal flora of the oropharynx and intestine.

    b. The most common **infection** caused by these organisms is **subacute bacterial endocarditis.**

    c. Identification of the viridans streptococci to the species level is a difficult task. Part of the reason for this is that there is not widespread agreement on a classification scheme. **Species** of viridans streptococci include *S. mutans, S. salivarius, S. sanguis, S. mitis,* **and** *S. milleri* (not beta hemolytic).

8. Nutritionally variant streptococci (NVS)

    a. The NVS subgroup of viridans streptococci are nutritionally deficient and have been isolated from patients who have **endocarditis** and **otitis media.** This subgroup is also known as **pyridoxal (vitamin B$_6$)–dependent, thiol-dependent, or symbiotic streptococci.** Pyridoxal is not present in most liquid and solid bacteriologic media. The NVS colonies are small, measuring 0.2–0.5 mm in diameter. When gram stained, the morphology can vary from classic gram-positive streptococci to gram-negative or gram-variable pleomorphic forms. As the optimal concentrations or required nutrients decrease, the cells become pleomorphic, even showing globular and filamentous forms. Bacteriologic media must include pyridoxal (vitamin B$_6$) to grow NVS.

    b. A clue to the presence of NVS is a positive Gram's stain but negative cultures.

9. Treatment of streptococcal and enterococcal infections. Most species of *Streptococcus* are susceptible to penicillin. *S. agalactiae* is less susceptible than is group A and may require a combination of ampicillin and an aminoglycoside. Group D is susceptible to penicillin, whereas *Enterococcus* is usually resistant. *Enterococcus* is often treated with a penicillin-aminoglycoside combination (synergy). Some isolates are resistant to this combination therapy. Although most pneumococcal isolates are susceptible to penicillin, some strains have shown resistance. Resistant streptococcal strains are often treated with erythromycin.

C. Streptococcus-like organisms

    1. *Aerococcus* (see Table 8-3) is very similar to *Enterococcus* on blood agar. It is susceptible to vancomycin and can be isolated from **tissue samples of endocarditis** and other varied infections.

    2. *Leuconostoc* is very similar to viridans streptococci on blood agar. It is found in the general environment. A Gram's stain shows gram-positive coccobacilli in pairs and short chains. *Leuconostoc* has been found in patients who have **meningitis** and **endocarditis.** It is resistant to vancomycin.

3. ***Pediococcus*** is also found in the general environment. A Gram's stain shows gram-positive cocci in pairs, tetrads, and clusters. *Pediococcus* is a rare isolate in patients who have septicemia.

D. **Laboratory identification**

1. **Hemolysis on blood agar** is an important characteristic (see Table 8-2).

2. **Bile solubility** measures autolysis of bacteria under the influence of a bile salt (sodium deoxycholate). ***S. pneumoniae*** is bile soluble.

3. **Optochin (ethylhydrocuprein hydrochloride)** susceptibility is measured by growing the organism on blood agar with a filter paper disk containing optochin. Results correlate with bile solubility; that is, optochin-susceptible isolates are bile soluble. ***S. pneumoniae*** is optochin susceptible.

4. **Bacitracin** susceptibility is a characteristic of ***S. pyogenes.*** The test is performed by placing a filter paper disk containing bacitracin on an inoculated blood agar plate.

5. Group A and B streptococci are resistant to **sulfamethoxazole-trimethoprim (SXT).** This resistance can be measured with a filter paper disk or by incorporating SXT into blood agar. The latter technique allows for selective isolation.

6. **Group B** streptococci **hydrolyze hippurate.** The glycine liberated can be detected by triketohydrindene hydrate (Ninhydrin), which imparts a purple color.

7. The **Christie, Atkins, and Munch-Petersen (CAMP) test** presumptively identifies **group B streptococcus** by measuring the enhanced hemolytic activity of staphylococcal beta-lysin by *S. agalactiae*. Group B streptococci demonstrate a characteristic arrow-shaped hemolysis pattern.

8. The ability of an organism to hydrolyze esculin is the basis of the esculin test. A positive result is a **black precipitate** in the agar surrounding the growth. Group D streptococci and *Enterococcus* are bile esculin positive.

9. *Enterococcus* is able to grow in nutrient broth containing **6.5% NaCl.**

10. Hydrolysis of **PYR** can be detected by the development of a red color on the addition of cinnamaldehyde reagent. This test is specific for ***Enterococcus*** and ***S. pyogenes.***

VII. MISCELLANEOUS GRAM-NEGATIVE BACILLI

A. ***Haemophilus***

1. Members of the genus *Haemophilus* are gram-negative, nonmotile bacilli and coccobacilli, which are often **pleomorphic.** Members of *Haemophilus* require **hemin (X factor)** or **nicotinamide adenine dinucleotide** (NAD; **V factor**) for growth.

2. ***H. influenzae*** is the most important species, causing **meningitis, otitis media, epiglottitis, pneumonia,** and contagious **conjunctivitis** (caused by *H. aegyptius*). Children, especially those who have not been immunized, are particularly at risk. *H. influenzae* is part of the normal upper respiratory tract flora. The most common capsular serotype of disseminated infections is type b.

Table 8-4. Differentiation of *Haemophilus* species

Species	Growth-Factor Requirement		Catalase	Fermentation of:		
	X	V		Glucose	Sucrose	Lactose
H. influenzae	+	+	+	+	−	−
H. parainfluenzae	−	+	V	+	+	−
H. ducreyi	+	−	−	−	−	−
H. aprophilus	−	−	−	+	+	+

V = variable; + = positive; − = negative.

3. ***H. ducreyi*** is the cause of **chancroid,** a sexually transmitted disease. Organisms enter through breaks in the skin and multiply locally. Approximately 1 week later, a small papule appears that soon develops into a painful ulcer. A Gram's stain of the lesion exudate may show small pleomorphic gram-negative bacilli in clusters ("school of fish" morphology).

4. ***H. parainfluenzae*** and ***H. aprophilus*** are seen primarily in endocarditis.

5. **Differentiation** of the *Haemophilus* species is summarized in Table 8-4.

   a. **X and V factor requirements** can be determined by placing X and V factor–impregnated filter paper strips onto a nutrient agar plate that has been inoculated with the unknown species. X and V requirements are determined by growth patterns (e.g., growth around X indicates a requirement for that factor).

   b. Growth can also be seen surrounding colonies of *S. aureus.* This is called the **satellite phenomenon** and is a result of the staphylococci providing required growth factors by secreting V factor and lysing RBCs in the medium, which releases X factor.

   c. The **porphyrin test** is a sensitive method to determine X factor requirements. Those species that do not require X factor yield a positive porphyrin test (e.g., *H. influenzae* is porphyrin negative).

   d. **Fermentation** of carbohydrates (glucose, sucrose, lactose) can identify the species.

   e. *H. influenzae* may be divided into **biotypes.** The site of infection by *H. influenzae* can be correlated with biotype. Biotypes are determined by an isolate's activity with **indole, urease,** and **ornithine decarboxylase.** The disease association and biochemical characteristics are summarized in Table 8-5.

6. **Antibiotic resistance.** Resistance to the penicillins is common due to **β-lactamases** and other mechanisms.

B. **Pasteurella multocida** is the most commonly encountered species in the *Pasteurella* genus. It is found as normal flora in the respiratory tract of

Table 8-5. *Haemophilus influenzae* Biotypes

Biotype	Indole	Ornithine	Urease	Infection Site
I	+	+	+	Meningitis
II	+	–	+	Eye, respiratory tract
III	–	–	+	Eye, respiratory tract
V	+	+	–	Ear, respiratory tract

+ = positive; – = negative.

animals, especially dogs and cats. Isolation of *P. multocida* is always a strong possibility in an **infected dog or cat bite or scratch.** This species appears as a **small gram- negative coccobacillus.** The key characteristics for differentiating *P. multocida* are listed in Box 8-1.

C. ***Bordetella*** species are **very small gram-negative bacilli.** There are three species that cause human infection: ***pertussis, parapertussis,*** and ***bronchiseptica.*** All cause respiratory tract infection, but ***B. pertussis*** causes the most serious infection, which is **whooping cough.**

   1. ***Bordetella pertussis,*** the cause of **pertussis** or **whooping cough,** is found worldwide and is spread via **droplets.**

      a. **Disease progression.** The disease begins with coldlike symptoms (i.e., runny nose, sneezing, malaise). This stage is the most infectious. After 1–2 weeks, the paroxysmal stage begins, with violent coughs that often make it difficult for the infected person to take a breath. Convalescence can take weeks to months, with secondary complications such as pneumonia, seizures, and encephalopathy possible.

      b. **Specimen collection and transport.** *B. pertussis* is very sensitive to drying and to trace toxic chemicals on swabs and in media. Specimen collection and transport must be done correctly for successful culture. Cotton swabs are toxic; calcium alginate or Dacron swabs should be used. The best specimen is a nasopharyngeal swab or aspirate. Immediate plating is preferred, because the organism does not readily survive transport. A swab should also be collected for a direct fluorescent antibody and Gram's stain of smears.

         (1) Growth can be accomplished with **Regan-Lowe** or **Bordet-Gengou** media. *B. pertussis* colonies are small and pearl-like in appearance after 3–4 days.

Box 8-1. Key Characteristics of *Pasteurella multocida*

Growth on blood agar (may have a musty or mousey smell)
No growth on MacConkey agar
Catalase positive
Indole positive
Oxidase positive
Penicillin susceptible (2-U disk)

(2) Identification is by microscopic and colonial morphology on selective media and reactivity with specific antiserum, usually in a direct fluorescence test.

   2. **B. parapertussis** can be found in patients who have respiratory tract illness that resembles a mild form of pertussis. This species grows on sheep blood agar within 1–2 days and is **urease positive.** *B. bronchiseptica* is rarely found in humans but causes respiratory tract disease in animals ("kennel cough").

   D. **Francisella tularensis** is the causative agent of **tularemia.** Isolation generally requires extended incubation on media enriched with **cystine** or **cysteine.** The organism is very small and stains poorly on Gram's stain. Identification is made with specific antisera (direct fluorescence). **This organism is very dangerous to work with in the laboratory. It should always be handled under a biologic safety hood, with safety precautions strictly observed.**

   E. Members of the genus **Brucella** cause disease in animals. Human disease is normally a result of contact with the animals or their waste, meat, hides, or secretions. There are four species responsible for the majority of human disease: **B. melitensis, B. abortus, B. suis,** and **B. canis.**

   1. The disease caused is **brucellosis** (also known as Bang's disease, undulant fever). It is characterized by fever, chills, fatigue, weakness, and internal organ lesions. It can be chronic.

   2. *Brucella* species are most often isolated from blood or bone marrow. The organism is **slow-growing,** and blood cultures may need to be incubated for 4–6 weeks before they are considered negative. A Gram's stain shows a faintly staining, small coccobacillus. **Serologic tests** (agglutination of the isolate) are valuable in **identification,** but the **CO_2 requirement,** along with **urease, hydrogen sulfide,** and growth in the presence of **thionin** and **basic fuchsin** can also be used. Table 8-6 summarizes the characteristics used in the identification of *Brucella*.

   F. **Actinobacillus actinomycetemcomitans** is a slow-growing, small, facultative bacillus associated with **endocarditis, bacteremia,** and **dental infections.** It may be associated with *Actinomyces*. It is **catalase positive** and **oxidase negative.**

Table 8-6. Differentiation of *Brucella* Species

Species	CO_2 Required	Urease	H_2S	Inhibition by: Thionine	Fuchsin
B. abortus	+	+	+	+	−
B. melitensis	−	+	+	−	−
B. suis	−	+	+	−	+
B. canis	−	+	−	−	+

H_2S = hydrogen sulfide; + = positive; − = negative.

Table 8-7. Differentiation of Gram-Negative Bacilli/Coccobacilli

Organism	Oxidase	Catalase	Cell Shape Coccoid	Cell Shape Fusiform	Indole
Actinobacillus actinomycetemcomitans	−	+	+	−	−
Capnocytophaga	+	+	−	+	−
Cardiobacterium hominis	+	−	Pleomorphic		+
Kingella kingae	+	−	+	−	−
Pasteurella multocida	+	+	+	−	+
Brucella	+	+	+	−	−

+ = positive; − = negative.

G. ***Kingella kingae*** is primarily associated with infections of bones and joints, as well as endocarditis in children and young adults. It grows on sheep blood agar and is beta hemolytic. A Gram's stain shows short, plump rods with square ends.

H. ***Capnocytophaga*** is normal oral flora in humans. It may cause serious infections in immunosuppressed patients. It has been associated with **dog bites** and is usually isolated from blood or cerebrospinal fluid. It grows on sheep blood agar but must have CO_2. Colonies are beige or yellow and show a haze of growth at the periphery as a result of **gliding motility.** Gram's stain shows a **fusiform** bacillus.

I. ***Cardiobacterium hominis*** is a **pleomorphic rod** that grows on blood but not MacConkey agar. It is normal human oral flora and is found in patients who have endocarditis and bacteremia. The colonies are small, and growth is slow. Differentiation of the miscellaneous gram-negative bacilli and coccobacilli is summarized in Table 8-7.

VIII. *NEISSERIA* AND *MORAXELLA CATARRHALIS*

A. **General characteristics**

1. Members of this group are **gram-negative cocci** that are often seen in pairs. The adjacent sides are flattened, producing a **kidney-bean shape.**

2. They are all **oxidase positive.**

3. Some of the pathogenic species may have fastidious growth requirements.

4. Proper **specimen collection** is essential for successful isolation. *N. gonorrhoeae* and *meningitidis* are especially sensitive to drying, cold, and chemicals (disinfectants and antiseptics). Dacron or rayon swabs are less inhibitory than calcium alginate and cotton and are preferred for collection. Plating should occur as soon as possible following collection.

B. *Neisseria gonorrhoeae*

1. **Infections**

a. **Gonorrhea** is a frequently seen venereal disease. The majority of infected men show symptoms such as burning and discharge from the urethra. Females may be asymptomatic, but infection in this gender may lead to pelvic inflammatory disease. Gonorrhea may cause sterility in males and females and disseminate to blood, skin, and joints.

b. **Ophthalmia neonatorum** is primarily a gonococcal infection of the conjunctiva of newborns as a result of passage through an infected mother's birth canal. It can be successfully treated at birth to prevent blindness.

c. **Penicillinase-producing *Neisseria gonorrhoeae*** are a common problem. A β-lactamase test should be done on each isolate to detect resistance.

2. **Direct microscopic examination** of gram stained urethral discharge from males is a valuable diagnostic procedure. The presence of **gram-negative intracellular diplococci** from a symptomatic male with discharge has a 95% correlation rate with culture and is strong presumptive evidence of gonorrhea. Correlation is much lower in females because of the normal flora.

3. **Culture** of *N. gonorrhoeae* can be accomplished with various enriched and selective media.

a. **Agar.** *N. gonorrhoeae* grows on chocolate agar but not on blood agar. In those cases in which normal flora may contaminate the medium, selective agars, which inhibit the growth of certain organisms other than *Neisseria* species, may be used.

   (1) **Selective media** include Thayer-Martin and modified Thayer-Martin (MTM), Martin-Lewis, and New York City.

   (2) These media are often packaged in self-contained transport/incubation systems that are inoculated at the site of collection. Examples include Transgrow, Gono-Pak, and JEMBEC plates.

b. **Culture and identification.** Plates are incubated at 35°C in a 3%–5% carbon dioxide, humidified atmosphere. Colonies of *N. gonorrhea* are flat, smooth, glistening, and gray to white. Identification/differentiation is outlined in Table 8-8. Various tests are available for direct detection of *N. gonorrhoeae* from clinical specimens. These include detection of cellular antigens and those that detect gonococcal nucleic acid.

Table 8-8. Differentiation of *Neisseria* and *Moraxella catarrhalis*

Organisms	Oxidase	Acid from Glucose	Acid from Maltose	DNAse	Growth on Nutrient Agar
N. gonorrhoeae	+	+	−	−	−
N. meningitidis	+	+	+	−	−
Other *Neisseria* species	+	+/−	V	−	+
M. catarrhalis	+	−	−	+	+

DNAse = deoxyribonuclease; V = variable; + = positive; − = negative.

C. *Neisseria meningitidis*

1. **Infections**

   a. Meningococcal **meningitis** is transmitted by respiratory droplets. Prolonged close contact is necessary for infection. The onset is abrupt, with headache, stiff neck, and fever. Petechial skin lesions may be present.

   b. **Meningococcemia** involves the blood vessels and various major organs. Petechial skin lesions are common. This condition may progress to DIC.

2. **Direct microscopic examination** of CSF sediment may reveal intracellular and extracellular gram-negative diplococci.

3. **Specimens** for **culture** include CSF, blood, joint fluid, and nasopharyngeal swabs to detect carriers. Specimens should be kept at room temperature and processed as soon as possible. Swabs should not be allowed to dry out. Growth is seen on blood and chocolate agar and is enhanced with increased carbon dioxide and humidity. Colonies of *N. meningitidis* are flat, smooth, glistening, and gray to white. Identification is outlined in Table 8-8.

D. *Moraxella catarrhalis* is part of the normal upper respiratory tract flora. It may cause **otitis media, sinusitis,** and **respiratory infections.** *M. catarrhalis* grows on blood, chocolate, and nutrient agars. Identification is outlined in Table 8-8.

E. **Other** *Neisseria* **species** only rarely cause clinical infection. These species may need to be differentiated from the pathogenic species, because they are normal flora at the same sites at which the pathogenic species are located.

IX. ENTEROBACTERIACEAE

A. **General characteristics**

1. The Enterobacteriaceae is the largest and most medically important family of gram-negative bacilli. Although there are numerous genera and species, more than 90% of the medically important isolates belong to just a few genera (Box 8-2).

2. The Enterobacteriaceae are found worldwide and are part of the normal flora of all animals. They are a common cause of nosocomial infections.

3. Commonly seen sites of infection with members of the Enterobacteriaceae are listed in Table 8-9.

Box 8-2. Medically Significant Enterobacteriaceae

Escherichia
Shigella
Salmonella
Klebsiella
Enterobacter
Serratia
Proteus

Table 8-9. Sites of Infections with Enterobacteriaceae

Site	Type of Enterobacteriaceae
Blood	*Escherichia* *Klebsiella* *Enterobacter*
Central nervous system	*Escherichia*
Gastrointestinal	*Escherichia* *Salmonella* *Shigella* *Yersinia*
Lower respiratory tract	*Klebsiella* *Enterobacter* *Escherichia*
Urinary tract	*Escherichia* *Proteus* *Klebsiella*

Table 8-10. Media Used to Isolate and Select *Salmonella* and *Shigella*

Media	Characteristic Result
Bismuth sulfite agar	*Salmonella typhi* shows black colonies surrounded by a black zone of precipitate
Brilliant green agar	*Proteus* colonies are red to pink *Salmonella* colonies are red to pink *Shigella* is inhibited
Gram-negative broth	The growth of most gram-negative rods is inhibited, whereas *Salmonella* and *Shigella* growth is enriched
Hektoen enteric agar	*Escherichia coli* gives orange to salmon pink colonies *Proteus* is usually inhibited *Salmonella* colonies are blue to blue-green, with black centers if hydrogen sulfide is produced *Shigella* colonies are green
Salmonella–Shigella agar	*E. coli* colonies are red *Proteus* colonies are colorless, with black centers *Salmonella* colonies are colorless, with or without black centers *Shigella* colonies are colorless
Selenite broth	*Salmonella* stool specimens are enriched Gram-positive organisms are inhibited
Xylose-lysine-deoxycholate agar	*E. coli* colonies are yellow *Proteus* colonies are clear or yellow *Salmonella* colonies are red, with black centers *Shigella* colonies are clear

Table 8-11. Media Used for the Isolation and Detection of Lactose Fermenters

Media	Characteristic Result
Eosin-methylene blue agar	*Escherichia coli* colonies are dark, with a green metallic sheen Gram-positive organisms are inhibited Lactose fermenters show pink to red colonies Lactose nonfermenters have colorless colonies
MacConkey agar	Gram-positive organisms are inhibited Lactose-fermenter colonies are pink to red Lactose-nonfermenter colonies are colorless

   4. All members **ferment glucose, reduce nitrates to nitrites,** and are **oxidase negative.** The oxidase reaction is especially important in making a rapid distinction between the Enterobacteriaceae and the majority of the gram-negative nonfermenters.

   5. Antigens of this group include the **O antigen** found in the cell wall, the **H or flagellar antigen,** and the **K or capsular antigen.**

B. Various **culture media** and **tests** are used for the **isolation, selection, differentiation,** and **identification** of the Enterobacteriaceae.

   1. Media used for isolation and selection of *Salmonella* and *Shigella,* along with expected reactions, are summarized in Table 8-10.

   2. Media used for the isolation and detection of lactose fermenters are summarized in Table 8-11.

   3. **Media and tests used for the identification of the Enterobacteriaceae** include the following.

      a. **Citrate.** A positive test turns the green agar slant to blue. Any growth on the slant is a positive test regardless of color.

      b. **Gelatin hydrolysis.** A slant of nutrient gelatin is inoculated by streaking. Incubation is at room temperature for several days. If incubation is at 35°C, the medium should be chilled in a refrigerator before reading test results. Liquefaction along the growth line indicates a positive test.

      c. **Decarboxylases.** The decarboxylation of lysine, ornithine, and arginine may be detected by inoculating the appropriate medium. The media are semisolid agar tubes that are inoculated by stabbing. A yellow color initially indicates that the organism is viable and ferments glucose and that the pH has been lowered enough to activate the decarboxylase enzymes. A positive test is a return to the original color of the uninoculated medium. This results from the release of amines from the decarboxylation reaction, which raises the pH.

      d. **Hydrogen sulfide (H_2S)** is indicated by a black precipitate in the medium being used. There are numerous media that indicate the production of H_2S [e.g., sulfide-indole motility agar, motility-indole-ornithine agar (MIO), Hektoen enteric agar, Salmonella-Shigella agar, triple sugar iron agar, lysine-ion agar].

      e. **Methyl red–Voges-Proskauer (MR-VP) broth.** Isolates are inoculated into MR-VP broth and allowed to grow for 48 hours. At that time, the broth is split into two fractions: one to measure methyl red and one for the Voges-Proskauer test.

(1) Those organisms that carry out mixed-acid fermentation produce vast amounts of acid that will convert the **methyl red** indicator to a red color (pH < 4.4).

(2) The **Voges-Proskauer test** measures the production of acetoin. The addition of potassium hydroxide followed by naphthol results in a red complex, which indicates a positive test.

f. **Nitrate reduction.** Nitrate test medium is inoculated and incubated overnight to determine the ability of microorganisms to reduce nitrates to nitrite. The presence of nitrites in the medium is detected by the addition of alpha-naphthylamine and sulfanilic acid. The formation of a red color after the addition of the two reagents indicates that nitrite is present (positive test). If a red color is not detected, all available nitrate may have been reduced to nitrite and then completely converted to ammonia, in which case no nitrite remains to react with the sulfanilic acid. This scenario can be detected by adding a small pinch of zinc dust to the tube (metallic zinc reduces nitrate to nitrite). With the formation of nitrite upon addition of zinc, the reactions can take place, resulting in the red color. A red color at this point indicates that nitrate was still present in the broth (negative test). Absence of red color after the addition of zinc indicates that no nitrate was left (positive test).

g. **Beta-galactosidase and the orthonitrophenyl galactosidase (ONPG) test.** Organisms that are late or slow lactose fermenters may appear as nonfermenters on primary media. The ONPG test determines if the organism is slow or late (i.e., lacks the permease that allows lactose to enter the cell but has β-galactosidase, which splits lactose). Lactose nonfermenters lack the β-galactosidase. Beta-galactosidase acts on ONPG to form a yellow compound (positive test), which indicates that the organism is a lactose fermenter.

h. **Phenylalanine deaminase.** The deamination of phenylalanine results in the production of phenylpyruvic acid. When ferric chloride is added, an intense green color forms (positive test).

i. **Urea.** Organisms that produce urea will split urea to form ammonia. The ammonia reacts in solution to form ammonium carbonate, which increases pH. This is detected by the phenol red in the medium and turns the medium a bright pink color (positive test).

j. **Triple sugar iron agar.** This medium differentiates gram-negative bacilli by their ability to ferment glucose, lactose, and sucrose and to produce hydrogen sulfide.

(1) **Nonfermenters** produce an alkaline slant and alkaline deep (no change in the red color of the medium).

(2) **Nonlactose fermenters** produce an alkaline slant (red) and acid (yellow) deep.

(3) **Lactose fermenters** produce an acid (yellow) slant and acid (yellow) deep.

4. The identification of the Enterobacteriaceae can be accomplished using the information presented in Table 8-12.

X. *CAMPYLOBACTER, HELICOBACTER,* AND *VIBRIONA-CEAE*

A. *Campylobacter*

1. **Diarrhea** is the primary disease caused by *Campylobacter*. It is often transmitted by means of contaminated water and animals, especially poultry and carcasses.

2. The most clinically relevant species are *C. jejuni, C. coli,* and *C. fetus.*

3. Characteristics of *Campylobacter* species are summarized in Box 8-3.

4. The **isolation** of *Campylobacter* is accomplished by inoculating the specimen (usually stool) to Campylobacter blood agar. This contains several antibiotics that suppress growth of normal flora. The plate is incubated in a microaerophilic atmosphere.

5. The **laboratory identification** of *Campylobacter* is summarized in Figure 8-2 and Table 8-13.

B. *Helicobacter* is an organism very similar to *Campylobacter*.

1. **Diseases** caused by *Helicobacter* include gastritis and ulcers.

2. The **identification** is made from gastric biopsy material. Isolates are strongly **urease positive.**

C. The **Vibrionaceae** include *Vibrio, Aeromonas,* and *Plesiomonas.*

1. The most commonly isolated species of *Vibrio* include *V. cholerae* (O-1 and non O-1), *V. parahaemolyticus, V. alginolyticus,* and *V. vulnificus.*

2. All of these species are found in water sources and are transmitted by contaminated food and water.

3. *Vibrio cholerae* is the cause of cholera, a disease in which vast quantities of fluid and electrolytes are lost from the intestinal tract. Cholera-causing isolates have a somatic antigen referred to as **O-1.** Non-O-1 isolates do not cause cholera but may cause other infections.

4. *Vibrio parahaemolyticus* and *Vibrio alginolyticus* usually cause gastroenteritis or wound infections following ingestion of raw or improperly handled seafood or exposure to sea water. They both require salt for growth (halophilic).

5. *Vibrio vulnificus* is an extremely virulent organism that causes rapidly progressive wound infections after exposure to contaminated water or septicemia after eating raw oysters.

6. The **laboratory isolation and identification of *Vibrio*** is summarized in Tables 8-14 and 8-15. The organisms are usually isolated from stool specimens. *V. cholerae* can be enriched by using alkaline peptone water (pH 8.4). This suppresses the growth of other organisms. All *Vibrio* species grow well on routine media. The differential medium of choice is TCBS agar. All isolates are **indole and oxidase positive.** The reactions of the various *Vibrio* species on TCBS are summarized in Table 8-14.

Table 8-12. Identification of the Enterobacteriaceae

Species	Indole	Methyl Red	V-P	Citrate	H₂S	Urea	PDA	LDC	ODC	Motility	Gelatin (22°C)	Lactose	DNAse (25°C)
Escherichia coli	+	+	−	−	−	−	−	+	V	+	−	+	−
Shigella serogroups A,B,C	V	+	−	−	−	−	−	−	−	−	−	−	−
S. sonnei	−	+	−	−	−	−	−	−	+	−	−	−	−
Salmonella, most serotypes	−	+	−	+	+	−	−	+	+	+	−	−	−
S. typhi	−	+	−	−	+	−	−	+	−	+	−	−	−
S. paratyphi A	−	+	−	−	−	−	−	−	+	+	−	−	−
Citrobacter freundii	−	+	−	+	V	V	−	−	V	+	−	−	−
C. diversus	+	+	−	+	−	V	−	−	+	+	−	V	−
Edwardsiella tarda	+	+	−	−	+	−	−	+	+	+	−	−	−
Klebsiella pneumoniae	−	−	+	+	−	+	−	+	−	−	−	+	−
K. oxytoca	+	V	+	+	−	+	−	+	−	−	−	+	−
Enterobacter aerogenes	−	−	+	+	−	−	−	+	+	+	−	+	−
E. cloacae	−	−	+	+	−	V	−	−	+	+	−	+	−
Hafnia alvei	−	V	V	−	−	−	−	V	+	+	−	−	−
Serratia marcescens	−	V	+	+	−	V	−	+	+	+	+	−	+
Proteus mirabilis	−	+	−	V	+	+	+	−	+	+	+	−	V
P. vulgaris	+	+	−	V	+	+	+	−	−	+	+	−	V
Providencia rettgeri	+	+	−	+	−	+	+	−	−	+	−	−	−
Morganella morganii	+	+	−	−	−	+	+	−	+	+	−	−	−
Yersinia enterocolitica	−	+	−	−	−	V	−	−	+	−	−	−	−
Y. pestis	−	V	−	−	−	−	−	−	−	−	−	−	−
Y. pseudotuberculosis	−	+	−	−	−	+	−	−	−	−	−	−	−

DNAse = deoxyribonuclease; H₂S = hydrogen sulfide; LDC = lysine decarboxylase; ODC = ornithine decarboxylase; PDA = phenylalanine deaminase; V = 10% to 89% are positive; V-P = Voges-Proskauer test; + = ≥90% are positive; − = ≤10% are positive.

Box 8-3. Characteristics of *Campylobacter*

> Gram negative
> Curved rods
> Darting motility
> Microaerophilic
> Oxidase positive
> Catalase positive

7. ***Aeromonas*** and ***Plesiomonas*** are found in fresh and salt waters. They may cause **diarrheal disease** as well as other miscellaneous infections. Normally, only patients who have underlying disease are treated. This type of diarrhea is usually a self-limiting disease. The role of *Aeromonas* and *Plesiomonas* in diarrheal disease is not well established. These organisms grow well on **blood and MacConkey agar,** are **oxidase positive,** and **ferment glucose.** Gram's stain reveals **gram-negative rods.** *Plesiomonas* may show long filamentous forms. Differentiation of *Aeromonas* and *Plesiomonas* is summarized in Table 8-16.

8. Differentiation of *Aeromonas, Plesiomonas,* and *Vibrio* is summarized in Table 8-17.

XI. GRAM-NEGATIVE NONFERMENTATIVE BACILLI

A. This large group of organisms uses biochemical pathways other than fermentation. They may be oxidizers, or they may be inert (nonoxidizers). Gram-negative nonfermentative bacilli account for approximately 15% of gram-negative rod-shaped bacteria isolated in the clinical laboratory. They are found in the environment and cause disease by infecting immunocompromised people. Virtually all of these organisms are opportunists. An isolate that grows on blood agar but not MacConkey agar should be suspected of being a nonfermenter. This is especially true if the isolate is also oxidase positive. Organisms that grow on MacConkey agar appear as lactose negative.

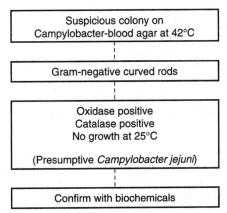

Figure 8-2. Identification of *Campylobacter* species.

Table 8-13. Characteristics of *Campylobacter* Species

Species	Growth at: 25°C	37°C	42°C	Hippurate Hydrolysis	Nalidixic Acid	Cephalothin
C. jejuni	−	+	+	+	S	R
C. coli	−	+	+	−	S	R
C. fetus	+	+	−	−	R	S

S = susceptible; R = resistant; + = positive; − = negative.

B. The most commonly isolated gram-negative nonfermentative rod-shaped bacteria are listed in Box 8-4.

C. The most frequently isolated gram-negative nonfermenter is ***Pseudomonas aeruginosa***. This organism is commonly seen in patients who have **serious burns** and **cystic fibrosis**. *P. aeruginosa* is also found to cause **urinary** tract infections, **endocarditis,** and **external otitis** (swimmer's ear). Infections may be difficult to control because of antibiotic resistance; this situation is usually only a problem in immunocompromised persons.

1. The **growth requirements** of *P. aeruginosa* are very simple. It has been found growing in distilled water. It also grows over a wide temperature range (4°C–42°C).

2. **Identification of *P. aeruginosa*** is not difficult and is summarized in Box 8-5. This organism grows well on most media.

D. Infections by ***Burkholderia (Pseudomonas) cepacia*** are primarily **nosocomial** infections related to **contaminated disinfectants** used for antisepsis. Community-acquired infections are rare except in **intravenous drug abusers.**

E. *Stenotrophomonas (Xanthomonas) maltophilia* is found in the environment and causes a wide range of nosocomial infections.

F. *Acinetobacter* species are opportunists found in soil and water. They cause pneumonia and urinary tract infections. On Gram's stain, this genus is characteristically a fat coccobacillus.

Table 8-14. Isolation of *Vibrio* Species on TCBS Agar

Species	Colony
V. cholerae O1	Yellow
V. cholerae non-O1	Yellow
V. alginolyticus	Yellow
V. parahaemolyticus	Dark blue-green
V. vulnificus	Dark blue-green

TCBS = thiosulfate-citrate-bile salts-sucrose.

Table 8-15. Identification of *Vibrio* Species

| Species | Growth in 8% NaCl | VP | Acid from: | | | Susceptible to O/129 | |
			Lactose	Sucrose	Arabinose	10 mg	150 mg
V. alginolyticus	+	+	−	+	−	−	−
V. cholerae	−	V	V	+	−	V	V
V. parahaemolyticus	+	−	−	−	+	−	+
V. vulnificus	−	−	+	V	−	+	+

V = variable; VP = Voges-ProsKauer; O/129 = 2,4,diamino-6,7-diisopropylpteridine phosphate; + = positive; − = negative.

    G. ***Flavobacterium meningosepticum*** is a cause of **neonatal meningitis.**

    H. ***Eikenella corrodens*** is found as normal mouth and nasopharyngeal flora. Trauma to the face or mouth, including dental work, may predispose to infection. Human bite wounds are another source of infection. This isolate is often found as part of a mixed infection. The name is derived from the corroding or pitting of the agar by the colonies.

    I. ***Moraxella*** species are normal flora of mucous membranes. They infrequently cause infection. **Conjunctivitis** is caused by ***M. lacunata.***

    J. The **antibiotic susceptibility** patterns of gram-negative nonfermentative bacilli are similar to that of the Enterobacteriaceae. Some are resistant to most of the antibiotics used.

    K. The **laboratory identification** of this group is summarized in Table 8-18.

XII. AEROBIC GRAM-POSITIVE BACILLI

    A. General characteristics

        1. The members of this group that are seen most frequently in the clinical laboratory are listed in Box 8-6.

        2. Except for *Corynebacterium diphtheriae*, these organisms are of low pathogenicity and usually require an immunocompromised host.

Table 8-16. Differentiation of *Aeromonas* and *Plesiomonas*

| Organism | Esculin Hydrolysis | Lysine Decarboxylase | Ornithine Decarboxylase | Acid from: | | |
				Mannitol	Arabinose	Sucrose
A. hydrophila	+	+	−	+	+	+
A. caviae	+	−	−	+	+	+
A. sobria	−	+	−	+	−	+
P. shigelloides	−	+	+	−	−	−

+ = positive; − = negative.

Table 8-17. Differentiation of Oxidase-Positive, Glucose-Fermentative, Gram-Negative Bacilli

Characteristic	*Aeromonas*	*Plesiomonas*	*Vibrio*
Susceptible to O/129:			
10 mg	−	+/−	+/−
150 mg	−	+	+/−
Ferment glucose	+	+	+
Gelatin	+	−	+
Growth on TCBS agar	−	−	+
NaCl requirement	−	−	+

TCBS = thiosulfate-citrate-bile salts-sucrose; O/129 = 2,4, diamino-6,7-diisopropylpteridine phosphate; + = positive; − = negative.

3. With the exception of *Bacillus*, these organisms are all pleomorphic rods, and most grow well on standard media.

B. ***Listeria monocytogenes*** is widespread in the environment. It causes a wide variety of infections, especially in neonates, pregnant women, and immuno-suppressed persons. **Meningitis** is a common outcome.

1. **Isolation** is usually from blood, CSF, or swabs of lesions. *L. monocytogenes* grows well on blood agar and **closely resembles group B streptococcus.** Growth occurs at 4°C. This allows the use of the **cold enrichment technique,** which requires inoculation of the specimen into broth medium, followed by incubation at 4°C for several weeks. This technique has limited clinical importance.

2. **Gram stain** shows a **coccobacillus.**

3. **Identification of this organism** is summarized in Box 8-7.

C. ***Erysipelothrix rhusiopathiae*** is an uncommon isolate. It is a **pleomorphic** rod that often forms long filaments. The usual route of infection is through the skin. It is **nonmotile, catalase negative,** and forms **hydrogen sulfide.**

D. The most important species of ***Corynebacterium*** are ***diphtheriae, jeikeium,*** and ***urealyticum.***

Box 8-4. Most Commonly Isolated Gram-Negative, Nonfermentative Rods

Pseudomonas aeruginosa
Burkholderia (Pseudomonas) cepacia
Stenotrophomonas (Xanthomonas) maltophilia
Acinetobacter
Flavobacterium meningosepticum
Eikenella corrodens
Moraxella

Box 8-5. Identification of *Pseudomonas aeruginosa*

Grows on most media

Colonies have a feathered, ground (frosted) glass appearance

Beta hemolytic

Corn tortilla odor (some prefer to describe it as a grapelike odor)

Blue-green pigment (pyocyanin)

Grows between 4°C and 42°C

Oxidase positive

1. All species are pleomorphic and resemble *C. diphtheriae* on Gram's stain. The morphology was therefore termed "diphtheroid." The morphology may also be described as "picket fence" or "Chinese letters."

2. ***C. diphtheriae*** is the cause of diphtheria. The disease has a presentation of local inflammation of the throat with a pseudomembrane caused by dead cells and exudate. The toxin damages major organ systems and results in a high mortality rate when infected persons go untreated. Diphtheria occurs in nonimmunized populations. Treatment is with an antitoxin.

   a. **Laboratory diagnosis** consists of culture and testing for toxin production. Media that have been developed for the growth and identification of *C. diphtheriae* are summarized in Table 8-19. Suspicious colonies from cystine-tellurite or Tinsdale's agar are gram stained. If the Gram's stain shows gram-positive rods with "diphtheroid" morphology, a urease test is done. A negative urease test is presumptive identification of *C. diphtheriae*.

   b. Toxin production may be determined by the **Elek test,** which detects toxin production by an isolate using an antitoxin-impregnated filter

Table 8-18. Identification of Nonfermentative, Gram-Negative Bacilli and Coccobacilli

Species	Oxidase	Catalase	Indole	Growth on MacConkey Agar	Motility	O/F Glucose
Acinetobacter baumanii	−	+	−	+	−	+
Acinetobacter lwoffi	−	+	−	+	−	−
Pseudomonas aeruginosa	+	+	−	+	+	+
Burkholderia cepacia	+	+	−	+	+	+
Stenotrophomonas maltophilia	−	+	−	+	+	+
Flavobacterium meningosepticum	+	+	+	+	−	+
Eikenella corrodens	+	−	−	−	−	−

O/F = oxidation/fermentation; + = positive; − = negative.

Box 8-6. Most Commonly Isolated
Aerobic Gram-Positive Bacilli

> *Bacillus*
> *Corynebacterium*
> *Erysipelothrix*
> *Listeria*
> *Nocardia*

paper strip that is laid perpendicular to lines of bacterial growth. Precipitin lines are formed if the antibody and antigen (diphtheria toxin) are present.

3. *C. jeikeium* (group JK) is an extremely virulent organism. It may cause infections following implantation of prosthetic devices, and it is resistant to a wide range of antibiotics. This organism is suspected in those patients who are immunocompromised or have undergone invasive procedures or in whom an isolate with typical diphtheroid morphology is found.

4. *C. urealyticum* is a urinary pathogen that is slow growing (48 hours) and strongly urease positive. Urease production occurs within minutes following inoculation on a urea slant.

5. **Differentiation between** *Corynebacterium, Erysipelothrix,* and *Listeria* is outlined in Table 8-20.

E. The two species of **Bacillus** that are of medical importance are **anthracis** and **cereus.** These organisms are spore formers that appear singly or in chains with a "boxcar" morphology on Gram's stain.

1. *B. anthracis* is the cause of **anthrax,** a rare disease in the United States. It usually appears in the cutaneous form as a result of wounds contaminated with anthrax spores. The lesion that is formed develops a characteristic center of necrosis, which has been termed a "black eschar" or "malignant pustule." **Handling of** *B. anthracis* **is extremely dangerous and should only be done within a biologic safety cabinet.**

2. *B. cereus* is a common cause of **food poisoning.**

3. **Laboratory identification** is accomplished by growth on blood agar. Colonies of both species are large and flat. The differentiation between *B. anthracis* and *B. cereus* is outlined in Table 8-21.

Box 8-7. Characteristics of *Listeria monocytogenes*

Umbrella motility pattern (motility agar tube) at room temperature
Hippurate hydrolysis positive
CAMP test positive
Esculin hydrolysis positive
Growth at 4°C
Catalase positive
Beta hemolytic (very similar to group B streptococcus)

Table 8-19. Media Used to Isolate *Corynebacterium diphtheriae*

Media	Reaction
Cystine-tellurite agar	Colonies are black or gray
Tinsdale's agar	Colonies are dark brown-to-black with brown-to-black halos
Loeffler agar	Supports growth and enhances pleomorphism

    F. *Nocardia asteroides* is the most commonly isolated member of *Nocardia*. This organism is usually found in immunocompromised patients as a chronic infection, particularly pulmonary. It is **pleomorphic** and **partially acid-fast.** Growth is slow (up to 6 weeks). The colonial morphology is dry and heaped, looking similar to a fungus. It also has a soil or musty-basement odor. Exudate may demonstrate "sulfur granules," which are masses of filamentous organisms with pus materials.

XIII. MISCELLANEOUS GENERA

    A. *Legionella* species are found worldwide in the environment. Most infections result from contaminated water sources. *Legionella pneumophila* is the most common isolate.

        1. Pneumonia is the most common infection caused by *Legionella*.

        2. Specimens for culture are generally from pulmonary sources.

        3. Various **staining** methods can be used to visualize *Legionella*. The organisms are small rods and stain weakly on **Gram's stain. Giemsa** stain may be used. A **direct fluorescent antibody** test is available and is very useful for detection from direct specimens.

        4. Culture can be accomplished using special media, because *Legionella* does not grow on blood agar. Cysteine is required for growth. The recommended medium for isolation is **buffered charcoal yeast extract agar.** After several days' incubation, the colonies are gray-white to blue-green. Definitive identification can be made with fluorescent antibody or DNA probes.

    B. *Chromobacterium* is characterized by a **purple pigment.** It is an extremely virulent organism that causes wound infections and bacteremia. *Chromobacterium* is found in soil and water in the southeastern United States.

Table 8-20. Differentiation of *Corynebacterium*, *Erysipelothrix*, and *Listeria*

Organism	Voges-Proskauer Test	Catalase	Growth at 4°C	Motility at Room Temperature	Esculin Hydrolysis	Hydrogen Sulfide H₂S
Corynebacterium spp.	−	+	−	−	−	−
Listeria monocytogenes	+	+	+	+	−	−
Erysipelothrix rhusiopathiae	−	−	−	−	−	+

+ = positive; − = negative.

Table 8-21. Differentiation of *Bacillus anthracis* and *B. cereus*

Species	10 U Penicillin	Motility	Beta-Hemolysis
B. anthracis	S	−	−
B. cereus	R	+	+

S = susceptible; R = resistant; + = positive; − = negative.

C. *Gardnerella vaginalis* is often associated with **bacterial vaginosis.** The organism is not thought to be the etiologic agent; however, isolation uses **human blood Tween agar,** which is incubated for 48 hours in 5%–10% carbon dioxide. Colonies are beta hemolytic. Gram's stain shows gram-variable or gram-negative small coccobacilli. A presumptive identification can be made when vaginal discharge shows squamous epithelial cells covered with tiny bacilli (i.e., **clue cells**).

D. *Streptobacillus moniliformis* is the agent of **rat-bite fever.** Gram's stain shows pleomorphic, long filamentous forms. In blood culture media, the organism grows as "fluff balls" or "bread crumbs."

XIV. *MYCOPLASMA* AND *CHLAMYDIA*

A. *Mycoplasma* species are very small free-living organisms that lack a cell wall. The three most common isolates are *M. pneumoniae, M. hominis,* and *Ureaplasma urealyticum. M. pneumoniae* is the cause of atypical or walking pneumonia. *U. urealyticum* and *M. hominis* are genital mycoplasmas that cause **nongonococcal urethritis** in males and **postpartum infections** in females. The organisms can be cultured on special media. The colonies are very small, requiring a dissecting microscope for observation, and they demonstrate what is often called a "fried-egg" appearance (raised center with flat edges).

B. *Chlamydia* are obligate intracellular bacteria. The three most common species are *C. trachomatis, C. pneumoniae,* and *C. psittaci.*

   1. *C. trachomatis* is the cause of trachoma, lymphogranuloma venereum, and various other sexually transmitted diseases. Trachoma is a leading cause of blindness worldwide.

   2. *C. pneumoniae* is an important cause of pneumonia and pharyngitis.

   3. *C. psittaci* is the cause of psittacosis, a respiratory tract disease seen in patients exposed to birds.

   4. **Laboratory diagnosis** can be accomplished several ways. **Cell lines** can be inoculated with specimens suspected of harboring *Chlamydia.* After 72 hours, staining with iodine shows darkly stained inclusion bodies within the cells. Other methods available include **immunofluorescence, enzyme immunoassay, nucleic acid probes,** and **polymerase chain reaction.**

XV. SPIROCHETES

A. **Three genera** cause human disease: *Treponema, Leptospira, Borrelia.*

B. *Treponema pallidum* is the etiologic agent of **syphilis.** It cannot be grown in vitro, so laboratory diagnosis must be from microscopy or serology. Syphilis progresses through three phases: primary, secondary, and late. Skin lesions are characteristic of primary and secondary syphilis. Fluid from these lesions can be used to perform **Darkfield microscopy,** in which the spiral-shaped organisms can be seen. Patient diagnosis is usually done by **serologic testing,** which requires either a nonspecific or specific treponemal test.

1. The **nonspecific tests** include the **rapid plasma reagin** and **Venereal Disease Research Laboratory tests.**

2. **Specific tests** include the fluorescent **treponemal antibody absorption test** and the **microhemagglutination test** for *T. pallidum.*

C. *Borrelia* is the cause of **relapsing fever (*B. recurrentis*) and Lyme disease (*B. burgdorferi*),** both of which are spread by ticks. Relapsing fever may be detected by noting spirochetes visible in stained blood smears. Lyme disease is determined by serologic means. Antibody in the patient's serum may be detected after the third week of the illness. Sensitivity of the various methods varies widely from poor to good.

D. *Leptospira interrogans* is the cause of **leptospirosis** or **Weil's disease.** The organism is transmitted via exposure to soil or water that has been contaminated with animal urine. The organism can be cultured using **Fletcher medium,** a semisolid tubed medium. Growth occurs in a ring just beneath the medium surface. Diagnosis may be made from microscopy or culture, but serology (slide agglutination) is the usual method.

XVI. MYCOBACTERIA

A. Members of this group are **aerobic bacilli.** The cell wall is rich in lipids, which makes them resistant to Gram's stain. Once stained, the bacilli are difficult to decolorize with acid solutions (i.e., they are acid-fast). Most members of this group **grow slowly,** dividing every 12–24 hours. Identification of a *Mycobacterium* species isolate is determined by the characteristics outlined in Box 8-8.

B. The most common **specimen collected and processed** is respiratory secretion, although mycobacteria can be recovered from virtually any body site. With sputum and other specimens collected from nonsterile sites, **digestion and decontamination** must be done before inoculation of growth media (Box 8-9).

C. Following treatment with one of the agents listed in Box 8-9, the suspension is diluted with buffer and centrifuged to **concentrate** any organisms present. The sediment is inoculated onto mycobacterial growth media and used to make a smear for acid-fast staining.

Box 8-8. Characteristics Used to Identify *Mycobacterium* Isolates

Colony morphology
Colony pigmentation
Growth rate
Growth temperature
Biochemical tests

Box 8-9. Decontamination and Digestion Agents

Sodium hydroxide
N-acetyl-L-cysteine
Benzalkonium chloride
Oxalic acid

1. **Mycobacterial growth media**
   a. The most commonly used **egg-based** medium is **Löwenstein-Jensen.**
   b. **Agar-based** media are variations of **Middlebrook 7H10** medium. All contain some inhibitory agents to suppress the growth of contaminating bacteria.
2. **Acid-fast stains**
   a. **Conventional** stains include **Ziehl-Neelsen and Kinyoun,** which use carbolfuchsin as the primary stain, acid alcohol for the decolorizing agent, and a methylene blue counterstain.
   b. The **fluorochrome** stains—**auramine and auramine-rhodamine**— are very sensitive and require a fluorescence microscope.
D. **Pigment groups** are helpful in a presumptive identification. To determine pigment groups, or **photoreactivity,** a specimen is inoculated to two tubes or plates of mycobacterial media.
   1. One is incubated in the **light,** and the other is incubated in the **dark.** Following growth, pigment production of each is noted. The medium initially incubated in the dark is incubated in bright light for several hours, and pigment production, if any, is noted.
   2. The **classification of mycobacteria according to photoreactivity** is summarized in Table 8-22. Pigment color may range from light yellow to a dark orange.
E. The **growth rate** is determined as rapid or slow. Rapid growers produce colonies in fewer than 7 days. Slow growers require longer than 7 days to produce colonies. Table 8-23 lists some of the medically significant mycobacterial species arranged according to pigment groups and growth rate.
F. The optimal **growth temperature** for most *Mycobacterium* species is 35°C–37°C. *M. marinum* grows best at 30°C, whereas *M. xenopi* grows best at 42°C.
G. There are several **biochemical tests** that are valuable in identification (Table 8-24). Most of these tests are performed only in those laboratories that do

Table 8-22. Characteristics of Mycobacterial Photoreactivity Groups

Group	Pigment Characteristics
Photochromogens	Produce pigment on exposure to light
Scotochromogens	Produce pigment in the light or dark
Nonchromogens	No pigment produced in the light or dark

Table 8-23. Medically Important Mycobacteria According to Pigment Group and Growth Rate

Group	Organism
Photochromogen	*Mycobacterium kansasii* *M. marinum* *M. simiae*
Scotochromogen	*M. gordonae* *M. scrofulaceum* *M. szulgai* *M. xenopi* *M. flavescens*
Nonchromogen	*M. tuberculosis* *M. avium–M. intracellulare**
Rapid growers	*M. chelonei* *M. fortuitum*

*Some isolates (15%) are pigmented.

complete identification. Some of the tests, like niacin and nitrate tests, are easy to perform and can give presumptive identification of *M. tuberculosis.*

1. **Niacin accumulation** is detected by measuring nicotinic acid, which reacts with cyanogen bromide in the presence of aniline to form a yellow compound.

2. **Nitrate reduction** is performed as with the method used for Enterobacteriaceae. The end product is a red pigment.

3. **Catalase** is determined by measuring the height of the column of bubbles when hydrogen peroxide is added. Catalase heat stability is determined by heating the specimen to 68°C for 20 minutes and then adding hydrogen peroxide.

4. **Tween hydrolysis** measures the presence of a lipase. Hydrolysis causes a pink color change.

5. **NaCl tolerance** is determined by using egg-based media with 5% NaCl and observing growth or no growth.

6. **Iron uptake** is determined by adding ferric ammonium citrate to the colonies and observing rusty-brown colonies as a result of the formation of iron oxide.

7. **Arylsulfatase** activity is detected by adding phenolphthalein to the colony/substrate mixture and observing the formation of a pink color.

8. The **urease** test is performed and read as a broth test. Urease-producing organisms hydrolyze urea to form ammonia, which produces an alkaline reaction. The increase in pH is detected by a change of color to red.

9. **Susceptibility to thiophen-2-carboxylic acid hydrazide** is determined by observing growth or no growth.

10. Identification of some species of mycobacteria by **nucleic acid amplification** is available. Specificity is very good, but use with clinical speci-

Table 8-24. Identification of Mycobacteria

Organism	Photo Reactivity Group	Niacin	Susceptible to TCH	Nitrate Reduction	Catalase	Tween Hydrolysis	Growth in 5% NaCl	Iron Uptake	Arylsulfatase	Urease
M. marinum	Photochromogen	+	–	–	–	+	–	–	–	+
M. kansasii	Photochromogen	–	–	+	+	+	–	–	–	+
M. simiae	Photochromogen	+	–	–	+	–	–	–	–	+
M. tuberculosis	Nonchromogen	+	–	+	–	–	–	–	–	+
M. bovis	Nonchromogen	–	+	–	–	–	–	–	–	–
M. avium–M. intracellulare	Nonchromogen	–	–	–	–	–	–	–	–	–
M. gordonae	Scotochromogen	–	–	–	+	+	–	–	V	–
M. scrofulaceum	Scotochromogen	–	–	–	+	–	–	–	V	+
M. szulgai	Scotochromogen	–	–	+	+	–	–	–	V	+
M. xenopi	Scotochromogen	–	–	–	–	–	–	–	+	V
M. flavescens	Scotochromgen	–	–	+	+	+	+	–	–	+
M. fortuitum	Rapid grower	–	–	+	+	V	+	+	+	+
M. chelonei	Rapid grower	V	–	–	+	V	V	–	+	+

TCH = thiophen-2-carboxylic acid hydrazide; V = variable; + = positive; – = negative.

Table 8-25. Summary of Clinical Infections Caused by Mycobacteria

Pigment Group	Organism	Clinical Infections
Photochromogen	*M. marinum*	Cutaneous infections from water exposure
	M. kansasii	Pulmonary disease
	M. simiae	Pulmonary disease (rare)
Nonchromogen	*M. tuberculosis*	Pulmonary disease; other sites
	M. bovis	Pulmonary disease (rare in US)
	M. avium–M. intracellulare	Pulmonary disease (especially AIDS patients)
Scotochromogen	*M. gordonae*	Common contaminant ("tap-water bacillus")
	M. scrofulaceum	Cervical lymphadenitis in children
	M. szulgai	Pulmonary disease
	M. xenopi	Pulmonary disease in immunosuppressed patients
	M. flavescens	Contaminant
Rapid grower	*M. fortuitum*	Pulmonary disease; other sites in immunosuppressed patients
	M. chelonei	Pulmonary disease; other sites in immunosuppressed patients

AIDS = acquired immunodeficiency syndrome.

mens may give false-negative results and so is not currently recommended.

H. Infections caused by mycobacteria are summarized in Table 8-25.

XVII. ANAEROBES

A. **Characteristics.** Anaerobes constitute the majority of bacteria found in and on the human host. They vary in their tolerance to oxygen and can be divided into moderate and strict anaerobes. The majority of medically significant anaerobes are moderate anaerobes. A list of the commonly isolated anaerobes with their gram morphology is listed in Table 8-26. Table 8-27 summarizes the microscopic characteristics of the more common isolates.

1. **Moderate anaerobes** can grow in an atmosphere containing low levels of oxygen (5%).

2. **Strict anaerobes** are killed by exposure to oxygen.

B. **Direct examination** of a specimen using **Gram's stain** is very helpful. Typical anaerobe morphology (pleomorphic rods; gram-positive, boxcar-shaped cells; thin rods with pointed ends) may be evident. Also, a positive Gram's stain with negative culture results may indicate the need for anaerobic culture. If culture has been performed, the negative results indicate a problem with collection, transport, or culture conditions. The Gram's stain can determine the culture conditions and media to be used.

C. The **media and tests** that are used to grow and identify anaerobes are as follows.

1. **Sheep blood agar** is a general growth medium for all anaerobes. It is supplemented with vitamin K and hemin, and the type of agar base may vary (e.g., Columbia, Schaedler, brain-heart infusion).

Table 8-26. Gram Morphology of Anaerobes

Gram Negative		Gram Positive	
Bacilli	**Cocci**	**Bacilli**	**Cocci**
Bacteroides	*Veillonella*	*Actinomyces*	*Peptostreptococcus*
Fusobacterium		*Bifidobacterium*	
Porphyromonas		*Clostridium*	
Prevotella		*Eubacterium*	
		Lactobacillus	
		Mobiluncis	
		Propionibacterium	

2. **Bacteroides bile esculin (BBE) agar** is used for the selection and presumptive identification of *Bacteroides fragilis*. It is inhibitory to other organisms. Colonies of *B. fragilis* appear as black colonies, with a black halo around the colonies.

3. **PEA** inhibits the gram-negative facultative bacilli, whereas most anaerobes show good growth.

4. **Kanamycin-vancomycin laked blood agar** selects for *Prevotella* and *Bacteroides*. Other gram-positive and gram-negative rods are inhibited.

5. **Egg-yolk agar** is used to determine if an isolate produces lecithinase or lipase. The lecithin in egg yolk is split by lecithinase, which results in an

Table 8-27. Microscopic Characteristics of Common Anaerobes

Organisms	Characteristics
Prevotella melaninogenica	Coccobacilli
Bacteroides fragilis	Pale-staining rods
Fusobacterium necrophorum	Pleomorphic rods with round to tapered ends; may be filamentous
F. nucleatum	Long, slender with sharply pointed or tapered ends
Clostridium	"Boxcar" rods with blunt ends
Actinomyces	Branching, thin filamentous rods
Bifidobacterium	Diphtheroid; coccoid or thin pointed; may be branching
Propionibacterium	Pleomorphic; diphtheroid
Eubacterium	Pleomorphic; diphtheroid
Peptostreptococcus	Pairs and chains
Veillonella	Clumps and short chains

opaque halo around the colony. Lipase is detected by observing an oily or "mother-of-pearl" margin surrounding the colony.

6. The **catalase** test for anaerobes uses 15% hydrogen peroxide instead of 3%.

7. A **spot indole test** is easily and quickly performed. This test uses *p*-dimethyl-aminocinnamaldehyde as the developing reagent. A blue color is produced when the test is positive.

8. **Antibiotic disks** can be very helpful. The susceptibility of anaerobes to colistin (10 μg), vancomycin (5 μg), and kanamycin (1 μg) varies.

9. Growth in 20% **bile** separates the bile-resistant *B. fragilis* group from *Prevotella*.

10. Susceptibility to a 1-mg sodium polyanethol sulfonate **(SPS) disk** is characteristic of *Peptostreptococcus anaerobius*.

11. A **reverse CAMP test** identifies *Clostridium perfringens*. In this test, the *Clostridium* isolate is streaked perpendicular to a known group B streptococcus. A positive test demonstrates characteristic arrowhead hemolysis.

D. The **characteristics** of the more commonly isolated anaerobes, including the types of infections caused by each, are as follows.

1. The **gram-negative bacilli** (Table 8-28) cause a wide variety of infections. These organisms are part of the normal flora in the gastrointestinal tract, the female genital tract, and the oropharynx.

   a. *Bacteroides fragilis* is the most common anaerobic isolate. It is **bile resistant;** therefore, it grows in broth with 20% bile. Growth occurs on BBE agar with characteristic black colonies.

   b. *Prevotella* and *Porphyromonas* are bile sensitive. Most of the clinically important species are pigmented.

   c. *Fusobacterium nucleatum* and *F. necrophorum* are normal flora in the respiratory and gastrointestinal tracts. A gram-negative isolate with characteristic morphology that is positive for indole and lipase is *F. necrophorum*.

2. The **gram-positive bacilli** are found as normal flora and are also widely distributed in the environment (e.g., *Clostridium* species).

   a. *Clostridium* **species** (Table 8-29) cause a wide variety of infections.

   (1) *C. botulinum* is the agent of botulism.

   (2) *C. tetani* causes tetanus. The clinical laboratory has little role in the diagnosis of either *C. botulinum* or *C. tetani*. The diagnosis is based on the clinical symptoms.

   (3) *C. difficile* infection often results in **antibiotic-associated diarrhea and pseudomembranous enterocolitis.**

   (a) Treatment with broad-spectrum antibiotics may suppress the normal intestinal flora.

   (b) *C. difficile,* which produces a toxin, is then able to proliferate, which results in diarrhea or colitis.

   (c) Tests to detect *C. difficile* toxin are available (e.g., tissue culture, latex agglutination, electroimmunoassay).

Table 8-28. Identification of the Anaerobic Gram-Negative Bacilli

Species	Vancomycin	Kanamycin	Colistin	Indole	Lipase	Esculin Hydrolysis	Growth in 20% Bile
Bacteroides fragilis	R	R	R	–	–	+	+
Prevotella intermedia	R	S	S	+	+	–	–
P. melaninogenica	R	R	R	–	–	–	–
Porphyromonas asaccharolytica	S	R	R	+	–	–	–
Fusobacterium nucleatum	R	S	S	+	–	–	–
F. necrophorum	R	S	S	+	+	–	–
F. mortiferum	R	S	S	–	–	+	+

R = resistant; S = susceptible; + = positive; – = negative.

Table 8-29. Identification of *Clostridium* Species

Organism	Lecithinase	Lipase	Esculin Hydrolysis	Double Zone Hemolysis	Reverse CAMP	Motility
C. perfringens	+	–	–	+	+	–
C. novyi	+	+	–	–	–	+
C. septicum	–	–	+	–	–	+
C. sporogenes	–	+	+	–	–	+

CAMP = Christie, Atkins, and Munch-Petersen; + = positive; – = negative.

> **(4)** *C. difficile* can be selectively grown on **cycloserine cefoxitin fructose egg-yolk agar. Gas gangrene (myonecrosis)** can be caused by *C. perfringens, C. septicum, C. sporogenes, and C. novyi.* Clostridial spores are introduced into tissue by trauma or surgery. The organisms produce gas and cause extensive muscle necrosis.
>
> **(5)** Detection of lecithinase may be achieved with **Nagler's test.** This test uses anti–*C. perfringens* antibody to neutralize lecithinase. The antitoxin inhibits the lecithinase reaction on egg-yolk agar. This test is not often performed in clinical laboratories.

> **b.** The **gram-positive, non-spore-forming bacilli** (Table 8-30) are normal flora in various body sites. Their significance in infections is secondary when compared with *Clostridium.*
>
> > **(1)** *Actinomyces israelii* is the most frequently isolated member of this genus. Infections often involve periodontal disease. **Sulfur granules** may be present in exudate.
> >
> > **(2)** *Bifidobacterium* are part of the normal intestinal flora. Identification is difficult unless laboratory personnel are experienced with anaerobes.
> >
> > **(3)** *Eubacterium* are normal intestinal flora that also are difficult to identify.
> >
> > **(4)** *Propionibacterium* are common on skin. *P. acnes* is the most common isolate. This organism is seen as a contaminant in much the same fashion as coagulase-negative staphylococci.

> **3.** Presumptive identification of the **anaerobic cocci** is simple.
>
> > **a.** An anaerobic isolate that is a **gram-negative coccus is** *Veillonella.*

Table 8-30. Presumptive Identification of Anaerobic Gram-Positive Bacilli

Organisms	Spores	Kanamycin	Vancomycin	Colistin	Indole	Catalase
Clostridium perfringens	+	S	S	R	–	–
Propionibacterium acnes	–	S	S	R	+	+
Eubacterium lentum	–	S	S	R	–	–

R = resistant; S = susceptible; + = positive; – = negative.

Table 8-31. Summary of Antimicrobial Tests

Procedure	Definition	Specimen Tested
Minimum inhibitory concentration	Lowest concentration of antibiotic that inhibits visible growth	Bacterial isolate
Disk diffusion (Kirby-Bauer)	Measure diameter of growth inhibition around filter paper disk containing antibiotic	Bacterial isolate
Minimum bactericidal concentration	Lowest concentration of antibiotic that kills 99.9% of the inoculum	Bacterial isolate
Synergy	Activity of multiple antibiotics	Bacterial isolate
Serum bactericidal titer	Dilution of serum that kills 99.9% of the inoculum	Peak serum; trough serum; bacterial isolate
Antibiotic level	Concentration of antibiotic in serum	Peak serum; trough serum

       b. An anaerobic isolate that is a **gram-positive coccus** is ***Peptostreptococcus. P. anaerobius*** is susceptible to an SPS disk; *P. asaccharolyticus* is resistant.

XVIII. ANTIMICROBIAL SUSCEPTIBILITY TESTING

    A. Background. The changing pattern of antimicrobial resistance of clinical isolates makes susceptibility testing of each isolate increasingly important. The in vitro results do not always give the complete picture. The antibiotic that should be used depends on other variables, such as host conditions, site of infection (e.g., CSF versus urine), route of administration, cost, and side effects.

    B. Standardization. An important part of any technique used is use of a standard inoculum of bacteria. The most common procedure is to compare with a **McFarland standard,** which correlates turbidity of a chemical precipitate with numbers per milliliter of bacteria. Regardless of the test used, each is highly standardized. The most commonly used tests are the Kirby-Bauer disk diffusion test and the minimum inhibitory concentration (MIC). A summary of these and other antimicrobial test procedures available for use is given in Table 8-31. There are areas of standardization that apply to both the Kirby-Bauer and MIC tests. These are summarized in Box 8-10.

    C. Interpretation of results. Results may be interpreted according to the following four categories:

       1. Susceptible. The organism should respond to the usual doses of the drug.

       2. Moderately susceptible. The isolate may be inhibited by concentrations of a drug that are achieved when the maximum parenteral doses are given.

       3. Intermediate. The results are equivocal or indeterminate.

Box 8-10. Areas of Standardization for Susceptibility Testing

Growth medium

pH (7.2–7.4)

Atmosphere (ambient air, no carbon dioxide)

Temperature (35°C)

Inoculum (McFarland 0.5 standard)

Antibiotics (store properly)

Quality control (use of stock cultures and regular control runs)

    4. **Resistant.** The bacterium is not inhibited by achievable concentrations of drug.

  D. The **MIC** is the lowest concentration of the agent that inhibits growth of the organism, as detected by lack of turbidity.

    1. The antibiotic is added to broth in **serial twofold dilutions** (e.g., 0.5 μg, 1.0 μg, 2.0 μg). The MIC is the concentration of the first well that shows no growth. Virtually all of the routine MIC tests use commercially prepared broth microdilution trays with antibiotics preselected.

    2. A **sterility well** monitors contamination and should have no growth. A **growth well** monitors organism growth and should have growth. If either the sterility well shows growth or the growth well shows no growth, the test is invalid and should not be read.

  E. The **Kirby-Bauer or disk diffusion method** measures the diameter of inhibition around the antibiotic-impregnated filter paper disk. As soon as the disk comes in contact with the agar surface, water is absorbed into the filter paper, and the antibiotic diffuses into the surrounding medium. The concentration of antibiotic decreases with increased distance from the disk. If the test is properly performed, the edges of the **zone of inhibition** are clear and easy to measure. There are times when the zone is not obvious.

    1. **Swarming** by *Proteus* may result in a thin film of growth beyond the outer margin. The zone of swarming should be ignored, and the outer margin should be measured.

    2. Occasionally, colonies grow within the zone of inhibition. This represents either resistant **mutants** or a mixed culture. If the inoculum is a pure culture, the colonies represent a mutant, and the isolate is considered resistant.

    3. The disks must be placed so that the zones of inhibition do not overlap. **Overlapping zones** may make accurate reading impossible.

    4. **Control plates** are performed weekly using stock cultures.

  F. The **minimum bactericidal concentration (MBC)** measures the lowest concentration of antibiotic that kills 99.9% of a bacterial isolate. It is used to demonstrate tolerance to an antibiotic. Tolerance is determined when the MBC endpoints are five or more twofold dilutions greater than the MIC.

  G. **Synergy** describes the effect of two drugs being significantly better than the combined action of each used separately. This is helpful information in those cases where two antibiotics are used in treatment (e.g., *Enterococcus*). A **checkerboard MIC plate** is used. Each antibiotic is tested separately and together at various concentrations to determine what concentration of each drug results in synergy.

H. The **serum bactericidal titer** tests the bacterial isolate from the patient with the patient's own serum (containing the antibiotic). The lowest dilution of patient serum that kills a standard inoculum is called the serum bactericidal level. The **Schlichter test** is the most commonly used protocol; however, it is not routinely performed.

I. **Antibiotic levels** in serum (e.g., gentamicin) are measured using immunoassay or other chemical methods.

Study Questions

Directions: Each of the numbered items or incomplete statements in this section is followed by answers or by completions of the statement. Select the ONE lettered answer or completion that is BEST in each case.

1. Which one of the following tests may be used to differentiate *Micrococcus* from *Staphylococcus*?

a. coagulase
b. bacitracin susceptibility
c. catalase
d. fermentation of mannitol

2. Which one of the following characteristics is common to members of the Enterobacteriaceae?

a. ferment glucose
b. oxidase positive
c. gram-negative pleomorphic bacilli
d. growth in 6.5% sodium chloride

3. A stool specimen demonstrated growth on Campylobacter blood agar at 42°C but not at 25°C. The isolate was tested, and the following results were obtained: oxidase positive, catalase positive, nalidixic acid susceptible, hippurate hydrolysis positive, hydrogen sulfide negative. The most likely identity of this isolate is

a. *Vibrio alginolyticus*
b. *Campylobacter coli*
c. *C. jejuni*
d. *Pleisomonas*

4. Thiosulfate-citrate-bile salts-sucrose (TCBS) agar is used to isolate and identify which one of the following genera?

a. *Aeromonas*
b. *Pseudomonas*
c. *Campylobacter*
d. *Vibrio*

5. An isolate from a urine culture demonstrated the following characteristics: gray, spreading colonies on blood agar; cream-colored colonies on MacConkey agar; indole negative; hydrogen sulfide positive; phenylalanine deaminase positive; ornithine decarboxylase positive; urea positive; citrate negative. The most likely identity of this isolate is

a. *Escherichia coli*
b. *Morganella morganii*
c. *Proteus vulgaris*
d. *P. mirabilis*

6. Which one of the following is a characteristic of *Pseudomonas aeruginosa*?

a. oxidase positive
b. nonmotile
c. no growth on MacConkey agar
d. ferments glucose

7. Which one of the following tests distinguishes *Streptococcus pyogenes* from *Streptococcus agalactiae*?

a. catalase
b. bile esculin
c. hippurate hydrolysis
d. 6.5% sodium chloride broth

8. The porphyrin test is a sensitive method to determine which one of the following requirements?

a. X factor requirement
b. V factor requirement
c. folic acid requirement
d. vitamin K requirement

9. A 4-year-old was bitten on her hand by her pet cat. Two days later, the bite area was swollen and had some drainage. A Gram's stain of the exudate revealed a small gram-negative coccobacillus. The most likely identity of this organism is

a. *Brucella* species
b. *Vibrio vulnificus*
c. *Pasteurella multocida*
d. *Francisella tularensis*

10. A Gram's stain of the cerebrospinal fluid of a 33-year-old man revealed many polymorphonuclear leukocytes and intra- and extracellular gram-negative diplococci. Culture and tests were as follows: small, flat, gray colonies on chocolate agar; oxidase positive; cystine trypticase agar (CTA) maltose positive; CTA lactose negative. The most likely identity of this isolate is

a. *Neisseria gonorrhoeae*
b. *N. meningitidis*
c. *Moraxella catarrhalis*
d. *Acinetobacter* species

11. The production of hydrogen sulfide is a characteristic used to differentiate which one of the aerobic gram-positive bacilli?

a. *Corynebacterium*
b. *Listeria*
c. *Erysipelothrix*
d. *Lactobacillus*

12. A sputum specimen from an AIDS patient was processed for mycobacteria. After 14 days' incubation at 37°C, buff-colored colonies were seen on Löwenstein-Jensen slants that had been incubated in the light. Tubes incubated in the dark also showed buff-colored colonies. Biochemical testing gave the following results: niacin negative, nitrate negative, Tween hydrolysis negative, catalase negative, urease positive, no growth on 5% sodium chloride agar. What is the most likely identity of this organism?

a. *Mycobacterium tuberculosis*
b. *M. avium-intracellulare*
c. *M. fortuitum*
d. *M. simiae*

13. A sputum specimen was processed for mycobacteria. After 20 days' incubation at 37°C, orange colonies were seen on Löwenstein-Jensen slants that had been incubated in the light. Tubes incubated in the dark also showed orange colonies. Biochemical testing gave the following results: niacin negative, nitrate negative, Tween hydrolysis positive, catalase positive, urease negative, iron uptake negative, no growth on 5% sodium chloride agar. The most likely identity of this organism is

a. *Mycobacterium scrofulaceum*
b. *M. szulgai*
c. *M. gordonae*
d. *M. flavescens*

14. Acid-fast staining of a smear prepared from a digested sputum showed slender, slightly curved, beaded, red mycobacterial rods. Growth on Middlebrook 7H10 slants produced buff-colored colonies after 14 days' incubation at 37°C. Niacin and nitrate reduction tests were positive. The most likely identification of this isolate is

a. *Mycobacterium tuberculosis*
b. *M. kansasii*
c. *M. bovis*
d. *M. ulcerans*

15. A gram-positive, spore-forming bacillus growing on blood agar anaerobically produces a double zone of beta hemolysis and is positive for lecithinase. What is the presumptive identification of this isolate?

a. *Bacteroides ureolyticus*
b. *B. fragilis*
c. *Clostridium perfringens*
d. *C. difficile*

16. The L-pyrolidonyl-β-naphthylamide (PYR) hydrolysis test is a presumptive test for which one of the following streptococci?

a. Groups A and B
b. *Streptococcus pneumoniae* and Group D
c. Group A and *Enterococcus*
d. Groups A and D

17. Obligate anaerobic gram-negative bacilli that do not form spores, grow well in 20% bile, and are resistant to kanamycin are most likely which one of the following organisms?

a. *Porphyromonas* spp.
b. *Bacteroides* spp.
c. *Fusobacterium* spp.
d. *Prevotella* spp.

18. A large gram-positive, spore-forming rod growing on blood agar as large, raised, beta-hemolytic colonies that spread and appear as frosted green-gray glass is most likely which one of the following organisms?

a. *Bacillus*
b. *Pseudomonas*
c. *Corynebacterium*
d. *Listeria*

19. A culture of a skin (hand) wound from a manager of a tropical fish store grew on Löwenstein-Jensen agar slants at 30°C in 10 days, but did not grow on the same medium after 20 days at 37°C. Biochemical testing yielded the following results: photochromogen, niacin negative, urease positive, catalase negative, nitrate negative, Tween hydrolysis positive. What is the most likely identification of this organism?

a. *Mycobacterium kansasii*
b. *M. marinum*
c. *M. avium*
d. *M. tuberculosis*

Directions: Each of the numbered items or incomplete statements in this section is negatively phrased, as indicated by a capitalized word such as NOT, LEAST, or EXCEPT. Select the ONE lettered answer or completion that is BEST in each case.

20. All of the following organisms are gram-positive anaerobic cocci EXCEPT

a. *Peptococcus*
b. *Peptostreptococcus*
c. *Streptococcus*
d. *Veillonella*

Answers and Explanations

1. The answer is b [V A 6]. A positive coagulase test result will differentiate *Staphylococcus aureus* from other *Staphylococcus* species. Coagulase-negative staphylococci will not be distinguished from *Micrococcus*. An 0.04-U bacitracin disk on blood agar will not differentiate the two genera. *Micrococcus* species are sensitive, whereas *Staphylococcus* species are resistant. Both genera are catalase positive. The majority of species from both genera, with the exception of *S. aureus* and a few others, do not ferment mannitol.

2. The answer is a [IX A]. Members of the Enterobacteriaceae all ferment glucose, and all are oxidase-negative, gram-negative rods. Unlike members of *Vibrio*, they do not grow in the presence of a high salt content.

3. The answer is c [X A]. Growth on Campylobacter blood agar at 42°C but not 25°C raises suspicion of a *Campylobacter* species. Colonies that are oxidase and catalase positive are confirmed with biochemicals. *C. jejuni* will be nalidixic acid susceptible, hippurate hydrolysis positive, and hydrogen sulfide negative.

4. The answer is d [X C]. Thiosulfate-citrate-bile salts-sucrose (TCBS) agar has an elevated pH for the cultivation of disease-producing vibrios. *Vibrio cholerae* and *V. alginolyticus* form yellow colonies, whereas *V. parahemolyticus* forms colonies with bluish green centers. *Aeromonas* and *Pseudomonas* form blue colonies.

5. The answer is d [Table 8-12]. *Escherichia coli* is lactose and indole positive. It is also urea and phenylalanine deaminase negative. *M. morganii* does not swarm (i.e., spread) on blood agar, and it is hydrogen sulfide negative. Both *Proteus vulgaris* and *P. mirabilis* swarm, but *P. mirabilis* is indole negative, and *P. vulgaris* is indole positive.

6. The answer is a [XI C]. *Pseudomonas aeruginosa* is an oxidase-positive, motile, gram-negative rod that grows well on MacConkey agar. It is a nonfermenter.

7. The answer is c [VI D]. Both *Streptococcus pyogenes* and *S. agalactiae* are catalase negative, bile esculin negative, and 6.5% sodium chloride negative. *S. agalactiae* hydrolyzes hippurate (i.e., hippurate hydrolysis positive), whereas *S. pyogenes* is hippurate hydrolysis negative.

8. The answer is a [VII A 5 c]. Species that do not require X factor give a positive porphyrin test (e.g., *Haemophilus influenzae* is porphyrin negative).

9. The answer is c [VII B]. *Pasteurella multocida* is found as normal mouth flora in dogs and cats. *Brucella* and *Francisella* are rarely found in domestic animals. *Vibrio vulnificus* is a water-borne organism.

10. The answer is b [VIII C; Table 8-8]. *Neisseria gonorrhoeae* and *Moraxella catarrhalis* are cystine trypticase agar (CTA) maltose negative. *Acinetobacter* species are oxidase negative.

11. The answer is c [XII C]. *Erysipelothrix* is the only aerobic gram-positive bacillus that produces hydrogen sulfide in triple sugar iron agar.

12. The answer is b [XVI A-G]. *Mycobacterium avium-intracellulare* is the most likely organism in the described culture. Negative nitrate and niacin tests eliminate *M. tuberculosis* as the correct answer. *M. fortuitum* is a rapid grower (i.e., grows in fewer than 7 days). *M. simiae* is a nonphotochromogen, but it is niacin positive.

13. The answer is c [XVI A-G]. *Mycobacterium scrofulaceum*, *M. szulgai*, and *M. flavescens* are urease positive. *M. flavescens* grows on 5% sodium chloride agar. *M. szulgai* and *M. flavescens* are nitrate positive. *M. scrofulaceum* is Tween hydrolysis negative.

14. The answer is a [XVI A-G]. *Mycobacterium kansasii* may cause pulmonary disease. However, *M. kansasii* is niacin negative. *M. bovis* is rarely seen in the United States. *M. ulcerans* produces skin infections.

15. The answer is c [XVII D 2]. *Bacteroides* is a gram-negative bacillus. *Clostridium perfringens* is the only member of the genus that yields a double zone of hemolysis.

16. The answer is c [VI B 2 d, 6 c]. Only two members of the Streptococcaceae are positive for the L-pyrolidonyl-β-naphthylamide (PYR) test: Group A (e.g., *Streptococcus pyogenes*) and *Enterococcus*.

17. The answer is b [XVII D 1]. *Bacteroides* is not sensitive to bile (i.e., no growth). *Prophyromonas* spp., *Fusobacterium* spp., and *Prevotella* spp. are all bile sensitive.

18. The answer is a [XII E]. Of *Bacillus*, *Pseudomonas*, *Corynebacterium*, and *Listeria*, *Bacillus* is the only genus that forms spores.

19. The answer is b [XVI A-G]. *Mycobacterium marinum* may cause skin infections, especially in persons who are exposed to salt water. This organism grows best at 30°C. *M. kansasii*, *M. avium*, and *M. tuberculosis* will not grow at 30°C.

20. The answer is d [XVII D 3 a]. *Veillonella* is a gram-negative coccus. *Peptococcus*, *Peptostreptococcus*, and *Streptococcus* are all gram-positive anaerobic cocci.

9

Clinical Parasitology, Mycology, and Virology

Lori Rice-Spearman

I. PARASITOLOGY

A. INTRODUCTION

1. **Definition.** Parasitism is a symbiotic relationship in which one animal, the host, is injured through the activities of the other animal, the parasite.

2. **Medical significance.** Parasites of medical significance belong to four phyla: **Protozoa, Platyhelminthes, Aschelminthes,** and **Arthropoda.**

B. Phylum protozoa.
The protozoa are eukaryotic (unicellular) and have organelles that function in nutrition or locomotion. The **trophozoites** (growing stage) feed by engulfing particles and move by flagella, cilia, or pseudopodia. The cyst stage is more resistant and typically is the form shed in stools and transmitted by the fecal-oral route.

1. **Sarcodina.** This subphylum of Protozoa includes *Amoeba,* which is a group of organisms that move by means of cytoplasmic protrusions called pseudopodia. *Entamoeba histolytica* is the most medically significant species in this group. *E. histolytica* is the agent of **amebic dysentery,** amebic liver abscess, and amebiasis. Other species such as *Entamoeba coli, Entamoeba hartmanni, Entamoeba gingivalis, Iodamoeba bütschlii,* and *Endolimax nana* are considered commensals. **Identifying structures** are summarized in Figure 9-1.

2. **Sporozoa.** This class is primarily **tissue parasites** with an involved life cycle that alternates between sexual and asexual generations. *Plasmodium* species are found as blood parasites and cause the disease **malaria.** *Toxoplasma, Pneumocystis,* and *Sarcocystis* species are spread throughout various organs and tissues. *Isospora* species colonize the intestinal mucosa.

   a. *Plasmodium.* The **anopheline** mosquitoes are definitive hosts of these malarial parasites. The female mosquito first must bite a human who is infected with malaria. Sexual reproduction occurs within the mosquito, with the development of **sporozoites.** Sporozoites enter the salivary glands of the mosquito and are inoculated into the next person bitten. The sporozoites enter the liver and begin an asexual maturation stage. After several

395

Stage	*Entamoeba histolytica*		*Entamoeba coli*	
	Morphology	Features	Morphology	Features
Trophozoite	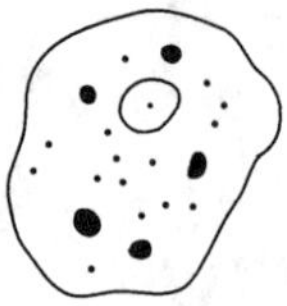	Nuclear chromatin fine and dispersed Sharp central karyosome 12-50 µm diameter; may have ingested erythrocytes	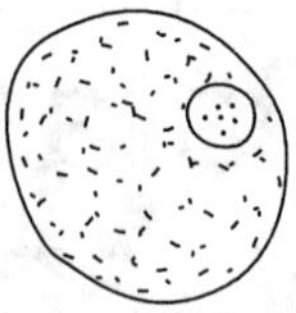	Nuclear chromatin coarse and clumped 20-30 µm; eccentric karyosome No ingested erythrocytes
Cyst	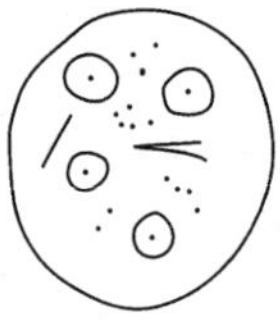	Chromatid bars with rounded ends One to four nuclei; chromatin and karyosome; similar to trophozoite	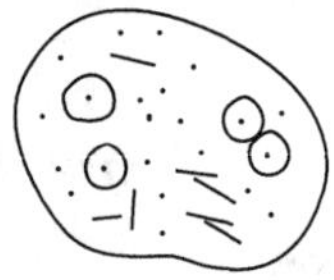	Chromatid bars with ragged ends One to eight nuclei; chromatin and karyosome; similar to trophozoite

Figure 9-1. Differentiation of *Entamoeba histolytica* and *E. coli*. (Reprinted with permission from Johnson AG, Ziegler RJ, Lukasewycz OA, et al: *Microbiology and Immunology*, 2nd ed. Baltimore, Williams & Wilkins, 1993, p 188.)

generations have developed, they invade the red blood cells (RBCs). The four species of Plasmodium are: **P. vivax** (benign tertian malaria), **P. falciparum** (malignant tertian or subtertian malaria), **P. malariae** (quartan malaria), and **P. ovale** (ovale malaria).

(1) Early forms of **P. vivax** in the RBC are trophozoites, which have a **signet-ring shape.** Later stages demonstrate fine red granules known as **Schüffner's dots.** RBCs continue to enlarge, and the mature trophozoites begin division (at this point, they are referred to as **schizonts**). Schizonts mature into merozoites. The infected RBCs finally rupture to release merozoites to infect more RBCs.

(2) **P. falciparum** gametocytes are elongated or **banana-shaped** compared to the ovoid morphology of the other *Plasmodium* species. The two stages observed are the young trophozoites and gametocytes. The young trophozoites are tiny ring forms. In later stages, **Maurer's dots** (coarse red granules) are formed. Gametocytes have a distinct crescent shape.

(3) **P. malariae** trophozoites demonstrate a **band form.** Schizonts mature into **merozoites.**

(4) **P. ovale demonstrates ovoid infected RBCs** with early ring forms. **Schüffner's dots** are present. In later stages, an average of **14–16 merozoites** are observed.

b. **Toxoplasma.** The definitive host is the **cat. Oocysts** (containing two sporocysts) are passed in the feces. Transmission to humans occurs from consumption or handling of infected meat or from contact with cat feces in litter pans or soil. Serology is used for differential diagnosis.

   c. ***Isospora belli*** is characterized by release of immature **oocysts** from the intestinal wall. Maturation of the oocyst occurs in the stool. The organism (30 μm) has an ellipsoid shape and contains two sporoblasts. Recovery is better with the zinc-sulfate concentration technique.

   d. ***Pneumocystis carinii*** is the cause of **pneumonia** in patients who have congenital and acquired immunologic disorders [e.g., acquired immuno-deficiency syndrome (AIDS)]. Demonstration of the organism in smears of **lung tissue** is obtained by open or brush biopsy and Gomori's stain **(silver methenamine technique).** The organism appears as a cyst (5–10 μm) that contains eight nuclei. Single ovoid organisms (2–4 μm) are also observed.

   e. ***Cryptosporidium parvum*** causes chronic diarrhea in immunocompromised hosts. Diagnosis of cryptosporidosis is based on observation of **oocysts** in the stool or biopsy material. Recovery of the **acid-fast** oocysts can be achieved by the sugar flotation procedure. Serologic testing allows for direct detection of the organism in fecal specimens.

3. Mastigophora. The organisms in this subphyla move by means of specialized **flagella** (Figure 9-2). The number and position of the flagella vary according to species. The ***Trypanosoma*** are the blood flagellates. The ***Leishmania*** are the tissue flagellates. ***Giardia*** and ***Dientamoeba fragilis*** are intestinal flagellates, and ***Trichomonas*** can be medically significant in the genitourinary tract. ***Chilomastix*** is typically considered commensal.

   a. ***Trypanosoma.*** The three medically significant hemoflagellates are *T. brucei gambiense* (West African sleeping sickness), *T. brucei rhodesiense* (East African sleeping sickness), and *T. cruzi* (Chagas' disease).

     (1) ***T. brucei gambiense*** is transmitted by ***Glossina*** (tsetse flies). The **trypomastigotes** reside in the blood stream, lymphatics, and cerebrospinal fluid (CSF). They are slender-bodied organisms with long, free flagella and an attached undulating membrane. A kinetoplast is posteriorly located, and the nucleus has a central karyosome.

Amastigote	Promastigote	Epimastigote	Trypanomastigote
Nonmotile, intracellular (mammalian host), replicative form; absent in *Trypanosoma brucei*, *T. brucei gambiense*, and *T. brucei rhodesiense*	Flagellated form with no undulating membrane; present in *Leishmania* life cycles in the sandfly	Short undulating membrane; present in tsetse fly or reduviid bugs in trypanosomal life cycles; absent in *Leishmania*	Full undulating membrane; form transmitted by tsetse fly or reduviid bug, which first gets into the blood; absent in *Leishmania*

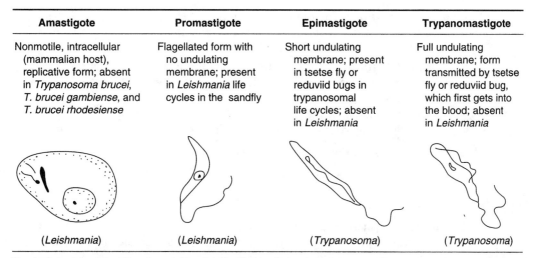

| *(Leishmania)* | *(Leishmania)* | *(Trypanosoma)* | *(Trypanosoma)* |

Figure 9-2. Hemoflagellate forms. (Reprinted with permission from Johnson AG, Ziegler RJ, Lukasewycz OA, et al: *Microbiology and Immunology*, 2nd ed. Baltimore, Williams & Wilkins, 1993, p 190.)

    (2) *T. brucei rhodesiense* is a **virulent** form of trypanosomiasis transmitted by *Glossina*. Its structure is difficult to distinguish from *T. gambiense*.

    (3) *T. cruzi.* The reservoir of this organism is infected wild rodents. An intermediate host is the **reduviid bug** contained in rodent feces (not from bites). The trypanosome in blood smears has a "C" or "S" shape, a large kinetoplast, and a delicate undulating membrane. The **amastigote** stage is observed in cardiac muscle and other tissues.

  b. *Leishmania.* The four major species (i.e., *L. tropica, L braziliensis, L. mexicana, L. donovani*) are transmitted by the intermediate host the **sandfly (*Phlebotomus* spp.).** The **amastigote form** is observed in man, and the **promastigote** form resides in the gut of the sandfly.

    (1) *L. tropica* (Old World leishmaniasis, cutaneous leishmaniasis, Oriental sore) has a round amastigote form that can be observed in monocytic cells. It also has a rod-shaped kinetoplast with a single nucleus.

    (2) *L. mexicana* (New World leishmaniasis or cutaneous leishmaniasis) has the same structure as *L. tropica.*

    (3) *L. braziliensis* (mucocutaneous leishmaniasis or espundia) is disfiguring.

    (4) *L. donovani* (**Kala-Azar** or visceral leishmaniasis) demonstrates diffuse parasitization of the **reticuloendothelial system.** The amastigote resides within phagocytic cells and causes enlargement of the spleen, liver, and lymph nodes.

  c. *Giardia.* *G. lamblia* (Figure 9-3) is the causative agent of giardiasis, the most common waterborne diarrheal disease in the United States.

    (1) The structure of the **trophozoite** is pear-shaped (9–16 μm); it contains four pairs of flagella; two prominent nuclei; an axostile; and an oval, concave-sucking disk ("old man with glasses"). Motility is described as **"falling leaf."**

    (2) The **cyst** (infective stage) is ovoid (9–12 μm) and contains two to four nuclei, as well as two longitudinal fibrils in the center.

  d. *Trichomonas.* The three morphologically similar species are *T. tenax, T. hominis,* and *T. vaginals.* Trichomonads appear only in the trophozoite form, which is the transmissible form.

    (1) *T. vaginalis* (see Figure 9-3) is one of the main causes of sexually transmitted **vaginitis.** Differential diagnosis requires a **saline wet mount** of genitourinary tract specimens.

    (2) Trophozoites are pear-shaped with an undulating membrane. They demonstrate a jerky, swift motility.

  e. *Chilomastix mesnili* is a commensal organism.

    (1) The trophozoite is pear-shaped with three anterior flagella and a nucleus.

    (2) The cyst is lemon-shaped with a large nucleus and a large karyosome.

4. Ciliata. *Balantidium coli* (see Figure 9-3) has short, bristle-like cilia. *B. coli* is the largest protozoan that infects humans; it causes balantidial dysentery.

  a. The trophozoite (60 μm) has two nuclei, and the cilia surrounds the organism.

Species	Morphology	Associated Diseases	Mode/form of Transmission	Diagnosis	Treatment
Entamoeba histolytica	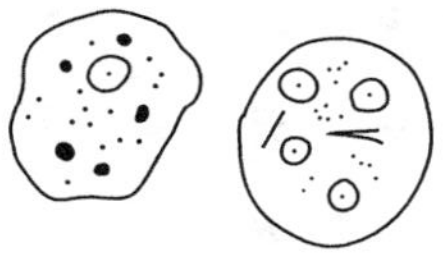	Amebiasis	Fecal-oral by water; fresh fruits and vegetables; via cysts	Trophozoites Cysts in stool; serology Pathology (inverted flask-shaped lesions)	Metronidazole followed by iodoquinol
Giardia lamblia	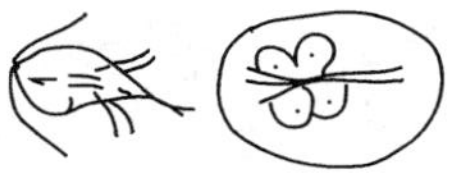	Giardiasis	Fecal (e.g., human, beaver, muskrat) by water, food, oral-anal sex; via cysts	Trophozoites Cysts in stool	Quinacrine hydrochoride
Cryptosporidium species	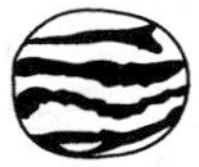	Cryptosporidiosis (transient diarrhea in healthy persons; severe diarrhea in immunocompromised persons)	Undercooked meat; via cysts	Acid-fast oocysts in stool Biopsy; dots (cysts) in intestinal glands	Spiramycin
Balantidium coli	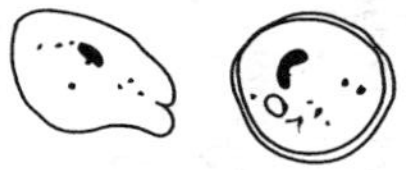	Dysentery; colitis; diarrhea to severe dysentery	Contaminated food or water; via cysts	Trophozoites Cysts in feces	Tetracycline
Trichomonas vaginalis	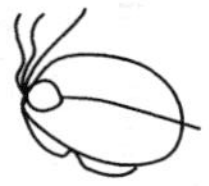	Trichomoniasis	Sexual contact; via trophozoites	Motile trophozoites and excessive neutrophils in methylene blue wet mount	Metronidazole

Figure 9-3. Intestinal and urogenital protozoan parasites. (Reprinted with permission from Johnson AG, Ziegler RJ, Lukasewycz OA, et al: *Microbiology and Immunology*, 2nd ed. Baltimore, Williams & Wilkins, 1993, p 187.)

    b. The cyst (50 μm) has a macronuclei and a micronuclei. Cilia surround the membrane.

C. Phylum Platyhelminthes. The Platyhelminthes, or **flatworms,** are multicellular animals characterized by a flat, bilaterally symmetric body. Generally, the flatworms are **hermaphroditic.** The two medically significant classes are the *Trematoda* and the *Cestoda.*

    1. Trematoda. The **flukes** are organisms that possess attachment organs in the form of **hooks** or cup-shaped **suckers.** The medically significant order is **Digenea.** The Digenea have life cycles that have at least one intermediate **molluscan host.**

        a. *Fasciolopsis buski.* Reservoirs are pigs, dogs, and rabbits; snails are intermediate hosts. Transmission is ingestion of metacercariae that are encysted on **freshwater vegetation,** such as bamboo shoots or water chestnuts, which are consumed raw. The ellipsoid egg is approximately 130 μm, with a small **operculum** at the pointed end.

        b. *Heterophyes heterophyes* and *Metagonimus yokogawai.* Transmission is through ingestion of **raw** or **pickled freshwater fish. Metacercariae** encyst under the scales or in the flesh of the fish. The egg is approximately 30 μm and possesses prominent **opercular shoulders.**

        c. *Clonorchis sinensis.* The **Chinese liver fluke** is approximately 30 μm. Transmission occurs with the consumption of **freshwater fish** containing the encysted metacercariae. The adult worm harbors in the liver and sheds eggs into the feces. The eggs resemble *Heterophyes* but have a **small comma-shaped process** at the abopercular end.

        d. *Fasciola hepatica.* The sheep liver fluke infection occurs following the consumption of **aquatic vegetation** (metacercariae encyst **watercress**). Eggs are observed in the feces and are difficult to distinguish from *Fasciolopsis.* The eggs are operculated and measure 130 μm.

        e. The three **medically significant schistosomes** that parasitize man are *Schistosoma mansoni, S. japonicum,* and *S. haematobium.* The schistosomes are not hermaphroditic, they are **diecious.** The eggs are not operculated; the hatched miracidium swim in search of the appropriate snail host. The **cercariae infect humans.** Schistosomes directly **penetrate the skin** to invade the circulatory system. The final locations differ in each host.

            (1) *S. mansoni.* Eggs are isolated from the feces. They are elongated, ovoid, and possess a **large lateral spine** that is shaped like a thorn and projects from the side of the egg near one end. These eggs measure approximately 150 μm.

            (2) *S. japonicum.* Eggs are isolated from the feces. They are spherical in shape and possess a **small lateral spine** (sometimes this is absent or very difficult to view). These organisms measure approximately 65 μm.

            (3) *S. haematobium* is the cause of **urinary schistosomiasis.** Eggs are isolated in urine or in a biopsy of the bladder. The eggs have a **terminal spine** and measure approximately 150 μm.

    f. *Paragonimus westermani*. The lung fluke is transmitted by the ingestion of raw or **improperly cooked crayfish or fresh-water crabs** encysted with the metacercarial stage. The eggs are discharged into the bronchi or bronchioles; they can be expectorated in **sputum** or, if swallowed, appear in the **feces**. The ovoid eggs have **raised opercular shoulders** and measure approximately 100 μm.

2. Cestoda. The **tapeworms** have elongated segmented (proglottid) bodies with a **scolex** (specialized attachment organ). They inhabit and gain nourishment from the small intestine. All cestodes of man have four muscular, cup-shaped suckers on the scolex, and a **rostellum** that can be armed with hooks. Transmission occurs when infective larvae are accidentally **ingested with food.**

    a. *Diphyllobothrium latum* selectively **absorbs vitamin B$_{12}$** from the host's intestinal tract. The **primary intermediate host** is the ciliated **coracidium larvae** (which has ingested the *D. latum* eggs). The larvae are ingested by **copepods** (*D. latum* develops and forms larvae). These infected copepods are then ingested by **fish,** and *D. latum* grows within the flesh of the fish to the plerocercoid larva stage. Only if the infected fish is ingested by man will the larva pass into the intestine and develop into adulthood.

      (1) The **adult worm** scolex is elongated, spoon shaped, and has two longitudinal grooves. The uterus, within the proglottid, has a unique morphology and forms a rosette.

      (2) The **eggs** are ovoid with an operculum and a thick, smooth shell. They are approximately 70 μm.

    b. *Taenia solium*. The **pork tapeworm** is transmitted by ingesting **cured or undercooked pork.** Embryonated eggs are ingested by the intermediate host (the pig) and develop into the infective larval stage or **cysticerci in the muscles.** Humans ingest the cysticerci; the larvae develop, and the scolex attaches to the intestinal wall and begins to develop proglottids **(cysticercosis).**

      (1) Structure. The **adult worm** scolex has four suckers and a **double crown of hooks** (armed rostellum). Differential diagnosis is by observation of **7–13 branches** of the central uterine stem in a gravid segment.

      (2) The **egg** contains the **oncosphere.** A thick coat, called the embryophore, is a dark color and is radially striated. Observation of *Taenia* eggs cannot differentiate *T. solium* from *T. saginata.*

    c. *Taenia saginata*. The **beef tapeworm** is transmitted by the ingestion of **raw or insufficiently cooked beef.** Embryonated eggs are ingested by cattle and develop in the flesh into the infective cysticercus stage. (*T. saginata* does not cause cystercosis of humans.)

      (1) The **adult worm** scolex has four suckers with a small rostellum that has **no hooks** (unarmed rostellum). The gravid segment is longer in *T. saginata*, and there are **15–20 branches** off of the central uterine stem.

      (2) Morphology of the eggs of *T. saginata* is similar to that of *T. solium.*

    d. *Echinococcus granulosus*. The **minute tapeworm** lives as an adult in the intestines of the ***Canidae*.** Intermediate hosts are typically herbivores (e.g., sheep, goats). The human is an accidental intermediate host. Humans can ingest the eggs, which hatch and develop into oncospheres. The oncospheres penetrate the intestinal mucosa, enter the circulation, and progress to the liver. A **hydatid cyst** begins to develop, with buds forming on the cyst. The cysts contain protoscolices, which appear as **hydatid sand** when the cyst begins to break down.

(1) The **adult worm** has a scolex (with six hooklets) and three proglottids.

(2) **Structure.** Eggs cannot be differentiated from *Taenia* eggs.

e. *Hymenolepis nana.* **The dwarf tapeworm** is transmitted to humans by ingestion of the egg, which develops into the adult worm in the intestines of the human. The reservoir is the house mouse.

(1) The **adult worm** has a scolex with four suckers and a rostellum armed with a circle of **hooks.**

(2) The **eggs** are ovoid and have a thin, smooth outer shell with **two polar thickenings or knobs** that have fine **filaments** (4–8) that are difficult to observe. The eggs are approximately 40 μm.

f. *Hymenolepis diminuta* transmission is through ingestion of **infected insects from flour** contaminated by the droppings of infected rats. Larvae grow into adults in the intestine of humans.

(1) **Adult worms** have a scolex with four suckers and an **"unarmed" rostellum.**

(2) **Eggs** are ovoid with a thick shell that also has **two polar knobs but no filaments.**

D. **Phylum Aschelminthes.** The medically significant class is **Nematoda,** the **roundworms.** They posses a stiff cuticle, and the **sexes are separate.** The roundworms can inhabit the intestines, the blood, or the tissues. The filariae are thread-like worms that inhabit the human lymphatic system, as well as subcutaneous and deep connective tissues. All of the filariae require an **arthropod intermediate host** for transmission of infection. Some species demonstrate **periodicity.** That is, they appear in the blood at specific times of the day.

1. *Ascaris lumbricoides.* The life cycle of *Ascaris* is complex. After the fully **embryonated eggs** are ingested, they hatch in the intestines and begin to **migrate** (up to 20 days) through the blood and lymphatic system. They finally reach the esophagus and once again enter the intestines, where the mature worm then begins to lay eggs.

a. **Adult worm**

(1) The adult female worm is 30 cm in length and is as thick as a lead pencil.

(2) The adult male worm is 25 cm in length and is slender with an "incurved tail."

b. The **eggs** are broadly oval with a rough outer coating, an albuminoid coat. They are referred to as **fertilized corticated** eggs. **Decorticated** eggs have a thick, smooth shell. **Infertile** eggs are narrow and have a thin shell (corticated or decorticated).

2. *Enterobius vermicularis.* The **pinworm** is the most common helminth parasite in modern countries. Transmission is by ingestion of the eggs, which pass to the intestine and begin development. The females migrate down the intestinal tract to pass out of the anus and deposit their eggs. The **cellophane**

tape preparation is useful for diagnosis. Typically, the eggs are **not observed in the feces.**

a. **Structure**

(1) The adult female worm can reach 13 mm in length. It has a long, thin, sharply pointed tail.

(2) The adult male worm reaches 5 mm in length.

b. The **eggs** are 50 μm and have a translucent shell that is **flattened on one side** (football appearance).

3. *Trichuris trichiura.* The **whipworm** is acquired through ingestion of embryonated eggs. It can cause rectal prolapse and nutritional deficiencies in children.

a. The female worm measures 3–5 cm and is typically longer than the male.

b. The eggs are 50 μm and have **bipolar plugs.**

4. *Ancylostoma duodenale.* The **Old World hookworm** eggs are deposited into moist sandy soil, and within 24–48 hours **rhabditiform** larvae develop and hatch. Further development transforms the larvae into the infective **filariform** larvae. The filariform penetrate the skin of humans. Humans may develop **ground itch** at the site of penetration. Hookworm infestation is associated with **iron deficiency anemia.**

a. **Adult worm**

(1) The **female** worm is grayish white with a buccal cavity that has four teeth.

(2) The **male** worm is smaller than the female worm and has a prominent copulatory bursa posteriorly.

b. The eggs of *A. duodenale* and *N. americanus* cannot be differentiated. The eggs are approximately 50 μm with a thin, smooth colorless shell. Clearly visible are the two-cell, four-cell, or occasionally eight-cell stage of embryonic cleavage.

5. *Necator americanus* is the **New World hookworm.**

a. **Adult worm**

(1) The female worm is 1 cm in length. The buccal cavity of *Necator* is armed with a pair of cutting plates.

(2) The male worm is smaller than the female worm.

b. **Eggs** (see I D 4 b)

c. Rarely, hookworm eggs can hatch and release the rhabditiform larvae. The larvae can be differentiated from *Strongyloides* larvae by observing the buccal cavities. The hookworm buccal cavity has a long capsule between the oral opening and the esophagus. The *Strongyloides* buccal capsule is comparatively short.

6. *Strongyloides stercoralis.* The **threadworm** is less prevalent than the hookworm and can exist as a free-living nematode. Transmission and life cycle are similar to the hookworm (see I D 4, 5).

a. **Adult worm**

(1) The **female** worm is longer than 2 mm and is **parthenogenic** (capable of unisexual reproduction, no fertilization required).

(2) The **male** worm is smaller, and it may be eliminated from the body early in infection.

b. **Structure.** Eggs of the threadworm cannot be distinguished from the hookworm eggs. The eggs hatch in the intestine to form the rhabditiform larvae and are usually passed in the feces. Occasionally, a few of these larvae transform into the filariform larvae, which penetrate the mucosa wall, enter the bloodstream, and begin the migratory cycle again. This is termed **autoreinfection.**

7. *Trichostrongylus* **spp.** This worm is very similar to the hookworm. The life cycle differs in that *Trichostrongylus* is transmitted by ingestion of contaminated food. The adult worms are much smaller than the hookworms. The eggs are much larger than the hookworm eggs (80 μm).

8. *Trichinella spiralis.* **Trichinosis** and **trichinellosis** are acquired by ingesting **uncooked pork** or **bear meat** that contains the encysted larvae. The larvae excyst and penetrate into the intestinal mucosa of the host and develop into adult worms. The male and female worms mate, and more larvae are produced (intestinal phase). The larvae enter the bloodstream and disseminate to the striated muscle, where they encyst. Diagnosis is based on observation of the encysted larvae in **biopsied muscle** or post-infection serologic testing.

9. *Dracunculus medinensis.* The **guinea worm** is a parasite of dogs and other carnivores in North America.

a. **Infection.** The larvae are ingested by the intermediate host—the **copepod** (crustacean)—and develop into the infective form. The infective larvae are ingested in drinking water and migrate in the host to the subcutaneous tissues. The larvae develop into the adult worm. The female worm migrates to the skin surface and forms a **papule** to discharge large numbers of larvae.

b. **Structure**

(1) The adult female worm is approximatly 800 mm in length and can be removed from the papule manually or excised surgically.

(2) The adult male worm is approximately 40 mm in length.

10. *Ancylostoma braziliense* or *A. caninum* are the **dog hookworms** that occasionally infect humans and cause **cutaneous larva migrans** or creeping eruptions. The larvae penetrate the skin and are unable to complete their migratory cycle; therefore, they begin to migrate through the subcutaneous tissues.

11. *Wuchereria bancrofti.* Bancroftian filariasis, **elephantiasis,** or Bancrofti's filariasis are associated diseases.

a. **Infection.** The infective larvae enter the human host through the proboscis of the *Culex* or *Anopheles* mosquito. They migrate to the lymphatics (lymph nodes), where mating occurs and microfilariae are produced (can be observed in a blood smear).

b. **Structure.** The microfilariae are sheathed. The anterior is rounded, and the posterior tapers to a point. There are no nuclei in the tail.

12. *Brugia malayi.* Malayan filariasis or elephantiasis is transmitted by the *Mansonia* or *Anopheles* mosquito.

    a. Infection. Migration occurs through the lymphatics. Microfilariae can be observed in the blood smear.

    b. Structure. The microfilariae are sheathed. There are two nuclei present in the tip of the tail.

13. *Loa loa.* The **African eyeworm** is transmitted by the ***Chrysops*** (fly) and migrates through the subcutaneous tissues (especially across the conjunctiva of the eye). Calabar swellings also occur. The microfiliariae can be observed in the blood. They are sheathed and have a continuous row of posterior nuclei.

14. *Onchocerca volvulus.* Onchocerca is transmitted by the ***Simulium*** fly and migrates through the subcutaneous tissues. They usually settle in groups of two and become encapsulated to form nodules. These nodules can occur anywhere, but are typically observed on the patient's scalp. The microfilariae can be observed in **"skin snips"** taken from the nodules. The microfilariae are unsheathed, with no terminal nuclei, and typically have straight tails.

15. *Mansonella*

    a. *M. ozzardi* is typically a nonpathogenic filaria. The microfiliariae have no sheaths and no nuclei in their tails.

    b. *M. streptocerca* (formerly *Dipetalonema streptocerca*) is pathogenic and transmitted by *Culicoides*. The microfilariae are observed only in tissue scrapings. They have no sheaths and have single nuclei in their tails.

    c. *M. perstans* (formerly *D. perstans*) is nonpathogenic. The microfilariae have no sheaths and have paired nuclei in their tails.

E. Specimen collection, transport, and processing

    1. Collection and transport for **fecal examination** should include the following precautions.

        a. The specimen should be collected in a clean container and must not be contaminated with urine.

        b. If not examined within 1 hour, part of the specimen should be preserved in polyvinyl alcohol fixative (PVA) or in 10% formalin.

            (1) PVA preserves cysts and trophozoites for permanent staining.

            (2) Formalin preserves eggs, cysts, and larvae for wet-mount examination and concentration.

        c. Three specimens every other day is the optimal number for recovery of parasites.

        d. Saline purges are satisfactory to obtain specimens; castor and mineral oils make examination for protozoa impossible.

        e. Specimens containing radiographic contrast media (e.g., barium salts) are inappropriate.

    2. Processing of specimens. The processing should include a macroscopic examination, a microscopic examination, and a concentration procedure.

        a. The process of **macroscopic examination** involves the following:

            (1) Noting the consistency of the specimen (i.e., soft stools suggest the presence of trophozoites or protozoa; formed stools suggest the presence of cysts)

(2) Examining the surface for tapeworm proglottids or adult pinworms

(3) Examining for blood and mucus

b. The **microscopic examination** should include a direct saline and/or iodine mount. A **calibrated ocular micrometer** should be used routinely. Size differences of various internal structures and of whole organisms are important in differential diagnosis.

c. A **fecal concentration technique** increases the possibility of detecting parasites when few are present in feces; this technique should be a routine part of the examination process.

(1) The **Ritchie formalin-ether method** is the most commonly used method for concentrating eggs and cysts.

(2) The **zinc sulfate flotation method** is not appropriate for operculated eggs, schistosomes, or infertile ascaris eggs. This method is recommended for recovery of oocysts.

3. The **trichrome technique** is a rapid procedure that gives good results for routine identification of intestinal protozoa in fresh fecal specimens. The specimen must be fixed with either PVA or Schaudinn's solution.

a. The cytoplasm of trophozoites and cysts appears light blue-green or light pink.

b. Karyosomes stain ruby red.

c. Degenerated organisms and the background material stain pale green.

II. MYCOLOGY

A. Introduction

1. **Definition.** The fungi are eukaryotic and commonly called yeasts, molds, and mushrooms.

2. **Characteristics** of fungi include the following.

a. **Hyphae** are filamentous subunits of molds and mushrooms.

(1) Hyphae may be dematiaceous (dark) or hyaline (colorless).

(2) Hyphae can be septate or aseptate

b. **Pseudohyphae** are a series of elongated blastoconidia that remain attached to each other and form a hyphal-like structure but with constrictions of the septations (characteristic of *Candida albicans*).

c. **Spores** may be formed by either an asexual or a sexual process.

(1) **Asexual spores**

(a) **Conidia** are asexual spores formed on the outside of the conidiophore.

(b) **Blastoconidia** reproduce by budding from a mother cell. They can elongate to form pseudohyphae.

(c) **Arthroconidia** fragment from the hyphal strand at the septation points.

(d) **Chlamydoconidia** are thick-walled survival conidia that can occur either at a terminal site (end), an intercalary site (within the hyphae), or a sessile site (on the sides).

(e) **Sporangiospores** are formed by internal cleavage of the contents of a sac called a sporangium.

(2) **Sexual spores**

(a) **Zygospores** are thick-walled zygotes formed by fusion of two hyphal tips.

(b) **Ascospores** are sexual spores that occur in multiples of four inside an ascus.

(c) **Basidiospores** are sexual spores that form on the outside of the basidium.

B. **Specimen collection and transport**

1. **Collection** of specimens for mycologic cultures must include:

   a. Sterile technique

   b. Adequate amount

   c. Sample from the area most likely affected

2. **Transport**

   a. **Blood and bone marrow** are collected into a brain heart infusion (BHI) broth for transportation to the laboratory. An alternative method is to collect blood and bone marrow into a sterile vacutainer tube and then process it by the membrane filter technique.

   b. **CSF** is aseptically collected and transported immediately to the laboratory.

   c. **Hair, nails,** and **skin** are initially cleaned with 70% alcohol to remove surface contaminants. Scrapings and plucked hairs are placed in a sterile Petri plate for transportation.

   d. **Respiratory tract specimens** (e.g., sputum) should be collected in the morning and put into a sterile container for transport.

   e. **Tissues** and **biopsy specimens** are aseptically collected and kept moist with sterile saline for transport.

   f. **Vaginal and cervical specimens** are typically collected on sterile swabs, then placed into transport media or broth.

   g. **Scrapings from wounds and lesions** may be placed into sterile saline for transport. Aspiration specimens can be collected from deep cysts or abscesses by needle and syringe.

C. **Media and tests**

1. **Sabouraud dextrose agar (SDA)** inhibits the growth of many bacteria because its pH is 5.6. However, this medium allows fungal contaminants and pathogenic fungi to grow.

2. **SDA** with **cycloheximide** and **chloramphenicol** is reserved for skin, hair, and nail specimens.

3. **BHI agar (BHIA)** is very nutritious and supports the growth of *Histoplasma* and *Nocardia.*

   a. **BHIA with blood** is recommended for converting dimorphic fungi from the mold to the tissue (yeast) phase.

   b. **BHIA with blood, cycloheximide, and chloramphenicol** is very nutritious but inhibits the growth of *Nocardia.* (NOTE: Chloramphenicol inhibits the yeast phase of dimorphic fungi.)

4. **Corn meal Tween 80 agar** (CMT 80) allows the demonstration of blastoconidia and pseudohyphae in the identification of *Candida* species and other yeasts.

5. **Germ tube media** (rabbit, fetal calf, or human serum) inoculated with test organisms collected within the past 24 hours and incubated for 3 hours may produce hyphae.

6. **Urea agar slant** is streaked with the test organism, incubated at room temperature, and observed for production of a pinkish purple color within 48 hours.

   a. *Trichosporon, Rhodotorula,* and *Cryptococcus* test positive in this medium.

   b. *Geotrichum, Saccharomyces,* and *Candida* test negative in this medium.

7. **Inhibitory mold agar** is used primarily to recover pathogenic fungi exclusive of dermatophytes.

8. **Mycosel agar** is used to recover dermatophytes.

D. **Microscopy of clinical specimens**

1. **Saline wet mounts** allow budding yeast, hyphae, conidia, and filaments to be observed.

2. **Lactophenol cotton blue stain**

   a. **Phenol** kills organisms.

   b. **Lactic acid** preserves the fungal structures.

   c. **Cotton blue** stains the chitin in the fungal cell walls.

3. **Potassium hydroxide** (KOH) is ideal for observing skin, hair, or nails. Ten percent potassium hydroxide dissolves the keratin and allows the fungi more visibility.

4. **Gram's stain.** The fungi appear gram-positive or blue.

5. **Acid-fast stain.** The modified Kinyoun acid-fast stain is recommended for staining *Nocardia*.

6. **India ink.** The Torula preparation is recommended for observing capsules around yeast, especially *Cryptococcus neoformans*.

7. **Periodic acid-Schiff** (PAS) stains fungi (except *Actinomycetes*) magenta against a light pink or green background.

8. **Calcofluor white stain** is observed under a fluorescent microscope. This stain is very sensitive, with any fungal elements flourescing against a dark background.

E. **Opportunistic mycoses** can cause a range of infections, from a mild self-limiting infection to a serious disseminated infection in severely compromised patients. Opportunistic mycoses are caused by endogenous organisms, and they are increasing as the number of compromised patients increases.

1. *Candida albicans* is part of the normal flora of the skin, mucous membranes, and gastrointestinal tract.

   a. *C. albicans* forms germ tubes, chlamydospores, blastoconidia, and pseudohyphae on CMT 80 agar.

   b. *C. albicans* assimilates the carbohydrate sucrose.

2. **Candidiasis** is an acute-to-chronic fungal infection that can involve the mouth, vagina, skin, nails, bronchi, lungs, alimentary tract, bloodstream, or urinary tract. Typically, the causative agent is *Candida albicans* or other species of *Candida*.

    a. **Oral thrush** is a yeast infection that forms white curd-like patches on the oral mucocutaneous membranes.

    b. **Vulvovaginitis** or vaginal thrush manifests as a thick yellow-white discharge. Diabetes, antibiotic therapy, oral contraceptives, and pregnancy predispose the patient to this condition.

    c. **Candidemias** occur in patients who have indwelling catheters.

3. ***Malassezia furfur*** septicemia occurs in patients who receive intravenous lipid emulsions.

    a. *M. furfur* requires a media overlayed with a **lipid,** such as olive oil.

    b. Microscopically, *M. furfur* appears as thick, round oval cells in clusters with hyphae (spaghetti and meatballs).

4. **Cryptococcosis** infections primarily involve the lungs and meninges and often occur in AIDS patients.

    a. *Cryptococcus neoformans* (yeast) has a capsule that is demonstrated with the **India ink** preparation.

    b. *C. neoformans* is associated with **pigeon** feces.

    c. The capsular material in the CSF can be detected with antigen latex agglutination test and is urea positive.

5. **Aspergilloses** are a variety of infections and allergic diseases caused by *Aspergillus fumigatus*.

    a. *A. fumigatus* is a ubiquitous fungus with airborne spores.

      (1) Hyphae are septate with dichotomous branching.

      (2) *A. fumigatus* produces conidial heads with numerous conidia.

      (3) *A. fumigatus* **grows at 45°C.**

    b. **Allergic aspergillosis** involves the organism colonizing the mucous plugs in the lung. A high titer of IgE antibody to *Aspergillus* is present.

    c. **Invasive aspergilloma** occurs in neutropenic patients. The patient has sinusitis, and dissemination throughout the body (e.g., brain) occurs.

6. **Zygomycoses,** also known as phycomycoses or mucormycoses, are infections caused by *Rhizopus, Absidia,* and *Mucor*. **Zygomycota** have nonseptated hyphae and grow rapidly. **Rhizopus** species are unbranched sporangiophores that arise opposite rhizoids. These species can cause zygomycosis or otomycosis. **Absidia** species are branching sporangiophores between the rhizoid nodes on the stolons. These species can cause zygomycosis or mycotic keratitis. **Mucor** species are single or branching sporangiophores that support round, spore-filled sporangia. No rhizoids or stolons are present. These species can cause zygomycosis, otomycosis, or allergies.

F. **Systemic mycoses** affect internal organs and may disseminate to multiple organs in the body. Typically, they are caused by **dimorphic** (fungi that grow as molds at 25°C or as yeast at 35°C) fungal pathogens.

1. **Histoplasmosis** is a granulomatous fungal infection caused by *Histoplasma capsulatum*, which is a noncapsulated fungus that is a facultative intracellular yeast localized in monocytic cells throughout the reticuloendothelial system.

   a. The **mold phase** is a large tuberculate macroconidia in soil enriched with bat or bird guano (inhalation transmission).

   b. The **major endemic region** is the Ohio, Missouri, and Mississippi River areas.

2. **North American blastomycosis** is caused by *Blastomyces dermatitidis*.

   a. **Transmission** is inhalation of the conidia.

   b. The **tissue (37°C) phase** is a yeast with a double refractile wall and broad-based buds.

   c. The **mold phase** is single oval conidia at the ends of short conidiophores.

   d. The **major endemic areas** are the St. Lawrence, Mississippi, and Ohio river beds.

3. **Coccidioidomycosis** is caused by *Coccidioides immitis* and is commonly known as "valley fever."

   a. **Transmission** is by inhalation of arthroconidia in sand and dirt.

   b. The **tissue phase** involves large spherules with endospores.

   c. **Diagnosis** is based on serologic and skin testing.

   d. The **major endemic area** is the San Joaquin Valley and the lower Sonoran Desert in the southwestern United States.

G. **Superficial mycoses** affect the outermost layer of skin and hair.

   1. **Pityriasis versicolor** infection is caused by *M. furfur* (see II E 3), which infects the stratum corneum epidermidis and causes hypopigmentation or hyperpigmentation on the trunk of the body.

   2. **Tinea nigra** is also an infection of the stratum corneum epidermidis caused by *Exophiala werneckii*.

      a. *E. werneckii* is dematiaceous.

      b. At room temperature, the colony grows black and yeasty and later develops short olive-gray mycelia.

      c. Microscopically, dark septate hyphae with one- or two-celled blastoconidia are demonstrated in clusters along the hyphae.

      d. *E. werneckii* hydrolyzes casein.

   3. **Piedra** is an infection of the hair shaft that produces hair breakage.

      a. *Trichosporon beigelli* forms soft nodules around the beard and mustache hairs. Microscopically, it forms hyaline hyphae with blastoconidia and arthroconidia on CMT 80 agar.

      b. Black piedra is caused by *Piedraia hortai*, which forms firmly attached hard, black nodules around the outside of scalp hairs. Microscopically, it produces dark thick-walled hyphae with swellings.

H. **Cutaneous mycoses** are typically caused by a group of filamentous fungi referred to as the **dermatophytes**. Some cutaneous mycoses can be caused by *Candida*. The cutaneous mycoses involve skin, hair, and nails. They may be acquired from animals (e.g., *Trichophyton rubrum, Microsporum canis*) or from humans (e.g., *Epidermophyton floccosum, Microsporum audouinii*). Diagnosis is made by microscopic examination of skin, hair, and nails with 10% KOH. The term **tinea,** or ringworm, is applied to the diseases caused by these dermatophytes.

1. **Tinea capitis** is ringworm of the scalp.

    a. **Epidemic tinea capitis** occurs in children and is extremely contagious. It is caused by *M. audouinii*, which fluoresces under a Wood's lamp.

    b. **Zoophilic tinea capitis** occurs primarily in children. Transmission of infection is through animals. It is most commonly caused by *Microsporum canis* (spindle-shaped macroconidia) or *Trichophyton mentagrophytes* (grape-like clusters of microconidia).

    c. **Black-dot tinea capitis** occurs in adults and is a chronic infection. The infectious agent is *Trichophyton tonsurans*.

    d. **Favus** (tinea favosa) is caused by *Trichophyton schoenleinii*.

2. **Tinea barbae** is an infection of the beard, neck, or face.

    a. *Trichophyton verrucosum* requires thiamine for growth and microscopically produces a three- to five-cell macroconidia with a rat-tail end.

    b. *T. mentagrophytes* (see II H 1 b)

    c. *Trichophyton rubrum* produces numerous club-shaped microconidia, which occur singly along a hypha and produce a deep red pigment on potato dextrose agar or corn meal agar.

3. **Tinea corporis,** which usually affects the inside skin folds, is typically caused by yeast (*Candida*) or *T. rubrum, T. mentagrophytes,* or *M. canis*.

4. **Tinea cruris** is a fungal infection of the groin caused by the following organisms:

    a. *Epidermophyton floccosum,* which produces two- to four-celled smooth, club-shaped macroconidia

    b. *T. rubrum* (see II H 2 c)

    c. *T. mentagrophytes* (see II H 1 b)

    d. *Candida* species

5. **Tinea pedis** is an infection of the feet, commonly called **athlete's foot,** that can be caused by the following organisms:

    a. *T. rubrum* (see II H 2 c)

    b. *T. mentagrophytes,* which is the most common cause of athlete's foot (see II H 1 b)

    c. *E. floccosum,* which causes epidemic tinea pedis in summer camps (see II H 4 a)

I. **Subcutaneous mycoses** typically result from traumatic implantation (e.g., via thorn, splinter) of a fungi into the cutaneous and subcutaneous tissues.

1. **Sporotrichosis** is caused by the dimorphic fungus *Sporothrix schenckii*.

    a. At 37°C, growth is a cigar-shaped budding yeast.

    b. At 25°C, a daisy head or flowerette of microconidia is produced at the end of unbranched conidiophores.

    c. *S. schenckii* is found on plant material such as rose thorn, sphagnum moss, and timbers.

    d. Diseases can be lymphocutanueous, fixed, or pulmonary.

  2. Eumycotic mycetoma is a disease characterized by swelling, sinus tract formation, and the presence of sulfur granules. It typically occurs in third world countries.

    a. *Pseudoallescheria boydii,* the sexual stage of *Scedosporium apiospermum*, is the most common cause of mycetoma in the United States.

    b. *Madurella* species (Madura foot) most commonly cause mycetoma in Africa.

  3. Chromoblastomycoses begin with traumatic implantation of the spore on a limb. The disease produces cauliflower-like lesions. Infection is caused by the dematiaceous fungi *Phialophora, Fonsecaea,* or *Cladosporium* and typically occurs in third world countries.

III. VIROLOGY

  A. Viruses (virions) are the smallest known form of infectious disease–causing agents.

    1. Size. Viruses are 1/10 the size of bacteria and 1/100 the size of eukaryotic cells. They cannot be observed with a light microscope.

    2. Structure. Viruses of humans are composed of nucleic acid [deoxyribonucleic acid (DNA) or ribonucleic acid (RNA)].

      a. The nucleic acid is surrounded by a protein matrix referred to as the **nucleocapsid.** The **capsid** surrounds the nucleocapsid and is composed of structural units called **capsomers.** Virus particles are either "naked" or have a lipoprotein structure, the **envelope,** which surrounds the capsid.

      b. Symmetry can be **helical, icosahedral** (20-sided polygon), or **complex.**

    3. Viral replication can occur only in living cells and involves many host-cell enzymes and functions. The steps of replication are as follows.

      a. Attachment or adsorption occurs when the virion comes in contact with the host cell.

      b. Penetration occurs when the virus passes through the plasma membrane.

        (1) Enveloped viruses penetrate via **fusion.**

        (2) Naked viruses can penetrate transversely. **Pinocytosis** is the process of pinching through the plasma membrane, which results in viruses entering within cytoplasmic vacuoles.

      c. Uncoating is typically mediated by cellular proteases and results in the separation of the capsid from the viral genome.

      d. Synthesis of early proteins. These proteins are involved in genome replication.

      e. Synthesis of late proteins. These proteins are used in the development of structural components of the virion.

      f. Assembly is the packaging of the new copies of the genome nucleic acid into the capsid proteins.

    g. Release or egress of the progeny virus is the final step. The lipid envelope is acquired along with the glycoproteins as the progeny viral nucleocapsid buds through the membrane.

B. Specimen collection, transport, and processing

  1. Time of collection. Specimens for viral identification are best collected during the time of **first presentation of symptoms.**

    a. Virus titers (concentration of virus) are usually highest in the early part of the illness.

    b. Serologically, **a fourfold rise** in the antibody titer between acute and convalescent sera has been used to identify a particular infectious agent as the cause of a recent disease.

  2. Viral culture. The type of viral illness and the disease symptoms influence the specimens of choice for viral culture. Viral specimens are typically divided into nonsterile sites and sterile sites.

    a. Nonsterile sites include the following:

      (1) Conjunctival

      (2) Skin (e.g., mouth, lips)

      (3) Vesicular

      (4) Nasal (aspirates or washes)

      (5) Throat/upper respiratory tract

      (6) Sputum

      (7) Urine

      (8) Genital (cervical, penile)

      (9) Stool/rectal swab

    b. Sterile sites include the following:

      (1) Autopsy

      (2) Biopsy

      (3) CSF

      (4) Fine needle aspirate

      (5) Blood

      (6) Bronchial alveolar (wash)

      (7) Pleural fluid

  3. The **procedure for specimen collection** is vital for recovery of the infectious virus.

    a. Specimens collected with a **dacron or rayon swab** (cotton swabs are not recommended for collection of viral samples because they are toxic to viruses) must not dry out during transport. The swab can be placed in a **modified Stuart transport medium** for transport to the laboratory.

    b. Nonsterile specimens that are not liquid, vesicular fluid, fine needle aspirates, or tissue biopsy specimens should be collected into **viral transport media** such as Hanks' balanced salt solution, 0.2 M sucrose-phosphate, or 2% fetal calf serum with Eagle's minimum essential medium. Some transport mediums contain the following ingredients:

      (1) Antibiotics to inhibit growth of normal bacterial or fungal flora

      (2) Gelatin media to stabilize protein

    c. Urine for viral culture should not be collected into containers with preservatives.

    d. Blood for viral culture should be collected into heparin or ethylenediamine tetra-acetic acid tubes.

    e. Stool specimens for viral culture should be collected into a clean container.

4. All specimens submitted for viral recovery regardless of source should be **transported** at refrigerated temperatures **(0°C–4°C).**

5. If the inoculation of the specimen into tissue culture media will **exceed 5 days,** the specimen should be quickly frozen at **−70°C.**

6. Tissue culture is the inoculation of patient specimens into cells to determine the growth of a viral agent.

    a. Cells derived directly from the donor (animal or human sources) are known as **primary cultures.**

        (1) Primary rabbit kidney is the first choice for herpes simplex viruses types 1 and 2.

        (2) Primary monkey kidney is the first choice for the following viruses:

            (a) Influenza types A and B

            (b) Parainfluenza viruses types 1, 2, and 3

            (c) Mumps

            (d) Measles

            (e) Rubella

            (f) Enteroviruses

        (3) Primary human embryonic kidney is the first choice for the following viruses:

            (a) Parainfluenza virus

            (b) Measles

            (c) Rubella

            (d) Adenoviruses

            (e) Rhinoviruses

            (f) Herpes simplex viruses types 1 and 2

            (g) Varicella zoster

    b. Cell lines are primary cultures that have been subcultured.

        (1) Cell lines that have at least 75% of the cells with a normal chromosome complement are referred to as **diploid** (e.g., diploid human fibroblast cell line). Diploid cell lines usually die after 30–50 passages. The choices for culturing cytomegalovirus (CMV) are WI-38, MRC-5, or IMR-90.

        (2) Cell lines that have a predominance of cells containing an abnormal number of chromosomes are designated as **heteroploid.** Typically, these cell lines are **continuous,** that is, they have an indefinite number of passages.

            (a) A549 cells, which are derived from a human lung carcinoma, are used to culture adenoviruses and varicella zoster.

            (b) HEp-2 cells, which are derived from a human laryngeal carcinoma, are used to culture respiratory syncytial virus (RSV) and adenoviruses.

(c) HeLa cells, which are derived from a human cervical adenocarcinoma, are used to culture RSV, rhinoviruses, and adenoviruses.

c. **Order of inoculation.** The diploid cell lines are inoculated first. The continuous cell lines are inoculated second. The primary cells are inoculated last.

d. **Viral adsorption** refers to the time point when the virus comes in contact with the tissue culture cells.

   (1) **Stationary adsorption** is the procedure of simply incubating the cell and virus for 30–60 minutes at 35°C.

   (2) The **roller drum method** refers to the gentle rotation of the culture tubes to enhance adsorption.

   (3) The **low-speed centrifugation method** requires that shell vials be centrifuged at 750 to 1000 × g for 30–40 minutes at 25°C.

e. **Viral detection** in the culture cells depends on virus replication in the cells. Virus may be detected by observing a **characteristic cytopathogenic effect,** such as swelling or inclusions.

7. **Direct examination** of clinical specimens for the presence of viral pathogens can be done by immunohistochemical staining, nucleic acid hybridization, or solid-phase immunoassay.

   a. **Immunohistochemical staining** uses fixed or fresh specimens incubated with chemically labeled (fluorescein) or enzymatically labeled (peroxidase) antibodies to detect viral antigens.

   b. **Nucleic acid hybridization** involves the detection of viral DNA or RNA sequences in nucleic acid extracted from specimens.

      (1) **Polymerase chain reaction** is a technique that allows the viral genes to be amplified to enhance detection.

      (2) **The Western blot (dot blot)** is a technique that employs single-stranded, complementary nucleic acid probes for detection of human immunodeficiency virus (HIV) in the blood of seronegative individuals.

   c. **Solid-phase immunoassays** use antibodies and radioimmunoassay or enzyme-linked immunosorbent assay (ELISA) to detect viral antigens.

D. **DNA viruses**

   1. The **naked DNA viruses** with an **icosahedral** symmetry are the *Parvoviridae, Papovaviridae, Adenoviridae,* and *Hepadnaviridae.*

      a. *Parvoviridae.* Parvovirus B19 is spread by close physical contact. It causes **erythema infectiosum,** or fifth disease.

      b. *Papovaviridae* have two significant genera, papillomavirus and papovavirus.

         (1) **Human papillomavirus** causes **warts** in humans and is associated with some genital cancers.

         (2) **Polyomavirus** produces histologically diverse tumors in various parts of the body.

      c. *Adenoviridae* have more than 35 serotypes of adenovirus. This virus causes infection of the respiratory tract (nasopharyngitis); the eye (keratoconjunctivitis); and the intestines (e.g., diarrhea, vomiting).

      d. *Hepadnaviridae* have a tropism for infection of the liver.

       (1) Hepatitis B virus is also known as serum hepatitis and chronic hepatitis.

         (a) Transmission of the virus is through the **parenteral route** (e.g., intravenous drug abuse and contaminated blood products) and **sexual intercourse.**

       (2) Hepatitis surface antigen (HBsAg) is present in early disease; anti-HBsAg indicates immunity.

2. The **enveloped DNA** virus with **icosahedral symmetry** is the *Herpesviridae,* which has three medically significant subfamilies: *Alphaherpesvirinae, Betaherpesvirinae,* and *Gammaherpesvirinae.* All have the ability to become **latent** after the primary infection.

  a. Within the group of *Alphaherpesvirinae* are herpes simplex 1 (HSV-1), herpes simplex 2 (HSV-2), and varicella zoster virus.

    (1) HSV-1 is usually seen on the lips or skin or as an eye lesion. It may be diagnosed by the Tzanck cell test.

    (2) HSV-2 affects the genital or lips area and is frequently transmitted sexually.

      (a) Neonatal herpes is a severe disease of the newborn caused by contact with the virus during passage through an infected birth canal.

      (b) HSV-2 disease can be primary or recurrent.

    (3) Varicella zoster virus causes a primary disease (chickenpox) and a recurrent disease (shingles).

      (a) Chickenpox is a mild, self-limiting, highly infectious disease that occurs mainly in children.

      (b) Shingles (or zoster) is caused by the reactivation of varicella zoster virus that has been latent in the neurons. Severely painful vesicles form on the trunk area.

  b. The significant viral pathogen in the *Betaherpesvirinae* is CMV.

    (1) CMV is typically an inapparent disease of childhood. In immunosuppressed patients, CMV can cause a generalized disease.

    (2) If CMV infection occurs in the uterus or soon after birth, it may cause fetal or infant death.

  c. The viral pathogen in the *Gammaherpesvirinae* group is the **Epstein-Barr virus (EBV).** EBV may cause **infectious mononucleosis** (IM) and is associated with **Burkitt's lymphoma.**

    (1) IM, or "kissing disease," produces **atypical lymphocytes** and immunoglobulin (IgM) **heterophile antibodies** that are detected by the monospot test.

    (2) Burkitt's lymphoma patients have elevated titers of EBV antibodies.

  d. The **human herpes virus type 6** causes a common **exanthem disease** (roseola infantum), or sixth disease.

3. The *Poxviridae* are **naked DNA** viruses with a **complex** symmetry. They include the human viruses vaccinia, variola, and molluscum contagiosum.

  a. Vaccinia is a variant of the variola virus and produces a mild disease. Vaccinia is used as the immunogen in smallpox vaccination.

    b. The **variola** virus is the causative agent of smallpox, a disease that the World Health Organization presumes to be eradicated.

    c. Molluscum contagiosum causes small wart-like lesions on the face, arms, buttocks, and genitals.

        (1) This virus can cause a disease that mimics genital herpes.

        (2) M. contagiosum forms eosinophilic inclusion bodies in infected cells.

E. RNA viruses

  1. The **enveloped RNA** viruses with **helical** symmetry are the *Orthomyxoviridae, Paramyxoviridae, Arenaviridae, Rhabdoviridae, Coronaviridae,* and *Bunyaviridae.*

    a. The **orthomyxoviruses** have a hemagglutinin, a neuraminidase, and a matrix protein associated with the envelope.

        (1) The **influenza viruses** are classified as types A, B, and C.

            (a) Types A and B are responsible for the epidemics of respiratory tract infections.

            (b) Reye's syndrome is associated with **influenza type B.**

            (c) Influenza is diagnosed by viral isolation or the hemagglutination inhibition test.

        (2) Antigenic drift is caused by a minor mutation in the hemagglutinin glycoprotein that leads to yearly epidemics.

        (3) Antigenic shift is caused by a major shift in the hemagglutinin glycoprotein that leads to intermittent pandemics.

    b. *Paramyxoviridae* are divided into three genera: paramyxoviruses, morbilliviruses, and pneumoviruses.

        (1) The **paramyxoviruses** are associated with the parainfluenza and mumps viruses.

            (a) Parainfluenza virus causes croup in infants.

            (b) The **mumps** virus results in a generalized disease associated with enlargement of the parotid glands.

        (2) The **morbillivirus** is associated with the **measles** virus and causes a maculopapular rash, fever, and **Koplik's spots** on the buccal mucosa.

        (3) The **pneumovirus** responsible for bronchiolitis and pneumonia in infants is RSV. RSV is rapidly diagnosed by demonstration of viral antigens in nasal washings with fluorescent antibody or immunohistochemical techniques.

    c. The *Arenaviridae* are not typically encountered in the United States. Included in this family are the **hemorrhagic fevers** (e.g., Junin, Machupo, and Lassa viruses) and the flu-like illness caused by the lymphocytic choriomeningitis virus.

    d. Rhabdoviruses are bullet-shaped viruses associated with the human pathogenic **rabies virus** and bovine **vesicular stomatitis virus (VSV).**

        (1) The rabies virus produces a fatal disease following inoculation by an **animal bite** or, occasionally, by inhalation.

            (a) The rabies virus produces specific cytoplasmic inclusion bodies called **Negri bodies** in infected cells.

            (b) Postexposure prophylaxis consists of passive immunization with human rabies immune globulin.

(c) **Diagnosis** is verified by biopsies from skin, cornea impressions, or postmortem examination of brain tissue.

(2) VSV is a mild disease associated with cattle.

e. The **coronaviruses** are the second most frequent cause of the common cold and have been implicated in infant gastroenteritis. These viruses typically are not diagnosed in the laboratory.

f. Members of the family ***Bunyaviridae*** are Hanta virus, LaCrosse virus, and California virus.

(1) The **Hanta virus** has been associated with severe life-threatening respiratory tract infections in the southwestern United States. Transmission has been through exposure to infected **deer mice droppings.**

(2) The **California** and **LaCrosse viruses** produce an encephalitis, mainly in the Mississippi and Ohio River Valleys. Transmission is via an infected mosquito bite.

2. The **enveloped RNA** viruses with **icosahedral** symmetry are *Togaviridae, Flaviviridae,* and *Retroviridae.*

a. The two medically significant genera in the ***Togaviridae*** are the alphavirus and the rubivirus.

(1) The **alphaviruses** are **arboviruses** with mosquito vectors and animal reservoirs, such as:

(a) Eastern equine encephalitis

(b) Western equine encephalitis

(c) Venezuelan equine encephalitis

(2) The significant **rubivirus** is the **rubella virus,** which causes **German measles,** a systemic infection characterized by lymphadenopathy and a morbilliform rash.

(a) The rubella virus can produce congenital infections that can cause severe birth defects.

(b) Diagnosis is by a serologic test for IgM antibodies.

b. The ***Flaviviridae*** include the dengue virus, hepatitis C, St. Louis encephalitis virus, and yellow fever virus.

(1) **Dengue virus** is an arbovirus transmitted by mosquitoes.

(2) **Hepatitis C** virus, also known as **non-A, non-B** virus, causes 90% of the hepatitis cases associated with blood transfusion or infected blood products.

(3) **St. Louis encephalitis virus** is an arbovirus transmitted by mosquitoes.

(4) **Yellow fever** virus is an arbovirus transmitted by mosquitoes.

c. The ***Retroviridae*** contain a **reverse transcriptase enzyme**—RNA–dependent DNA polymerase. This family is classified into three genera: lentiviruses, spumaviruses, and oncoviruses.

(1) The **lentivirus** genus contains HIV-1 and HIV-2, which are the causative agents of **AIDS.**

(a) **Transmission** is through sexual intercourse, intravenous drug use, or transplacental from mother to child.

(b) AIDS is preceded by **AIDS-related complex,** which is characterized by anorexia.

       (c) **Full-blown AIDS** is characterized by Kaposi's sarcoma, *Pneumocystis carinii* pneumonia, CMV, and AIDS-related dementia.

       (d) Diagnosis is by **ELISA** and is confirmed with the **Western blot** test.

    (2) **Human T-cell leukemia virus I** (HTLV-I) is classified within the Type C **oncoviruses.**

       (a) HTLV-I causes a neurologic degenerating disease.

       (b) Transmission is the same as for HIV.

       (c) **Long-term effects** include debilitation and paralysis.

3. The **naked RNA viruses** with **icosahedral** symmetry are *Picornaviridae* and *Reoviridae.*

  a. The medically significant **picornaviruses** are classified as enteroviruses or rhinoviruses.

    (1) The **enteroviruses** include the polioviruses, coxsackievirus types A and B, echoviruses, enteroviruses, and the hepatitis A virus.

       (a) The **poliovirus** can cause a mild illness, aseptic meningitis, or **poliomyelitis** (poliovirus types 1, 2, or 3).

         (i) Spinal cord motor neurons are killed, and flaccid paralysis results.

         (ii) Diagnosis is through serologic testing or cultivation of the virus from throat culture or feces.

       (b) **Coxsackievirus type A** infections are associated with the following diseases: hand-foot-and-mouth disease, hemorrhagic conjuctivitis, aseptic meningitis, and colds.

       (c) **Coxsackievirus type B** infections are associated with the following diseases: herpangina, viral heart disease, and Bornholm disease (pleurodynia).

       (d) **Echovirus** primarily infects the enteric tract but can cause a range of diseases from the common cold to meningitis and hemorrhagic conjunctivitis.

       (e) **Enterovirus** infections are associated with respiratory tract infections, central nervous system disease, and hemorrhagic conjunctivitis.

       (f) **Hepatitis A** virus (HAV) is also referred to as **infectious hepatitis.**

         (i) Transmission is via the **fecal-oral route.**

         (ii) Infections can cause epidemics.

         (iii) HAV is diagnosed serologically by a rise in IgM as detected by ELISA.

    (2) The **rhinoviruses** are the most frequent cause of the **common cold.** More than 100 serotypes exist.

  b. The primary pathogen in the *Reovirus* group is the rotavirus, which is the primary cause of **acute infantile diarrhea.** Diagnosis is by demonstration of virus in the stool or by serologic testing (e.g., ELISA).

F. Chlamydia

  1. Chlamydia are **obligate intracellular parasites** that resemble gram-negative bacteria.

    a. The **elementary body** is the infectious form.

     b. The **reticular body** is the intracellular reproductive form.

  2. The medically significant species are *Chlamydia psittacci* and *Chlamydia trachomatis.*

     a. *C. psittaci* causes a wide spectrum of human respiratory tract diseases associated with birds.

     b. *C. trachomatis*

        (1) **Subtypes A, B, and C** cause **keratoconjunctivitis,** which can lead to conjunctival and corneal scarring.

        (2) **Subtypes D to K** cause nongonococcal urethritis , which is a sexually transmitted disease.

        (3) **Subtype L** causes a sexually transmitted disease called **lymphogranuloma venereum.**

  3. **Diagnosis** is based on clinical symptoms or the presence of **elementary bodies in exudates.**

G. Rickettsia

  1. Rickettsia are **intracellular** bacteria that cause zoonotic diseases in which arthropods are vectors of human disease.

  2. The four relevant species are *R. prowazekii, R. typhi, R. rickettsii,* and *R. akari.*

     a. **Epidemic typhis** is transmitted by lice and caused by *R. prowazekii.*

     b. **Endemic typhus,** also called **murine typhus,** is transmitted by rat fleas and caused by *R. typhi.*

     c. **Rocky mountain spotted fever** is transmitted by the tick and is caused by *R. rickettsii.*

     d. **Rickettsial pox** is carried by mites and is caused by *R. akari.*

  3. **Q fever** is transmitted by inhalation of infected dust or ticks and is caused by *Coxiella burnettii.*

  4. **Diagnosis** is determined by comparing acute and convalescent sera, using agglutination reactions, and cross-reacting *Proteus vulgaris* antigens.

Study Questions

Directions: Each of the numbered items or incomplete statements in this section is followed by answers or by completions of the statement. Select the ONE lettered answer or completion that is BEST in each case.

1. The cellophane tape preparation for the recovery of parasitic ova is most frequently used to aid in the identification of which one of the following organisms?

a. *Giardia lamblia*
b. *Onchocerca volvulus*
c. *Enterobius vermicularis*
d. *Entamoeba histolytica*

2. Banana-shaped or crescent-shaped gametocytes are present in human infections with which one of the following organisms?

a. *Plasmodium vivax*
b. *Plasmodium ovale*
c. *Plasmodium malariae*
d. *Plasmodium falciparum*

3. The finding of ingested red blood cells (RBCs) in the cytoplasm of a trophozoite is presumptive evidence that the organism is

a. *Dientamoeba fragilis*
b. *Trichomonas vaginalis*
c. *Giardia lamblia*
d. *Entamoeba histolytica*

4. Which one of the following filariae is referred to as the African eyeworm?

a. *Brugia malayi*
b. *Loa loa*
c. *Onchocerca volvulus*
d. *Wuchereria bancrofti*

5. Which one of the following diseases is a subcutaneous fungal disease characterized by swelling of the sinus tracts and the presence of sulfur granules?

a. sporotrichosis
b. eumycotic mycetoma
c. coccidioidomycosis
d. histoplasmosis

6. The tissue form of which one of the following organisms is a large yeast with a thick cell wall and broad-based buds?

a. *Blastomyces dermatitidis*
b. *Aspergillus fumigatus*
c. *Histoplasma capsulatum*
d. *Sporothrix schenckii*

7. Tinea versicolor is caused by which one of the following organisms?

a. *Candida albicans*
b. *Microsporum gypseum*
c. *Epidermophyton floccosum*
d. *Malassezia furfur*

8. Which one of the following organisms is a dimorphic fungi that grows well on brain-heart infusion agar with blood and has a mold phase that is a large tuberculate macroconidia?

a. *Blastomyces dermatitidis*
b. *Histoplasma capsulatum*
c. *Cryptococcus neoformans*
d. *Sporothrix schenckii*

9. Which one of the following diseases results from traumatic implantation of a fungal spore on a limb and produces cauliflower-like lesions?

a. sporotrichosis
b. eumycotic mycetoma
c. chromoblastomycoses
d. histoplasmosis

10. A specimen for viral culture is collected on Friday and must be held for processing until the following Thursday. What would be the optimal temperature for holding this specimen?

a. 35°C
b. −70°C
c. 4°C
d. 25°C

11. The influenza viruses vary from year to year, producing epidemics. This variation is a result of

a. antigenic drift
b. antigenic shift
c. gene splicing
d. gene mutation

Directions: Each of the numbered items or incomplete statements in this section is negatively phrased, as indicated by a capitalized word such as NOT, LEAST, or EXCEPT. Select the ONE lettered answer or completion that is BEST in each case.

12. The zinc sulfate flotation method is inappropriate for all of the following parasitic forms EXCEPT

a. operculated eggs
b. schistosomes
c. infertile ascaris eggs
d. oocysts

13. All of the following are methods of viral penetration EXCEPT

a. fusion
b. egress
c. pinocytosis
d. transverse

14. All of the following statements concerning *Diphyllobothrium latum* are correct EXCEPT

a. the adult worm scolex has a crown of hooks
b. the eggs hatch into a ciliated form that is ingested by copepods
c. the adult worm has a uterus with a unique rosette morphology
d. humans obtain the parasite by ingesting raw fish

Answers and Explanations

1. The answer is c [I D 2]. The cellophane tape preparation is useful for diagnosis of *Enterobius vermicularis* because typically the eggs are not observed in the feces.

2. The answer is d [I B 2]. *Plasmodium falciparum* gametocytes are elongated or banana-shaped compared to the ovoid morphology of the other *Plasmodium*. This is sometimes referred to as a crescent shape.

3. The answer is d [I B 1; Figure 9-1]. The *Entamoeba histolytica* trophozoite is 10–20 mm and contains ingested red blood cells (RBCs). The other species of *Entamoeba* do not ingest RBCs.

4. The answer is b [I D 13]. *Loa loa* is the African eyeworm. It is transmitted by the *Chrysops* (fly) and produces calabar swellings.

5. The answer is b [II I 2]. Eumycotic mycetoma is characterized by swelling sinus tract formation and the presence of sulfur granules. The most common cause of mycetoma in the United States is *Pseudoallescheria boydii*, which is the sexual stage of *Scedosporium apiospermum*.

6. The answer is a [II F 2]. *Blastomyces dermatitidis* in the tissue phase (37°C) produces a yeast with broad-based buds.

7. The answer is d [II E 3, G 1]. *Malassezia furfur* causes pityriasis (tinea) versicolor. The fungi requires a media that is rich with a lipid source, such as olive oil.

8. The answer is b [II F 1]. *Histoplasma capsulatum* is a dimorphic fungi that in the mold phase (25°C) produces a large tuberculate macroconidia. This form is found in soil enriched with bat or bird guano.

9. The answer is c [II I 3]. Chromoblastomycoses is an infection caused by the dematiaceous fungi *Phialophora*, *Fonsecaea*, or *Cladosporium*.

10. The answer is b [III B 5]. If the inoculation of the specimen into tissue culture media will exceed 5 days, the specimen should be quickly frozen at −70°C.

11. The answer is a [III E 1 a (2)]. Antigenic drift is caused by a minor mutation in the hemagglutinin glycoprotein that leads to yearly epidemics.

12. The answer is d [I E 2 c (2)]. The zinc sulfate flotation method is recommended for the recovery of oocysts, but is not recommended for the recovery of operculated eggs, schistosomes, and infertile ascaris eggs.

13. The answer is b [III A 3 b]. Penetration occurs when the virus traverses the plasma membrane or passes through by fusion or pinocytosis.

14. The answer is a [I C 2 a (1)]. The adult worm scolex of *Diphyllobothrium latum* is elongated, spoon-shaped, and has two longitudinal grooves.

10

Urinalysis and Body Fluids

Joel D. Hubbard
Sally Becker

I. THE URINARY SYSTEM

A. Structure and function

1. **Components** (Figure 10-1). The urinary system consists of two bean-shaped **kidneys;** the **ureters,** which carry urine into the **bladder** for storage; and the **urethra,** which transports urine outside the body.

2. **Kidneys.** Each kidney weighs approximately 150 g and measures 5 cm by 12 cm.

   a. **Structure**

   (1) Each kidney contains 1–1.5 million **nephrons,** which are the functional units of the kidney (Figure 10-2). A nephron is composed of the **glomerulus,** the filtering unit, and the **renal tubules,** which are 30–40 mm in length.

   (a) The **glomerulus** is made up of a tuft of blood vessels (i.e., plexus) formed from the **afferent** (entering) and **efferent** (exiting) arterioles.

   (b) The **renal tubules** include **Bowman's (glomerular) capsule,** the **proximal convoluted tubule,** the **loop of Henle,** and the **distal convoluted tubule.**

   (2) The **cortex** contains the **glomerulus** and the **proximal convoluted tubules.**

   (3) The **medulla** consists of the **loop of Henle,** the **distal convoluted tubules,** and the **collecting tubules.**

   (4) The **calyx** is the area where the collecting tubules come together and empty freshly formed urine into the **renal pelvis.** From there, the urine flows into the **ureters,** then to the bladder.

   b. **Function.** The kidneys maintain homeostasis by regulating body fluids, acid-base balance, and electrolyte balance. They also excrete waste products and help to maintain blood pressure and erythropoiesis.

B. Urine formation. In an adult, urine volume ranges from 400–2000 mL per day.

1. **Overview.** Approximately 1200 mL of blood per minute (i.e., 20%–25% of the blood volume) is supplied to the kidneys through the renal artery, which branches into the afferent arterioles and efferent arterioles.

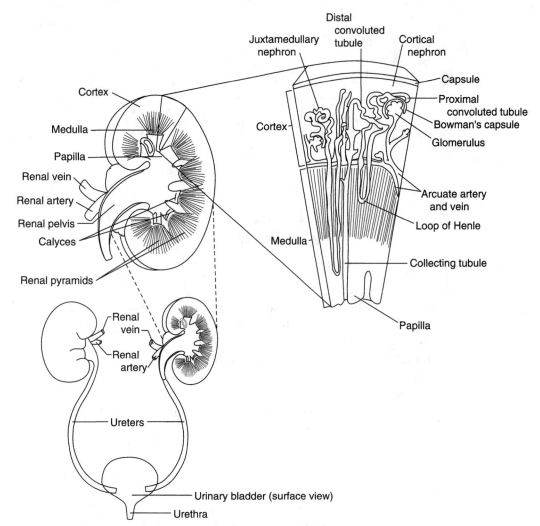

Figure 10-1. Structure and components of the urinary system. (Reprinted with permission from Strasinger SK: *Urinalysis and Body Fluids.* Philadelphia, F.A. Davis, 1989, p 14.)

a. **Glomerular filtration** is accomplished through the thin walls of the afferent and efferent arterioles. The difference in the size of the lumen of these two vessels produces an increase in the hydrostatic pressure within these capillaries. This pressure increase forces the **filtrate** through the thin capillary epithelium and into the space of **Bowman's capsule,** which surrounds the glomerulus.

(1) The glomerulus functions as a **sieve** or filter. The capillaries retain blood cells and serum proteins, whereas smaller molecules (e.g., ions, amino acids, glucose, urea, creatinine, uric acid, ammonia, or dissolved solutes with a molecular weight less than 70,000) and water filter into **Bowman's space.**

(2) Approximately 20% of the volume of plasma (i.e., 120 mL/min) that passes through the glomerular tuft is caught in Bowman's space and is called the **glomerular filtrate.** At this point, the filtrate is

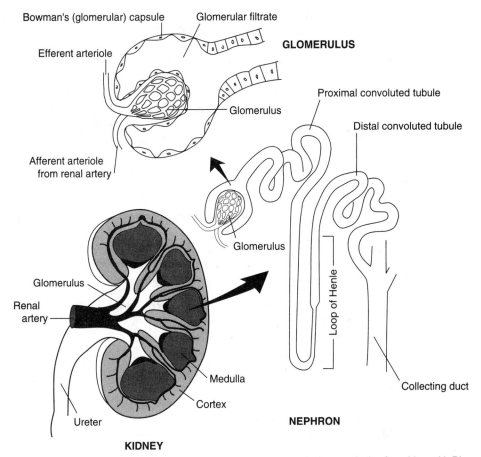

Figure 10-2. Structure of the nephron and the glomerulus. (Reprinted with permission from Linne JJ, Ringsrud KM: *Basic techniques in clinical laboratory science,* ed 3, St. Louis, 1992, Mosby, p. 320.)

iso-osmotic with plasma and is called an **ultrafiltrate.** It has a **specific gravity of 1.010 +/−0.002** and a **pH of 7.4.**

(3) The ultrafiltrate then passes into the **tubular system,** which consists of the proximal convoluted tubule, the loop of Henle, and the distal convoluted tubule.

b. **Cellular transport mechanisms.** Obviously, the body cannot lose 120 mL of water and essential substances every minute. Thus, when the ultrafiltrate enters the **proximal convoluted tubule (PCT),** cellular transport mechanisms begin to **reabsorb essential substances and water.** Cellular mechanisms involved in tubular reabsorption can be **active** or **passive.**

(1) **Active transport** occurs when substances to be reabsorbed combine with a carrier protein contained in the membranes of the renal tubular cells. Electrochemical energy produced by this interaction transfers the substance across the cell membrane back into the bloodstream. Substances reabsorbed by active transport are: **glu-**

cose, amino acids, and salts in the PCT; chloride in the ascending loop of Henle; and sodium in the distal convoluted tubules.

(2) **Passive transport** moves molecules across a membrane based on physical differences, concentration, or electrical potential. **The ascending loop of Henle is impermeable to water;** therefore, passive reabsorption of **water** takes place in all other parts of the nephron. **Urea** is passively reabsorbed in the PCT and the ascending loop of Henle. **Sodium** is passively reabsorbed in the ascending loop of Henle.

C. **Normal constituents of urine**

1. **Urine** is continuously formed by the kidneys. Depending on dietary intake, physical activity, body metabolism, and endocrine function, concentrations of normal urine constituents vary.

   a. **Urea** normally accounts for half of the total dissolved solids in urine (6–18 g/24 h). It is a metabolic waste product that results from the breakdown of protein and amino acids by the liver.

   b. Other organic compounds in urine are **creatinine** (0.3–0.8 g/24 h) and **uric acid** (0.08–0.2 g/24 h). A fluid can be identified as urine if it contains a high concentration of **urea** and **creatinine.**

   c. **Chloride** (100–250 mEq/24 h) is the major inorganic solid dissolved in urine, followed by **sodium** (100–200 mEq/24 h) and **potassium** (50–70 mEq/24 h).

2. A small amount of **protein,** mainly albumin, is normally excreted (150 mg/d). **Urobilinogen** is normally present at a concentration of 1 mg/dL [i.e., 1 Ehrlich unit (EU)].

3. In the urinary sediment, it is normal to find a **few squamous, transitional, and renal epithelial cells** per high-power field (40X) as well as **one to two red blood cells** (RBCs) or **one to five white blood cells (WBCs). Mucus and one to two hyaline casts** per low-power field are common. **Sperm cells** can be normally found in a urine specimen from a female but not a male. Amorphous **urate** and **phosphate crystals** are common, especially in refrigerated specimens.

II. THE URINE SPECIMEN

A. **Routine urinalysis** describes a series of screening tests that are capable of **detecting a variety of renal, urinary tract,** and **systemic diseases.** Urine is readily available and easy to collect.

1. When there is **disease of the kidney or bladder,** kidney function may be impaired. Substances that are normally retained by the kidney may be excreted, and substances that are normally excreted may be retained. The routine urinalysis is a good screening test for the detection of abnormally excreted substances.

2. **Metabolic or systemic diseases** may lead to the excretion of substances such as abnormal amounts of metabolic end products or substances specific for a particular disease that can be detected in urine.

3. All body fluid specimens should be considered **infectious** and collected, transported, and handled according to safety protocols.

4. Urine specimens should be **analyzed within 1 hour of collection,** or they must be stored in a dark refrigerator between 4°C and 7°C to preserve chemical and cellular constituents.

B. **Quality control in urinalysis**

1. **Definition.** Quality control is a **system for monitoring analytic testing to ensure the reliability or accuracy of each measurement performed** on a patient specimen. Quality control procedures detect analytic or technical errors during analysis as well as defects in the reagents or equipment to prevent reporting of incorrect patient results or values.

2. **Monitoring.** Analytic methods are monitored by **analyzing control material** (i.e., substances with constant concentrations) and then comparing the observed values with the known or expected values for the control. The control material is analyzed exactly like the patient sample for the particular testing procedure.

   a. **Numeric or qualitative limits** are determined for each control. When tested, they must fall within the control limits to ensure that the analytic system is functioning properly.

   b. Every testing method has a characteristic inherent variability. Thus, a **control has a mean value ± two standard deviations,** which is the 95% confidence limit of parametric statistics.

3. **Each day that a method is performed, quality control material must be analyzed.** This is a regular responsibility of clinical laboratory scientists. The quality control material can be a frozen pooled sample, commercially available lyophilized pooled material, or commercially available paper strips that are placed in a tube of distilled water and mixed for a period of time to suspend the control material into a solution for testing.

   a. It is important to **follow the manufacturer's instructions** when preparing and using quality control material.

   b. The control should be labeled with the **date of preparation,** its **expiration date,** and the **initials of the person who prepared the control material.**

   c. The control material is analyzed as a **"known"** substance during the testing of **"unknown"** patient samples.

   d. Two to three different levels of control substances are usually tested.

      (1) A **normal** control contains constituents at concentrations within nondisease reference ranges.

      (2) An **abnormal** control contains analytic constituents at concentrations outside of the reference range.

   e. A **three-level control system** usually contains a low, normal, and high reference range when medically significant decisions are made at each level.

   f. **The clinical laboratory scientist must assure that the control material has validated the testing procedure before any patient values are reported.**

g. This data should be **permanently recorded** with the date and name of the clinical laboratory scientist who has done the testing as well as an interpretation of the data (e.g., "in control" or "out of control").

4. In the urinalysis laboratory, the first quality control measure is to **assure the identity and proper collection and handling of the submitted specimen.**

    a. Proper performance of the refractometer or other **specific gravity method, dipsticks** for chemical testing, and any **confirmatory testing** methods must be compared with quality control materials. The results must be recorded.

    b. All controls and reagents have a **lot number** and **expiration date. No reagents or controls are used past their expiration dates,** even if they seem to be functioning properly.

    c. Any reagent that looks unusual or reacts outside of the reference or control range should not be used.

    d. Whenever a reagent is opened for the first time, the **date and initials of the person** placing the control or reagent in use must appear on the container.

    e. All **lot numbers** and **expiration dates** are recorded on the quality control record.

5. **Dipsticks,** which are plastic strips impregnated with chemicals for reagent strip testing, are subject to deterioration caused by **moisture, heat, or light exposure.** Dipsticks are packaged in opaque containers that contain a desiccant. They should be **stored in a cool, dry place** and checked each day of use with at least two levels of a control material.

    a. Strips that are brown or discolored indicate that there has been contamination.

    b. The container should be recapped promptly after removing the number of strips needed for immediate testing.

    c. The chemical testing areas should not be touched.

    d. The strip should be dipped into a well-mixed specimen (control or patient) to moisten all test areas. The strip should be removed promptly, drawing it along the edge of the urine container to remove excess urine, and placing it horizontally on a clean piece of paper. Excessive dipping or keeping the strip vertical can cause the reagents from one area to flow into another.

    e. The strip should be held close to the color chart on the container when the technician is reading results, and observations should be made in a well-lit area.

    f. Whenever a **new container of strips or a new control** is opened, the dipstick strips should be tested with the control material. All lot numbers and expiration dates should be recorded.

    g. Any **questionable reactions** with the dipsticks should be checked with the confirmatory tests. Interfering substances in the urine specimen or improper technique can lead to inaccurate results.

h. The clinical laboratory scientist should be aware of the limitations and interfering substances for each dipstick reaction.

6. To check the function of the **refractometer,** the specific gravity of **distilled water** (reference range, 1.000 ± 0.001), **5% NaCl** (1.022 ± 0.001), **3% NaCl** (1.015 ± 0.001), **9% sucrose** (1.034 ± 0.001), or other known substances should be measured. The results should be recorded.

   a. The specific gravity of a **normal and abnormal control** substance should be measured and the results recorded.

   b. **Verification should be made** that the results are all in range and that the ranges are for that particular lot of control. The reference ranges will vary from lot to lot.

7. Whenever a **confirmatory test** is performed [e.g., a Clinitest for reducing substances, Ictotest for bilirubin, sulfosalicylic acid (SSA) test for protein], the reagents must be checked with the normal and abnormal quality control material. Results must be recorded and verified as being "in control" before any patient samples can be analyzed.

8. Some commercially available control materials can be used to assess the **microscopic portion of urinalysis** testing. The package insert lists the expected ranges for the elements that should be found in the sediment of the control.

9. If a quality control result is out of control or out of the acceptable limits of the control range, **the problem must be identified and corrected before any patient testing can be performed.**

10. The following steps are useful in identifying problems:

    a. A newly opened bottle of reagent should be tested with the controls. If the new reagent is acceptable, the old reagent can be discarded, and testing can continue with the new reagent.

    b. If the new reagent is also out of the control range, a new control can be opened. If the reactivity is now within range, the old control can be discarded, and testing can continue.

    c. If the reactivity is also out of the control range for the new reagent and the new control, the supervisor should be notified before the work is continued.

    d. All problems and resolutions should be noted in the quality control logbook.

11. In general, the **potential inaccuracies** that may occur in urinalysis testing may be attributed to:

    a. Failure to maintain the identity of a specimen throughout the testing phases

    b. Failure to follow recommended procedures of the laboratory and manufacturer regarding reagents and control material

    c. Failure to use color charts for dipstick and Clinitest testing

    d. Expecting tests based on different methodologies to agree

    e. Lack of good control procedures

C. **Types of urine specimens**

1. To assess a patient's metabolic state, it is often necessary to **regulate certain aspects of urine specimen collection, such as the time, length,** and **method of collection,** as well as the patient's dietary and medicinal intake.

2. Types of urine specimens include: **random, first morning, fractional,** and **timed.**

D. **Methods of collection**

1. The **random specimen** is the most commonly encountered specimen.

   a. To obtain a **random void** specimen, the patient merely voids urine from his/her bladder into a container. The container, usually a 100–200 mL cup, should be sterile in case a bacterial, fungal, or viral culture may be needed. A random specimen may be collected at any time of the day and is an ideal specimen to screen for many abnormalities.

   b. A random midstream **"clean catch,"** in which contamination from the external genitalia and vagina is minimized, is desirable if a bacterial culture is to be performed. Before this specimen is collected, the glans penis of the male or the urethral meatus of the female is thoroughly washed and rinsed. To collect the specimen, the patient begins to void a few milliliters of urine into the toilet, then collects the midstream flow of urine into a sterile container. Any remaining urine is passed into the toilet.

   c. A **catheterized** specimen is obtained after a sterile catheter is inserted through the urethra into the bladder, which allows the urine to flow down the catheter into a collection bag. These specimens can be random or timed. They are used for routine testing and microbial cultures.

   d. A **suprapubic aspiration** involves collecting urine directly from the bladder by puncturing the abdominal wall and entering the bladder with a sterile needle and syringe. The normally sterile urine is aspirated into the syringe and sent to the laboratory for analysis. This specimen can be used to diagnose bacterial infections of the bladder, especially anaerobes, as well as for cytology studies and routine testing. This technique may be used with infants to avoid fecal contamination of the specimen.

2. A **first morning specimen** is collected immediately on arising and should be delivered to the laboratory as quickly as possible. It is used to evaluate orthostatic proteinuria and detect low levels of human chorionic gonadotropin (hCG). Substances are more concentrated in a first morning specimen than in most random specimens because the urine is retained in the bladder overnight.

3. **Fractional specimens** involve at least two voided collections. Most commonly, a series of blood and urine samples are collected at specific time intervals to compare the concentration of a substance in urine with its concentration in blood. This aids in the evaluation of renal threshold values and in the diagnosis of diseases such as diabetes.

4. **Timed collections** enable quantitation of various analytes in urine. Circadian or diurnal variations in the excretion of various substances as well as the effect of exercise, metabolism, and hydration may necessitate collection

of urine specimens at specific times, or for a specific amount of time (usually 2, 12, or 24 hours). **Accurate timing** is essential to ensure valid results. Depending on the substance being measured, a urine preservative, as well as dietary restrictions, may be necessary.

III. PHYSICAL EXAMINATION OF THE URINE

A. **Color and transparency indications in a urine sample** (Table 10-1). Observations of urine color and transparency should always be performed on a **well-mixed, unspun specimen.**

1. **Variations in color.** Urine color can vary from **colorless to black.**

   a. **Normal urine color.** Throughout the day, an individual's normal urine color can be a **pale straw or yellow-amber color to a dark amber color,** depending on the concentration of the urine. High fluid intake results in a dilute urine, which is pale in color. Darker urine results from reduced fluid intake. Normal urine color is produced by the presence of three pigments:

      (1) **Urochrome,** which is a yellow pigment that is present in the highest concentration

      (2) **Uroerythrin,** which is a red pigment

      (3) **Urobilin,** which is an orange-red pigment

   b. **Abnormal urine** color can result from pathologic conditions or normal circumstances, such as medications and diet. Some dyes used to color food may cause changes in normal urine color, as can the ingestion of rhubarb and beets in genetically susceptible individuals.

      (1) **Red or red-brown** is the most commonly seen abnormal urine color. A red color usually indicates the presence of **blood (hematuria)** or **hemoglobin (hemoglobinuria).**

         (a) If this color is seen in the urine of a female, menstrual contamination should be suspected.

         (b) Other causes of a red-colored urine include myoglobin (myoglobinuria), porphyrins (porphyrinuria), food dyes, or ingestion of rhubarb or beets.

      (2) **Dark brown to black** urine can be caused by alkaptonuria or malignant melanoma.

         (a) **Alkaptonuria** is a rare disorder caused by a lack of the enzyme homogentisic acid oxidase. This enzyme is required for the catabolism of tyrosine and phenylalanine. In this disorder, **homogentisic acid** is excreted into the urine. The urine is normal in color when freshly voided but turns black on standing or when alkalinized.

         (b) Patients who have **malignant melanoma** excrete **melanogen** into their urine. On exposure to light, this chromogen is converted to melanin, which is black.

      (3) **Yellow-brown to yellow-green** urine results from the excretion of **bilirubin or bile pigments** into the urine of patients who have **obstructive jaundice.**

2. Urine **appearance, transparency, clarity, or character** indicates the presence of particulate matter.

Table 10-1. Summary of Possible Causes of Urine Color and Appearance

Appearance	Cause	Remarks
Colorless	Very dilute urine	Polyuria; diabetes insipidus
Cloudy	Phosphates, carbonates	Soluble in dilute acetic acid
	Urates, uric acid	Dissolve at 60°C and in alkali
	Leukocytes	Insoluble in dilute acetic acid
	Red blood cells ("smoky")	Lyse in dilute acetic acid
	Bacteria, yeasts	Insoluble in dilute acetic acid
	Spermatozoa	Insoluble in dilute acetic acid
	Prostatic fluid	
	Mucin, mucous threads	May be flocculent
	Calculi, "gravel"	Phosphates, oxalates
	Clumps, pus, tissue	
	Fecal contamination	Rectovesical fistula
	Radiographic dye	In acid urine
Milky	Many neutrophils (pyuria)	Insoluble in dilute acetic acid
	Fat	
	Lipiduria, opalescent	Nephrosis, crush injury—soluble in ether
	Chyluria, milky	Lymphatic obstruction—soluble in ether
	Emulsified paraffin	Vaginal creams
Yellow	Acriflavine	Green fluorescence
Yellow-orange	Concentrated urine	Dehydration, fever
	Urobilin in excess	No yellow foam
	Bilirubin	Yellow foam if sufficient bilirubin
Yellow-green	Bilirubin-biliverdin	Yellow foam
Yellow-brown	Bilirubin-biliverdin	"Beer" brown, yellow foam
Red	Hemoglobin	Positive ⎫
	Erythrocytes	Positive ⎬ reagent strip for blood
	Myoglobin	Positive ⎭
	Porphyrin	May be colorless
	Fuscin, aniline dye	Foods, candy
	Beets	Yellow alkaline, genetic
	Menstrual contamination	Clots, mucus
Red-purple	Porphyrins	May be colorless
Red-brown	Erythrocytes	
	Hemoglobin on standing	
	Methemoglobin	Acid pH
	Myoglobin	Muscle injury
	Bilifuscin (dipyrrole)	Result of unstable hemoglobin
Brown-black	Methemoglobin	Blood, acid pH
	Homogentisic acid	On standing, alkaline; alcaptonuria
	Melanin	On standing, rare
Blue-green	Indicans	Small intestine infections
	Pseudomonas infections	
	Chlorophyll	Mouth deodorants

(Reprinted with permission from Henry JB (ed): *Clinical Diagnosis and Management by Laboratory Methods.* Philadelphia, WB Saunders, 1991, pp 394.)

a. **Normal urine** is essentially clear, although a cloudy urine does not necessarily indicate a pathologic condition.

b. **Turbidity** is often caused by crystal precipitation, referred to as **amorphous** material, when a specimen is refrigerated. Other causes of turbid urine include the presence of bacteria, yeast, WBCs, RBCs, mucus, squamous epithelial cells, spermatozoa and prostatic fluid, or lipids.

B. **Odor indications in a urine sample**

1. **Normal odors.** Urine normally has a **faint, aromatic odor** caused by the presence of volatile acids produced by the ingestion of various foods. **Distinctive** odors may result after ingestion of certain foods (e.g., asparagus, garlic, onions).

2. **Abnormal odors** may indicate pathologic conditions, improper handling, or improper storage of the urine specimen. If allowed to stand, especially unrefrigerated, bacteria in a urine specimen break down urea to form **ammonia.**

    a. **Urinary tract infections.** Large numbers of bacteria present in urine specimens from patients who have urinary tract infections can result in a **putrid, foul** odor.

    b. **Ketone bodies.** Increased ketone bodies excreted by diabetic or young women who are on starvation diets give the urine a **fruity** odor.

    c. **Tubular necrosis.** A **lack of odor** may indicate acute tubular necrosis.

    d. **Amino acid disorders** produce characteristic smelling urines.
       (1) **Phenylketonuria** is associated with a **mousy**-smelling urine.
       (2) **Tyrosinuria** produces a **rancid** odor.
       (3) **Maple syrup urine disease** produces a **maple syrup**-smelling urine.
       (4) **Methionine malabsorption** causes urine to smell like **cabbage or hops.**
       (5) **Isovaleric acid and glutaric acid** in urine give it a **sweaty feet** smell.
       (6) **Trimethylaminuria** makes urine smell like **rotting fish.**

C. **Specific gravity, refractive index, and osmolality** measurements of urine indicate the amount of dissolved solids in urine or its concentration.

1. **Specific gravity** is a measure of the **weight** of a substance compared with an equal volume of pure, solute-free water at the same temperature. **Urine is water that contains dissolved substances, primarily urea, sodium, and chloride.** The specific gravity of urine is a measure of its density, and it is influenced by the number and size of the particles present. Because the specific gravity of water is 1.000, and the specific gravity of urine is compared with it, the number is a ratio and has no units. For urine, the specific gravity is reported to the third decimal place and normally ranges from **1.003–1.035.**

2. Specific gravity reflects the **ability of the kidney to concentrate and dilute urine.** Ordinarily, the specific gravity of urine is inversely proportional to the volume. With disease of the kidney, this ability is lost, and the specific gravity is **fixed at 1.010** (similar to the initial plasma filtrate concentration of the glomerulus) and is termed **isothenuria.**

3. There are **four basic methods for determining the specific gravity** of urine: by **urinometer, refractometer, reagent strip,** and the **falling drop** method.

   a. The **urinometer** is a glass float weighted with mercury, with an air bubble above the weight and a graduated stem on top (Figure 10-3). The weighted float displaces a volume of liquid equal to its weight and is calibrated at a **specific temperature** to sink to a level of 1.000 in distilled water. Dissolved substances in urine provide additional mass that causes the float to displace a smaller volume of urine than distilled water. The specific gravity measurement is read at the bottom of the meniscus on the stem of the urinometer. Urinometry is considered an **inaccurate method** that has four major **disadvantages.**

      (1) A **large volume** of urine (10–20 mL) is required to perform the measurement.

      (2) The measurement may need to be **corrected if the temperature of the urine is not the same as the temperature at which the urinometer was calibrated.**

         (a) **Colder.** If the urine is at a temperature colder than the calibrated temperature, **0.001 must be subtracted** from the reading for **every 3°C** that the urine is lower than the calibrated temperature.

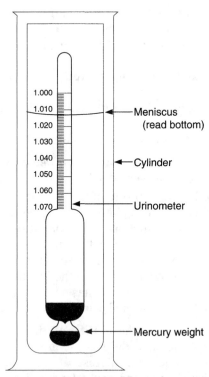

Figure 10-3. Urinometer used to measure specific gravity. (Reprinted with permission from Linne JJ, Ringsrud KM: *Basic techniques in clinical laboratory science,* ed 3, St. Louis, 1992, Mosby, p. 334.)

       (b) Warmer. If the urine is at a temperature higher than the calibrated temperature, **0.001 is added for every 3°C** that the specimen is higher than the calibrated temperature.

    (3) Corrections should be made for the presence of glucose and protein in a specimen.

       (a) Protein. For each gram of protein, 0.003 is subtracted per 100 mL of urine.

       (b) Glucose. For each gram of glucose, 0.004 is subtracted per 100 mL of urine.

    (4) Urinometry is a **time-consuming** procedure.

  b. A **refractometer** measures the **refractive index** of a solution, which is the **ratio of the velocity of light in air to the velocity of light in a solution.** The velocity depends on the number of dissolved particles in the solution and determines the angle at which light passes through the solution. The clinical refractometer measures the angle and mathematically converts this angle to specific gravity, which is read from a scale in the handheld instrument (Figure 10-4). Refractometers should be **calibrated each day of use.** Distilled water and sodium chloride or sucrose solutions of known concentration, as well as commercial controls, should be measured and recorded.

    (1) The major **advantages of the refractometer** method are: a **small volume of specimen** is needed (1–2 drops); **no temperature corrections** are required; it is **simple to operate;** and it gives **rapid, reliable results.**

    (2) Disadvantages include **required corrections for large amounts of glucose and protein,** as with the urinometer, and a scale **reading maximum of 1.035.** Very concentrated specimens or urine samples contaminated with radiographic dyes need to be diluted and remeasured.

  c. Reagent strips can be dipped into urine to measure the concentration of ions. The **results are not identical to specific gravity because not all substances in urine ionize.** Glucose, urea, and radiographic dyes do not contribute to the measurement. Most normal waste constituents of urine do ionize and will be measured.

    (1) Interfering substances. Ketones, which elevate the value, interfere with the reagent strip method. **Highly buffered alkaline urines** decrease the value because the method contains an indicator that changes color when acid groups of the polyelectrolyte on the reagent strip dissociate in proportion to the number of ions in the urine.

    (2) The **disadvantage** of the reagent strip compared with the urinometer and refractometer is that **readings are in 0.005 intervals** and must be **compared to a color chart.** The strips need to be checked each day of use with commercially available control urines and whenever a new container is opened.

  d. The falling drop method is used by most automated urinalysis instruments to assess specific gravity of urine. The instrument measures the **amount of time it takes a drop of urine to fall a fixed distance** through an insolvent liquid and converts this time to specific gravity.

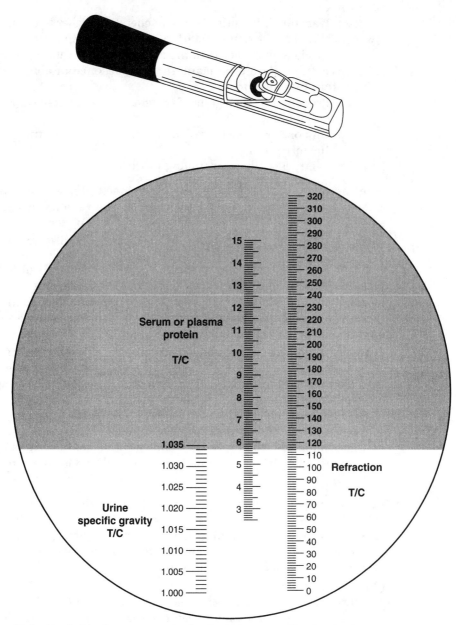

Figure 10-4. Handheld refractometer and refractive index scale. (Reprinted with permission from Linne JJ, Ringsrud KM: *Basic techniques in clinical laboratory science,* ed 3, St. Louis, 1992, Mosby, p. 336; and Strasinger SK: *Urinalysis and Body Fluids.* Philadelphia, F.A. Davis, 1989, p 49.)

4. **Osmolality** is a measure of the **number of solute particles per unit of solvent.** It is affected only by the **number of particles present and not their density.** It is used to assess the renal concentrating ability.
   a. **Evaluation.** When evaluating renal concentration ability, small molecules (primarily sodium and chloride) are of interest. Urea is of no interest and contributes more to the specific gravity than do sodium and chloride. Because all three of these molecules contribute equally to the osmolality

of a urine specimen, a more representative measure of renal concentrating ability can be obtained by measuring serum and urine osmolality.

    b. Specific gravity and osmolality have a **good correlation in nondisease states,** but if a patient has a renal disease, osmolality measurements are preferred because high-molecular-weight substances (e.g., protein and sugar, which are excreted in various disease states) contribute to the specific gravity measurement.

D. Urine volume

    1. Urine volume normally ranges from 400–2000 mL per day in a healthy adult.

        a. Oliguria is a decrease in the normal daily urine output and commonly accompanies states of dehydration, such as vomiting, diarrhea, perspiration, or severe burns.

        b. Anuria is no urine flow and may result from serious damage to the kidneys or from a decrease in the flow of blood to the kidneys.

        c. Nocturia is an increase in the nocturnal excretion of urine.

        d. Polyuria is an increase in the normal daily urine output and is seen in individuals who have diabetes mellitus and diabetes insipidus, or this condition can be induced with diuretics, caffeine, or alcohol consumption.

IV. CHEMICAL EXAMINATION OF THE URINE

    A. Chemical abnormalities detected in urine. Testing of a urine specimen should be done as soon as possible. Chemicals and cellular elements are not stable at room temperature in an unpreserved specimen sitting in light (Table 10-2). The **most common** chemical abnormalities detected in urine are **increased amounts of sugars** (e.g., glucose, galactose), **protein, RBCs, WBCs, bilirubin, ketones,** and **urobilinogen.**

    B. Reagent strip screening tests (Table 10-3)

        1. Urinalysis usually includes initial testing with **reagent multitest strips (dipsticks),** which are plastic strips impregnated with chemicals. Depending on the manufacturer or the desires of the testing laboratory, strips are available to test between 1 and 10 analytes. Chemical strip testing usually includes tests for urine **pH, specific gravity, blood, protein, glucose, ketones, bilirubin, urobilinogen, leukocytes,** and **nitrates** (Table 10-4).

        2. Procedure. The reagent strip is dipped into the urine specimen and, at the specified time for each test (determined by the manufacturer), the color reaction of each test area is compared to a color chart on the side of the dipstick container. It is important to **read each test at the time stated by the manufacturer** by comparing the reaction colors to the chart on the container. **Highly pigmented urines may cause difficulty in reading the colored reactions.** The reagents incorporated into each test area vary, depending on the manufacturer.

        3. Test methodologies may vary with each lot of strips. Therefore, it is important to **read the package information sheet enclosed with all reagents before using them.** Knowledge of each test methodology is

Table 10-2. Possible Changes in an Unpreserved Urine Specimen
When Left at Room Temperature in Light

Constituent	Possible Change	Comments
Red blood cells, white blood cells, epithelial cells, casts	Decrease	Rapid decomposition in alkaline and hypotonic specimens
Glucose	Decrease	Utilized by cells and bacteria
Ketones	Decrease	Volatilized or utilized
Bilirubin and urobilinogen	Decrease	Unstable in light and acid urines

Bacteria	Increase	• Most enteric bacteria double every 20 minutes
		• Can alter other urinary constituents:
		    Produce peroxidase, which interferes with blood dipstick reaction
		    Urea-splitting bacteria produce ammonia, which makes pH alkaline
		• Increase turbidity

pH	Increase	Urea-splitting bacteria produce ammonia, which makes pH alkaline and interferes with specific gravity and protein dipstick reaction; may cause precipitation of crystals
Protein	Increase	Bacterial proliferation
Nitrates	Decrease	Reduced to nitrites by bacteria
Trichomonad	Decrease	Become immobile or die; possible misidentification as white blood cells
Crystals	Increase	Precipitation enhanced by standing and cooling, which causes an increase in turbidity

needed to evaluate results and to select confirmatory testing methods, if necessary.

4. **The pH** level is a measure of the kidney's ability to maintain normal **hydrogen ion concentration** in plasma and extracellular fluid. The tubular cells exchange hydrogen for sodium, and the urine becomes acidic.

   a. **Test methodology** involves test strips coated with substances that can function either as **proton donors or proton acceptors** and that absorb radiant energy differently in these two different forms. Indicators in the test area react to the different forms, changing color according to the hydrogen ion content of the urine.

   b. **The pH of urine in a normal healthy adult ranges from 4.6–8,** depending on dietary intake. High protein intake results in an acidic urine; a diet high in vegetables and fruits (particularly citric fruits) makes the urine more alkaline.

Table 10-3. Summary of the Reagents, Test Principle, Sensitivity, and Factors That Can Affect Reagent Strip Testing

Test	Reagents	Principle	Sensitivity	Affecting Factors
pH	Indicators: methyl red and bromthymol blue	Substances act as either proton acceptors or proton donors	5–9	Bacterial growth and metabolism may cause marked increase
Specific gravity	Polyelectrolyte, bromthymol blue indicators; buffers	pK_a change of pretreated polyelectrolyte	0.005 increments between 1.000 and 1.030	Alkaline urine, add 0.005 for pH > 6.5; protein may increase value
Blood	H_2O_2, tetramethylbenzidine, or orthotoluidine	Catalase and peroxidase activity of heme; myoglobin and red blood cells causing oxidation of chromogen	5–20 red blood cells; 0.05–0.3 mg/dL hemoglobin	Oxidizing contaminants, ≥ 5 mg/dL ascorbic acid may inhibit reaction
Protein	Citrate buffer at pH 3; tetrabromphenol blue indicator	"Protein error" of indicators; indicator combines with protein, which alters its spectral absorption	5–20 mg/dL albumin	Highly buffered alkaline urine may cause a false-positive result; protein may normally be increased with exercise or dehydration
Glucose	Glucose oxidase; peroxidase; o-toluidine, potassium iodide, or aminopropylcarbazol	Glucose + O_2 → gluconic acid + H_2O_2; H_2O_2 + chromogen → oxidized chromogen + H_2O	0.1 g/dL; more sensitive than Clinitest	≥ 50 mg/dL ascorbic acid may inhibit reaction
Ketones	Sodium nitroprusside	Acetoacetic acid + sodium nitroprusside → purple	5–10 mg/dL	Highly volatile; bacteria can degrade
Bilirubin	Dichloroaniline or dichloro-benzene-diazonium tetrafluoroborate	Diazo reaction: bilirubin + diazonium salt → tan to purple	0.4–0.8 mg/dL; less sensitive than Ictotest	Unstable in light; large amounts of ascorbic acid or nitrite lower results
Urobilinogen	Dimethylaminobenzaldehyde	Urobilinogen + dimethylaminobenzaldehyde → yellow to brown-orange	0.2–8 Ehrlich units	Urobilinogen is unstable in urine; fresh specimen is required
Leukocytes	Indoxylcarbonic acid ester, diazonium salt	Indoxylcarbonic acid ester + leukocyte esterases → indoxyl + diazonium salt + purple	5–15/hpf intact or lysed leukocytes with esterases	High levels of glucose and protein inhibit reaction; false-positive with histiocytes and trichomonads
Nitrite	Para-arsanilic acid, tetrahydrobenzo(h)-quinolin-3-ol	Nitrite + para-arsanilic acid → diazonium + tetra-hydrobenzo(h)-quinolin-3-ol → pink	≥ 10^5 bacteria/mL	Bacteria without reductase do not react; ≥ 25 mg/dL ascorbic acid may inhibit reaction; less than 4-hour retention of urine in bladder; lack of dietary nitrate.

H_2O_2 = hydrogen peroxide; hpf = high-powered field; pK_a = negative log of dissociation constant.

Table 10-4. Clinical Significance of Chemical Dipstick Reactions

Test	Clinical Significance
pH	Kidney's ability to excrete excess acid; distal tubular dysfunction; acidic with persistent metabolic and respiratory acidosis; persistent alkalinity with metabolic alkalosis and urinary tract infection
Specific gravity	Diabetes insipidus (deficient antidiuretic hormone); isothenuria (loss of tubular concentrating ability)
Blood	Bleeding in the urogenital tract as the result of trauma or irritations, such as cystitis (bladder infection), glomerulonephritis (inflammation of the glomerulus), pyelonephritis (inflammation of the kidney), burns, tumors, or exposure to toxic chemicals; transfusion reactions; menstruation; myoglobin
Protein	Glomerular membrane damage, defective tubular reabsorption, immunoglobulin light chains in multiple myeloma (Bence Jones protein), diabetic nephropathy; transient elevation with fever, exercise, dehydration, acute phase of illness, pregnancy, and orthostatic or postural proteinuria following long periods of standing
Glucose	Diabetes mellitus, pregnancy, impaired tubular reabsorption
Ketones	Diabetes mellitus, starvation diets
Bilirubin	Liver damage such as hepatitis or cirrhosis; obstruction of the bile duct
Urobilinogen	Liver damage such as hepatitis or cirrhosis; red blood cell lysis; prophyrinuria
Leukocytes	Urinary tract infections: cystitis, pyelonephritis
Nitrite	Cystitis, pyelonephritis

5. **The specific gravity reagent test area method** is based on the **pK$_a$ change of a pretreated polyelectrolyte** (e.g., polymethylvinyl ether/maleic acid) in relation to ionic concentration, where pH is the negative logarithm of the hydrogen ion concentration, and the pK$_a$ is the negative dissociation constant K$_a$ of H_2CO_3. An increased concentration of electrolytes or many ions in urine decreases the pK$_a$ of the polyelectrolytes in the test area, causing a decrease in pH. The change in pH caused by increasing ion concentration is related to an increase in specific gravity.

   a. An **increased specific gravity** can be caused by the presence of **glucose or protein** in the urine. Radiographic dyes do not affect the dipstick method. Persons with **diabetes mellitus** who are spilling glucose into their urine often have polyuria, which leads to a **pale-colored urine with a high specific gravity.**

   b. **Diabetes insipidus** is a condition in which there is **insufficient antidiuretic hormone (ADH).** This condition is also accompanied by polyuria and a pale urine, but the specific gravity is low.

   c. A **fixed specific gravity of 1.010 (isothenuria)** indicates a loss of the concentrating abiltity of the glomerulus (see III C 2).

6. **Blood** in the urine may be in the form of intact **RBCs or hemoglobin** from lysed RBCs. **Myoglobin** will also react with the blood test area.

   a. The dipstick method is based on the **catalase** and **peroxidase** activity of heme, myoglobin, and red blood cells, which cause **oxidation of orthotoluidine or tetramethylbenzidine** and produces a green to dark-blue color.

   b. The dipstick **sensitivity is 5–20 RBCs, or 0.05–0.3 mg/dL hemoglobin** and should normally be **negative.**

7. **Protein** is normally excreted into the urine at a concentration of **150 mg/ 24 h.** Approximately one third is albumin, with the remainder being small globulins with molecular weights less than 50,000.

   a. The test is based on the **"protein error" of indicators.** The strip contains a **citrate buffer at a pH of 3 and a tetrabromphenol blue indicator.** At this pH, the indicator is yellow. Proteins present in the sample combine with the indicator, **altering the spectral absorption of the dye;** a yellow-green, green, or blue color results, depending on the concentration of protein.

   b. The test detects **albumin** but not larger proteins.

   c. Highly buffered **alkaline urine** specimens may produce a **false-positive** result with this method.

8. **Glucose** is not normally detectable in urine. It is excreted into the urine when the plasma level exceeds the **kidney threshold of 150–180 mg/dL** or when there is a defect in its reabsorption mechanism.

   a. **The test strip is specific for glucose.** The sensitivity is **100 mg/dL.**

   b. In the first of a double sequential enzyme reaction, **gluconic acid** and **hydrogen peroxidase** are formed from the oxidation of glucose by **glucose oxidase.** In the second reaction, peroxidase catalyzes the reaction of hydrogen peroxidase with potassium iodide chromogen, which produces color from blue to green, orange, or brown, depending on the quantity of glucose in the specimen.

9. **Ketones** are the products of incomplete fat metabolism, and their presence in urine indicates acidosis. The three ketone bodies present in urine are **acetoacetic (diacetic) acid, acetone, and 3-hydroxybutyrate.**

   a. The test method is based on the reaction of **sodium nitroprusside** with acetoacetic acid. The test does not detect acetone or 3-hydroxybutyrate, but if one ketone is excreted, all are excreted. Positive reactions produce a **maroon** color.

   b. The test sensitivity is **5–10 mg/dL of acetoacetic acid.**

10. **Bilirubin** is not normally detectable in urine. The reagent strip method can detect **0.4–0.8 mg/dL bilirubin** with the **diazo reaction,** in which **2,4 dichloroaniline diazonium salt** reacts with bilirubin to produce a **tan-to-purple** color.

11. **Urobilinogen** is normally present in urine in small amounts up to 4 mg/ 24 h.

   a. **Paradimethylaminobenzaldehyde** (Ehrlich's reagent) reacts with urobilinogen (and porphobilinogen, depending on the brand of reagent strips) to form colors ranging from light yellow to brown-orange.

b. In a random urine specimen, the **normal concentration** on the **test strip reflects 0.2 and 1.0 EU.** Increased concentrations can be detected by the strip method, but the method is **not suitable for detecting decreases in concentration.** Fresh specimens should be used for testing because **urobilinogen is unstable in urine.**

12. Leukocytes can be detected in urine with the **leukocyte esterase reaction.** Granulocytic leukocyte esterases catalyze the hydrolysis of the derivative pyrrole-N-tosyl-L-alanine ester to form pyrrole alcohol. The alcohol then reacts with a diazonium salt to produce a **purple** color.

a. The test strip can detect **5–15 leukocytes per high-power field** and is even **sensitive to lysed granulocytes.**

b. Vaginal contamination or trichomonads can cause a false-positive result.

13. The **nitrite** test provides a rapid screen for the **detection of bacteria that are capable of reducing nitrates to nitrite.**

a. The test results should normally be negative.

b. False-negative reactions may occur if:

(1) The bacteria in the specimen do not have the enzymes necessary to reduce nitrates.

(2) The diet of the individual is deficient in nitrates.

(3) The bacteria reduce the nitrate beyond the nitrate state to nitrogen or ammonia.

(4) The urine has not been in the bladder at least 4 hours, so the bacteria did not yet reduce the nitrates.

C. Other chemical tests used for determining abnormalities in urine

1. Glucose and other reducing substances, such as other disaccharides (e.g., fructose, galactose, lactose, pentose) and other reducing substances (e.g., ascorbic acid) in the urine can be detected with the **copper reductase test (Clinitest).**

a. The test uses the reagents **copper sulfate, sodium hydroxide, sodium carbonate, and citric acid incorporated into a tablet.**

b. In the **five-drop method,** five drops of urine are added to 10 drops of distilled water in a test tube. One Clinitest tablet is added, and the solution begins to boil. **Copper sulfate reacts with reducing substances in urine, converting cupric ions to cuprous ions** in an exothermic process.

(1) After 15 seconds, the tube is gently mixed and compared to a color chart. A negative reaction is **blue.** Depending on the concentration of reducing substance(s), the solution changes from green-blue to orange.

(2) It is important to watch the reaction because if a **high glucose concentration is present (> 2 g/dL),** the color reaction will pass from orange to a brownish color and back to blue (**"pass-through" phenomenon**). If this occurs, the urine must be retested at a lower concentration with a two-drop method (same procedure as the five-drop method, except two drops of urine are added to the test tube).

c. The test **sensitivity is 150 mg/dL,** which is **less sensitive than the dipstick method.**

(1) Thus, at low glucose concentrations, it is **possible to have a positive dipstick test and a negative Clinitest.**

(2) It is also possible to have a **positive Clinitest and a negative dipstick** test if the sugar present is one other than glucose, or the urine contains another reducing substance (e.g., ascorbic acid).

    (a) **Nonglucose mellituria** can occur in various situations. Inherited enzyme deficiencies can cause the accumulation of lactose, fructose, galactose, pentose, or sucrose in plasma. All of the sugar cannot be reabsorbed, and it appears in urine.

    (b) **Lactosuria** can occur during late pregnancy or during lactation.

    (c) **Pentosuria** can occur following ingestion of certain fruits.

    (d) **Fructosuria** can occur with parenteral feedings with fructose.

(3) **Sucrose** is not a reducing sugar, so it **does not react** in the Clinitest.

2. **Precipitation tests for protein** are more sensitive than are the reagent strip methods and detect other proteins besides albumin.

    a. An aliquot (usually 1 mL) of **3% SSA or trichloroacetic acid** is added to an equal amount of urine in a test tube and mixed by inversion. The tube is allowed to stand for 10 minutes and then is inverted twice.

    b. **The degree of precipitation is graded according to the following criteria:**

        (1) **Negative:** no turbidity, ≤ 5 mg/dL protein

        (2) **1+:** faint turbidity but no discrete granulation; ≈ 50 mg/dL protein

        (3) **2+:** turbidity with granulation but no flocculation; ≈ 200 mg/dL protein

        (4) **3+:** turbidity with granulation and flocculation; ≈ 500 mg/dL protein

        (5) **4+:** clumps of precipitation; ≥ 1.0 g/dL protein

    c. The test **sensitivity is 5–10 mg/dL** and **detects albumin, globulins, glycoproteins, and Bence Jones protein. Radiographic dyes** react with this method. When the radiographic dyes are present, the specific gravity of the urine is usually > 1.035, and typical crystals are seen on the microscopic examination of the urine specimen.

3. The **Ictotest** is a sensitive test for the detection of bilirubin in urine in which **2,4-dichloro-benzene-diazonium tetrachlorozincate, sodium bicarbonate, and sulfosalicylic acid** are combined into a tablet.

    a. Five drops of urine are placed on an **asbestos cellulose test pad,** which concentrates the specimen so that much smaller concentrations of bilirubin **(0.05–0.1 mg/dL)** can be detected as compared with the dipstick method.

    b. The urine is allowed to absorb into the pad for 1 minute, and then a reagent tablet is placed on the wet area of the pad.

    c. One drop of distilled water is placed onto the tablet. After 5 seconds, a second drop of distilled water is placed on the tablet so that the drops run down the side of the tablet onto the test pad.

    d. The tablet is removed, and the test pad is observed within 1 minute for a **purple** color, which indicates the **presence of bilirubin.** A pink or red color is a negative reaction.

V. MICROSCOPIC EXAMINATION OF THE URINE

A. Urine sediment preparation

1. To ensure the accuracy and reproducibility of the urine microscopic examination, each laboratory must establish a protocol for the preparation of the urine sediment. Factors that must be considered in urinalysis to help **standardize the microscopic examination** include the following:

   a. **Appropriate specimen collection, preservation, and handling.** It is best to examine a specimen within 1 hour of patient voiding because many aspects of the chemical and microscopic examination may change as the urine stands, especially at room temperature.

   b. A **standard amount of urine,** usually 12 mL, is placed in a conical tube and centrifuged for a **uniform amount of time and speed,** usually 5 minutes at a relative centrifugal force of 400.

   c. The spun tube is decanted, which leaves approximately **1 mL of fluid in which to resuspend the urinary sediment.** If a stain is used, it should be added at this time.

   d. A small drop of well-mixed sediment is placed onto a microscope slide and shielded with a coverslip. **Slides with uniform wells and coverslips** are available for the microscopic examination of urine. Drop size determines the amount of sediment viewed.

   e. A **consistent method should be used to examine the urinary sediment.** The slide is first viewed on high power to assess the overall composition of the specimen and to observe and count casts. The light must be very low to see hyaline casts. Other elements are counted on high power. An average range count of 10–20 fields is usually reported.

   f. **Microscopic results should be correlated with the color, appearance, and dipstick reactions for each specimen.**

2. **Microscopic sediment stains (supravital stains)** can be used to aid the identification of formed elements.

   a. The most commonly used stain is the **Sternheimer-Malbin** stain, which consists of crystal violet and safranin O. This stain provides a more detailed visualization of the internal structure of cells and casts.

   b. Another supravital urine sediment stain is **0.5% toluidine blue.** It differentially stains various cell components (e.g., the nucleus, cytoplasm) to help distinguish cells that may be similar in size, such as leukocytes and renal cells.

   c. **Sudan III or oil red O** stains are used to confirm the presence of neutral lipids. Lipids or fats within renal cells or histiocytes (oval fat bodies) or free-floating triglycerides stain red or orange with these two stains.

   d. The **Prussian blue** stain is used to confirm the presence of hemosiderin (iron) in epithelial cells and casts, as well as hemosiderin that is free-floating. The iron turns a characteristic blue color.

   e. **Hansel stain** consists of methylene blue and eosin-Y in methanol. It is used to identify eosinophils.

    f. One to two drops of **2% acetic acid** added to a few drops of urine sediment can be used to differentiate RBCs from yeast cells, small WBCs, or epithelial cells. The RBCs lyse; the yeast cells remain intact. The internal structures of WBCs and the epithelial cells are accentuated.

B. Normal and abnormal cells in urine (Figure 10-5)

    1. RBCs are small biconcave disks without a nucleus. They are 7–10 μm in diameter. In a hypertonic urine they become **crenated,** appearing to have a crinkled border. In a hypotonic, alkaline urine, the RBCs swell and may lyse. These lysed cell membranes are called **ghost or shadow cells** and appear as faint, colorless circles. Normally, a urine specimen can contain 0–3 RBCs; increased numbers indicate renal bleeding or glomerulonephritis.

    2. WBCs, usually **neutrophils,** are larger than RBCs **(10–15 μm diameter) and contain a distinct nucleus.** A normal urine sample contains 0–8 WBCs. An increase is called **pyuria** and indicates the presence of an infection or inflammation in the genitourinary tract. Frequent causes of pyuria include bacterial infections (e.g., cystitis, pyelonephritis, prostatitis, urethritis) or nonbacterial disorders (e.g., glomerulonephritis, lupus erythematosus, tumors). In dilute alkaline urines, WBCs can lyse or swell and become **glitter cells,** in which brownian movement of their internal granules produces a sparkling appearance.

        a. Eosinophils in a urine specimen are identified with the **Hansel stain** and indicate acute interstitial nephritis caused by **hypersensitivity reactions to medications** such as penicillin derivatives.

        b. Mononuclear cells (histiocytes, lymphocytes, or plasma cells) indicate an **inflammatory** process or **renal transplantation rejection.**

    3. There are three types of **epithelial cells found in urine: squamous, transitional, and renal.** They are derived from the linings of the urogenital tract. A few of each type can normally be found in urine because of normal sloughing of old cells.

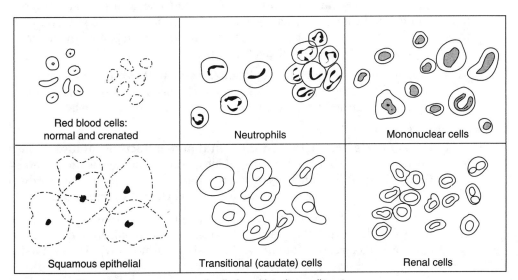

Figure 10-5. Characteristic appearance of cells found in urine sediment.

a. **Squamous cells** are derived from the lining of the vaginal tract and lower portions of the female and male urethras. They are the **most frequently seen** but least significant epithelial cell. Increased numbers in a female urine specimen indicate that the specimen was not collected using the midstream clean-catch technique. Squamous cells are **30–40 μm in diameter and contain abundant cytoplasm with a small (7 μm in diameter) centrally located nucleus.** Their **cytoplasmic borders are irregular,** and they are often folded over on themselves in a urine specimen.

b. **Transitional or caudate epithelial cells** line the urinary tract from the renal pelvis to the proximal two thirds of the urethra. They measure **12–20 μm** and are characteristically **round or pear-shaped with a centrally located nucleus.** Unless present in large numbers with unusual morphology, transitional cells are seldom pathologic. When unusual or in large numbers, samples of these cells should be referred for cytologic examination and may indicate renal transplantation rejection, acute tubular necrosis, ischemic injury to the kidney, or renal carcinoma.

c. **Renal tubular epithelial cells** line each portion of the renal tubules. **Cells from the proximal or distal convoluted tubules are relatively large (20–60 μm).** They are oblong or round to oval and contain an eccentric nucleus. Increased numbers in urine are the result of acute tubular necrosis from heavy metals or drug toxicity.

d. **Renal tubular cells from the collecting ducts range from 12–20 μm and are cuboidal, polygonal, or columnar.** They have a **single, large, dense nucleus** that takes up approximately two thirds of its interior. Large numbers in urine are caused by all types of renal diseases and are often accompanied by granular, waxy, or renal tubular cell casts and an increased number of blood cells.

e. Renal tubular cells containing fat are called **oval fat bodies.** They can be stained with Sudan III or oil red O. When visualized with **polarized light, these fat globules display a maltese cross.** Oval fat bodies often indicate glomerular dysfunction with renal tubular cell death. When present in a urine specimen, these cells are accompanied by increased amounts of protein and cast formation.

4. **Tumor cells, platelet, or epithelial cells with viral inclusions** may be found in urine sediment. Cytologic techniques are more sensitive than conventional urine microscopy in detecting these kinds of cells.

C. **Urine casts** (Figure 10-6)

1. Urinary **casts are formed in the distal and collecting tubules.** Except for a few hyaline or granular casts, which can accompany strenuous exercise (**athletic pseudonephritis**) or severe stress, casts are not normally present in the urine. The presence of urinary casts is termed **cylindroiduria.**

2. **Tamm-Horsfall** protein, which is a mucoprotein secreted only by renal tubular cells, forms the matrix of casts. As the tubular lumen contents become concentrated (often due to stasis of urine flow), Tamm-Horsfall

Type	Appearance	Clinical Significance
Hyaline	Colorless, homogeneous protein matrix with rounded ends; various sizes and shapes 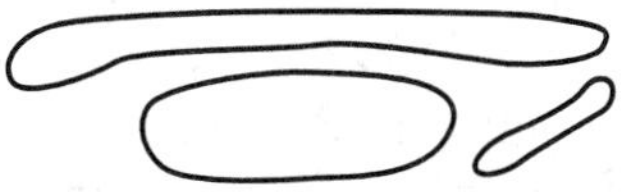	Strenuous exercise, stress Inflammation of the urogenital tract Often found with other casts
Red blood cell	Protein matrix filled with red blood cells; often many free red cells in microscopic field 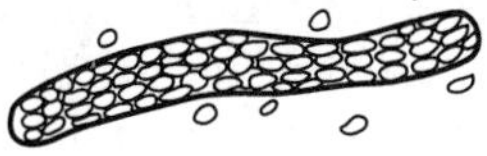	Glomerulonephritis Acute interstitial nephritis Strenuous exercise
White blood cell	Protein matrix filled with white blood cells 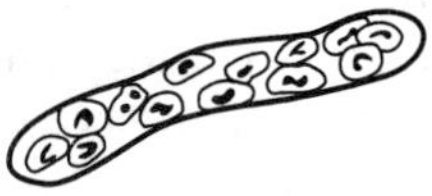	Pyelonephritis Kidney infection (accompanied by bacteria, protein, red blood cells) Glomerulonephritis (accompanied by red blood cell casts)
Epithelial cell	Protein matrix filled with renal epithelial cells 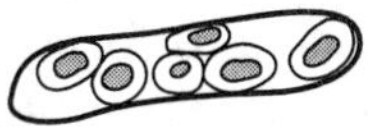	Renal tubular damage
Fine or coarsely granular	Protein matrix filled with degenerating cells, amorphous crystals, or bacteria; colorless to yellowish; many shapes and sizes 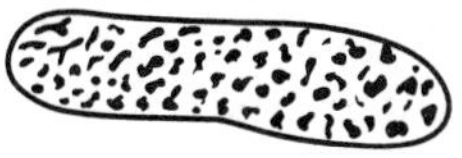	Urine flow stasis Urogenital tract infections Strenuous exercise, stress
Fatty	Protein matrix containing oval fat bodies 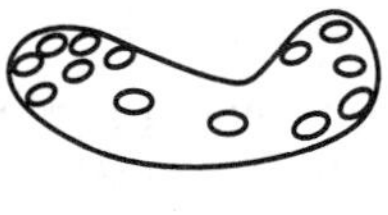	Nephrotic syndrome Renal tubular cell death Severe crush injury with disruption of body fat accompanied by significant proteinuria
Waxy or broad	Homogeneous with waxy, thick appearance, often with blunt, uneven, brittle-looking edges 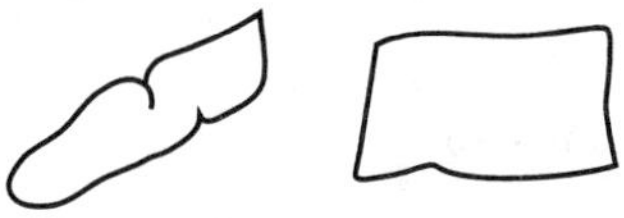	Tubular obstruction or disease with extreme urine flow stasis Severe nephron damage Nephrotic syndrome Poor prognosis with large numbers present
Pigmented	Hyaline matrix with coloration due to pigment incorporation 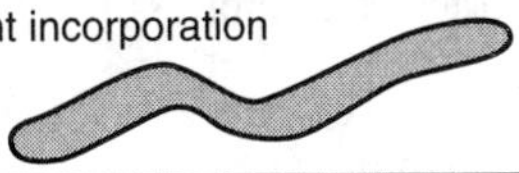	Incorporated bilirubin (golden-brown) Hemoglobin or myoglobin (yellow to red-brown)
Mixed	Two or more cell types enmeshed in a protein matrix; part granular and part waxy Any combination is possible	Two cell types in filtrate during cast formation; initial cast formation in one tubule, followed by stasis in another wider lumen and further cast formation

Figure 10-6. Types of urinary casts: their appearance and clinical significance.

protein forms fibrils that attach it to ductal cells and hold it temporarily in place. As it is held in the tubule, it enmeshes into its matrix any cellular or chemical substance that is present in the filtrate at the time it is formed. Eventually, the cast detaches from the tubular epithelial cells and is flushed into the urine.

3. Because casts form in the tubules, they are **cylindrical with parallel sides and rounded ends.** Casts formed in the collecting ducts are broader than those formed in the proximal and distal convoluted tubules.

4. The **number and type of casts reflect the extent of renal tubule involvement in disease processes.** They are classified by the composition of their matrix and the type of substance enmeshed within them. Hyaline casts are the hardest to view because they do not contain any inclusions. Also, they consist primarily of a homogeneous Tamm-Horsfall protein matrix with a low refractive index similar to urine. They must be viewed with subdued light when using bright-field microscopy.

5. Casts in urine are often accompanied by **proteinuria.**

D. **Crystals** are commonly found in urine sediment but are rarely clinically significant. Precipitated crystals appear in various forms or as amorphous material. **Crystal identification is based on microscopic appearance and urine pH.** Normal crystals (Table 10-5) can be found in acid, alkaline, or neutral urine.

1. **Normal crystals** found in **acidic urine** (Figure 10-7) are **urates** (i.e., **uric acid, amorphous urates**) and **calcium oxalate.** Microscopically, all urates appear yellow to reddish-brown.

   a. **Uric acid crystals** appear in many shapes, including four-sided and flat; yellow or reddish-brown forms; rhombic plates or prisms; ovals with pointed ends; rosettes; wedges; and needles. They are **best identified with polarized light, under which they are multicolored.**

   b. **Amorphous urates** are yellow-brown granules, often found in clumps that may obscure other elements present in the urine sediment. When

Table 10-5. Summary of Normal Urinary Crystals

Crystal	pH	Color	Solubility
Uric acid	Acid	Yellow-brown	Alkali or heat
Amorphous urates	Acid	Brick dust or yellow-brown	Alkali and heat
Calcium oxalate	Acid, neutral, alkaline	Colorless (envelopes)	Dilute HCl
Amorphous phosphate	Alkaline, neutral	White-colorless	Dilute acetic acid
Calcium phosphate	Alkaline, neutral	Colorless	Dilute acetic acid
Triple phosphate	Alkaline	Colorless (coffin lids)	Dilute acetic acid
Ammonium biurate	Alkaline	Yellow-brown (thorny apples)	Acetic acid with heat
Calcium carbonate	Alkaline	Colorless (dumbbells)	Gas from acetic acid

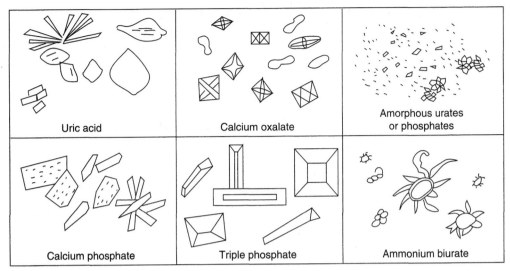

Figure 10-7. Appearance of normal urinary crystals.

present in **large amounts, they make the gross urine specimen appear pink-orange or reddish-brown and turbid.** They are easily made soluble by heating the urine specimen.

c. **Calcium oxalate** crystals can be seen in acidic or neutral urine. On rare occasions, they are found in alkaline urine. These crystals usually appear under the microscope as small, **colorless octahedrals that resemble envelopes.** They look like they have a cross on their surface. They can also appear in a dumbbell shape.

2. **Normal crystals** found in **alkaline urine** (see Table 10-5 and Figure 10-7) are predominantly **phosphates,** which include triple phosphate, amorphous phosphates, and calcium phosphate. Other crystals found in alkaline urine are **ammonium biurate and calcium carbonate.**

a. **Triple phosphate** crystals have a distinct colorless, three- to six-sided prism shape with oblique ends and are often called **coffin lids.**

b. **Amorphous phosphates** are granular in appearance. When present in large numbers, they give the urine specimen a **white turbidity.** They can mask other elements present in the urine sediment. Dilute acetic acid dissolves some of the crystals, but can also lyse any RBCs that may be present.

c. **Calcium phosphate** appears as **colorless, thin prisms, plates, or needles.** These crystals are not frequently seen in urine, but when present can be confused with sulfonamide crystals, which are abnormal. The two are distinguished by adding dilute acetic acid to the urine sediment. Calcium phosphate is soluble; sulfonamides are insoluble.

d. **Ammonium biurate** crystals are **yellow-brown spheres with irregular projections or thorns** and are referred to as **thorny apples.**

e. **Calcium carbonate** crystals are **small, colorless dumbbells or spheres.** They often appear in clumps and can be confused with amorphous phosphates. They are distinguished by the **formation of carbon dioxide gas after the addition of acetic acid.**

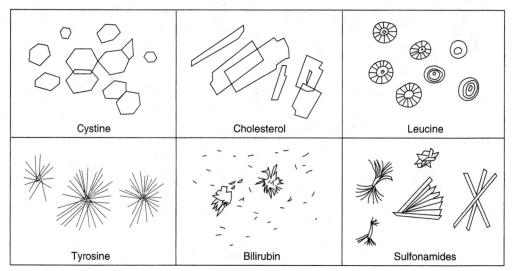

Figure 10-8. Appearance of abnormal urinary crystals.

3. **Abnormal crystals are found in acidic or neutral urine and have characteristic shapes** (Figure 10-8; Table 10-6). No abnormal crystals are found in alkaline urine. Abnormal crystals found in urine are **cystine, cholesterol, leucine, tyrosine, bilirubin, sulfonamides, ampicillin, and radiographic dyes.** It is important to check the drug therapy of patients when unusual crystals are found in their urine specimens.

a. **Cystine crystals** are **colorless hexagonal plates** that precipitate in acidic urine. They result from an inherited metabolic defect that prevents the reabsorption of cystine by the proximal convoluted tubule.

b. **Cholesterol crystals** in acidic urine resemble **rectangular plates with a notch** in one or more corners. They are seen when urine specimens have been refrigerated.

Table 10-6. Summary of Abnormal Urinary Crystals

Crystal	pH	Color	Solubility
Cystine	Acid	Colorless	Ammonia, dilute HCl
Cholesterol	Acid	Colorless (notched rectangles)	Chloroform
Leucine	Acid, neutral	Yellow	Alkali and heat, alcohol
Tyrosine	Acid, neutral	Colorless-yellow	Alkali or heat
Bilirubin	Acid	Yellow	Acetic acid, HCl, NaOH, ether, chloroform, acetone
Sulfonamides	Acid, neutral	Colorless, yellow-brown	
Ampicillin	Acid, neutral	Colorless	
Radiographic dye	Acid	Colorless	10% NaOH

    c. **Leucine** appears as yellow-brown oily looking **spheres** that contain concentric circles with radial striations.

    d. **Tyrosine crystals** look like **sheaths of fine needles.** They are rare, but can occur in individuals who have severe liver disease. They are found in acidic or neutral urine.

    e. **Bilirubin** can precipitate in acidic urine as **yellowish spheres with spicules.**

    f. **Sulfonamides** most often look like colorless or yellow-brown **bundles of wheat** with central bindings in acidic or neutral urine that has been refrigerated. Depending on the form of the drug the patient is taking, these crystals can appear as rosettes, arrowheads, needles, petals, or round forms with striations. They usually appear when patients are not adequately hydrated.

    g. **Ampicillin crystals** appear as long, fine colorless **needles** or form coarse **sheaves** after refrigeration.

    h. **Radiographic dyes** (contrast media) may have many colorless forms and can be confused with uric acid crystals. **When radiographic dyes are present in a urine specimen, the specific gravity is very high (>1.040).**

E. Microorganisms, artifacts, and miscellaneous

    1. **Bacteria** may or may not be significant, depending on the method of specimen collection and how soon after collection the specimen is examined. If **WBCs are also present** in the sediment with bacteria, an infection may exist.

    2. **Yeasts** are usually found in the urine of patients who have diabetes, but may also have gained access into the urine from places they usually reside (e.g., skin, vaginal tract) as the urine is voided. Airborne yeasts may also contaminate a urine specimen if it is left uncovered. Unless they are budding, yeasts can be confused with RBCs. To differentiate RBCs and yeast, it is best to add a drop of dilute acetic acid to the urine sediment and re-examine it. RBCs lyse; yeast cells remain intact. Occasionally, mycelial forms of *Candida* are seen.

    3. The parasite ***Trichomonas vaginalis*** (8–20 μm) is seen in urine specimens as the result of vaginal contamination. Small species can be confused with WBCs, but the parasite has a characteristic undulated flagella.

    4. Ova of the parasite ***Schistosoma haematobium*** are shed directly into urine. These are large (30 $\times$ 80 μm) ovals with a lateral spine.

    5. Occasionally, amoebae can find their way to the bladder through the lymphatics. ***Entamoeba histolytica*** (cyst 10–20 μm) is usually accompanied by erythrocytes and leukocytes.

    6. ***Enterobius vermicularis*** (pinworm) eggs or ova (30 $\times$ 50 μm) can contaminate urine when the female migrates to the perianal fold to lay its eggs. Other intestinal parasites can be seen in urine that has been contaminated with feces.

    7. **Artifacts** seen in urine include muscle fibers and vegetable cells seen with fecal contamination and hair, cotton fibers from diapers or other cloth

materials, wood from wooden sticks used to mix urine specimens, starch granules from surgical gloves, and oil droplets from lubricants used as catheter lubricants or vaginal creams.

8. **Mucus,** a protein material produced by glands and epithelial cells in the urogenital tract, is commonly observed in urine specimens, but has no clinical significance. Microscopically, mucus appears as threadlike structures with low refractive indexes, which requires subdued light for observation. The irregular appearance of mucus helps to differentiate it from hyaline casts.

9. **Spermatozoa** may be found in a female urine specimen after sexual intercourse and are considered vaginal contaminants. Spermatozoa may be found in the urine of men after nocturnal emission or ejaculation.

10. Unstained **hemosiderin** granules appear as coarse yellow-brown granules and are the result of ferritin degradation following a severe hemolytic episode. Hemosiderin can be confused with amorphous crystals. The **Prussian blue** stain is used to identify hemosiderin granules (see V A 2 d).

VI. METABOLIC PRODUCTS IN THE URINE

A. **Homogentisic acid** is excreted in the urine of patients who have **alkaptonuria** [see III A 1 b 2 (a)]. Two screening tests are used to detect homogentisic acid: the **ferric chloride** test and the **silver nitrate** test.

1. A transient, dark blue color is seen as two drops of 10% **ferric chloride** are added to 2 mL urine.

2. A black color develops after several drops of 10% ammonium hydroxide are added to 0.5 mL urine containing 4 mL of 3% **silver nitrate.**

B. A second metabolic pathway for **tyrosine** is responsible for the production of **melanin.** When melanin and its precursors are present in urine, the **urine turns dark, even black,** with exposure to light or air. To distinguish melanin from homogentisic acid, two tests can be performed.

1. In the **ferric chloride tube test,** a gray or black precipitate will form with melanin.

2. A red color is produced with melanin and **sodium nitroprusside.**

C. **Phenylketonuria (PKU)** is a well-known aminoaciduria. It occurs in approximately **1 in every 15,000 births,** and most states require that newborn infants be tested for this disease. If undetected, this condition results in severe **mental retardation.** Increased amounts of phenylalanine metabolites in urine give it a characteristic **mousy odor.**

1. **Cause.** PKU is caused by the failure to inherit the gene for production of the enzyme phenylalanine hydrolase (Figure 10-9).

2. **Dietary restrictions** that eliminate phenylalanine can prevent damage.

3. The disease is usually **first detected in blood** because urinary accumulation of phenylpyruvic acid takes 2–6 weeks.

4. The newborn must have adequate ingestion of dietary phenylalanine, which is a major constituent of milk, prior to blood collection.

5. The best known test for PKU is the **bacterial inhibition test developed by Guthrie.**

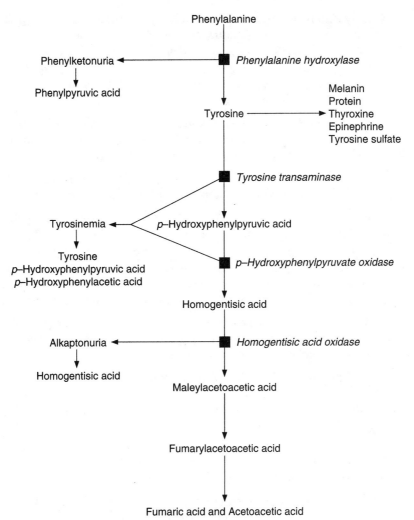

Figure 10-9. Metabolism of phenylalanine and tyrosine. (Reprinted with permission from Strasinger SK: *Urinalysis and Body Fluids.* Philadelphia, F.A. Davis, 1989, p 120.)

    a. Blood is collected on filter paper disks.

    b. The blood-impregnated disks are placed on culture media streaked with ***Bacillus subtilis*** bacteria.

    c. If increased amounts of phenylalanine are present in the blood, this will counteract the action of an inhibitor present in the media, and *Bacillus subtilis* will grow around the disk.

  6. Phenylpyruvic acid can be detected in urine with the **ferric chloride** reaction. Phenistix reagent strips are available for the detection of PKU. When dipped into urine containing phenylpyruvic acid, a permanent blue-gray to green-gray color is produced.

D. Disorders of **tyrosine** metabolism (see Figure 10-9) can result from inherited or metabolic defects. If tyrosine derived from the diet or from the metabolism of phenylalanine is not metabolized, it accumulates in the serum up to 100 times normal, producing **tyrosinemia** and overflow into the urine **(tyrosyluria).**

1. Cirrhosis of the liver, renal dysfunction, and rickets are the principal clinical findings in **hereditary tyrosinemia,** which is rare. More often, transient tyrosinemia, and thus tyrosyluria, occur in low-birth-weight infants and must be distinguished from PKU.

2. Precipitated **tyrosine crystals may be seen in urine sediment.** A screening test to detect tyrosine in urine uses nitrosonaphthol, which forms red complexes with tyrosine and tyramine, but is nonspecific.

3. **Chromatography** should be used to confirm the presence of increased levels of tyrosine because normal urine contains some tyrosine.

E. **Maple syrup urine disease (MSUD) is one of a group of disorders associated with abnormal branched-chain amino acids.**

1. Failure to inherit the gene for the enzyme necessary to produce oxidative decarboxylation of the keto acids in the metabolic pathways of **leucine, isoleucine, and valine** results in their accumulation in the blood and urine. These excess keto acids give the urine a characteristic **maple syrup odor.**

2. The most commonly used screening test for keto acids is the **2,4-dinitrophenylhydrazine (DNPH)** reaction. Addition of DNPH to urine containing keto acids produces a yellow turbidity or precipitate.

F. **Miscellaneous tests for metabolic products**

1. Dysfunction in the metabolism of **tryptophan** can result in an increase of **indican or 5-hydroxyindoleacetic acid (5-HIAA)** in the urine.

   a. In certain **intestinal disorders,** including obstruction, the presence of abnormal bacteria, malabsorption syndromes, or a rare inherited disorder (Hartnup disease), increased amounts of tryptophan are converted to **indole** in the intestine.

   b. The excess **indole** is then reabsorbed into the blood and converted to **indican** by the liver and excreted into the urine.

   c. **Indican** in urine, when exposed to air, is oxidized to **indigo blue.**

   d. Urinary indican is detected by an acidic ferric chloride solution, which reacts with indican to form a deep-blue or purple color.

2. In another metabolic pathway, **tryptophan** is converted to **serotonin** in the **argentaffin cells of the intestine.**

   a. Malignant tumors of the argentaffin cells produce excess amounts of serotonin, which results in elevated levels of the urinary **degradation product 5-HIAA.**

   b. 5-HIAA can be detected in urine with the addition of 1-nitroso-2-naphthol, which produces a purple to black color, depending on the concentration of 5-HIAA.

3. **Cystinuria** is characterized by **defective tubular reabsorption** of cystine and the amino acids arginine, lysine, and ornithine after glomerular filtration.

   a. The demonstration of multiple amino acids not being reabsorbed rules out the possibility of an error in metabolism, although the condition is inherited. Approximately 65% of individuals who have cystinuria **tend to form calculi.**

   b. **A fresh, first morning urine specimen** should be examined for cystine crystals.

   c. A chemical screening test for urinary cystine uses the **cyanide-nitroprusside** test. Sodium cyanide reduces cystine, and the free sulfhydryl groups then react with nitroprusside to produce a red-purple color.

  4. **Homocystinuria** is caused by deficiency of the liver enzyme cystathionine β-synthase. Homocysteine is rapidly oxidized to homocystine, which accumulates and is excreted in the urine. Children afflicted with this disease may have **seizures** and **thromboses,** and they may become **mentally retarded.**

   a. **A fresh urine specimen** should be tested for homocystine because it is labile.

   b. The **cyanide-nitroprusside** reaction is positive.

G. Urine calcium

  1. **Sulkowitch's test** is a quick qualitative test for increased levels of urinary calcium. Sulkowitch's reagent consists of oxalic acid, ammonium oxalate, and glacial acetic acid. When reacted with urinary calcium, calcium oxalate precipitates, producing turbidity that is graded on a scale from 0–4.

  2. Increased levels of urinary calcium may be seen in patients who have hyperparathyroidism, osteoporosis, or multiple myeloma.

H. Urine porphyrins

  1. **Porphyrins** are **intermediate compounds in the production of heme.**

  2. **Porphyrias** are a group of disorders resulting from **defects in the heme synthesis pathway** (Figure 10-10).

   a. **Inherited enzyme deficiencies** and **lead poisoning** interrupt the heme synthesis pathway and produce porphyrins, which result from the spontaneous and irreversible oxidation of their respective porphyrinogens.

   b. **These porphyrins cannot re-enter the heme synthesis pathway and must be excreted.**

   c. Porphyrias are **rare disorders.** The most common type in North America is cutanea tarda.

  3. The principle porphyrins include **uroporphyrin, coproporphyrin, and protoporphyrin.**

  4. Porphyrin **precursors** commonly found in urine are **porphobilinogen and α-aminolevulinic acid (ALA).**

  5. In their oxidative forms, uroporphyrin, coproporphyrin, and protoporphyrin are dark red or purple and fluorescent. The oxidative form of porphobilinogen—porphobilin—is dark red. Thus, **urine containing porphobilinogen and porphobilin may look dark red,** often referred to as **"port wine."**

  6. If test results are negative for blood in a red-colored urine, and the patient is not taking medication that could color the urine, the specimen should be tested for **porphyrinuria.**

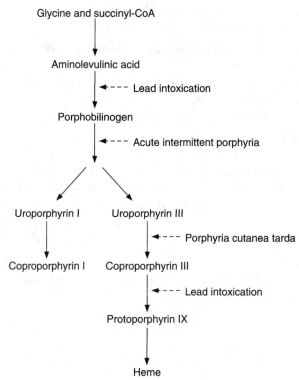

Figure 10-10. Heme synthesis pathway, with major disruptions indicated. (Reprinted with permission from Strasinger SK: *Urinalysis and Body Fluids.* Philadelphia, F.A. Davis, 1989, p 127.)

7. There are two **screening tests** for porphyrinuria: **the Ehrlich's reaction and fluorescence under ultraviolet light from a Wood's lamp.**

8. **Urobilinogen** and **porphobilinogen** react with *p*-**dimethylaminobenzaldehyde (Ehrlich's reagent)** to produce a cherry-red color.

9. To detect ALA, acetylacetone is added to the specimen before testing to convert ALA to porphobilinogen. Addition of Ehrlich's reagent produces a cherry-red color in a specimen that yields positive test results. Increased **urinary ALA** is a common screening test for **lead poisoning.**

10. If a cherry-red color is produced by a urine specimen after the addition of Ehrlich's reagent, the **Watson-Schwartz test** is performed to **differentiate urobilinogen and porphobilinogen based on solubility differences.**

    a. **Chloroform** is added to the tube to **extract urobilinogen,** and porphobilinogen remains in the aqueous phase. The tube is shaken vigorously, and the phases are allowed to separate.

    b. If the red color resides only in the **chloroform layer,** increased amounts of **urobilinogen** are present. If the **aqueous layer** is red, **porphobilinogen** or other Ehrlich-reactive substances are present.

11. **Fluorescence screening** detects the presence of **urobilinogen, coproporphyrin, and protoporphyrin.**

a. These porphyrins must be extracted into a mixture of glacial acetic acid and ethyl acetate.

b. The **solvent layer** is then examined with a **Wood's lamp.**

c. If **it tests positive,** the solvent layer **fluoresces as pink, violet, or red,** depending on the concentration of porphyrins present.

VII. DISEASES OF THE KIDNEY

A. Glomerular diseases

1. **Morphologic changes.** Four distinct morphologic changes of the glomeruli are recognized: **cellular proliferation, leukocyte infiltration, glomerular basement-membrane thickening,** and **hyalinization with sclerosis.**

   a. **Leukocyte infiltration** results from local chemotactic response or cellular proliferation. **Neutrophils and macrophages** can readily infiltrate glomeruli in response to chemotactic factors.

   b. **Cellular proliferation** causes increased numbers of epithelial cells, mesangial cells, and **endothelial cells,** which compose the capillary endothelium and accumulate in the glomerular tuft.

   c. **Glomerular basement-membrane thickening** usually results from **deposition of precipitated proteins** (e.g., immune complexes, fibrin).

   d. **Hyalinization of glomeruli results** from the accumulation of a homogeneous, eosinophilic extracellular material in the glomeruli, which causes them to lose their structural detail and become sclerotic.

2. **Immunologic disorders are the primary cause of glomerular injury. Circulating immune complexes** created in response to either endogenous (e.g., cellular) or exogenous antigens (e.g., microorganisms) become trapped in the glomeruli. A second immune response involves **antibodies that react directly with antigens on the glomerular tissue.** These may be cross-reacting antibodies formed against exogenous antigens. Glomerular injury results from the toxic substances (e.g., proteases, oxygen-derived free radicals, and arachidonic acid metabolites) produced by the complements, neutrophils, monocytes, platelets, and other factors at the site of antibody deposition.

   a. **Clinical features** of glomerulonephritis include some or all of the following: **hematuria, proteinuria, oliguria, azotemia, edema, and hypertension.**

   b. **Acute glomerulonephritis** refers to a disease characterized by the rapid onset of symptoms (e.g., fever, malaise, nausea, oliguria) caused by an **inflammatory process in the glomerulus. Blood, protein, and casts,** particularly **RBC casts,** are detected in the urine.

      (1) **Poststreptococcal glomerulonephritis** is most frequently seen in children or young adults following a respiratory tract infection caused by **group A streptococci** (e.g., *Streptococcus pyogenes*) in which treatment either did not occur, or it failed. As the bacteria proliferate and the body forms antibodies to them, opsonized bacteria form immune complexes that deposit on the glomerular membrane.

(2) Approximately 95% of children and 60% of adults recover spontaneously or with minimal therapy. The remainder of patients recover more slowly or develop chronic glomerulonephritis.

3. **Crescentic (rapidly progressive) glomerulonephritis** is a more serious type of glomerulonephritis, which often terminates in renal failure.

   a. It is characterized by **cellular proliferation of epithelial cells** inside Bowman's capsule to form **"crescents,"** which cause pressure changes in the glomerular tuft and can even occlude the entrance to the proximal tubule, because there is fibrin deposition and leukocyte infiltration.

   b. Urinalysis findings include **hematuria; proteinuria; oliguria; RBCs; and hyaline, granular, RBC, and WBC casts.**

4. **Chronic glomerulonephritis** results from continual or permanent damage to the glomerulus associated with irreversible loss of renal tissue and chronic renal failure.

   a. Clinical signs include **edema, hypertension, anemia, metabolic acidosis, and oliguria that progresses to anuria.**

   b. Urinalysis findings include **hematuria; proteinuria; isothenuria; and many types of casts, including broad or waxy.**

   c. Blood urea nitrogen (BUN), serum creatinine, phosphorous, and potassium levels are elevated; serum calcium levels tend to be decreased.

5. **Membranous glomerulonephritis** is characterized by **thickening of the glomerular capillary basement membrane,** which is usually caused by **immune complex deposition.**

   a. The **clinical course** of this disease is variable, but may progress to a nephrotic syndrome.

   b. Urinalysis findings include **hematuria** and **proteinuria.**

6. **Mesangiocapillary (membranoproliferative) glomerulonephritis** is characterized by **cellular proliferation** and **leukocyte infiltration** that leads to thickening of the glomerular basement membrane.

   a. **Immune complex deposition** and **complement activation** over many years leads to **chronic renal failure.**

   b. Laboratory findings may include **hypocomplementemia, hematuria, and proteinuria.**

7. In **focal glomerulonephritis,** only a **certain number of glomeruli are sclerotic.** Characteristic findings include immune complex deposition with **hematuria and proteinuria.**

8. **Minimal change disease** produces little cellular change in the glomeruli.

   a. Frequently, **children** are affected, probably through an **allergic reaction.**

   b. The disease is usually transient and is characterized by **edema, heavy proteinuria, lipiduria, and hematuria.**

B. **Tubular and interstitial diseases**

   1. **Acute tubular necrosis** results from **destruction of renal tubular epithelial cells,** which is caused by decreased perfusion of the kidneys and

ischemia or toxic agents (e.g., hemoglobin, myoglobin, drugs) or toxins (e.g., heavy metals, poisons, organic solvents) that produce ischemia.

   a. The resulting **oliguria** leads to **acute renal failure.**

   b. Urinalysis findings include **proteinuria, hematuria, pyuria, and many types of casts,** depending on the phase of the disease.

2. Tubular dysfunction can be a primary renal disease or secondary to some other disease process.

   a. Fanconi's syndrome is any condition that is characterized by a **generalized proximal tubular dysfunction.** As a result, the reabsorption of water, glucose, phosphorus, potassium, calcium, and amino acids is decreased. Therefore, these substances are excreted into the urine.

   b. Cystinosis is an inherited trait that results in the **intracellular deposition of cystine.** Every cell in the body is affected, including the proximal and distal tubular cells. The kidney can no longer concentrate or acidify urine. The extensive renal cell damage eventually requires dialysis or transplantation.

3. Tubulointerstitial disease results from other diseases that affect the renal tubules and eventually involve the interstitium. Causes of tubulointerstitial diseases are **infections; toxins (e.g., drugs, heavy metals); vascular or metabolic diseases; irradiation; neoplasms; and organ transplantation rejection.**

4. Urethritis is infection of the urethra. **Cystitis** is infection of the bladder. **Pyelitis** is infection of the renal pelvis. **Pyelonephritis** is infection of the renal pelvis and the interstitium.

5. Urinary tract infections (UTIs) are more common in women, and 85% of UTIs are caused by gram-negative enteric bacteria. The most common pathogen is *Escherichia coli.*

   a. UTIs cause pain or **burning on urination (dysuria).**

   b. Urinalysis findings include: **pyuria (i.e., presence of WBCs)** and **bacteriuria. Hematuria** and **proteinuria** are possible as well.

6. Acute pyleonephritis is an acute infection of the renal tubules, interstitium, and renal pelvis.

   a. There are **two possible mechanisms** leading to acute pyelonephritis.

      (1) Bacteria can ascend the ureters from a lower urinary tract infection.

      (2) Bacteremia can occur, with bacteria localizing in the kidney.

   b. Bacteria multiply in the kidney, which causes inflammation that spreads to the tubules. Large numbers of neutrophil enzymes and bacterial toxins can cause necrosis of the tubules.

   c. Urinalysis findings include **pyuria with WBCs, often in clumps; large numbers of bacteria; leukocyte casts** (and possibly granular, renal cell, or broad casts); **proteinuria;** and **hematuria.**

7. Yeast infections of the urinary tract usually result from inoculation of these organisms into the urinary tract by catheters or from the bloodstream if it is infected with yeast.

8. **Chronic pyelonephritis** is a chronic inflammation of the tubulointerstitial tissues and results in **permanent scarring.**
   a. Urinalysis findings include **pyuria and proteinuria.** Bacteria and casts may or may not be present.
   b. **Polyuria** and **nocturia** develop as tubular function is lost, which results in **low specific gravity.**
9. **Acute interstitial nephritis** is a condition of renal injury that results from various drugs and toxins.
   a. Drugs such as penicillin and sulfonamides can cause an immediate allergic reaction in the renal interstitium.
   b. Heavy metals and aminoglycosides can cause direct damage to tubules.
10. **Acute renal failure** results from tubular necrosis. Typical symptoms produced by acute renal failure include:
    a. Decreased glomerular filtration rate and oliguria
    b. Lack of renal concentrating ability
    c. Increased serum BUN and creatinine levels
    d. Normal urinalysis findings
11. **Chronic renal failure** results from a progressive loss of renal function. Urinalysis findings consist of **isothenuria at 1.010, significant proteinuria, hematuria, and all types of casts** (particularly broad and waxy).

C. **Other renal-related diseases**
1. **Systemic diseases** producing glomerular damage include systemic lupus erythematosis (SLE), amyloidosis, and diabetes mellitus.
   a. In patients who have **SLE,** immune complexes (e.g., DNA and anti-DNA) are deposited in the glomerular membrane.
      (1) Complement is activated, inflammatory cells are called to the area, and the cellular proteases destroy the surrounding tissue.
      (2) Disease progression may lead to recurrent hematuria, acute nephritis, or nephrotic syndrome.
      (3) Chronic renal failure is a leading cause of death in SLE patients who have renal involvement.
   b. **Amyloidosis** is characterized by deposition of amyloid between cells in any organ or tissue of the body. Amyloid is a substance composed of 90% fibril protein and 10% glycoprotein.
      (1) The deposition of amyloid within the glomeruli eventually destroys them.
      (2) Clinical findings include **proteinuria** and **nephrotic syndrome.** Eventually, **renal failure** and **uremia** occur as more and more glomeruli are destroyed.
   c. **Diabetes mellitus** can result in renal disease.
      (1) Prolonged glucosemia is toxic to the kidney, particularly the glomerulus, and causes thickening of the basement membrane.
      (2) These patients have an excessive thirst (**polydipsia**), which leads to high volume urine with a high specific gravity because of the glucose it contains.

       (3) After 10–20 years, pronounced cellular proliferation causes glomeru-losclerosis (i.e., scarring).

       (4) Chronic renal failure eventually develops, with persistent protein-uria.

   2. Nephrotic syndrome is characterized by **pronounced proteinuria** (i.e., ≥ 3.5 g/d).

     a. Many plasma proteins, particularly albumin, are excreted into the urine because of increased permeability of the glomeruli.

     b. Other clinical findings include hypoproteinemia (particularly albumin), hyperlipidemia, lipiduria, and edema.

     c. Decreased plasma immunoglobulins and other low-molecular-weight molecules (e.g., complement components, coagulation factors) make these patients more susceptible to infections and thrombosis.

     d. Urinalysis findings include marked **proteinuria; lipiduria; hematuria; and fatty, waxy, and renal cell casts.**

     e. Systemic diseases that can lead to nephrotic syndrome include:

       (1) SLE

       (2) Amyloidosis

       (3) Diabetes mellitus

       (4) Malignant neoplasms

       (5) Infections

     f. Nephrotoxic agents such as drugs and poisons can also lead to ne-phrotic syndrome.

   3. Calculi are solid aggregates of mineral salts that form within various glands. Calculi of the urinary tract are called kidney **stones.** They can be found in the renal calyces, pelvis, ureters, or bladder.

     a. Composition. Calculi are usually composed of a mixture of elements. Most renal calculi contain **calcium** and **oxalate.** Other frequently seen components are phosphates, uric acid, and cystine.

     b. Causes of calculi formation include underlying metabolic or endocrine disorders, infections, or a fixed urinary pH. When the urine pH is optimal, and the urine becomes supersaturated with a particular chemical compo-nent, renal calculi tend to form.

D. Renal endocrinology and pharmacology

   1. ADH, also called **vasopressin,** is a hormone produced by the posterior pituitary. This hormone controls water reabsorption by the distal convoluted and collecting tubules of the kidney.

     a. Increased levels of ADH cause increased water reabsorption, which leads to a small amount of concentrated urine.

     b. Decreased ADH levels induce **polydipsia** (i.e., excessive thirst) and **polyuria,** which produces a large volume **(diuresis)** of **very dilute urine with a low specific gravity.**

     c. Diabetes insipidus is a disease characterized by polyuria and polydipsia resulting from **inadequate ADH secretion or inability of the renal tubules to respond to this hormone.**

      d. Causes of inadequate ADH secretion include adrenal insufficiency; toxic drugs; pulmonary disorders (e.g., tuberculosis, pneumonia); and cerebral disorders caused by trauma or neoplasms.

   2. Renin is a proteolytic enzyme formed and stored by juxtaglomerular cells of the kidney and released into the lymph and the renal venous blood. **Renin** converts angiotensinogen into **angiotensin products,** which **directly stimulate the synthesis and secretion of aldosterone** by the adrenal cortex.

      a. Low plasma volume and a low sodium level stimulate renin secretion, resulting in **aldosterone release,** which **causes sodium retention and reabsorption** and potassium loss.

         (1) This results in water retention, which increases extracellular fluid volume and elevated blood pressure.

         (2) As systemic pressure increases, renin production decreases. This produces a decrease in angiotensin and aldosterone levels.

         (3) Potassium loss stimulates aldosterone secretion and suppresses renin release, whereas increased potassium decreases renin and aldosterone levels.

      b. Lesions found in the kidney or its vascular supply can lead to increased renin levels, resulting in increased aldosterone production and subsequent changes in sodium and potassium excretion as well as possible hypertension.

      c. Chronic renal failure can result in low, high, or normal renin levels.

      d. Increased aldosterone levels can result from adrenal adenoma, low renin levels, potassium wastage, sodium retention, nephrosis, cirrhosis, and heart failure.

VIII. PREGNANCY TESTING

  A. Molecular characteristics of hCG

   1. Pregnancy testing is not a direct test for pregnancy (i.e., detection of a fetus) but rather is a test **to detect the presence of hCG.**

   2. The hormone hCG, which is a mucoprotein, is **produced by the cytotrophoblastic cells of the placenta approximately 10 days after conception.** The molecule consists of two noncovalently bound polypeptide **subunits: alpha and beta.**

      a. The **alpha subunit** of hCG is **nearly identical to the alpha subunit of luteinizing hormone** (LH) and **follicle-stimulating hormone** (FSH). Therefore, it **cross-reacts** with LH in bioassay systems to give **false-positive results.**

      b. The beta subunit determines the biologic and immunologic specificity of hCG.

   3. A rapid rise of hCG begins at approximately 5 weeks' gestation and peaks at 10 weeks, as illustrated in Figure 10-11.

  B. Methodologies for pregnancy testing

   1. General considerations

      a. Methods testing the presence of hCG must be standardized.

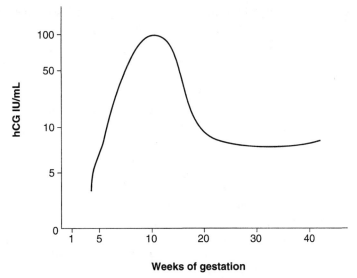

Figure 10-11. The increase of hCG in urine begins at approximately 5 weeks' gestation and peaks at 10 weeks' gestation.

    (1) The hCG values, expressed as **IU/mL, represent the amount of gonadotropic activity contained in 0.0013 mg of dried hCG standard** distributed as an international reference preparation.

    (2) Currently, various kits are standardized to test for either hCG-complete, hCG-α, or hCG-β.

    (3) The methods with the highest sensitivity test for β-hCG.

  b. Criteria. Each laboratory must select the best testing method for its purposes. The usefulness of any diagnostic test depends, in part, on the incidence of the condition it detects in the population tested. The following criteria must be considered:

    (1) Diagnostic specificity

    (2) Sensitivity

    (3) Diagnostic accuracy

2. Bioassays were the first methods used to determine pregnancy.

  a. Aschheim and Zondek reported a method in which they injected 21-day-old mice with urine. Four days later, the ovaries of the injected mice were examined for corpus luteum formation in the presence of hCG.

  b. Friedman's test was based on the principle of injecting mature female rabbits with human female urine. The rabbit ovaries were examined 48 hours later for corpus luteum formation and hemorrhagic follicles in the presence of hCG.

  c. The **Lancelot Hogben method** was based on the principle of injecting human female urine into a female South African clawed toad (i.e., *Xenopus laevis*). Four hours later, the toad would extrude eggs if hCG was present in the urine sample.

3. Hemagglutination inhibition immunoassays are a common methodology of testing today.

    a. The majority of immunoassays use either hemagglutination inhibition or latex particle inhibition, but the basic principle is the same as illustrated in Figure 10-12.

        (1) Human anti-hCG or anti-β-hCG is prepared by injection of the antigen into rabbits.

        (2) The antibody is added to the urine or serum specimen and allowed to preincubate. If hCG is present in the specimen, the antibody binds and forms a complex.

        (3) Particles (such as RBCs or latex beads) coated with the antigen, hCG, or β-hCG are then added to the specimen-antibody mixture.

        (4) Visible agglutination indicates that antigen was not present in the sample in sufficient amounts to bind all the antibody, so the antibody binds to the indicator particle, which causes agglutination.

        (5) The **absence of agglutination indicates that increased levels of hCG were present in the patient's sample,** thus preventing secondary agglutination. **The absence of agglutination indicates positive test results.**

    b. Generally, latex tests are more rapid but not as sensitive.

  4. Other methods are now more suitable for today's laboratory.

    a. Radioimmunoassay methods are dependent on β-hCG antibodies binding competitively with unlabeled antigens and radionuclide-tagged antigens. These methods have a high sensitivity.

    b. Immunoradiometric assays use a radiolabeled anti-hCG. A second antibody is immobilized on a solid phase.

    c. Immunoenzymetric assays are easily used for the semi-quantitative determination of hCG and currently are one of the most popular methodologies for detecting β-hCG in laboratories.

        (1) The method employs two different monoclonal antibodies, which react with two different regions of an hCG molecule in a **double-tagging, or sandwich, method.**

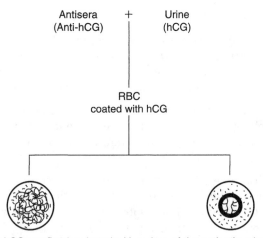

Figure 10-12. Antisera to hCG are first incubated with a drop of the patient's urine. In the presence of hCG, the antigen (i.e., hCG) will bind to the antibody. The subsequent addition of RBCs coated with hCG will yield a nonagglutination pattern.

(2) The first antibody is bound to a solid phase.

(3) The second antibody is **linked to an indicator enzyme.**

(4) If hCG is present in sufficient quantities in the specimen, the hCG molecule is "sandwiched" between the two antibodies, which links the enzyme-tagged antibody to the solid phase.

(5) Color is developed in the area of solid binding because of the presence of the enzyme. Color intensity is directly proportional to the amount of hCG present in the specimen.

IX. URINARY CALCULI ANALYSIS

A. Classification of urinary calculi

1. **Urinary calculi are classified by location and chemical nature.** In the United States, most urinary calculi are found in kidneys or ureters. Multiple calculi and bladder calculi are less common.

2. **Calcium calculi** are the most common in the United States.

B. Inspection of calculi

1. **Size** can range from 1 mm to several cm in diameter.

2. **Shapes** may be spherical, ellipsoidal, or tetragonal, and calculi are sometimes given descriptive names (e.g., mulberry, hempseed, staghorn, or jackstone).

3. **Colors** range from white to almost black.

4. **Texture** can range from smooth and highly reflective to rough and covered with large crystals.

5. **Many calculi exhibit an internal structure** such as concentric laminations or bands.

C. Techniques for analyzing calculi include the following methods:

1. Chemical analysis

2. Polarizing microscopy

3. Radiographic diffraction

4. Infrared spectroscopy

5. Electron microscopy

D. Reasons for calculi analysis

1. **Knowledge of calculi chemical composition** can aid in identifying the underlying disease or condition.

2. **Factors that predispose to calculi formation** include the following physiologic abnormalities:

a. Metabolic, nutritional, or idiopathic disturbances (e.g., gout)

b. Endocrinopathy (e.g., hyperparathyroidism)

c. Urinary obstruction

d. Infection with urea-splitting organisms

e. Mucosal changes (e.g., dietary deficiency)

f. Extrinsic and environmental factors (e.g., dehydration, alkali excess, chemotherapy)

     g. Isohydruria with fixation of urinary pH and loss of normal acid and alkaline "tides"

  3. It is estimated that calculi occur in 9 persons per 10,000 population.

E. Causes of various calculi

  1. Calculi of calcium composition are caused by the following diseases or physiologic conditions:

    a. Idiopathic hypercalciuria

    b. Primary hyperparathyroidism

    c. Bone disease

    d. Excessive milk, alkali, or vitamin D intake

    e. Renal tubular acidosis

    f. Sarcoidosis

    g. Berylliosis

  2. Calculi of calcium oxalate composition are caused by the following diseases or physiologic conditions:

    a. Oxaluria

    b. Incomplete catabolism of carbohydrates

    c. Isohydria at pH 5.5–6.0

    d. Excessive glycogen breakdown

  3. Calculi of calcium-phosphate composition are caused by the following diseases or physiologic conditions:

    a. Same conditions as for calcium oxalate

    b. Alkaline infection (urea-splitting)

    c. Persistently alkaline urine

  4. Calculi of magnesium ammonium phosphate hexahydrate composition are caused by alkaline infection with urea-splitting bacteria.

  5. Calculi composed of uric acid and urate are caused by the following diseases or physiologic conditions:

    a. Gout

    b. Polycythemia

    c. Leukemia

    d. Lymphoma

    e. Liver disease

    f. Acid isohydria

    g. Theophylline and thiazide therapy

    h. Conditions associated with rapid protein catabolism

  6. Calculi of cystine composition are caused by the following diseases or physiologic conditions:

    a. Transient acute phases of chronic renal diseases

    b. Heavy metal nephrotoxicity

    c. Aminoaciduria

    d. Renal tubular acidosis syndromes

F. pH correlations can be associated with calculi formation.

    1. Urine consistently acid with a pH lower than 5.5 favors the formation of uric acid, cystine, or xanthine calculi.

    2. Urine consistently acid with a pH between 5.5 to 6.0 favors the formation of calcium oxalate and apatite calculi.

    3. Urine consistently alkaline with a pH of greater than 7.0 favors the formation of magnesium ammonium phosphate, or calcium phosphate calculi.

X. SEROUS BODY FLUIDS

A. Origin and anatomic relationships of body fluids

    1. The cavities of the body that hold abdominal organs, lungs, and the heart are lined with a thin layer of connective tissue of mesothelial cells, which forms a sac around the organs.

        a. The peritoneum encloses abdominal organs. The fluid contained between the visceral and parietal membranes is known as **peritoneal fluid.**

        b. The pleural cavity encloses the lungs. Fluid from this cavity is called **pleural fluid.**

        c. The pericardium encloses the heart and is filled with **pericardial fluid.**

    2. Normally, 1–10 mL of fluid is found in each cavity. This fluid functions to lubricate between cavities and to allow free movement.

    3. Specimen collection of serous fluids is known as paracentesis and refers to the percutaneous puncture of a body cavity for the aspiration and removal of fluid.

        a. Thoracentesis is the collection of pleural fluid.

        b. Peritoneocentesis is the collection of peritoneal fluid.

        c. Pericardiocentesis is the collection of pericardial fluid.

    4. Abnormal accumulation of fluid in any body cavity is termed **effusion** and indicates an abnormality.

        a. Transudates result from filtration of blood serum across a physically intact vascular wall because of systemic diseases such as congestive heart failure, hepatic cirrhosis, or nephrotic syndrome.

        b. Exudates are the active accumulation of fluid within body cavities in association with inflammation and vascular wall damage. Exudates, which are closer to serum in chemical composition, are caused by the following conditions:

            (1) Inflammatory disorders

            (2) Malignancies

            (3) Infections

B. Routine analysis of body fluids

1. **Chemical examination** of the fluid helps to confirm and differentiate between an exudate and a transudate (Table 10-7). The following tests may be ordered.

   a. **A total protein evaluation and fluid-to-serum ratio** can help distinguish between the physiologic basis of different fluids.

   b. **A lactate dehydrogenase (LDH) test with a fluid-to-serum ratio** can also be used to confirm the formation of the fluid.

   c. **Transudate glucose levels** are equivalent to the plasma glucose levels; however, exudate glucose levels are low compared to plasma glucose levels.

   d. **Amylase** determination aids in the diagnosis of pancreatitis, bowel perforation, or metastasis.

   e. **Triglyceride** testing can confirm a chylous effusion.

   f. **A pH value for pleural fluids** is helpful for identifying parapneumonic effusions with abnormally low pH values.

   g. **Carcinoembryonic antigen (CEA)** determination is useful in evaluating effusions from patients who have a past or current diagnosis of a CEA-producing tumor.

2. **Fluid specimens can be sent to microbiology** for Gram's stain, bacterial culture, and sensitivity studies.

3. **Hematologic examination** includes a cell count and differential, if necessary.

   a. Cells found in normal serous fluid include the following:

      (1) Lymphocytes
      (2) Monocytes and macrophages
      (3) Mesothelial lining cells

Table 10-7. Comparison of Exudates and Transudates Based on Laboratory Profile

Laboratory Value	Exudate	Transudate
Clarity	Cloudy	Clear
Color	Yellow-green	Yellow
Common cell type	Segmented neutrophils	Mononuclear cells
White blood cell count (μL)	> 1000 (pleural) > 500 (peritoneal)	< 1000 (pleural) < 300 (peritoneal)
Clottable fibrinogen	Yes	No
Glucose	$\leq$ plasma	Equal to plasma
Total protein	> 50% of plasma value	< 50% of plasma value
Fluid-to-plasma total protein ratio	> 0.5	< 0.5
Lactate dehydrogenase	> 60% of plasma value	< 60% of plasma value

    b. Nonmalignant cells found in disease states include the following:

        (1) Neutrophils can be found in an exudate during the early stage of inflammatory diseases.

        (2) Eosinophils found in serous fluids are associated with infections, malignancy, myocardial infarction, and hypersensitivity reactions.

        (3) RBCs can occur in association with hemorrhage, malignancy, or traumatic puncture.

    c. Malignant cells can be found in serous fluids in patients who have leukemia, lymphoma, or metastatic tumors.

C. Synovial fluid

    1. Synovial fluid is present in free-moving joints, with the largest amounts in the knee. This fluid **functions to lubricate the joints and to provide the sole nutrient source for the joint tissue.**

    2. Indications for synovial fluid analysis include the following conditions:

        a. Arthritis and other joint diseases can be better diagnosed with a synovial fluid examination. Joint disorders are classified as noninflammatory, inflammatory, septic, and hemorrhagic.

        b. The degree of joint inflammation can be better assessed with a synovial fluid analysis.

        c. Synovial fluid can be removed from a joint to provide therapeutic benefit (i.e., to remove transudate, exudate, or blood from an inflamed joint).

    3. Routine synovial fluid analysis

        a. Microscopic examination consists of color, clarity, viscosity, and clot formation observations (Table 10-8).

        (1) Color abnormalities of red or brown are associated with joint trauma. Infections can produce a greenish joint fluid.

        (2) Clarity can be altered by RBCs, WBCs, crystals, bacteria, fibrin, or cellular debris.

        (3) Viscosity is related to the concentration of the mucoprotein **hyaluronic acid.**

            (a) Viscosity can be estimated by expelling a drop of the synovial fluid from a syringe. Synovial fluid of high viscosity (i.e., normal fluid) forms a "string" of 3–6 cm before breaking.

            (b) Viscosity can be decreased in inflammatory conditions.

        (4) Clot formation indicates the presence of fibrinogen when the synovial membrane is damaged or when there is hemorrhage or blood contamination during a traumatic tap.

        b. Microscopic examination of synovial fluid includes a count of RBCs and WBCs, a differentiation of the types of WBCs, and a wet preparation examination for crystals (see Table 10-8 for normal values).

        (1) An increase in RBCs indicates joint hemorrhage or traumatic tap.

        (2) A **WBC count greater than 2000/μL,** with a predominance of neutrophils, is associated with **bacterial arthritis, acute gouty arthritis, or rheumatoid arthritis.**

        (3) Eosinophils may be present in cases of rheumatic fever or parasitic infestation.

Table 10-8. Normal Synovial Fluid Parameters

Parameter	Typical Result
Volume	Up to 3.5 mL
Color	Straw to yellow
Clarity	Clear
Viscosity	High
Clot formation	None
Red blood cell count	< 2000 μL
White blood cell count	< 200 μL
Differential:	
Monocyte/macrophage	50%–70%
Lymphocytes	20%–40%
Neutrophils	5%–15%
Crystals	None
Glucose	Equal to plasma
Uric acid	Equal to plasma
Total protein	1–3 g/dL
Lactic acid	Equal to plasma
Hyaluronic acid	0.3–0.4 g/dL

    (4) The presence of **crystals can be diagnostic of joint disease.**
        (a) Monosodium urate monohydrate crystals are fine, needle-like crystals associated with **gouty arthritis.**
        (b) Calcium pyrophosphate dihydrate crystals are rodlike or rhombic crystals associated with **pseudogout.**
        (c) Cholesterol crystals are flat, platelike crystals with notched corners. These are seen in conditions of chronic **rheumatoid arthritis.**
        (d) Calcium hydroxyapatite crystals can also be present, but can be seen only with an electron microscope.

  c. Chemical examination of synovial fluid includes only a few diagnostically useful tests (see Table 10-8 for normal values).
    (1) A **decrease in synovial glucose** that exceeds a plasma-fluid difference of 25 mg/dL **indicates an inflammatory condition or sepsis.**
    (2) Increased protein levels indicate synovium permeability changes and damage to the synovial membrane.
    (3) An increase in fluid uric acid levels helps diagnose gout when fluid crystals are not found.

(4) **Increased lactate concentration** is thought to occur from conditions of increased anaerobic glycolysis in the synovium, which is associated with severe inflammatory conditions such as **septic arthritis. Gonococcal arthritis** produces normal-to-low lactate levels.

d. **A microbiologic examination** can aid in the differential diagnosis of joint disease.

(1) A Gram's stain and a culture are performed.

(2) The majority of infectious agents in septic arthritis are bacterial (i.e., **streptococcal infections**), but can also include fungal, mycobacterium, or viral infections.

XI. SEMINAL FLUID ANALYSIS

A. **Seminal fluid physiology**

1. **Composition.** Seminal fluid is comprised of secretions from the testes, epididymis, seminal vesicles, and prostate gland.

a. **Spermatozoa cells form approximately 5% of the ejaculate by volume.**

b. Seminal fluid is a complex solution of **proteins and enzymes** that include the following components:

(1) Acid phosphatase (i.e., unique to prostatic fluid)

(2) Citric acid

(3) Zinc

(4) Fructose

(5) Fibrinogen-like coagulable proteins

2. **Function in the fertilization process.** Seminal fluid has the following mechanisms in fertilization:

a. Activation of spermatozoal motility

b. Provision of nutritive substances

c. Conveyance of the spermatozoa to the female egg

d. Provision of enzymes necessary to penetrate the ovum wall and achieve fertilization

3. **Spermatozoa maturation takes place in the testes.**

a. Spermatozoa have a haploid complement of chromosomes.

b. **FSH** is necessary for the initiation of spermatogenesis.

c. **Testosterone** is necessary for the subsequent stages of maturation.

d. The **stages of cellular maturation** from the **youngest to the most mature** stage are as follows:

(1) Spermatogonia

(2) Spermatocytes

(3) Spermatids

(4) Spermatozoa

B. **Indications for seminal fluid analysis** vary.

1. Seminal fluid examination should be one of the first tests performed in any **infertility investigation.**

2. **Qualification of donors for artificial insemination programs** requires a complete seminal analysis.

3. Analysis can provide the necessary information for the **documentation of completeness for a vasectomy.**

4. **Evaluation of semen quality is necessary for semen and sperm banking.**

5. Seminal fluid analysis often is necessary for **forensic studies in sexually related crimes,** such as rape.

6. Forensic studies of seminal fluid can also be necessary with **paternity allegations.**

C. **Routine analysis of seminal fluid involves a physical, chemical, and microscopic examination of the specimen.**

1. **Physical examination** includes an assessment of the appearance, volume, and viscosity of the ejaculate.

   a. The normal appearance is gray-white and opalescent, although a brown or red color may indicate blood.

   b. Normal volume for an ejaculate is **2–5 mL. Volumes outside this range can be associated with infertility.**

   c. Viscosity can be estimated by observing the formation of droplets that form when the fluid is expelled with a Pasteur pipette.

      (1) A specimen of normal viscosity is watery after liquefaction and easily forms droplets on a flat surface.

      (2) **Increased viscosity is seen when the fluid forms a string** as the drop is expelled from the pipette.

      (3) A normal semen specimen should liquefy approximately 30 minutes after ejaculation.

2. **A microscopic examination** is vital for fertility studies and includes a determination of motility, sperm count, sperm morphology, viability, and an examination of cells other than sperm that may be present.

   a. **Motility** is evaluated as an important indicator of fertility.

      (1) **Motility is directly proportional to the anatomic integrity of spermatozoa as well as fertility.**

      (2) Sperm are evaluated microscopically in a counting chamber (e.g., **Makler chamber**).

      (3) The slide is prewarmed to 37°C, and sperm are examined with a high-dry objective.

      (4) At least 100 spermatozoa in at least 10 different fields are evaluated on a 0–4+ scale. **Motility rankings** are based on the following **criteria**:

         (a) **0:** Immobile
         (b) **1:** Mobile; no forward progression
         (c) **2:** Mobile; slow nondirectional motility
         (d) **3:** Mobile; moderate linear progression
         (e) **4:** Mobile; strong linear progression

(5) Normal motility is defined as 50% or more of the sperm with a ranking of 3 or 4.

b. **Sperm counts** can be obtained from a counting chamber by the same method that is used to get a manual WBC or RBC count.

   (1) A **normal** sperm count is **between 20 million and 200 million** sperm per milliliter.

   (2) Infertility is highly associated with counts lower than 20 million.

c. Spermatozoa **morphology** is also routinely assessed.

   (1) Normally, at least 50% of the sperm should have normal morphology.

   (2) More than 50% morphologically abnormal sperm could be related to infertility.

d. **Viability** is observed using supravital staining of a sample of fresh semen with an eosin stain. A smear is then made of the stained solution.

   (1) Viable sperm do not take up the stain, whereas dead sperm have damaged membranes and absorb the stain.

   (2) One hundred sperm are counted and evaluated.

   (3) The percentage of dead sperm should not exceed the percentage of immobile sperm.

   (4) Normally, 50% or more of the sperm should be viable.

e. The stained seminal fluid smear should also be **examined for the presence of cells other than spermatozoa.**

   (1) An ejaculate may **normally contain leukocytes and urethral epithelial cells.**

   (2) An increase of **leukocytes greater than one million per milliliter of ejaculate is suggestive of an inflammation.**

   (3) The presence of **RBCs or bacteria** indicates a pathologic process, and this should be reported.

3. **A chemical analysis** of seminal fluid is of limited usefulness. However, measurement of the pH, fructose level, and acid phosphatase activity can provide diagnostic information.

   a. **The pH** should be obtained from a **fresh seminal specimen.**

      (1) A pH greater than 7.8 could indicate an infectious process.

      (2) A **pH lower than 7.0** indicates either **successful vasectomy** or that the seminal fluid is entirely prostatic fluid, which indicates **tubule blockage or inflammation.**

   b. **Fructose** is produced and secreted by the **seminal vesicles.**

      (1) Normal. A normal fructose level of greater than 13 μmol per ejaculate reflects normal secretory function.

      (2) Low. Ejaculatory duct obstruction or pathology of the vas deferens produces low fructose levels.

   c. **Acid phosphatase activity** can determine secretory function of the **prostate gland,** because this gland uniquely secretes high levels of this enzyme. Determination of this enzyme in forensic studies can be used to determine the presence of seminal fluid.

    d. Citric acid and zinc levels can be determined to evaluate prostate gland function. **Low levels of both substances are associated with prostatitis.**

XII. CEREBROSPINAL FLUID (CSF) ANALYSIS

  A. Anatomy of CSF location and formation

    1. The central nervous system (CNS) is bathed by a network of reservoirs containing CSF. The anatomic areas that form the CNS include the following:

      a. Cerebral hemispheres

      b. Cerebellum

      c. Brain stem

      d. Spinal cord

    2. The CSF functions to protect and cushion the CNS, provide nutrients to neural tissue, and remove metabolic waste.

    3. CSF is circulated through a canal system comprised of an inner **ventricular system** and an outer **subarachnoid system** that covers the entire surface of the brain and spinal cord. The ventricular system is a connected series of the following reservoirs:

      a. Two lateral ventricles deep within the cerebral hemispheres

      b. The third ventricle located in the midline of the brain

      c. A fourth ventricle located between the brain stem and the cerebellum

      d. The central spinal cord

    4. CSF is produced by the choroid plexus.

      a. This tissue consists of villous tufts of blood vessels covered by a single layer of epithelium.

      b. Choroid plexus tissue is found in the two lateral ventricles.

      c. Approximately 500 mL/d of CSF is produced, with a total volume of 140–170 mL in adults.

  B. Specimen collection is only for diagnosis or for the treatment of disease.

    1. Ventricular puncture to obtain CSF can be performed by a neurosurgeon in special circumstances.

    2. Lumbar puncture between L2 and L3 or between the L3 and L4 interspace is the most common collection technique.

    3. Routinely, three specimen tubes are collected and labeled as 1, 2, and 3. Each tube is uniquely used for specific testing.

      a. Tube 1 is used for CSF chemistry analysis.

      b. Tube 2 is used for microbiology studies.

      c. Tube 3 is used for a hematology cell count and differential.

    4. All testing on CSF specimens should be performed immediately because of rapid cellular degeneration.

  C. Pathologic diseases detected by and involving the CSF include the following conditions:

1. **Subarachnoid or intracerebral hemorrhages** (i.e., strokes)

2. **Infections such as meningitis** (e.g., bacterial, fungal, parasitic, or viral); epidural and intracerebral **abscesses; and encephalitis**

3. **Malignant processes** such as primary brain tumors, metastatic brain tumors, or leukemias and lymphomas

D. **Routine CSF analysis typically includes a physical, chemical, and microscopic analysis.**

1. **Gross examination** includes a report of color and clarity of the specimen.

    a. **Normal CSF is clear and colorless.**

    b. **Turbidity** is most often produced by the increased presence of WBCs (> 200 cells per milliliter), by increased RBCs (> 400 RBCs per milliliter), or by microorganisms. Cellular turbidity is known as **pleocytosis.**

    c. **Abnormal specimen color** is most commonly caused by a disease process.

       (1) **Pink or red CSF is the result of RBC lysis** and can be seen 4–10 hours after a subarachnoid hemorrhage.

       (2) **Xanthochromic (i.e., yellow) specimens** result from the following conditions:

          (a) After **pathologic bleeding** caused by breakdown of hemoglobin and bilirubin formation in CSF

          (b) When CSF **protein** is increased greater than 250 mg/dL

          (c) **Liver disease** caused by increased total bilirubin levels

       (3) **Brown CSF specimens** are the result of the following conditions:

          (a) Presence of **methemoglobin**

          (b) Subdural or intracerebral **hematoma**

          (c) Presence of **melanin** caused by a melanoma

    d. **Distinguishing between pathologic bleeding and traumatic tap,** and therefore the presence of RBCs, is often necessary. The following criteria can be used to distinguish between the two:

       (1) **A serial decrease in RBCs in each tube** is seen with a traumatic tap.

       (2) **A clotted specimen or clumped RBCs** on microscopic examination indicates traumatic tap.

       (3) The color of the supernatant of a bloody specimen after centrifugation can be suggestive. **A clear supernatant indicates a traumatic tap,** whereas a **pink, yellow, or brown supernatant indicates pathologic bleeding.**

       (4) A ratio of > **500 RBCs for every WBC** indicates traumatic tap.

2. **Chemical examination** can include many analytes, but only a few have any diagnostic value on a routine basis.

    a. **Total protein in CSF** represents a combination of prealbumin, albumin, transferrin, and trace amounts of immunoglobulin G (IgG).

       (1) **Normally, CSF protein ranges between 20 and 50 mg/dL,** with albumin representing 50%–70%.

       (2) A CSF protein level **provides information as to the integrity of the blood-brain barrier.**

(3) Increased protein levels can be the result of the following conditions:
  (a) **Contamination with peripheral blood** on obtaining the specimen
  (b) **Obstruction** of CSF circulation (e.g., hematoma)
  (c) **Tissue degeneration**
  (d) **Increased permeability of the blood-brain membrane** caused by toxic factors or infection
  (e) **Chronic bleeding** and hemolysis
(4) Recognizing increases in individual protein constituents in the CSF can be important.
  (a) **Prealbumin** is uniquely found in CSF specimens.
  (b) **Albumin** is not produced by the choroid plexus; therefore, all albumin present in a specimen is from the passage of plasma albumin across the blood-brain barrier. **CSF albumin is increased when the permeability of the blood-brain barrier is compromised** (i.e., normal CSF/serum albumin index < 9.0).
  (c) **IgG is present in trace amounts** but can originate from production in the CSF or can come across the blood-brain barrier.
    (i) **A CSF/serum IgG index < 0.77 is normal.**
    (ii) An IgG CSF/serum **index > 0.77 is highly indicative of multiple sclerosis.**
  (d) **CSF protein electrophoresis** can be a useful tool to distinguish protein content.
    (i) A normal electrophoretic pattern has as the first band **prealbumin and then albumin, followed by two transferrin bands.** Faint bands of α_1-antitrypsin and IgG may also be present.
    (ii) The **prealbumin and transferrin bands are unique to CSF** protein electrophoresis tracings.
    (iii) **Abnormal oligoclonal bands** in the gamma region of the tracing are comprised of IgG and are **highly diagnostic of multiple sclerosis.**
  (e) **Myelin basic proteins** may be present with **multiple sclerosis.**
b. **Glucose** is in equilibrium with plasma glucose.
  (1) **Normal values** in the CSF range from **50–80 mg/dL or approximately two thirds of plasma glucose levels.**
  (2) Levels are **decreased in bacterial meningitis and fungal infections.**
  (3) Levels are **increased in hyperglycemia** and in cases of a traumatic tap.
c. **CSF enzyme levels** can be detected and are elevated in a variety of pathologic conditions.
  (1) **LDH concentrations** can be elevated in the following conditions:
    (a) Bacterial and viral meningitis
    (b) Subarachnoid hemorrhage
    (c) Lymphomas
    (d) Leukemias
    (e) Metastatic tumors

       (**2**) **Creatine kinase (CK) levels** can be elevated in the following conditions:

          (**a**) Stroke

          (**b**) Multiple sclerosis

          (**c**) Degenerative disorders

          (**d**) Primary brain tumors

          (**e**) Viral and bacterial meningitis

          (**f**) Epileptic seizure

       (**3**) **Aspartate aminotransferase (AST) levels** can be elevated in the following conditions:

          (**a**) Intracerebral hemorrhage

          (**b**) Subarachnoid hemorrhage

          (**c**) Bacterial meningitis

   d. **CSF lactic acid** concentrations are unrelated to plasma values.

       (**1**) The **normal concentration ranges from 10–22 mg/dL.**

       (**2**) Lactate is increased with any disorder associated with increased metabolism or ischemia in the CNS.

   e. CSF electrolytes reflect basically the same values as in serum, and their measurement in CSF is of no diagnostic advantage.

  3. **Cell count and differential** normally reflect low numbers of cells.

   a. Normally, **mononuclear cells (i.e., lymphocytes, monocytes) predominate** in a low concentration of **0–10 cells per microliter.**

       (**1**) Neutrophils compose 0%–6%.

       (**2**) Monocytes compose 15%–45%.

       (**3**) Lymphocytes compose the majority of cell types: 40%–80%.

   b. RBCs should be absent. **The presence of RBCs indicates either cerebral hemorrhage or traumatic tap.**

   c. Cell counts **must be performed within 1 hour of collection.**

   d. If increased WBCs are found, a **cytospin** smear is prepared, and the smear undergoes Wright's stain to determine the differential.

   e. Any other cell type or a change in differential percent could indicate a serious disorder.

       (**1**) An **increase in neutrophils** is indicative of **bacterial meningitis.**

       (**2**) An **increase in lymphocytes** can be found in cases of **viral, tubercular, or fungal meningitis.**

       (**3**) **Plasma cells** may be found in patients who have **multiple sclerosis or chronic inflammatory conditions.**

       (**4**) An **eosinophilia** may be associated with **parasitic or fungal disorders.**

       (**5**) **Macrophages** can be found in CSF in association with **hemorrhage.** The presence of **ferritin granules** in the cytoplasm of CSF macrophages may indicate an older or chronic hemorrhagic condition.

       (**6**) Malignant cells can be present as a result of a CNS tumor or a leukemic process.

  4. **Microscopic examination** consists of a Gram's stain or acid-fast stain, as well as a culture and sensitivity determination. Viral studies or fungal cultures can also be performed.

5. **Immunologic examination** can detect several bacterial and fungal organisms that cause meningitis.

a. **Assay methodologies** can include latex agglutination, radioimmunoassay, and counterimmunoelectrophoresis.

b. **Meningitis-causing organisms** that can be easily detected using immunologic assays include the following:

(1) *Cryptococcus* spp.

(2) *Coccidioides immitis*

(3) *Mycobacterium tuberculosis*

(4) *Haemophilus influenzae*

(5) *Neisseria meningitidis*

(6) *Streptococcus pneumoniae*

XIII. GASTRIC ANALYSIS

A. **Physiology of gastric secretion and digestion**

1. **Three physiologic functions of the stomach**

a. The stomach acts as an expandable reservoir for ingested food.

b. Initiation of protein digestion by pepsin occurs in the stomach.

c. The gastric mucosa secretes intrinsic factor for binding and absorption of vitamin B_{12} in the ileum.

2. **Three general phases of gastric secretion**

a. The **cephalic (i.e., neurogenic) phase** involves vagal nerve stimulation caused by stimuli such as taste, smell, or sight. Anticipation of food (i.e., hunger response) has four effects on the stomach.

(1) **Gastrin** is secreted into the blood by specialized **G cells** in the pyloric gland and stomach, and by the **delta cells of the pancreas.**

(2) Gastrin causes **secretion of hydrochloric acid by parietal cells** of the gastric glands in the proximal body and fundus and **secretion of pepsin by the chief cells.**

(3) Vagal excitation lowers the threshold of parietal cells to gastrin stimulation.

(4) Gastric peristalsis and emptying is promoted.

b. The **gastric phase** involves gastric distention and continued gastric secretion of digestive juices.

c. The **intestinal phase** involves digestion in the small intestines.

(1) Secretion of **gastrin** by G cells is **inhibited by gastric inhibitory polypeptide (GIP),** which is secreted by the duodenal glands in the small intestine.

(2) Gastrin secretion is reduced at a pH $\leq$ 3.0 and stops completely at a pH $\leq$ 1.5. When **K cells** located in the distal duodenum and proximal jejunum come in contact with fats, glucose, or amino acids, gastric GIP is produced.

B. **Chemical composition of gastric fluid**

1. **Hydrochloric acid** (HCl) is present in varying amounts.

a. HCl is **secreted by parietal cells** in the fundus of the stomach.

    b. HCl functions to **convert pepsinogen to pepsin and to hydrolyze polypeptides and disaccharides.**

  2. Pepsin, which catalyzes proteolysis at a pH of 1.6–3.6, is also present.

  3. Mucus is present to protect the mucosa of the stomach from autodigestion.

  4. Miscellaneous substances are present such as various enzymes, proteins, and intrinsic factor.

C. Gastric analysis may be necessary for the diagnosis of digestive disorders or ulcers.

  1. Gastric acidity may fall into one of several categories.

    a. Anacidity refers to the failure of the stomach acidity to fall lower than 6.0 in a stimulation test.

    b. Hypochlorhydria refers to the physiologic failure of pH to fall below 3.5, although it decreases 1.0 pH unit or more upon gastric stimulation.

    c. Achlorhydria is the physiologic failure of pH to fall below 3.5 or 1.0 pH unit **with gastric stimulation.**

  2. Evaluation of gastric fluid acidity may be performed to determine the proper surgical procedure to be used for peptic ulcer treatment.

  3. Gastric analysis may aid in the diagnosis of Zollinger-Ellison syndrome, which usually results from a neoplasm of the pancreas and causes increased gastric secretion of acid, secretory volume, and very high blood gastrin levels.

  4. Determination of gastric acid secretion in response to insulin-induced hypoglycemia can be beneficial to assess the completeness of surgical vagotomy.

D. Gastric analysis and collection of gastric fluid can be performed using several methods.

  1. The **basal gastric secretion test** measures fasting levels of gastric production.

    a. The gastric secretion collected represents the amount of secretion during a 15-hour fast.

    b. Four 15- or 30-minute specimens are collected. On each gastric specimen, the volume, pH, titratable acidity, and calculated acid output is determined.

  2. Maximal stimulation tests involve a subcutaneous dose of histamine acid phosphate. This test has been replaced by the **pentagastrin test,** in which pentagastrin is used to stimulate maximal secretion.

  3. Insulin-induced hypoglycemia test is often used to test for the completeness of vagotomy.

    a. Hypoglycemia stimulates the vagus to stimulate gastric acid secretion within 2 hours after insulin injection.

    b. Blood glucose measurements are also taken every 30 minutes (i.e., pre- and post-insulin injection) to make sure that glucose falls to 50 mg/dL or lower.

   4. Tubeless gastric analysis is a noninvasive method to determine gastric acidity.

   a. Dianex blue, which is a carboxylic acid cationic resin with an indicator dye (i.e., azure A) coupled to it, is given orally to the patient.

   b. Hydrogen ions in gastric secretion combine with the resin and release the azure A ions, which are absorbed into the bloodstream in the small intestine and excreted in the urine.

E. A routine physical evaluation of gastric fluid includes the following measurements:

   1. Appearance (i.e., normal is translucent, pale gray, and slightly viscous)

   2. Volume (i.e., normal is 50–75 mL)

   3. Odor (i.e., normal is faintly pungent)

   4. Mucus (i.e., normal quantity varies)

   5. Microscopic examination

   6. Measurement of gastric acid and pH

XIV. FECAL ANALYSIS

A. Abnormal fecal formation is often secondary to gastrointestinal disease.

   1. Diarrhea is defined as an increase in volume, liquidity, and frequency of bowel movements as compared with normal.

   a. Secretory diarrhea is caused by increased intestinal secretion of a solute. This condition can be caused by the following circumstances:

   (1) Endotoxin-producing bacteria
   (2) Mucosal damage
   (3) Drugs (e.g., caffeine, prostaglandins)

   b. Osmotic diarrhea results from the increased ingestion of osmotically active solutes that draw fluid into the gastrointestinal tract. This is seen in the following conditions or treatments:

   (1) Maldigestion caused by a **lactase deficiency** or a **lipase deficiency**
   (2) Malabsorption (i.e., celiac disease, tropical sprue)
   (3) Laxative use
   (4) Parasitic infections
   (5) Small bowel resection

   c. Increased intestinal motility is caused by the following conditions:

   (1) Parasympathetic nervous activity (e.g., stress)
   (2) Laxatives (e.g., castor oil)
   (3) Cardiovascular drugs (e.g., digitalis)

   2. Steatorrhea is defined as fecal fat excretion exceeding 3 g/d.

   a. Dietary fat has only a small effect on the total amount of fecal fat.

   b. With steatorrhea, feces appear pale, greasy, bulky, spongy, or pasty in consistency and have a very strong odor.

   c. Steatorrhea can occur in combination with diarrhea.

   d. This condition can result from either maldigestion or malabsorption.

      (1) Maldigestion can result from decreased levels of pancreatic enzymes (e.g., pancreatitis, pancreatic cancer) or decreased bile-acid formation (e.g., obstructive jaundice).

      (2) Malabsorption can result from diseases that damage intestinal mucosa (e.g., tropical sprue, celiac disease)

B. Specimen collection generally follows rules of common sense.

  1. Patients must be instructed how to obtain a proper specimen.

  2. A specimen container can be any clean, nonbreakable, leakproof container that is large enough to contain the specimen.

  3. The type and amount of fecal specimen depends on the type of test ordered.

    a. For fecal occult blood, WBCs, or qualitative fat, only a small specimen is required.

    b. Quantitative fecal fat analysis requires a 3-day specimen.

  4. The technologist must be aware of contaminants such as urine, water, or paper.

C. Macroscopic examination includes observation of specimen color, consistency, and form.

  1. Color changes of the stool specimen can result from gastrointestinal irregularities. Color changes of stool and their indications include the following:

    a. Brown (i.e., normal)

    b. Gray (i.e., fecal obstruction or barium)

    c. Red (i.e., blood or food dyes)

    d. Black (i.e., blood from upper gastrointestinal tract, iron therapy, or charcoal treatment)

    e. Green (i.e., vegetables, biliverdin)

  2. Consistency can demonstrate the following variety:

    a. Formed (i.e., normal)

    b. Hard (i.e., constipated)

    c. Watery (i.e., diarrhea or steatorrhea)

  3. Form of the stool specimen and changes in form can also be caused by gastrointestinal irregularities. The types of fecal form and their indications include the following:

    a. Cylindrical (i.e., normal)

    b. Ribbon-like (i.e., intestinal strictures)

    c. Small, round (i.e., constipation)

    d. Bulky (i.e., steatorrhea)

    e. Mucus (i.e., colitis, constipation)

D. Chemical examination typically includes an examination for only blood, fat, or carbohydrates.

  1. Fecal blood determination is important as an early detector of colorectal cancer.

    a. The physician must be aware that any bleeding from the gums to the anus can result in positive fecal blood.

        (1) Melena is defined as large amounts of fecal blood (i.e., 50–100 mL/d) that turn the stool black.

        (2) Occult blood refers to small amounts of fecal blood (i.e., 30–50 mL/d).

    b. Testing principles are designed for sensitivity and turnaround times.

        (1) Hemoglobin-reduction methods are based on the reaction of hemoglobin (Hb) with hydrogen peroxide (H_2O_2) and an indicator. These methods are popular and very common because of their ease of operation and short testing time. The chemical reaction formula is demonstrated as follows:

$$H_2O_2 + \text{Indicator} \xrightarrow{\text{(Hb)}} \text{Oxidized indicator} + H_2O$$
$$\text{(blue-green color)}$$

            (a) The following are **common indicators** that are used (most sensitive to least sensitive):

                (i) Benzidine (i.e., carcinogenic)

                (ii) Orthotoluidine

                (iii) Guaiac (i.e., most common)

            (b) There are a variety of **interfering factors** that can cause false-positive or false-negative test results.

                (i) False-positive results are seen with a diet of rare-cooked meats; some vegetables (e.g., turnips, broccoli); some fruits (e.g., cantaloupes, bananas); and drugs (e.g., aspirin).

                (ii) False-negative results can be caused by vitamin C (i.e., ascorbic acid).

            (c) There are **limitations to the sensitivity and specificity** of this method.

                (i) More than one fecal site needs to be tested for accuracy.

                (ii) If Hb has been degraded on standing or in the gastrointestinal tract, its pseudoperoxidase activity has been lost, and it will not react with the indicator.

        (2) HemoQuant test principle is based on the conversion of nonfluorescent heme to fluorescent porphyrins.

            (a) This method detects total fecal Hb (i.e., degraded and nondegraded).

            (b) A higher degree of specificity is obtained as compared to conventional methods (i.e., is not affected by common interfering substances).

        (3) Immunodiffusion and enzyme immunoassay using an anti-human Hb are the most sensitive methods.

  2. Fetal hemoglobin (Hb F) in feces must sometimes be determined, because differentiation between fetal and maternal blood is critical.

    a. Newborns may excrete stools containing blood originating from maternal blood that was ingested during delivery.

    b. Maternal RBCs can be distinguished from fetal RBCs in a stool sample with the **Apt test.**

      (1) The test **principle** is based on the **alkaline resistance** of fetal Hb.

      (2) A fecal suspension is made, and 5 mL of the supernatant is mixed with 1 mL of 0.25 mol/L sodium hydroxide.

    c. If the pink color of the blood changes to yellow or brown in 2 minutes, the Hb present is Hb A (i.e., adult, maternal).

    d. If the pink color remains, the Hb present is Hb F (i.e., fetal).

  3. Quantitative fecal fat is a definitive test for steatorrhea.

    a. Two days before collection, the patient is put on a normal diet to include adequate fat and caloric intake.

    b. A 3- to 6-day fecal collection is obtained.

    c. The test principle is based on the determination of fat content by either **titrimetric or gavimetric methods.**

    d. The procedure involves first weighing the sample and then homogenizing it.

      (1) Analysis by the **titrimetric method** involves the following basic steps:

        (a) Lipids are converted to free fatty acids before extraction with a solvent.

        (b) The extracted free fatty acids are titrated against sodium hydroxide.

        (c) This method measures up to 80% of the total fat content.

      (2) The **gravimetric method of analysis** quantitates up to 100% of fats.

    e. Normal values range between 1 and 6 g/d of fecal fat.

    f. Percent fat retention can be calculated using the following formula:

$$\% \text{ Fat retention} = \frac{\text{Dietary gram fat} - \text{fecal fat}}{\text{Dietary gram fat}}$$

  4. Fecal carbohydrate analysis may be necessary to differentiate disaccharidase enzyme deficiencies.

    a. If disaccharides from the diet are not enzymatically reduced to monosaccharides, **they will remain in the intestine and be osmotically active, producing an osmotic diarrhea.**

    b. Causes of osmotic diarrhea due to an increase of disaccharides in the gastrointestinal tract include the following disorders:

      (1) Hereditary disaccharidase deficiency is rare.

      (2) Acquired disaccharidase deficiency occurs from malabsorption diseases (e.g., tropical sprue) or from drug effects (i.e., neomycin).

      (3) Lactose intolerance is the most common cause, and it is seen most often in African or Asian populations.

    c. Osmotic diarrheal stools characteristically **have an acid pH between 5.0 and 6.0.** Normal feces are alkaline (i.e., greater than 7.0).

Table 10-9. Maldigestion and Malabsorption Differentiation

Cause	First Slide (Neutral Fat)	Second Slide (Free Fatty Acids)
Malabsorption	Normal	Increased
Maldigestion	Increased	Normal or increased

    d. Analysis for disaccharidase deficiency includes the following testing methods:

        (1) Clinitest can be used to test for reducing sugars, but the specific disaccharide is not identified, and sucrose cannot be detected [see IV C 1 c (3)].

        (2) Determination of specific enzyme deficiencies can be made by an **oral tolerance test using specific sugars** (e.g., lactose, sucrose).

            (a) Normally, the disaccharide is converted to a monosaccharide (e.g., glucose, galactose) in the small intestine.

            (b) An increase in the patient's blood glucose or galactose 30 mg/dL greater than the fasting level indicates adequate enzyme activity.

E. Microscopic examination is necessary to identify stool WBCs or the presence of increased fecal fat.

    1. A determination of fecal WBCs aids in the differential diagnosis of diarrhea.

        a. The presence of **stool WBCs indicates an infectious or inflammatory intestinal mucosal wall.**

        b. The finding of stool WBCs can indicate the following disorders:

            (1) Ulcerative colitis

            (2) Dysentery (bacterial)

            (3) Ulcerative diverticulitis

            (4) Intestinal tuberculosis

            (5) Abscesses

    2. The presence of fecal fat can also be determined microscopically.

        a. Sudan III, Sudan IV, or oil red O stains all **stain fecal triglycerides** orange to red in suspension.

            (1) A suspension of the fecal preparation can also be placed on a slide with several drops of ethanol.

            (2) Stain is added to the slide, and the wet preparation is shielded with a cover slip and observed for stained fat globules.

            (3) Normal stool contains more than 60 globules per high-power field.

            (4) To a second slide, HCl and heat can be added, which also causes free fatty acids to be stained. An increase in the number of fat globules is normally observed.

            (5) An **increased number of globules greater than 100** per high-power field, **and large globules measuring 40 to 80 μm, are indicative of steatorrhea.**

      b. Differentiation. Cases of maldigestion can be differentiated from malabsorption by comparing results from both slide preparations (Table 10-9).

  3. The increased presence of meat fibers can be diagnostically significant.

      a. An **increase in fecal meat fibers (creatorrhea)** indicates **impaired digestion and/or rapid intestinal transit.**

      b. Meat fibers are identified microscopically as rectangular or cylindrical fibers with cross striations.

Study Questions

Directions: Each of the numbered items or incomplete statements in this section is followed by answers or by completions of the statement. Select the ONE lettered answer or completion that is BEST in each case.

1. The filtering unit of the kidney is the

a. tubule
b. nephron
c. glomerulus
d. ureter

2. Approximately how many milliliters of blood are filtered through the kidneys each minute?

a. 200
b. 900
c. 1200
d. 2000

3. A doctor sent the laboratory a sample of a fluid he aspirated from the abdomen of one of his patients. To determine if this fluid is urine, the clinical laboratory scientist should measure which one of the following groups of substances?

a. urea, creatinine, sodium, and chloride
b. glucose, protein, blood, and nitrates
c. urochrome, urobilin, bilirubin, and urobilinogen
d. glucose, protein, urea, and chloride

4. Reagent dipsticks in their original container should be stored in which one of the following locations?

a. in the refrigerator
b. in a cool, dry place
c. in a warm, humid place
d. in direct sunlight

5. The type of urine specimen routinely required for a microbial culture is

a. random void specimen
b. midstream "clean catch"
c. catheterized
d. suprapubic

6. Normal urine color is produced by the presence of

a. uroporphyrin, coproporphyrin, and protoporphyrin
b. urobilinogen, bilirubin, and hemoglobin
c. porphobilinogen and urobilinogen
d. urochrome, uroerythrin, and urobilin

7. A urine with a fruity odor most probably contains which one of the following substances?

a. phenylalanine
b. ammonia
c. ketones
d. tyrosine

8. The specific gravity of urine is best described by which one of the following statements?

a. It reflects the ability of the kidney to concentrate and dilute urine.
b. It is a measure of the number of solute particles per unit of solvent.
c. It is a measure of the weight of a substance compared with an equal volume of saline.
d. It is equal to the amount of dissolved substances in plasma.

9. A urine specimen is too concentrated to read on the refractometer scale. It is diluted by taking one drop of the specimen and adding it to three drops of distilled water. The diluted sample now reads 1.012 on the refractometer scale. The specific gravity of this sample should be reported as

a. 1.012
b. 1.036
c. 1.048
d. 3.036

10. A 25-year-old man who has a normal food and fluid intake excreted 4000 mL of urine in 24 hours. This urine volume can best be described as

a. pyuria
b. polyuria
c. anuria
d. oliguria

11. An unpreserved urine specimen was at room temperature for 4 hours in an unsterile container. Which one of the following sets of actions can occur?

a. bacteria decrease, ketones decrease, glucose decreases, pH decreases
b. bacteria decrease, ketones increase, glucose decreases, pH increases
c. bacteria increase, ketones decrease, glucose decreases, pH increases
d. bacteria increase, ketones increase, glucose decreases, pH decreases

12. A reagent strip test impregnated with 2,4-dichloroaniline diazonium salt reacts with urine, producing a purple to tan color. The detected substance most likely is

a. bilirubin
b. glucose
c. protein
d. urobilinogen

13. Which one of the following groups of crystals is normally found in alkaline urine?

a. uric acid, calcium oxalate, cystine
b. cholesterol, bilirubin, calcium carbonate
c. calcium oxalate, triple phosphate, and leucine
d. triple phosphate, ammonium biurate, and calcium carbonate

14. Patients who have diabetes mellitus produce urine that has

a. increased volume with a low specific gravity
b. decreased volume with a low specific gravity
c. decreased volume with a high specific gravity
d. increased volume with a high specific gravity

15. Nephrotic syndrome is characterized by pronounced

a. glucosuria
b. proteinuria
c. hematuria
d. bilirubinuria

16. A positive test result for β-hCG and pregnancy using a standard latex procedure would visually appear as what type of reaction?

a. hemolysis
b. no agglutination (i.e., smooth)
c. agglutination (i.e., clumped)
d. fluorescent

17. Kidney stone formation of calcium composition is most commonly caused by

a. primary hyperparathyroidism
b. chronic renal tubular acidosis
c. idiopathic hypercalciuria
d. all of the aforementioned

18. A serous fluid that results from filtration of serum across a physically intact vascular wall, which is caused by a systemic disease such as congestive heart failure, is known as

a. a transudate
b. an osmolite
c. an exudate
d. synovial fluid

19. Viscosity in synovial fluid is related to the concentration of which one of the following substances?

a. fluid protein
b. fluid uric acid
c. hyaluronic acid
d. calcium hydroxyapatite

20. A seminal fluid pH lower than 7.0 could indicate which one of the following situations?

a. unsuccessful vasectomy
b. seminal tubule blockage or inflammation
c. prostatitis
d. the presence of increased leukocytes

21. Three separate tubes of cerebrospinal fluid (CSF) are routinely collected in a lumbar puncture procedure. What type of testing is performed on tube 3?

a. microbiology
b. immunology
c. chemistry
d. hematology

22. A cerebrospinal fluid (CSF) protein electrophoresis can be a good test to aid in obtaining a diagnosis of central nervous system (CNS)–related disorders. If oligoclonal bands of IgG are found, their presence is diagnostic of

a. multiple myeloma
b. bacterial meningitis
c. cerebral tumor
d. multiple sclerosis

23. Zollinger-Ellison syndrome refers to which one of the following conditions?

a. a condition caused by the accumulation of uric acid in the synovial fluid of joints
b. the physiologic failure of gastric pH to fall lower than 3.5 with gastric stimulation
c. a neoplasm of the pancreas causing increased secretion of gastrin and gastric secretion of acid
d. a condition of chronic osmotic diarrhea caused by a genetic disaccharidase deficiency

24. The most sensitive indicator that can be used in the hemoglobin reduction method for detecting fecal blood is

a. benzidine
b. orthotoluidine
c. guaiac
d. peroxidase

25. The presence of stool white blood cells (WBCs) indicates which one of the following intestinal disorders?

a. disaccharidase deficiency
b. lactose intolerance
c. colorectal cancer
d. infectious or inflammatory bowel disease

Answers and Explanations

1. The answer is c [I A 2 a (1), B 1 a]. The glomerulus is comprised of a tuft of thin-walled capillaries. Blood flows into the capillary plexus from the relatively wider afferent arteriole and exits through the smaller efferent arteriole. The difference in the size of the lumen of these two vessels produces an increase in hydrostatic pressure within these capillaries, which forces the filtrate through the capillary epithelium and into Bowman's capsule.

2. The answer is c [I B 1]. Approximately 1200 mL of blood is supplied to the kidneys each minute.

3. The answer is a [I C 1 a–c]. Substances normally found in the urine include urea, creatinine, uric acid, chloride, sodium, and potassium.

4. The answer is b [II B 5]. Dipsticks are subject to deterioration caused by moisture, heat, or light exposure. Therefore, they should be stored in a cool, dry place.

5. The answer is b [II D 1 b]. A random midstream "clean-catch" urine specimen is desirable for microbial cultures so that contamination from the external genitalia and the vagina is minimized.

6. The answer is d [III A 1 a]. Normal urine color is produced by the presence of urochrome (a yellow pigment), which is present in the highest concentration; uroerythrin (a red pigment); and urobilin (an orange-red pigment).

7. The answer is c [III B 2 b]. Increased ketone bodies excreted during periods of starvation or by diabetic patients give the urine a fruity odor.

8. The answer is a [III C 2]. The specific gravity of urine reflects the ability of the kidney to concentrate and dilute urine. It is a measure of the weight of a substance compared with an equal volume of pure, solute-free water at the same temperature. Specific gravity is a measure of the amount of dissolved substances in urine.

9. The answer is c [III C 3 b]. Specific gravity relates the density of urine to the density of an equal volume of water. Because the value is a ratio, it is always greater than 1.000. Normal specific gravity of urine ranges from 1.002–1.035, which reflects the kidney's ability to concentrate the urine. Occasionally, urine specimens may have an extremely high specific gravity value that exceeds physiologically possible values (e.g., >1.040). Most often, a high-molecular-weight substance, such as a radiopaque contrast dye, has been excreted into the urine. The refractometer scale has a maximum value of 1.035. Urine with a specific gravity greater than 1.035 must be diluted. Because this specimen was diluted 1/4, the decimal portion of the 1.012 reading must be multiplied by 4. Therefore, $0.012 \times 4 = 0.048$, and the specific gravity of the sample is reported as 1.048.

10. The answer is b [III D 1 d]. The normal daily urine volume of an adult ranges from 400–2000 mL. A substantial increase in this volume (such as to 4000 mL) is termed polyuria. Anuria implies no urine production, oliguria is an increase in urine production, and pyuria is an increase in white blood cells (WBCs) in the urine.

11. The answer is c [IV A; Table 10-2]. As a urine sample stands at room temperature in light, a number of changes can occur in its constituents. Bacterial counts will increase as the bacteria proliferate. As these bacteria convert urea to ammonia, the pH will become more alkaline and therefore rise. Ketones are volatile or can be used by bacteria, so they will decrease. Glucose will also decrease because of utilization by bacteria and other cells that may be present in the specimen.

12. The answer is a [IV B 10]. A reagent test strip impregnated with 2,4-dichloroaniline diazonium salt reacts with bilirubin to produce a tan-to-purple color. This is called the diazo reaction. Bilirubin is coupled with a diazonium salt in an acid medium to form azobilirubin, a colored compound. The glucose dipstick reaction for urinary glucose is based on a double sequential enzyme reaction using glucose oxidase. Tests for urinary protein are based on the principle of protein error of indicators. Urobilinogen detection traditionally employs Ehrlich's aldehyde reaction. Urobilinogen reacts with *p*-dimethylaminobenzaldehyde in concentrated hydrochloric acid to form a colored aldehyde, which is usually a cherry-red color.

13. The answer is d [V D 2]. Normal crystals found in alkaline urine are predominantly phosphates, which include triple phosphate, amorphous phosphates, calcium phosphate, ammonium biurate, and calcium carbonate. Crystals are usually identified on the basis of morphology and urinary pH. Crystals precipitate out of solution (urine) when the salt concentration is greater than the solubility threshold for that salt. Thus, crystals are more likely to precipitate out of concentrated urine specimens.

14. The answer is d [VII C 1 c (2)]. Patients who have diabetes mellitus develop polydipsia and produce large volumes of urine with a high specific gravity because glucose is present in the urine. Patients who have diabetes insipidus produce large amounts of urine with a low specific gravity and normal glucose because of a deficiency in antidiuretic hormone production or secretion. Therefore, these patients are unable to concentrate urine.

15. The answer is b [VII C 2]. Nephrotic syndrome is characterized by pronounced proteinuria (i.e., $\geq$ 3.5 g/d). It generally results from excessive permeability of the glomerulus to plasma proteins, which results in immense proteinuria and lipiduria.

16. The answer is b [VIII B 3 a (5)]. Most latex methods for pregnancy testing are particle-inhibition procedures. Visible agglutination indicates that antigen was not present in the sample in sufficient amounts to bind all the antibody, so the antibody binds to the indicator particle, which causes agglutination. The absence of agglutination indicates that increased levels of human chorionic gonadotropin (hCG) were present in the patient's sample, thus preventing secondary agglutination. The absence of agglutination indicates a positive pregnancy test result.

17. The answer is d [IX E 1]. Calculi formation of calcium composition can occur as a secondary manifestation of disorders or conditions that increase the amount of excretable calcium in the blood. Such predisposing factors include idiopathic hypercalciuria; primary hyperparathyroidism; bone disease; excessive milk, alkali, or vitamin D intake; renal tubular acidosis; sarcoidosis; and berylliosis.

18. The answer is a [X A 4 a; Table 10-7]. Transudates result from filtration of blood serum across a physically intact vascular wall, which can be caused by a systemic disease such as congestive heart failure, hepatic cirrhosis, or nephrotic syndrome. Exudates are the active accumulation of fluid within body cavities in association with inflammation and vascular wall damage. Exudates, which are closer to serum in chemical composition, are caused by inflammatory disorders, malignancies, and infections. Synovial fluid, which is found in joints such as the knee, is not involved in congestive heart failure.

19. The answer is c [X C 3 a (3)]. Synovial fluid should have a high viscosity because of the presence of hyaluronic acid. This viscosity is important for the lubrication of the joints. Hyaluronic acid is a high-molecular-weight protein that contributes to synovial fluid viscosity far greater than do proteins. Uric acid or calcium hydroxyapatite should not be found in healthy synovial fluid.

20. The answer is b [XI C 3 a (2)]. An acidic seminal fluid (i.e., pH < 7) could indicate seminal tubule blockage or inflammation. By contrast, infectious processes are associated with an alkaline (i.e., pH > 7) seminal fluid.

21. The answer is d [XII B 3]. Of the three tubes of cerebrospinal fluid (CSF) that are routinely collected, a cell count and differential are performed on tube 3. Tube 1 is for chemistries, and tube 2 is for microbiology studies.

22. The answer is d [XII D 2 a (4) (d) (iii)]. Cerebrospinal fluid (CSF) normally contains proteins such as prealbumin, albumin, and IgG in small amounts. A normal electrophoretic pattern demonstrates the first band as prealbumin, then albumin, followed by two transferrin bands. Faint bands of α_1-antitrypsin and IgG may also be present. Abnormal bands composed of increased amounts of IgG are known as oligoclonal bands. The presence of these bands is diagnostic of multiple sclerosis. Multiple myeloma, bacterial meningitis, and cerebral tumor may increase CSF protein levels, but oligoclonal bands are usually not found in patients who have these conditions.

23. The answer is c [XIII C 3]. Zollinger-Ellison syndrome usually results from a neoplasm of the pancreas, which causes increased gastric secretion of acid and secretory volume, and very high blood gastrin levels.

24. The answer is a [XIV D 1 b (1) (a)]. Benzidine is the most sensitive indicator but is seldom used because of its carcinogenic nature. Guaiac is the least sensitive indicator but is the one that is most commonly used.

25. The answer is d [XIV E 1]. The presence of stool white blood cells (WBCs) indicates an infectious or inflammatory intestinal mucosal wall. The finding of stool WBCs can suggest an investigation for disorders such as ulcerative colitis, bacterial dysentery, ulcerative diverticulitis, intestinal tuberculosis, and colorectal abscesses. Disaccharidase deficiency, lactose intolerance, or colorectal cancer usually result in diarrhea.

Case Studies

■ CASE 1: *[Chapter 1]*

A 25-year-old man was admitted to the hospital after being found unconscious by his girlfriend. When he was first seen at the emergency department, blood was drawn for laboratory analysis, and the following results were obtained: serum glucose, 420 mg/dL; sodium, 146 mEq/L; potassium, 4.8 mmol/L; chloride, 95 mmol/L; and bicarbonate, 10 mmol/L. Blood pH was 7.2; PCO_2 was 20 mm Hg. The patient was severely dehydrated, weak, and complaining of abdominal pain. Urinalysis included positive results for glucose, ketones, and acetone.

Questions

- What is the cause of this patient's condition?
- What is the mechanism that results in elevated blood glucose?
- What type of acid-base imbalance is present?

Discussion

The condition of this patient is most likely caused by diabetes, or the elevation of blood glucose. The patient is in a state of ketoacidosis made evident by the presence of glucose and ketones in the urine. Diabetic ketoacidosis occurs when there is deficiency of insulin, which causes an inability of the body tissues to uptake glucose and leads to elevated blood glucose levels or hyperglycemia. In addition, the liver begins to produce ketones as an alternative fuel, which in turn causes metabolic acidosis (low blood pH and PCO_2). The elevated levels of blood glucose and ketones produce dehydration through osmotic diuresis and eventually lead to a decrease in blood pressure. The osmotic diuresis induces urinary losses of potassium, sodium, and bicarbonate; low levels of potassium cause muscle weakness. The ketosis is thought to lead to abdominal pain, although the cause of pain is unclear. The elevated blood and urine glucose levels and elevated urine ketone levels confirm the diagnosis of diabetic ketoacidosis.

Questions

- Why is glucose present in this patient's urine?
- What is responsible for the presence of ketones in the urine?

Discussion

The renal threshold for glucose is 180 mg/dL. Any serum glucose elevation greater than this level "spills over" into the urine. The renal threshold of a substance is defined as the plasma concentration of a substance above which the amount of the substance exceeds the ability of the renal tubules to reabsorb it, thus causing excretion in the urine. Glucose, under normal conditions, is not excreted in the urine but is reabsorbed by the proximal tubule of the kidney. When the renal threshold is reached for glucose, it appears in the urine. The higher the concentration of glucose in the plasma, the higher the amount excreted.

Ketones, acetoacetate, and acetone are common serum ketone bodies or ketoacids. These ketone bodies are intermediary products of fat metabolism and typically provide energy to the brain, kidneys, and striated muscle. In the normal, nondiabetic individual, the formation of ketoacids from 3-hydroxyl-3-methylglutaryl coenzyme A (HMG CoA) is a minor pathway. However, in persons who have Type I diabetes, the lack of insulin and the excess glucose causes the mobilization of fatty acids from triglyceride to be used as a source of energy for cells. Excess acetyl CoA is produced in the degradation of fatty acids and in turn produces high levels of ketoacids. Excess ketoacids in the serum lower blood pH and produce acidosis through the elevation of serum hydrogen. The ketone bodies are excreted by the kidneys, with loss of sodium and potassium.

■ CASE 2: *[Chapter 1]*

A 10-year-old girl exhibited the following symptoms at her pediatrician's office: failure to gain height, obvious weight gain with no change in diet, lethargy, weakness, and some impairment of school performance. Following thyroid hormone analysis, the following results were obtained: decreased thyroxine (T_4) level, decreased triiodothyronine (T_3) level, decreased T_3 uptake, elevated thyrotropin [also referred to as thyroid-stimulating hormone (TSH)], and a positive thyroid microsomal antibody titer of 1:3000. On physical examination, the thyroid gland was observed to be enlarged.

Questions
- What is the most likely diagnosis of this patient's disease?
- What mechanisms regulate the production and release of serum T_4 and TSH?

Discussion

The condition of this patient is most likely induced by the presence in the thyroid gland of lymphocytes and circulating thyroid autoantibodies, a condition known as Hashimoto's thyroiditis. This disorder is a form of progressive autoimmune thyroiditis that affects women eight times more often than men. Clinically, there is an enlarged thyroid gland and the presence of hypothyroidism. The massive infiltration of white blood cells (WBCs) into the gland leads to the inadequate synthesis of the thyroid hormones. Serum TSH levels can increase from 3–100 times the normal value because of the lack of circulating thyroid hormones. A positive erythrocyte hemagglutination test result for antithyroglobulin antibodies is diagnostic of Hashimoto's disease.

All steps involved in the synthesis of thyroid hormones (T_3 and T_4) are regulated by TSH, which interacts with the follicular cells of the thyroid gland to stimulate production and release of T_3 and T_4. TSH also causes an increase in the size and number of follicular cells. Protracted exposure to TSH leads to hypertrophy and enlargement of the thyroid gland, a disorder known as goiter. TSH is released in response to two factors. Thyrotropin releasing hormone (TRH) is synthesized in the hypothalamus and causes the pituitary gland to produce and release TSH. TRH, in turn, can be affected by the serum level of thyroid hormone. A decrease in T_3 and T_4 in the blood activates the hypothalamus to release TRH, which then induces release of TSH. The other factor that affects TSH release from the pituitary gland is the serum level of the thyroid hormones. An increase in circulating T_3 and T_4 inhibits the release of TSH from the pituitary. In the case of Hashimoto's thyroiditis, decreased levels of T_3 and T_4 caused by blocked synthesis in the thyroid gland stimulate the hypothalamic release of TRH, which then stimulates the synthesis and release of TSH. Serum TSH levels increase, which leads to goiter. The decreased levels of T_3 and T_4 cannot "shut off" the pituitary release of TSH.

Questions

- What other conditions can lead to an increase in serum TSH levels?
- Why is the T_3 uptake test abnormal in this patient?

Discussion

Serum TSH is a useful marker in the confirmation of hypothyroidism, in which the concentration of TSH is elevated even in unclear cases. In addition, primary hypothyroidism caused by defects in the thyroid gland can be differentiated from secondary hypothyroidism caused by pituitary dysfunction through the examination of serum TSH levels. In primary hypothyroidism, TSH is increased, whereas in secondary hypothyroidism, TSH levels are decreased along with T_3 and T_4 levels. Many laboratories consider TSH assays as important as free T_4 assays in the diagnosis of thyroid disorders. There are few disorders that demonstrate an increase in serum TSH levels other than primary hypothyroidism. In certain cases of thyrotoxicosis, TSH-secreting tumors lead to hyperthyroidism, with elevated serum TSH levels present despite elevated T_4 levels. Increased TSH release can also be observed in rare cases involving increased secretion of TRH from the hypothalamus.

The T_3 uptake assay analyzes the number of binding sites that are available for thyroid hormone to bind to the thyroxine-binding proteins, particularly thyroglobulin. Patient serum is added to a radioactive T_3 tracer and a T_3-binding resin. The amount of radioactive T_3 bound to the resin is inversely proportional to the number of available binding sites on the protein. In hypothyroidism, the binding sites on the thyroglobulin molecule are not bound by thyroid hormone. This results in a decreased amount of radioactive T_3 being bound to the resin, which leads to a decreased T_3 resin uptake.

■ CASE 3: *[Chapter 2]*

A 90-year-old woman was found unconscious in her bedroom by a neighbor. Paramedics were called to the scene. Before taking the woman to the hospital, one of the paramedics discovered an open box of rat poison in the bathroom. Rat poison contains a coumarin derivative, warfarin. The emergency department physician believes that a blood test should be performed to confirm or rule out poisoning with rat poison.

Questions
- What is the best single test for demonstrating coumarin's effect on this patient's blood?
- What other coagulation factors may be affected at a later time?
- Would the Stypven time test be of any use in confirming this patient's diagnosis? Why, or why not?

Discussion

The prothrombin time (PT) test is the single best test to show the effect of coumarin on a patient's blood. Warfarin is a coumarin derivative that expresses its pharmacologic effect by blocking vitamin K metabolism. This results in loss of activity of coagulation factors II, VII, IX, and X. The PT is prolonged by a deficiency in factor VII; therefore, the PT test is the best test to demonstrate coumarin's effect.

A decline in factor VII activity occurs quickly because factor VII has the shortest half-life (4–6 hours) of all the coagulation factors. A subsequent decline in factors II, IX, and X also occurs.

The Stypven time test would confirm the diagnosis of a factor VII deficiency. The addition of Russell's viper venom instead of lipoprotein reagent activates factor X directly, bypassing factor VII. In this case, the Stypven time would be normal.

■ CASE 4: *[Chapter 2]*

A 44-year-old woman with a history of heart disease and high blood pressure was thought by her physician to be anemic. However, she recently also complained of frequent bleeding from mucosal areas, headaches, fevers, and blackouts. The woman was hospitalized so that testing and a laboratory blood work-up could be performed. Significant laboratory results were: platelet count of 17,000/mm^3; anemia, with a high red cell distribution width (RDW) on her complete blood cell count (CBC); and polychromasia on her blood smear.

Questions

- Based on the given history and test results, would the best preliminary diagnosis for this patient be disseminated intravascular coagulopathy (DIC), thrombotic thrombocytopenic purpura (TTP), idiopathic thrombocytopenic purpura (ITP), or Glanzmann's thrombasthenia?
- What follow-up testing should be performed to confirm the diagnosis?
- What are the physiologic mechanisms responsible for the diagnosis?
- Based on the CBC results and case history, what seems to be a pre-existing condition in this patient?

Discussion

The case study concerns a woman who has an extremely low platelet count. The case history provides significant clues of heart problems and neurologic complications. Approximately 60% of patients who have TTP also have complications of neurologic symptoms and anemia.

To confirm the type of hemolytic anemia, the direct antiglobulin test should be performed. The coagulation profile for prothrombin time, activated partial thromboplastin time, and fibrin degradation products should be performed to eliminate the possibility of DIC. Platelet aggregation studies should be performed to ensure that the platelet disorder is not also functional. Physiologic mechanisms that cause thrombocytopenia include endothelial cell damage, an increase in platelet-aggregating factors or a deficiency of a platelet-aggregating factor inhibitor, a decrease in prostacyclin or an increase in prostacyclin degradation, or an absence of a plasminogen activator.

Based on the patient's CBC results and medical history, a pre-existing condition seems to be microangiopathic anemia, which is evident in more than half of patients who have TTP. The high RDW and polychromasia on the smear in relationship to the anemia and cardiovascular history are suggestive of microangiopathic anemia.

■ CASE 5: *[Chapter 2]*

A 35-year-old woman in labor was admitted to the obstetrics unit at 1:00 AM. Her history and physical examination revealed no significant abnormalities. At the time of admission, she was having irregular contractions. In the delivery room, bleeding became extensive. A hemoglobin and hematocrit, type and cross-match for 4 U of blood, and a coagulation profile were immediately ordered. The patient's laboratory data are given in Case Table 5–1.

Questions

- What is the most probable disorder causing the extensive bleeding in this woman?
- What is the most probable underlying physiologic cause of this woman's disorder?
- Why can a heparin overdose be ruled out as a possible cause?
- Why can a factor VIII deficiency or inhibitor be ruled out as a possible cause?

Case Table 5-1. Patient's Laboratory Data

Hemoglobin	10 g/dL (normal, 12.5–15.5 g/dL)
Hematocrit	27% (normal, 37%–48%)
Platelet count	75,000/mm^3
Bleeding time	19 minutes
Activated partial thromboplastin time	65 seconds
Prothrombin time	19 seconds
Thrombin time	24 seconds (normal, 18–22 seconds)
Fibrinogen	90 mg/dL (normal, 200–400 mg/dL)
Fibrinogen split products (fibrin degradation products) screen	Positive; >40
Protamine sulfate test	Positive

Discussion

Disseminated intravascular coagulation (DIC) is the most likely cause of this woman's bleeding. The patient is in a high-risk condition for DIC, and her bleeding is acute. Furthermore, her coagulation results indicate combined consumption of platelet and coagulation factors. In addition, her fibrin split products (FSP) are increased, which indicates excess fibrin and fibrin degradation.

The release of placental tissue or amniotic fluid into the maternal circulation is the most probable underlying physiologic cause of DIC. These tissue fluids are rich in lipoprotein and act like a massive influx of tissue factor into the circulation, which activates coagulation on a systemic scale.

Heparin administration does not usually result in an acute thrombocytopenia of this magnitude. In addition, heparin would not result in a low level of fibrinogen and a high level of FSP, because heparin functions by blocking thrombin (i.e., factor IIa) and factor Xa.

A factor VIII deficiency or inhibitor can be ruled out because more than the intrinsic clotting pathway is affected. The prothrombin time (PT) and thrombin time (TT) test results are also elevated, which indicates involvement of the extrinsic and common pathways. The elevated FSP level indicates an additional involvement of the fibrinolytic pathway. Also, a factor VIII disorder typically gives a normal bleeding time.

■ CASE 6: *[Chapter 2]*

Laboratory results for a patient who has a severe bleeding problem are given in Case Table 6–1.

Case Table 6-1.   Laboratory Results for Patient with a Severe Bleeding Problem

Platelet count	193,000/mm^3
Bleeding time	15 minutes
Prothrombin time	12.0 seconds (control, 12.0 seconds)
Activated partial thromboplastin time	92.0 seconds
Substitution tests with the activated partial thromboplastin time	
Normal plasma	Correction
Adsorbed plasma	Correction
Aged serum	No correction
Platelet aggregation studies	
Adenosine diphosphate	Normal aggregation
Collagen	Normal aggregation
Epinephrine	Normal aggregation
Ristocetin	No aggregation

Questions

- These results are consistent with a probable diagnosis of what coagulation disorder?
- What factors are missing from the aged serum that failed to correct?
- Why are factors of the common pathway not a possibility?
- What will likely happen to factor VIII:C levels when cryoprecipitate is administered as treatment?

Discussion

The coagulation results of this patient are consistent with von Willebrand's disease (vWD). The prothrombin time (PT) and activated partial thromboplastin time (APTT) results indicate a disorder of a factor in the intrinsic pathway. The platelet count is normal, but the bleeding time is increased, which indicates a platelet functional disorder. Aggregation studies indicate normal function except by restitution, which activates aggregation through VIII:R or von Willebrand's factor (vWF). In many cases, the blood concentrations of VIII:C (antihemolytic factor) will also be low; therefore, the APTT will be elevated.

Aged serum lacks factors I, II, V, and VIII. In this case, the patient's plasma was also deficient in factor VIII; therefore, a correction of the APTT was not obtained by mixing the patient's plasma and aged serum.

Factors of the common pathway are not a possibility because the PT was not elevated. The common pathway consists of factors I, II, V, and X, which are "common" to both the intrinsic (i.e., tested by the APTT) and the extrinsic pathway (i.e., tested by the PT).

The treatment response is different from patients who have hemophilia A. With hemophilia A, the increase in plasma VIII:C levels following cryoprecipitate treatment is entirely proportional to the amount of cryoprecipitate infused. Cryoprecipitate infusion given to patients with vWD stimulates production of factor VIII:C, because the defect is not in factor VIII:C but in the factor VIII:R portion. Levels of VIII:C will slowly peak between 4 and 24 hours to levels greater than the amount of VIII:C infused from the cryoprecipitate.

■ CASE 7: [Chapter 4]

A 26-year-old woman with a lifelong history of cardiac disease was initially seen with a murmur of mitral insufficiency. A recent history of chronic, low-grade menstrual bleeding exaggerated her anemia and compounded her cardiac problems. Treatment of the anemia was initiated, and blood work was obtained a few days after treatment began. A laboratory work-up and Coulter S-VI histogram revealed the results shown in Case Figure 7–1 and Case Table 7–1.

Questions

- This patient is most likely suffering from what type of anemia?
- What is the most likely cause of the appearance of the red blood cell (RBC) histogram in this particular patient?
- If this patient's current RBC distribution and histogram were compared with her RBC histogram before treatment, what would be the difference in patterns, if any?

Discussion

The patient has a long history of chronic blood loss. Her low serum iron level and percent saturation values indicate an iron deficiency. The RBC histogram has a dual peak, which indicates two populations of RBCs. One peak is in the microcytic range,

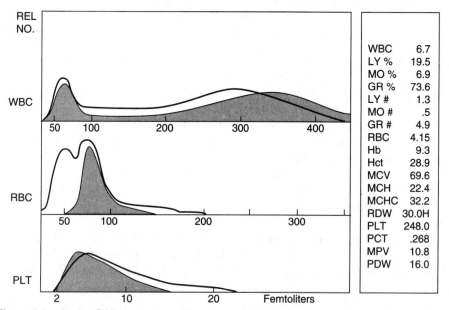

WBC	6.7
LY %	19.5
MO %	6.9
GR %	73.6
LY #	1.3
MO #	.5
GR #	4.9
RBC	4.15
Hb	9.3
Hct	28.9
MCV	69.6
MCH	22.4
MCHC	32.2
RDW	30.0H
PLT	248.0
PCT	.268
MPV	10.8
PDW	16.0

Case Figure 7-1. Coulter S-VI histogram and hemogram (shaded area represents a normal histogram).

Case Table 7-1. Patient's Laboratory Data

Serum iron	21 μg/dL
Total iron-binding capacity (TIBC)	350 μg/dL
Percent TIBC saturation	7%
Hemoglobin electrophoresis	Normal percentages
Peripheral blood smear	
Anisocytosis	2+
Hypochromasia	2+
Poikilocytosis	2+
Polychromasia	2+
Microcytosis	2+

and one peak is in the normal range. Because this woman is being treated for her anemia, a population of her original microcytic RBCs and a population of normocytic RBCs that are responding to the treatment are seen. The polychromasia on her blood smear supports the evidence that the rate of new RBC release from the marrow is increased. In an iron-deficient marrow, only microcytic RBCs would be produced.

■ CASE 8: *[Chapter 4]*

A 60-year-old white woman was admitted for evaluation of a painful, swollen right lower leg and marked leukocytosis. A physical examination revealed a distended abdomen and marked splenomegaly. The entire right lower leg was markedly swollen with tense edema, and the leg was warm and tender when palpated. There was no lymphadenopathy. Case Table 8–1 shows admission laboratory data.

Bone marrow biopsy and aspiration were obtained with some difficulty, with the results often coming up "dry." Sheets of abnormal cells resembling large, primitive monocytoid cells with abundant light blue cytoplasm filled the marrow. Erythroid and normal myeloid elements were greatly decreased. Serum muramidase levels were markedly increased, and cytogenetic studies revealed a translocation [i.e., t(9;11)].

Questions
- Based on the previous description and laboratory results, into what FAB classification would this patient's leukemia most likely fall?
- Immunologic monoclonal cluster differentiation (CD) marker studies were performed on this patient to confirm the diagnosis. The majority of these abnormal cells in the blood and marrow would type positive with what CD marker?
- The patient was treated with a course of cytosine arabinoside and achieved remission. A follow-up bone marrow aspiration revealed red blood cell (RBC) precursors with megaloblastoid characteristic morphology. What is causing the abnormal RBC precursor morphology?
- What was the physiologic cause of the microcytic/hypochromic RBC morphology in this patient?

Case Table 8-1. Admission Laboratory Data

Hemoglobin	9.4 g/dL
Hematocrit	27%
White blood cell count	60,000/mm³
Reticulocyte count	1%
Platelet count	19,000/mm³
Differential:	
Segmented neutrophils	5%
Lymphocytes	17%
Monocytes	22%
Promonocytes	23%
Monoblasts	33%
Red blood cell morphology	Microcytic/hypochromic

Discussion

The patient has a markedly elevated white blood cell (WBC) count but is anemic and thrombocytopenic. She has an absolute monocytosis with immature monocytes and blast cells. The high number of blast cells indicates an acute leukemia. Acute monocytic leukemia (AML-M5) is categorized as more than 20% promonocytes and monocytes, and less than 20% granulocytes and their precursors. Because all stages of monocytic maturation are seen, the proper diagnosis is well-differentiated monoblastic leukemia. Her cytogenetic data support this diagnosis. CD11 would be the marker that would type positive with abnormal cells in the blood and marrow.

Cytosine arabinoside is a deoxyribonucleic acid (DNA) inhibitor. The drug's effects are similar to those of a vitamin B_{12} or folate deficiency, which results in dyserythropoiesis and megaloblastic anemia. The microcytic/hypochromic RBCs appear secondary to the monocytic leukemia. The origin of her microcytic anemia may be similar to the etiology of an anemia of chronic inflammation. The malignant monocytes are not recycling stored iron, which could have been determined by obtaining serum iron, total iron-binding capacity, and ferritin levels. Another possible diagnosis is chronic blood loss due to the severely depressed platelet count.

■ CASE 9: *[Chapter 4]*

A 22-year-old man was initially seen with visual symptoms that were subsequently diagnosed as being secondary to a retinal hemorrhage. The patient works in a pesticide manufacturing plant and also recently had a tattoo applied on his right arm. A complete blood cell count (CBC) was obtained and analyzed on a flow cytometry system. The patient's hemogram and five-part differential results are shown in Case Table 9–1.

Case Table 9-1. Hemogram and Five-Part Differential Results

White blood cell count	$0.95 \times 10^3/mm^3$
Red blood cell count	$2.42 \times 10^6/mm^3$
Hemoglobin	6.0 g/dL
Hematocrit	18.5%
Mean corpuscular volume	87.0 fL
Mean corpuscular hemoglobin	29.9 pg
Mean corpuscular hemoglobin concentration	34.2 g/dL
Red cell distribution width	16.4
Platelet count	$13 \times 10^3/mm^3$
Mean plasma volume	6.8 fL
Differential ($\times 10^3/mm^3$)	
Segmented neutrophils	0.42 (56.7%)
Lymphocytes	0.24 (32.2%)
Monocytes	0.03 (3.9%)
Eosinophils	0.01 (1.4%)
Basophils	0

Questions

- Are the patient's differential results abnormal?
- What is the most probable type of anemia that this young man should be diagnosed as having?
- What is the most likely underlying or predisposing cause of this patient's anemia?
- What relationship or connection does the patient's retinal hemorrhage have to the symptoms and type of anemia from which he is suffering?

Discussion

Although this patient's differential indicates a normal percent of segmented neutrophils and lymphocytes, the absolute value must always be taken into account. His total white blood cell (WBC) count was only $0.95 \times 10^3/mm^3$. His segmented neutrophils were 56.7% (i.e., 950/mm³ × 56.7% = 538 segments per cubic millimeter). His lymphocytes were 32.2% (i.e., 950/mm³ × 32.2% = 306 lymphocytes per cubic millimeter). He has an absolute neutropenia and lymphocytopenia. The patient's hemapoiesis is significantly depressed in all three cell lines. In addition, his case history puts him in a high-risk category for aplastic anemia. This man has been chronically exposed to pesticides. In addition, he is at high risk for hepatitis because he recently received a tattoo. Both pesticide exposure and tattooing are known to be predisposing factors for aplastic anemia and marrow suppression. Such a low platelet count would result in an increased bleeding time and spontaneous hemorrhage.

■ CASE 10: *[Chapter 4]*

A 32-year-old white man was admitted in the early morning with complaints of acute abdominal pain. The patient was pale and demonstrated malaise and fatigue. He had a history of frequent headaches and one episode of deep vein thrombosis. Urinalysis test results showed mild hemoglobinuria. Laboratory data are shown in Case Table 10–1.

Case Table 10-1. Laboratory Data

White blood cell count	$3.2 \times 10^3/mm^3$
Red blood cell count	$2.20 \times 10^6/mm^3$
Hemoglobin	6.1 g/dL
Hematocrit	19.0%
Mean cell volume	86 fL
Mean corpuscular hemoglobin	26.8 pg
Mean corpuscular hemoglobin concentration	32.1 g/dL
Platelets	$70 \times 10^3/mm^3$
Red blood cell distribution width	12.5
Differential	
Segmented neutrophils	30%
Lymphocytes	59%
Monocytes	9%
Eosinophils	2%
Red blood cell morphology	1 + polychromatophilia
Bone marrow	30% cellularity
Myeloid/erythroid ratio	1 : 1
Additional tests ordered	
Direct antiglobulin test	Negative
Methemalbumin	Positive
Haptoglobin	Absent
Bilirubin	2.5 mg/dL
Coagulation screen	Normal

Questions

- The laboratory data suggests which disorder?
- Which disorder is the least likely to be considered from the previous test results?
- The peripheral smear shows normocytic, normochromic anemia; slight polychromatophilia; and no other morphologic abnormalities. Which diagnosis should be pursued?
- A reticulocyte count was not ordered. Based on the patient's admission blood results and the diagnosis, the reticulocyte count should be what?
- Further testing of the patient's red blood cells (RBCs) revealed that he had a normal osmotic fragility curve but had positive (increased RBC lysis) Ham test and sugar-water test results. Based on this additional information, what is the definitive diagnosis?

Discussion

The patient has a severe normocytic anemia with erythroid hyperplasia in his marrow. His bilirubin is high, and his serum haptoglobin is absent (or used up). The values indicate increased intravascular hemolysis. Hb AS disease, microangiopathic hemolytic anemia, autoimmune hemolytic anemia (AIHA), and paroxysmal nocturnal hemoglobinuria (PNH) are examples of hemolytic anemia, but because his direct antiglobulin test (DAT) is negative, AIHA is eliminated as a cause. The mean cell volume (MCV) indicates a normocytic anemia, and the red blood cell distribution width (RDW) is normal. An RBC morphology evaluation of his blood smear indicated fairly normal RBC populations, except for possibly an increased reticulocyte count. Chronic blood loss and β-thalassemia are microcytic anemias. Sickle cell anemia demonstrates a high RDW and abnormal RBC morphology. Therefore, an RBC membrane disorder or metabolic hemolytic anemia remain as the only possible diagnoses. Polychromasia suggests an elevated reticulocyte count. The marrow indicates erythroid hyperplasia. Also, the majority of hemolytic anemias demonstrate reticulocytosis. Positive Ham and sugar-water test results indicate PNH.

■ CASE 11: *[Chapter 4]*

An 82-year-old woman was initially seen with fatigue, weight loss, and fever. She had small nodes palpable in the head and neck region. Her spleen and liver were slightly enlarged. The laboratory results are shown in Case Table 11–1.

The bone marrow showed 40% lymphocytes and erythroid hyperplasia. The woman began prednisone therapy and was discharged 2 weeks later, with a hematocrit (Hct) of 35%. After 4 weeks receiving prednisone, her Hct was 42%. All medication was discontinued at that time. One month later, the patient was readmitted for fatigue and "blackout spells." Physical examination was the same as before; however, laboratory data were different (Case Table 11–2).

The patient restarted prednisone and also received chlorambucil treatments daily. After 2 weeks, her Hct increased to 38%, and her white blood cell (WBC) count decreased to 47,000. For 6 months she was followed up in the clinic for drug treatment three times a week.

Case Table 11-1. Initial Laboratory Results

White blood cell count	58,000/mm^3
Red blood cell count	2.51 × 10^6/mm^3
Hemoglobin	8.0 g/dL
Hematocrit	25.5%
Platelets	327,000/mm^3
Reticulocyte count	7.0%
Differential	
Segmented neutrophils	16%
Lymphocytes	82%
Monocytes	2%
Red blood cell morphology	Normocytic/normochromic
Bilirubin	2.9 mg/dL
Direct antiglobulin test	4+ positive

Case Table 11-2. Laboratory Results After 1 Month

White blood cell count	158,000/mm^3
Red blood cell count	2.41 × 10^6/mm^3
Hemoglobin	6.0 g/dL
Hematocrit	20%
Platelets	246,000/mm^3
Reticulocyte count	28.0%
Differential	
Segmented neutrophils	8%
Lymphocytes	92%
Bilirubin	8.5
Direct antiglobulin test	4+ positive

Questions

- Based on the patient's history, physical examination, and laboratory results, what is the diagnosis?
- What complication is present?
- What four laboratory results indicate that a hemolysis is present?
- With a 4+ positive antiglobulin test, how can the Hct remain normal?
- If this patient were typed with immunologic surface markers, which cluster differentiation (CD) marker would most likely be the strongest positive marker in the majority of cells?

Discussion

An elderly woman is initially seen with a significantly elevated WBC count and an absolute lymphocytosis. She has a normocytic anemia. Lymphocytic infiltration into her marrow, lymphadenopathy, and splenomegaly indicate a leukemic, malignant condition. The cells were identified as lymphocytes, not blasts or immature lymphocytes. Therefore, chronic lymphocytic leukemia is the best preliminary diagnosis. Her positive direct antiglobulin test result indicates that an immunoglobulin is attached to her red blood cells (RBCs), which suggests autoimmune hemolytic anemia (AIHA). Hemolysis is a survival disorder. Because her direct antiglobulin test (DAT) result is positive, her RBCs probably have an autoantibody attached. Therefore, they will be destroyed by phagocytosing monocytes and macrophages in the spleen and circulation, which will result in a high degree of intravascular hemolysis. The increased bilirubin level indicates increased RBC destruction. This results in anemia, as indicated by the hemoglobin and Hct. The reticulocyte count is greatly elevated, which indicates a marrow erythroid hyperplasia and increased erythropoiesis in response to RBC loss. The prednisone treatment suppresses the activity of the immune system and the phagocytic activity of the monocytes and macrophages, destroying immunoglobulin-bound RBCs.

■ CASE 12: *[Chapter 5]*

A 33-year-old woman received the first unit of a 2-U cross-match that had been ordered by her physician after surgery. Approximately 1 hour after the unit was transfused, the patient complained of a headache and nausea. Her temperature was slightly elevated, and she began to complain of a chill. An investigation into the transfusion reaction showed that the patient was O-positive, and her pretransfusion antibody screen had been negative. A post-transfusion specimen was tested, and the same results were obtained. The donor unit in question was retested and found to be O-positive with a negative antibody screen. The cross-match was compatible.

Questions

- What type of reaction did this patient experience?
- How common is this type of reaction?
- What is the probable cause of this reaction?
- What can be done to help prevent future reactions of this type in this patient?

Discussion

This patient experienced a febrile transfusion reaction, which is the most common type of transfusion reaction. One case occurs in every 200 transfusions. Usually, these febrile reactions are caused by an immunologic response to human leukocyte class I antigens on granulocytes or platelets. The use of leukocyte filters or the administration of washed red blood cells (RBCs) or deglycerolized RBCs can help reduce the likelihood of this patient experiencing another febrile transfusion reaction.

■ CASE 13: *[Chapter 5]*

A 62-year-old man was admitted to the emergency department of the local hospital with hematemesis. He had a long-standing history of ethanol abuse and four previous admissions for gastric bleeding. He had undergone transfusion on several occasions. Plans were made for immediate surgery, and 6 U of packed red blood cells (RBCs) were ordered. His antibody screen results were positive in the antiglobulin phase. An antibody identification panel was performed (Case Figure 13–1).

Cell	D	C	E	c	e	M	N	S	s	Le^a	Le^b	P$_1$	K	k	Fy^a	Fy^b	Jk^a	Jk^b	IS	37	IAT	enzyme
1	0	+	0	+	+	+	0	0	+	0	+	0	0	+	0	+	0	+	0	0	0	
2	+	+	0	0	+	+	+	+	+	0	+	+	0	+	+	0	0	+	0	0	0	
3	+	+	0	+	+	+	0	+	+	+	0	+	+	0	+	+	+	0	0	0	2+	
4	+	+	0	0	+	+	0	+	0	0	+	+	0	+	0	+	+	+	0	0	0	
5	0	0	0	+	+	+	0	+	+	0	+	0	0	+	+	+	+	+	0	0	0	
6	0	0	0	+	+	0	+	+	0	0	+	+	+	+	+	+	+	0	0	0	2+	
7	+	0	0	+	+	0	+	+	+	0	+	+	0	+	0	0	+	+	0	0	0	
8	+	0	+	+	0	0	+	0	+	+	0	+	0	+	0	+	0	+	0	0	0	
9	+	0	+	+	+	+	+	0	+	0	+	+	0	+	+	+	+	+	0	0	0	
10	0	0	0	+	+	+	+	+	+	0	0	+	0	0	+	+	0	+	0	0	0	
																	auto		0	0	0	

Case Figure 13-1. Antibody identification panel.

Questions
- What antibody was identified?
- What is the most likely source of this antibody?
- What is the next step in transfusing this patient?
- How difficult would it be to find antigen-negative units?

Discussion

The panel identified the antibody as anti-Kell. The patient most likely acquired this antibody through one of his previous transfusions. Donor units must be screened for the Kell antigen. Cross-matches should be performed on units found to be negative for the Kell antigen. Because fewer than 10% of the population has the Kell antigen, it should be relatively easy to find enough Kell-negative units to cross-match.

■ CASE 14: *[Chapter 5]*

A 23-year-old, group-O woman gave birth to a full-term, group-A infant, her first child. Approximately 36 hours after delivery, the infant appeared slightly jaundiced. The serum bilirubin level was slightly increased, and the direct antiglobulin test (DAT) was negative. The infant's peripheral blood smear showed increased numbers of spherocytes and nucleated red blood cells (RBCs).

Questions
- What is this infant's most likely diagnosis?
- What is the most likely cause?
- What is the basis for diagnosis?
- What other tests should be performed?

Discussion

This infant has hemolytic disease of the newborn (HDN), which has resulted from an ABO incompatibility between the mother and the infant. ABO-HDN occurs most frequently when the mother is group O, and the infant is group A. Without knowing the mother's and infant's Rh type, there is other evidence to support ABO-HDN as a diagnosis, rather than Rh-HDN. The increase in the bilirubin level is mild and delayed, the DAT is negative, and there are large numbers of spherocytes on the peripheral blood smear. All of these results indicate ABO-HDN rather than HDN caused by Rh incompatibility. An elution should be performed on the infant's blood to look for anti-A, anti-B, or anti-AB alloantibodies.

■ CASE 15: *[Chapter 5]*

The transfusion service receives a request for 2 U of packed red blood cells (RBCs) for a 62-year-old woman who has a diagnosis of multiple myeloma. Records show no history of pregnancy or previous transfusion. She is O-positive. The results of her antibody screen and cross-match are given in Case Table 15–1.

Case Table 15-1. Results of Antibody Screen and Cross-Match

	Immediate Spin	37°C	Antihemoglobin
Screening cells I	1+	1+	0
Screening cells II	1+	1+	0
Autocontrol	1+	1+	0
Donor unit 1	1+	1+	0
Donor unit 2	1+	1+	0

Questions

- What is the next step that should be taken?
- What is the most probable cause of the immediate spin results and 37°C incompatibilities?
- Why are the rouleaux not present in the antiglobulin phase?

Discussion

Based on the information presented in this case, the next step should be examining the antihemoglobin (AHG) tubes microscopically for agglutination. If there is no agglutination, and the Coombs' control cells are present, the negative AHG test results are valid. Patients who have multiple myeloma have increased serum proteins that can cause rouleaux. After incubation at 37°C, the patient's RBCs are washed with saline. If done properly, the excess protein is removed from the RBCs, and there is no rouleau formation.

■ CASE 16: *[Chapter 5]*

Two units of packed red blood cells (RBCs) are requested for a 25-year-old woman who has a history of three previous pregnancies. Her antibody screen results were positive. The results of an antibody panel are shown in Case Figure 16–1.

Questions

- What antibody or antibodies were identified?
- What could be done to confirm the presence of anti-Kell?
- What is the probable source of this patient's antibodies?

Discussion

The results of this patient's antibody panel are consistent with anti-c and anti-E antibodies. Anti-Kell cannot be ruled out. Treatment of cells with 2-aminoethylisothiouronium (AET) bromide or dithiothreitol plus cysteine-activated papain (ZZAP) would inactivate the Kell antigens and help determine if anti-Kell is present. Anti-c, anti-E, and anti-Kell antibodies may develop after transfusion or pregnancy.

Cell	D	C	E	c	e	M	N	S	s	Le^a	Le^b	P_1	K	k	Fy^a	Fy^b	Jk^a	Jk^b	IS	37	IAT	enzyme
1	0	+	0	+	+	+	0	0	+	0	+	0	0	+	0	+	0	+	0	0	1+	
2	+	+	0	0	+	+	+	+	+	0	+	+	0	+	+	0	0	+	0	0	0	
3	+	+	0	+	+	+	0	+	+	+	0	+	+	0	+	+	+	0	0	0	2+	
4	+	+	0	0	+	+	0	+	0	0	+	+	0	+	0	+	+	+	0	0	0	
5	0	0	0	+	+	+	0	+	+	0	+	0	0	+	+	+	+	+	0	0	1+	
6	0	0	0	+	+	0	+	+	0	0	+	+	+	+	+	+	+	0	0	0	2+	
7	+	0	0	+	+	0	+	+	+	0	+	+	0	+	0	0	+	+	0	0	1+	
8	+	0	+	+	0	0	+	0	+	+	0	+	0	+	0	+	0	+	0	0	2+	
9	+	0	+	+	+	+	+	0	+	0	+	+	0	+	+	+	+	+	0	0	2+	
10	0	0	0	+	+	+	+	+	+	0	+	0	0	+	+	0	+	0	0	0	1+	
																	auto		0	0		

Case Figure 16-1. Results of an antibody panel.

■ CASE 17: *[Chapter 6]*

A 48-year-old woman was seen by her family physician complaining of malaise, fatigue, and anorexia. Her husband had noticed that the "whites of her eyes looked yellow." She denied a history of drug use. She had no other social risk factors for hepatitis. However, 2 months earlier she had received a blood transfusion during an emergency dilatation and curettage. Laboratory tests indicated an elevated alanine aminotransferase level. Serologic test results for hepatitis B were negative.

Questions
- What is the most likely diagnosis for this patient?
- What is the basis for the diagnosis?
- How could an infected donor unit fail to be identified in routine donor testing?
- What is the prognosis for this patient?

Discussion

The patient described in this case probably has hepatitis C infection. Although the tests for hepatitis B were negative, this patient's clinical symptoms indicate some type of hepatitis infection. The woman had a history of previous transfusion, and the hepatitis C virus is the causative agent of more than 90% of all post-transfusion non-A, non-B hepatitis. Often, there is a long period of time between infection and seroconversion. Also, a significant number of persons infected with the hepatitis C virus never seroconvert. Approximately 20% of individuals infected with hepatitis C will develop a chronic form of the disease. And, 20% of these chronically infected persons will eventually develop hepatocellular carcinoma.

■ CASE 18: *[Chapter 6]*

A 17-year-old male was seen by his family physician complaining of sore throat, fever, and malaise. He also reported that he was extremely tired. Physical examination revealed splenomegaly and cervical lymphadenopathy. His white blood cell (WBC) count was 18 × 10⁹/L. The WBC differential showed 62% lymphocytes with 25% reactive lymphocytes.

Questions

- What is this young man's probable diagnosis?
- What commonly used test could be performed to confirm the suspected diagnosis?
- What causes this disease?
- What antibodies are present in this disease?
- How long after the infection will these antibodies persist?

Discussion

This patient probably has infectious mononucleosis. The Monospot test is commonly used to confirm a diagnosis of infectious mononucleosis, which is caused by the Epstein-Barr virus. Heterophile antibodies, anti-viral capsid antigen (VCA) antibodies, early antigen (EA) antibodies, and Epstein-Barr nuclear antigen (EBNA) antibodies are present during infectious mononucleosis infections. Immunoglobulin M (IgM) heterophile antibodies usually persist between 4 and 8 weeks after infection. IgM anti-VCA antibodies persist for 2–4 months after infection. Immunoglobulin G (IgG) anti-VCA antibodies persist for life. Anti-EA antibodies usually disappear within 3 months after infection. IgG EBNA antibody levels will remain at detectable levels indefinitely.

■ CASE 19: *[Chapter 8]*

A 62-year-old male alcoholic was admitted to the hospital with fever and shock. His wife told the admitting physician that they had eaten raw oysters at a restaurant the evening before. Blood cultures gave the following results: aerobic growth after overnight incubation; colonies subcultured to blood agar were flat and gray. Further characterization gave the following results: gram-negative, slightly curved rod; oxidase positive; fermentative growth in oxidation-fermentation glucose; green colonies on thiosulfate citrate bile salts sucrose agar; lysine decarboxylase positive; no growth in 0%, 8%, and 10% NaCl nutrient broth; growth in 1% and 6% NaCl nutrient broth.

Questions

- Based on the medical history, what organism should be suspected in this case?
- Based on the laboratory results, what is the identity of the blood isolate?

Discussion

There are several clues to indicate that *Vibrio* is a likely cause. First, the patient was exposed to shellfish. *Vibrio* infections, as well as some caused by *Yersinia* species, can often be traced to exposure to contaminated seawater via shellfish consumption. Second, the patient had a history of cirrhosis from alcoholism. Decreased liver function is a common finding in *V. vulnificus* septicemia. The rapid and progressive nature of the patient's infection is suggestive of *V. vulnificus*.

The Gram's stain is suggestive of *Vibrio*. Lack of growth in 0% NaCl broth eliminates *Plesiomonas* and *Aeromonas* species. The remaining laboratory results indicate *Vibrio vulnificus*.

■ CASE 20: *[Chapter 8]*

A 26-year-old woman complained of back pain, fever, and dysuria of 3 days' duration. A urinalysis revealed many white blood cells (WBCs), moderate red blood cells (RBCs), and presence of nitrate. Gram's stain of the urine revealed 5–10 gram-negative rods per high-power field as well as 5–10 neutrophils. A urine culture gave the following results:

Blood agar: >100,000 colonies per milliliter
MacConkey agar: dark pink, dry colonies

Characterization of the isolate gave the following results:

Indole positive
Citrate negative
Hydrogen sulfide negative
Urea negative
Motile

Questions

- What organism(s) is(are) most likely to cause a urinary tract infection?
- What is the most likely identity of this isolate?

Discussion

Escherichia, Klebsiella, Proteus, Staphylococcus saprophyticus, and other coagulase-negative staphylococci are commonly isolated from urinary tract infections. A lactose-positive isolate with dark pink, dry colonies on MacConkey agar is suggestive of *E. coli*. The positive indole results, negative citrate and urea results, and a positive motility test makes the most likely identification *E. coli*.

■ CASE 21: *[Chapter 8]*

A 70-year-old woman who has stage IV Hodgkin's disease sought medical treatment because of fever and headache of several days' duration. Her headache had become progressively worse, and her temperature was 103°F. A complete blood count revealed a white blood cell count of 11,000/mm³ with normal distribution. The urinalysis results were normal. Lumbar puncture was performed, and the laboratory results shown in Case Table 21–1 were obtained from the cerebrospinal fluid (CSF).

The Gram's stain did not reveal any microbial forms. The CSF was processed for culture. Two days later, a beta-hemolytic, short, gram-positive bacillus grew on blood and chocolate agars. Biochemical characterization revealed the following:

Catalase positive
Motile
Esculin positive
Hippurate hydrolysis positive
Cyclic adenosine monophosphate positive
Hydrogen sulfide negative

Questions

- Based on the medical and laboratory data before microbiologic analysis, what organism(s) might be responsible for this patient's infection?
- Based on the bacteriologic evidence, what is the most likely identity of this isolate?

Discussion

This patient may be immunosuppressed as a result of the advanced Hodgkin's disease. This broadens the possibilities of infectious agents. There were no petechiae, as is often seen with *Neisseria meningitidis*. The CSF chemistry results were classic for a bacterial meningitis (increased protein, decreased glucose levels). The CSF cell count was elevated, with an increase in mononuclear cells. Generally, meningitis caused by *Streptococcus pneumoniae, Haemophilus influenzae, Neisseria meningitidis,* and *Escherichia coli* results in a more pronounced cellular response, with a pronounced increase in polymorphonuclear leukocytes. The lack of bacterial forms with a Gram's stain is not the usual case with these organisms. Infection of a compromised host, the presence of mononuclear cells, lack of microbial forms in the CSF, and this particular CSF chemistry profile are consistent with a *Listeria monocytogenes* infection. The data are not unique for *L. monocytogenes*, however. The colonial

Case Table 21-1. Laboratory Results from Cerebrospinal Fluid

White blood cell count	250/mm³ (60% mononuclear cells)
Cerebrospinal fluid glucose	33 mg/dL (serum level: 105 mg/dL)
Cerebrospinal fluid protein	180 mg/dL

morphology and the Gram's stain may cause confusion with *S. agalactiae*. However, a closer look at the Gram's stain reveals that the bacteria are short rods rather than cocci. A positive catalase test result excludes *Streptococcus* species, whereas the remaining results are consistent with *L. monocytogenes*.

■ CASE 22: *[Chapter 9]*

A 31-year-old male leukemia patient was referred for evaluation of diarrhea. Two months before admission, the patient had sought experimental treatment in Mexico for his leukemia. On returning, he noted the onset of vague, crampy abdominal pain with profuse watery diarrhea that had continued to persist intermittently until presentation. His work-up included a normal flexible sigmoidoscope examination and negative stool culture results for bacterial pathogens. Parasitology studies demonstrated pear-shaped trophozoites 14 μm in length, with two bilateral nuclei and some ovoid cysts that had 2–4 nuclei and two fibrils in the center.

Questions

- What is the identity (genus and species) of the parasite?
- If motility would be expected on the wet mount, how could it be described?
- Which fecal concentration technique should be performed?

Discussion

The most likely infective parasite in this patient is *Giardia lamblia*. Motility on a wet mount of *G. lamblia* is described as "falling leaf." The fecal concentration technique that should be performed is the Ritchie formalin-ether method.

■ CASE 23: *[Chapter 9]*

An 8-year-old boy was admitted to the hospital with fever, malaise, loss of appetite, and a nonproductive cough. The patient was nearing completion of chemotherapy for acute lymphocytic leukemia. He was treated with broad-spectrum intravenous antibiotics and had a central venous catheter placed for administration of the chemotherapy. The fever persisted; therefore, blood cultures and cultures of the tip of the central line were ordered. Both grew an organism that was ovoid and reproduced by budding. This organism was subsequently shown to form germ tubes and produce blastoconidia, chlamydospores, and pseudohyphae on corn meal Tween 80 agar.

Questions

- What organism (genus and species) is most likely infecting this boy?
- Is this organism part of normal flora in humans?
- How did treatment with broad-spectrum antibiotics predispose the patient to infection with this organism?

Discussion

The organism most likely infecting this patient is *Candida albicans*, which is a part of the normal flora of the skin, mucous membranes, and gastrointestinal tract. Patients who are receiving broad-spectrum antibiotics are considered to be immunocompromised. Therefore, the boy was predisposed to infection.

■ CASE 24: *[Chapter 10]*

A 52-year-old man submitted a urine specimen during his routine physical examination. The results of the urinalysis are shown in Case Table 24–1.

Case Table 24-1. Results of Urinalysis

Appearance	Clear
Red blood cell/high-powered field	35–40
Color	Amber-brown
White blood cell/high-powered field	15–20
Specific gravity	1.008
Epithelial cells/high-powered field	5–10 squamous, 2–5 transitional
pH	6.0
Protein	Trace
Sulfosalicylic acid	Negative
Bacteria/high-powered field	1+
Blood	Small
Casts/low-powered field	5–10 hyaline, 1–2 finely granular
Glucose	1+
Clinitest	Negative
Ketones	Negative
Crystals/low-powered field	30–40 triple phosphate
Bilirubin	Negative
Urobilinogen	0.1 Ehrlich units
Other Yeast	1+
Nitrates	Negative
Leukocyte esterase	Negative

Questions

- Which of the previously mentioned test results are questionable?
- What are three possible causes for the discrepant results?
- What is the renal threshold for glucose?
- Explain the discrepancy between the glucose oxidase method and the Clinitest.
- List the sugars measured by each method and any interfering substances.
- Describe a situation in which the results of the Clinitest would be positive, but the reagent strip test results would be negative.

Discussion

A clear appearance of urine with many elements in the sediment is suspect. If there are numerous red blood cells (RBCs), white blood cells (WBCs), epithelial cells, and many crystals, a well-mixed specimen should look cloudy. An amber-brown color with a negative bilirubin result is also questionable. Bilirubin imparts a brownish color to urine. An acidic pH does not correlate with many triple phosphate crystals, which are formed in alkaline urine. The specimen was not well mixed. The specimen could have been incorrectly identified, or the dipsticks could have been expired or contaminated. In addition, the centrifuged specimen on which the microscopic examination was performed may not have been the same specimen on which the dipstick results were performed. The renal glucose threshold is 150–180 mg/dL. A glucose-oxidase (dipstick) result of 1+ and a copper-reductase (Clinitest) negative result can occur together, because the dipstick is more specific for glucose than the Clinitest. The dipstick is sensitive to 100 mg/dL; the Clinitest sensitivity is 150 mg/dL. The dipstick measures only glucose, although ≥ 50 mg/dL of ascorbic acid (vitamin C) can interfere with the method by falsely reducing the glucose results. The Clinitest measures reducing substances and all sugars (glucose, lactose, fructose, galactose, pentose) except sucrose. Ascorbic acid is measured by this method because it is a reducing substance. Either the sugar present is one other than glucose, or the urine contains another reducing substance, such as ascorbic acid.

■ CASE 25: *[Chapter 10]*

A 17-year-old male was taken to his family physician by his parents because he had complained of a headache for 4 days. His physician noted other symptoms such as neck stiffness, a chronic lack of energy, and a 101°F temperature that had existed for 3 days. The patient was admitted to the hospital for further testing. Fasting blood chemistries and a lumbar puncture were ordered. His blood and cerebrospinal fluid (CSF) results are shown in Case Table 25–1.

Questions

- Are there any abnormal findings in this case?
- Based on the aforementioned results, what is the most likely diagnosis?
- If lymphocytes were the predominate cell type instead of neutrophils (i.e., segmented), what would be the best diagnosis?
- What are the physiologic mechanisms that could result in the low CSF glucose value shown in this patient?

Case Table 25-1. Blood and Cerebrospinal
Fluid Results

Blood chemistry	
Glucose	105 mg/dL
Total protein	7.5 g/dL
Albumin	4.3 g/dL
Electrolytes	All in normal range
Cerebrospinal fluid	
Color	Colorless
Clarity	Turbidity (2+)
Total protein	125 mg/dL
Glucose	41 mg/dL
Lactate	29 mg/dL
White blood cell count	8700/mm³
Differential	
Segmented neutrophils	91%
Monocytes	7%
Lymphocytes	2%

Discussion

Abnormal findings in this patient's CSF examination include the specimen turbidity, white blood cell (WBC) count, neutrophilia, total protein, glucose, and lactate. The patient's symptoms and the CSF neutrophilia, low glucose level, and high protein and lactate levels are indicative of bacterial meningitis. A lymphocytosis in combination with the same symptoms would be indicative of viral meningitis. In patients who have bacterial meningitis, increased glycolysis is found within the central nervous system because of the increased leukocytes and the presence of bacteria. This decreases the level of glucose in the CSF.

Comprehensive Examination

Directions: Each of the numbered items or incomplete statements in this section is followed by answers or by completions of the statement. Select the ONE lettered answer or completion that is BEST in each case.

1. Most clinically significant antibodies against blood group antigens are of which one of the following immunoglobulin (Ig) types?

a. IgA
b. IgD
c. IgG
d. IgM

2. Prozone occurs when which one of the following conditions exists?

a. antibody molecules are in excess of antigen
b. antigen is in excess of antibody
c. equal amounts of antigen and antibody are present
d. either antigen or antibody is absent

3. Which one of the following is the formula for coefficient of variation?

a. $\dfrac{\text{standard deviation} \times 100}{\text{standard error}}$

b. $\dfrac{\text{mean} \times 100}{\text{standard deviation}}$

c. $\dfrac{\text{standard deviation} \times 100}{\text{mean}}$

d. $\dfrac{\text{variance} \times 100}{\text{mean}}$

4. A thrombocytopenia resulting from ineffective platelet production in the marrow is seen in which one of the following conditions?

a. splenomegaly
b. lymphoma
c. vitamin B_{12} deficiency
d. chronic alcohol consumption

5. The American Association of Blood Banks (AABB) requires that patient samples for compatibility testing be stored for at least

a. 3 days after transfusion
b. 7 days after transfusion
c. 10 days after transfusion
d. 14 days after transfusion

6. The immunoglobulin (Ig) class associated with Type I hypersensitivity reactions and parasitic infections is which one of the following?

a. IgA
b. IgG
c. IgM
d. IgE

7. An acute increase in intravascular hemolysis results in an increase in which one of the following plasma substances?

a. haptoglobin
b. indirect bilirubin
c. hemopexin
d. conjugated bilirubin

8. The purpose of a quality assurance program is to

a. ensure that a laboratory's results are reliable
b. ensure that a particular analyzer is working properly
c. ensure that only certified technologists are hired
d. ensure that instrumentation is updated

9. Which one of the following immunoglobulin G (IgG) classes binds complement most efficiently?

a. IgG1 and IgG2
b. IgG2 and IgG3
c. IgG3 and IgG1
d. IgG4 and IgG1

10. The finding of ingested red blood cells (RBCs) in the cytoplasm of a trophozoite is presumptive evidence that the organism is which one of the following?

a. *Dientamoeba fragilis*
b. *Trichomonas vaginalis*
c. *Giardia lamblia*
d. *Entamoeba histolytica*

11. On which one of the following specimens should observations of urine color and transparency be performed?

a. a centrifuged specimen
b. a well-mixed specimen
c. a 24-hour specimen
d. a fractional specimen

12. The bacterial cell structure(s) that serves as an osmotic barrier and is a site of action for some antibiotics is which one of the following?

a. cell wall
b. cell membrane
c. capsule
d. pili

13. The D^u test is performed by incubating the patient's red blood cells (RBCs) with which one of the following substances?

a. several different dilutions of anti-D serum
b. anti-D serum followed by washing and antihuman globulin (AHG) reagent
c. anti-D^u serum
d. AHG reagent

14. The rapid rise, elevated level, and prolonged production of antibody following a repeat exposure to an antigen is known as which one of the following?

a. hypersensitivity
b. immunization
c. secondary response
d. primary response

15. The term molarity describes which one of the following?

a. the charge carried by ions per kilogram of solution
b. the number of grams of solute per liter of water
c. the number of moles of solute per liter of solution
d. the number of moles of solute per kilogram of water

16. Thrombotic thrombocytopenic purpura (TTP) is known to be caused by which one of the following conditions?

a. antiplatelet antibodies
b. a deficiency in prostaglandin I_2 (PGI_2)
c. a chronic viral disorder
d. systemic lupus erythematosus (SLE)

17. Most cases of autoimmune hemolytic anemias (AIHA) are which one of the following types?

a. cold AIHA
b. warm AIHA
c. drug-induced AIHA
d. mixed-type AIHA

18. A yellow-brown urine results from the excretion of which one of the following substances?

a. hemoglobin
b. bilirubin
c. urobilin
d. uroporphyrin

19. The formation of intranuclear inclusions in tissue culture cells infected with virus particles is an example of which one of the following?

a. cytopathic effect
b. hemagglutination inhibition
c. interference
d. toxic effect

20. Six units of blood have been ordered for a 29-year-old man who is actively bleeding. He is AB negative. Which one of the following types available for cross-match would you choose?

a. AB positive
b. A negative
c. A positive
d. O negative

21. A patient was admitted to the hospital with a suspected anemia. A complete blood cell count (CBC) was performed, and the following values were reported:

Red blood cell count: $3.00 \times 10^6/mm^3$
Hemoglobin: 9.5 g/dL
Hematocrit: 27%
Reticulocyte count: 13.4%

If, because of anemia, the reticulocyte maturation time in the circulation is now twice as long, what is this patient's absolute reticulocyte count, and how many times greater than normal is this count?

a. 100,000/mm^3; normal number of reticulocytes per day
b. 1,000,000/mm^3; twice as many reticulocytes per day
c. 50,000/mm^3; half as many reticulocytes per day
d. 400,000/mm^3; four times as many reticulocytes per day

ing proce-
ne of the

27. Surface immunoglobulin M (IgM), surface immunoglobulin D (IgD), and crystallizable fragment (Fc) receptors are found in which one of the following types of cells?

a. B stem cells
b. pre-B cells
c. immature B cells
d. mature B cells

rmination,
rmula for
ɔn?

tration

28. Under the Clinical Laboratories Improvement Act guidelines, all written procedures must be

a. signed by all laboratory personnel
b. signed by the hospital administrator
c. signed by the shift supervisor
d. signed by the laboratory director

29. Which one of the following is a fluorescent stain used to detect bacteria in blood and other body fluids?

ons would
idiopathic

a. Kinyoun acid-fast stain
b. methylene blue stain
c. calcofluor white stain
d. acridine orange stain

yocyte
egakaryo-

ocyte

30. To prevent graft-versus-host disease, which one of the following types of transfusion products should be administered?

d. absence of bone marrow megakaryocyte

a. saline-washed red blood cells (RBCs)
b. irradiated RBCs
c. frozen and deglycerolized RBCs
d. fresh whole blood

25. Which one of the following reasons best describes why the Embden-Meyerhof (EM) pathway is vital in red blood cell (RBC) metabolism?

a. it handles 25% of RBC energy production
b. it produces the adenosine triphosphate (ATP) needed to maintain membrane ion pumps and membrane stability
c. it is fueled by free fatty acids
d. it binds thymidine for deoxyribonucleic acid (DNA) replication

31. Blood collected in heparin must be transfused within which one of the following periods of time?

a. 24 hours
b. 72 hours
c. 1 week
d. 2 weeks

26. Which one of the following antibodies is typically enhanced by treatment with proteolytic enzymes?

a. M
b. N
c. Duffy
d. Kidd

32. Which one of the following pairs of lipoprotein classes is involved in the transport of the majority of triglycerides from the small intestine through the circulation to various tissues?

a. chylomicron and very low-density lipoproteins (VLDL)
b. VLDL and high-density lipoproteins (HDL)
c. low-density lipoproteins (LDL) and HDL
d. HDL only

33. Which one of the following components in citrate-phosphate-dextrose-adenine (CPDA-1) binds calcium?

a. citrate
b. phosphate
c. dextrose
d. adenine

34. Which one of the following bacterial species is commonly found as normal flora on the skin and may be seen as a contaminant in blood cultures?

a. *Escherichia*
b. *Bacteroides*
c. *Staphylococcus*
d. *Enterococcus*

35. Each unit of platelet concentrate transfused should increase the platelet count by which one of the following amounts?

a. $2.5-5 \times 10^9/L$
b. $5-10 \times 10^9/L$
c. $10-12 \times 10^9/L$
d. $12-15 \times 10^9/L$

36. At low or absent levels, which one of the following hormones has the ability to produce hyperglycemia?

a. glucagon
b. insulin
c. thyroid hormone
d. parathyroid hormone

37. In the Monospot assay for infectious mononucleosis (IM), beef erythrocytes absorb only the

a. heterophile antibody of the Forssman type
b. heterophile antibody of IM
c. guinea pig kidney antigen
d. horse erythrocytes

38. Which one of the following statements is true regarding a cerebrospinal fluid (CSF) specimen received for microbiological analysis?

a. it should be processed immediately
b. it should be refrigerated and processed when possible
c. it should be frozen and processed when possible
d. it may be held at room temperature and processed any time within 24 hours without loss of organism viability

39. Which one of the following is the most common cause of false-negative results in the antiglobulin test?

a. dirty glassware
b. contaminated antihuman globulin (AHG) reagent
c. overincubation
d. inadequately washed red blood cells (RBCs)

40. Which one of the following conditions must exist in blood used for exchange transfusion between mother and fetus?

a. it must be the same Rh type as the mother
b. it must be the same ABO type as the mother
c. it must be negative for the antigen against which the mother's immunoglobulin G (IgG) antibody is made
d. it must be negative for the antigen against which the mother's immunoglobulin M (IgM) antibody is made

41. When interpreting a white blood cell (WBC) differential, a shift to the left indicates which one of the following?

a. a decrease in the hemoglobin-oxygen affinity
b. an increase in the percent of band neutrophils and other immature myeloid forms
c. an increase in the percent of lymphocytes greater than the percent of segmented neutrophils
d. an increase in the number of hypersegmented neutrophils

42. If the autocontrol and all antibody panel cells agglutinate at room temperature but react less strongly at 37°C and in the antihuman globulin (AHG) phase, which one of the following conditions should be suspected?

a. warm autoantibody
b. multiple antibodies
c. antibody to high-frequency antigen(s) on the panel cells
d. cold-reacting autoantibody

43. A 12-year-old female who is scheduled for a tonsillectomy is found to have the following laboratory findings:

Platelet count: 325,000/mm^3
Prothrombin time (PT): normal control = 11.5 seconds; patient = 23.4 seconds
Activated partial thromboplastin time (APTT): normal control = 30 seconds; patient = 58 seconds

The complete blood count was within normal limits. The APTT results of the patient's plasma plus aged normal serum were 30 seconds. The APTT results of the patient's plasma plus fresh absorbed plasma were 60 seconds. Assuming normal platelet factor 3 activity, in which one of the following factors is this patient deficient?

a. VII
b. VIII
c. IX
d. X

44. A patient is typed as O positive and cross-matched with 6 units of red blood cells (RBCs). The antibody screen and two cross-matched units are incompatible in the antiglobulin testing phase, and the autocontrol is negative. Which one of the following is the most likely cause of the incompatibility?

a. recipient alloantibody
b. recipient autoantibody
c. donor units have positive direct antiglobulin tests
d. rouleaux

45. Unsheathed microfilariae that are recovered from a "skin snip" are which one of the following organisms?

a. *Dipetalonema perstans*
b. *Onchocerca volvulus*
c. *Mansonella ozzardi*
d. *Wuchereria bancrofti*

46. Which one of the following terms best describes urine with a fixed specific gravity equal to 1.010?

a. anuric
b. polysteric
c. oliguric
d. isothenuric

47. A 25-year-old man with a normal food and fluid intake excreted 1400 mL of urine in 24 hours. Which one of the following terms best describes this urine volume?

a. lower than normal
b. normal
c. lower limit of normal
d. above normal

48. Which one of the following examples best describes Lewis antibodies?

a. Immunoglobulin (Ig) M antibodies that react on immediate spin
b. IgG antibodies that react on immediate spin
c. IgM antibodies that react in antihuman globulin (AHG)
d. IgG antibodies that react in AHG

49. When stored at $-18°C$, fresh frozen plasma (FFP) can safely be stored for which one of the following periods of time?

a. 90 days
b. 6 months
c. 1 year
d. 2 years

50. Absorption of vitamin B_{12} in the stomach and gut requires the presence of which one of the following substances?

a. folic acid
b. secretin
c. gastrin
d. intrinsic factor

51. Resistance to a 5-mg novobiocin disk is a characteristic used to identify which one of the following?

a. *Staphylococcus aureus*
b. *Staphylococcus epidermidis*
c. *Staphylococcus saprophyticus*
d. *Micrococcus* spp.

52. Which one of the following antistreptolysin-O (ASO) test results indicates a recent streptococcal infection?

a. <25 Todd units
b. <50 Todd units
c. >100 Todd units
d. >200 Todd units

53. The acute phase protein primarily responsible for an increased erythrocyte sedimentation rate (ESR) is

a. fibrinogen
b. haptoglobin
c. ceruloplasmin
d. C-reactive protein

54. A unit of whole blood collected from an adult should contain approximately which one of the following amounts?

a. 550 mL of blood
b. 500 mL of blood
c. 450 mL of blood
d. 475 mL of blood

55. For a red blood cell (RBC) to perform its function in the circulation and survive 120 days, it requires a membrane that has a high degree of which one of the following characteristics?

a. lipid-to-protein ratio
b. impermeability
c. rigidity
d. flexibility (deformability)

56. A 52-year-old man went to his doctor for a physical examination. The patient was overweight and had missed his last two appointments because of his business dealings in the insurance industry. His blood pressure was elevated, his cholesterol was 210 mg/dL, and his triglyceride level was 150 mg/dL. A high-density lipoprotein (HDL) cholesterol test was performed, and the result was 23 mg/dL (normal range is 29–60 mg/dL). Which one of the following would be this patient's calculated low-density lipoprotein (LDL) cholesterol value?

a. cannot be determined from the information given
b. 157 mg/dL
c. 137 mg/dL
d. 55.4 mg/dL

57. The immunoglobulin (Ig) class of anti-M antibodies is best described by which one of the following characteristics?

a. frequently a mixture of IgG and IgM
b. frequently a mixture of IgA and IgG
c. IgG only
d. IgM only

58. An individual who secretes A and H substances in his saliva must possess which one of the following genes?

a. A, O, and Se
b. A and H
c. A and Se
d. A, H, and Se

59. Which one of the following is the test most widely used to detect human immunodeficiency virus (HIV) antibodies?

a. radioimmunoassay (RIA)
b. Western blot
c. immunofluorescence (IF)
d. enzyme-linked immunosorbent assay (ELISA)

60. An unconscious young man known to have consumed large amounts of alcohol was admitted to the emergency department. The patient's breathing was shallow, and his color was poor. The acid-base status of this patient is likely to be which one of the following?

a. respiratory acidosis
b. metabolic acidosis
c. respiratory alkalosis
d. metabolic alkalosis

61. Which one of the following characteristics describes hepatitis A?

a. chronic infection transmitted by fecal-oral route
b. chronic infection transmitted by chronic carriers
c. acute infection transmitted by fecal-oral route
d. chronic infection transmitted by direct inoculation

62. Analysis of an isolate from cerebrospinal fluid (CSF) yielded the following characteristics: alpha-hemolytic on blood agar, catalase negative, gram-positive cocci, susceptible to optochin. Which one of the following is the most likely identity of this isolate?

a. *Streptococcus agalactiae*
b. *Streptococcus pyogenes*
c. viridans streptococci
d. *Streptococcus pneumoniae*

63. Which one of the following statements best describes characteristics of the ABO blood group antibodies?

a. they are naturally occurring and are mostly immunoglobulin M (IgM)
b. they are reactive only at 37°C
c. they are naturally occurring and are mostly immunoglobulin G (IgG)
d. they are mostly of immune origin

64. What would be the calculated anion gap for the following electrolytes?

Na	148 mmol/L
K	5.8 mmol/L
Cl	87 mmol/L
CO_2	24 mmol/L

a. 42.8 and normal
b. 42.8 and decreased
c. 42.8 and increased
d. 0 and normal

65. Afibrinogenemia is caused by which one of the following conditions?

a. a genetic decrease of prothrombin
b. a genetic decrease of fibrinogen
c. a functional abnormality of fibrinogen
d. snake venom bites

66. Anti-Sd^a antibodies should be suspected if which one of the following conditions exists?

a. the patient has recently undergone transfusion
b. the agglutination is mixed field
c. the patient is in group A or B
d. antibody screening cell test results are negative

67. Methemoglobin contains which one of the following?

a. ferric form of iron (Fe^{3+})
b. ferrous form of iron (Fe^{2+})
c. carbon monoxide molecule attached to the heme iron
d. defect in the beta-globin molecules

68. The D^u antigen is best described by which one of the following characteristics?

a. it is a weakened form of the D antigen
b. it can only be detected at room temperature
c. it is not detectable in the indirect antiglobulin test
d. it is clinically insignificant

69. Hepatitis B is best described by which one of the following characteristics?

a. it has no chronic stage of infection
b. it was formerly known as "the Australia antigen"
c. it is transmitted by a fecal-oral route
d. it is often seen with hepatitis A

70. Immunity to rubella is indicated by a titer of at least

a. 8
b. 16
c. 32
d. 64

71. Hydrolysis of L-pyrrolidonyl-β-naphthylamide (PYR) is a characteristic of which one of the following?

a. *Streptococcus pyogenes* and *enterococcus*
b. *Streptococcus pyogenes* and *Streptococcus agalactiae*
c. *Streptococcus pneumoniae* and *enterococcus*
d. *Streptococcus agalactiae* and *enterococcus*

72. Sputum from a patient with pneumonia was cultured on Sabouraud's media at 24°C and 37°C. A white, fluffy mold grew that microscopically demonstrated barrel-shaped arthrospores. A tissue biopsy of the lung demonstrated large spherules containing endospores. This fungus was which one of the following?

a. *Histoplasma capsulatum*
b. *Geotrichum candidum*
c. *Coccidioides immitis*
d. *Cryptococcus neoformans*

73. An unpreserved urine specimen was at room temperature for 4 hours in an unsterile container. Which one of the following dipstick reactions is most likely to be reliable?

a. pH
b. blood
c. ketones
d. bilirubin

74. Consider the following results:

Patient cells with anti-A: 4+
Patient cells with anti-B: 0
Patient serum with A_1 cells: 1+
Patient serum with B cells: 4+
Patient cells with patient serum: 2+

Of the following, which one is the most likely cause of the ABO typing discrepancy?

a. A_2 with anti-A_1
b. acquired A phenomenon
c. cold autoantibody
d. acquired B phenomenon

75. A positive antibody screen, negative autocontrol, and positive major cross-match may be caused by which one of the following factors?

a. ABO typing error
b. donor unit with a positive direct antiglobulin test (DAT)
c. recipient autoantibody
d. recipient alloantibody to donor cell antigens

76. The physiologic catabolism of glucose to pyruvate for adenosine triphosphate (ATP) production is referred to as which one of the following functions?

a. glycogenesis
b. glycolysis
c. glycogenolysis
d. gluconeogenesis

77. A gram-negative coccobacillus was isolated from an infected cat bite. The isolate grew on blood agar with a musty smell, but did not grow on MacConkey agar. It was catalase, indole, and oxidase positive and susceptible to a 2-U penicillin disk. Which one of the following is the most likely identity of this isolate?

a. *Haemophilus influenzae*
b. *Bordetella bronchiseptica*
c. *Pasteurella multocida*
d. *Brucella* spp

78. Which one of the following statements best describe anti-Fy^a antibodies?

a. they are usually cold-reacting
b. they are more reactive with enzyme-treated cells
c. they are capable of causing hemolytic transfusion reactions (HTR)
d. they are predominantly immunoglobulin M (IgM)

79. Paroxysmal nocturnal hemoglobinuria is a disorder of chronic intravascular hemolysis because

a. an autoantibody is produced against the red blood cell's (RBC) Rh surface antigens
b. the RBCs are rendered hypersensitive to complement C3 binding
c. there is an abnormal β-globin amino acid substitution that results in hemoglobin precipitation and premature hemolysis
d. there is an inherited glucose-6-phosphate dehydrogenase deficiency

80. Which one of the following tests aids in evaluating the respiratory burst of neutrophils?

a. neutrophil aggregation test
b. Boyden chamber assay
c. anti-neutrophil antibody assay
d. nitroblue tetrazolium (NBT) reductase test

81. Acute hemolytic transfusion reactions (HTR) are usually caused by which one of the following conditions?

a. human leukocyte antigen (HLA) class I antigens
b. bacterial contamination of donor unit
c. ABO incompatibility
d. recipient antibodies against donor red blood cells (RBCs)

82. Anaphylactic transfusion reactions are usually caused by antibodies against which one of the following?

a. Immunoglobulin (Ig) A
b. IgG
c. IgD
d. IgM

83. Which one of the following identifies large, multi-segmented, smooth-walled macroconidia occurring singly or in clusters of two to three?

a. *Epidermophyton floccosum*
b. *Trichophyton verrucosum*
c. *Microsporum canis*
d. *Fusarium moniliforme*

84. An isolate from a dog bite grows on blood agar in the presence of carbon dioxide only. The colonies are yellow and show a haze of growth at the periphery. Gram's stain reveals a gram-negative fusiform bacillus. Which one of the following genera is the most likely identity of this isolate?

a. *Actinobacillus*
b. *Kingella*
c. *Cardiobacterium*
d. *Capnocytophaga*

85. The reagent strip method used to detect protein in urine is based on which one of the following factors?

a. the pKa change of a polyelectrolyte
b. reduction of copper ions to cupric ions
c. the protein error of indicators
d. interaction of protein with sodium nitroprusside

86. Which one of the following is incompatible in the major cross-match?

	Recipient	Donor
a.	A positive	A negative
b.	A positive	O positive
c.	A positive	AB positive
d.	A negative	A positive

87. Which one of the following is a test specific for *Treponema pallidum?*

a. rapid plasmin reagin
b. Venereal Disease Research Laboratory (VDRL)
c. microhemagglutination-*Treponema pallidum* (MHA-TP)
d. reagin screening test

88. Complement is bound by which of the following classes of immunoglobulins (Ig)?

a. IgG and IgA
b. IgM and IgE
c. IgA and IgM
d. IgG and IgM

89. During a state of low blood volume and decreased extracellular sodium level (as in cardiac failure), which one of the following conditions occurs?

a. renin is produced by the adrenal glands, leading to vasoconstriction and production of antidiuretic hormone (ADH) by the pituitary gland, which increases fluid volume by causing water retention
b. aldosterone is produced by the kidneys, leading to the release of renin, which increases kidney reabsorption of sodium
c. ADH produced by the kidneys stimulates the production of aldosterone by the adrenal gland, which increases reabsorption of sodium and retention of water
d. renin is produced by the kidneys and is converted to angiotensin, which induces the secretion of aldosterone by the adrenal gland, which in turn increases reabsorption of sodium and retention of water

90. Laboratory findings of erythrocytosis, reticulocytosis, increased plasma erythropoietin levels, and normal leukocyte and platelet counts suggest the presence of which one of the following conditions?

a. polycythemia vera
b. refractory anemia
c. secondary polycythemia
d. hemoconcentration of pregnancy

91. Antibodies to Rh, MNS, Kell, or Duffy antigens may cause which one of the following reactions?

a. acute hemolytic transfusion reaction (HTR)
b. febrile transfusion reaction
c. delayed HTR
d. allergic transfusion reaction

92. Which one of the following groups of human leukocyte antigen (HLA) is most frequently associated with organ transplantation rejection?

a. HLA-A, HLA-B, HLA-C
b. HLA-A, HLA-B, HLA-DR
c. HLA-DP, HLA-DQ, HLA-R
d. HLA-B, HLA-C, HLA-DR

93. Antimitochondrial antibodies are often found in which one of the following conditions?

a. primary biliary cirrhosis
b. chronic active hepatitis
c. cytomegalovirus infection
d. infectious mononucleosis (IM)

94. Most immunodeficiencies are associated with primary defects of which one of the following cells?

a. T cells
b. T and B cells
c. B cells
d. phagocytic cells

95. The number and type of casts found in urine sediment reflect which one of the following?

a. the extent of renal tubular involvement in disease processes
b. the amount of Tamm-Horsfall protein contained in the tubule
c. no need of quantitation during sediment examination
d. the ability of the kidney to concentrate urine

96. Examination of an isolate on MacConkey agar yields the following results: oxidase negative, dark-pink colonies, indole positive, citrate negative. Which one of the following organisms is the most likely identity of this isolate?

a. *Klebsiella pneumoniae*
b. *Citrobacter diversus*
c. *Escherichia coli*
d. *Enterobacter cloacae*

97. Rh antibodies have been associated with which one of the following clinical conditions?

a. erythroblastosis fetalis
b. thrombocytopenia
c. hemophilia A
d. paroxysmal nocturnal hemoglobinuria

98. Severe skin photosensitivity, excretion of excessive amounts of uroporphyrin I and coproporphyrin I, and fatality early in life are characteristic of which one of the following porphyrias?

a. acute intermittent porphyria
b. congenital erythropoietic porphyria
c. lead poisoning
d. coproporphyria

99. Which one of the following best describes the red blood cell distribution width (RDW) value in patients who have disseminated intravascular coagulation (DIC)?

a. decreased
b. normal
c. increased
d. no significance

100. Which one of the following statements describes nonrespiratory (metabolic) acidosis?

a. increase in CO_2 content with a decreased pH
b. decrease in CO_2 content with an increased pH
c. increase in CO_2 content with an increased pH
d. decrease in CO_2 content with a decreased pH

101. *Mycoplasma pneumoniae* infections can sometimes be associated with which one of the following antibodies?

a. anti-P antibodies
b. anti-M antibodies
c. anti-I antibodies
d. anti-i antibodies

102. The D antigen of the Fisher-Race nomenclature corresponds to which one of the following antigens of the Wiener nomenclature?

a. Rh_o
b. rh'
c. rh''
d. hr'

103. Examination of an isolate from a urine culture yielded the following characteristics: oxidase positive, colorless colonies on MacConkey agar, and colonies are beta-hemolytic on blood agar, with a feathered margin and a corn-tortilla or grapelike odor. Further characterization showed the isolate to be nonfermentative. Which one of the following organisms most likely describes this isolate?

a. *Pseudomonas aeruginosa*
b. *Acinetobacter* spp.
c. *Stenotrophomonas maltophilia*
d. *Flavobacterium* spp.

104. The Widal reaction is used primarily to detect which one of the following diseases?

a. Q fever
b. typhoid fever
c. rickettsial diseases
d. babesiosis

105. Hepatitis B is considered most infectious when which one of the following markers is detectable?

a. HBeAg
b. HBsAg
c. HBcAg
d. HBsAb

106. In the direct antiglobulin test, the antiglobulin reagent is used for which one of the following reasons?

a. to detect in vivo antibodies or complement on red blood cells (RBCs)
b. to detect in vitro antibodies or complement on RBCs
c. to precipitate antibodies
d. to fix complement

107. Which one of the following coagulation tests serves as the most sensitive and earliest detector of coagulation abnormalities of chronic liver disease?

a. activated partial thromboplastin time
b. prothrombin time
c. thrombin time
d. substitution testing

108. The common, basic defect in megaloblastic anemias is indicated by which one of the following conditions?

a. folate deficiency
b. impaired DNA thymidine synthesis
c. vitamin B_{12} deficiency
d. iron excess

109. A synovial fluid was received in the laboratory for a 23-year-old man who had a recent football injury. In the days following the injury, he reported progressively increasing pain and swelling. The final laboratory report was as follows:

Color: brownish green
Clarity: turbid
Viscosity: low to absent
Fibrin clots: present
Total cells per microliter: 124,000
Differential: 93% segmented neutrophils; 7% lymphocytes
Plasma-synovial glucose difference: 45 mg/dL
Culture and staining: positive/*Staphylococcus aureus*
Based on the laboratory results, which one of the following diagnoses is the most probable?

a. septic inflammation
b. rheumatoid arthritis
c. meningitis
d. trauma with hemorrhage to knee joint

110. Polyspecific reagents used in the antiglobulin test should react with which one of the following?

a. Immunoglobulin (Ig) G and IgA
b. IgG and C3d
c. IgM and IgA
d. IgM and C3d

111. If agglutination occurs when Coombs' control cells are added to a negative antiglobulin test, which one of the following facts is confirmed?

a. the negative antiglobulin test was really negative
b. the patient's red blood cells (RBCs) were not washed thoroughly before the antihuman globulin (AHG) reagent was added
c. the Coombs' control cells are contaminated
d. the AHG reagent is contaminated

112. Regarding enzyme kinetics, which one of the following statements best defines first-order kinetics?

a. the reaction rate of an enzymatic reaction is directly proportional to the concentration of the substrate
b. the reaction rate of an enzymatic reaction is directly proportional to the concentration of enzyme
c. if enzyme concentration is exceeded by substrate concentration, the velocity of the reaction is proportional to the enzyme concentration
d. increased temperature increases the rate of an enzymatic reaction by increasing the probability of molecular collisions

113. A 41-year-old man is seen with a history of bleeding following mild trauma. Coagulation screening produced the following results:

Thromboplastin time: 25.0 seconds

Prothrombin time (PT): 21.0 seconds

Activated partial thromboplastin time (APTT): 58.0 seconds
    Patient + control APTT: 36.0 seconds
    Patient + aged serum APTT: 61.0 seconds
    Patient + adsorbed plasma APTT: 34.0 seconds

Bleeding time: 8 minutes

This patient most likely has which one of the following conditions?

a. lupus anticoagulant
b. factor IX deficiency
c. factor X deficiency
d. factor I deficiency

114. A patient complaining of weight loss, fever, and increased bruising was admitted to the hospital. Initial examination, which consisted of a physical examination as well as hemoglobin and hematocrit measurements, indicated splenomegaly and anemia. A complete blood count revealed a white blood cell (WBC) count of 200,000/mm³, and the differential showed 50% segmented neutrophils, 15% band neutrophils, 5% lymphocytes, 5% metamyelocytes, 20% myelocytes, 3% promyelocytes, and 2% blasts. Bone marrow aspiration results revealed the marrow to be hypercellular, with all stages of myeloid maturation increased. The leukocyte alkaline phosphatase (LAP) score was 5. Which one of the following would be the most likely diagnosis for this patient?

a. acute myelogenous leukemia (AML)-M2
b. chronic lymphocytic leukemia (CLL)
c. chronic myelogenous leukemia (CML)
d. polycythemia vera (PV)

115. Hemolytic disease of the newborn (HDN) is an example of which one of the following hypersensitivities?

a. immediate-type hypersensitivity
b. cytotoxic-type hypersensitivity
c. immune complex-type hypersensitivity
d. delayed-type hypersensitivity

116. Occupational Safety and Health Act guidelines for universal precautions are based on which one of the following principles?

a. Individuals are basically careless and must follow established guidelines for safety practices
b. all laboratory procedures must contain a section on safety
c. laboratory administration does not care about employees' safety, so it is up to the federal government to protect them
d. laboratory personnel must treat all human blood and body fluids as if they were infected with human immunodeficiency virus (HIV) or hepatitis B virus (HBV)

117. Cerebrospinal fluid (CSF) analysis showed a small gray isolate on blood agar that had a narrow zone of beta hemolysis. The isolate was hippurate hydrolysis and cyclic adenosine monophosphate positive. Which one of the following is the additional test that should be performed before a presumptive identification is reported?

a. coagulase
b. pyruvate
c. catalase
d. growth on nutrient agar

118. A low semen volume containing a sperm count of 15,000 would indicate which one of the following conditions?

a. virility
b. infertility
c. prostate cancer
d. prostatitis

119. The major cross-match involves testing of which one of the following?

a. donor serum and patient cells
b. donor cells and patient serum
c. patient serum and screening cells
d. patient cells and known antiserum

120. When a patient has undergone previous transfusion or has been pregnant within the past 3 months, the oldest a specimen can be for use in a cross-match is

a. 2 weeks old
b. 24 hours old
c. 48 hours old
d. 72 hours old

121. An 8-year-old girl is seen by her pediatrician with the following symptoms: failure to gain weight, lethargy, weakness, and some impairment of school performance. Following thyroid hormone analysis, the following results were obtained: decreased thyroxine (T$_4$), decreased triiodothyronine (T$_3$), elevated thyroid-stimulating hormone (TSH). Which one of the following would be the most likely cause of her disease?

a. Graves' disease
b. pituitary tumor
c. Hashimoto's thyroiditis
d. thyroid carcinoma

122. The alternate complement pathway is activated by which one of the following?

a. polysaccharides of target cells
b. Immunoglobulin (Ig) A
c. IgM and IgG
d. other complement components

123. In Type I hypersensitivity reactions, immunoglobulin (Ig) E attaches to basophils or tissue mast cells and triggers the release of

a. antihistamines
b. cytokines
c. histamines
d. lysozyme

124. Sputum was processed for staining and culture of acid-fast bacilli. An isolate with the following characteristics was grown on Löwenstein-Jensen agar: colonies buff-colored, dry, and heaped up; niacin, nitrate, and urease positive. Growth required 23 days at 35°C. Which one of the following organisms is the most likely identity of this isolate?

a. *Mycobacterium avium*
b. *Mycobacterium kansasii*
c. *Mycobacterium bovis*
d. *Mycobacterium tuberculosis*

125. An acute myelogenous leukemia (AML) patient demonstrated 40% blast cells on both peripheral and bone marrow Wright-stained smears. For the pathologist to differentiate between AML-M4 and AML-M5 or between AML-Ml and AML-M5, what two cytochemical stains must be performed?

a. Sudan black and peroxidase
b. chloroacetate esterase and alpha-naphthyl acetate esterase
c. chloroacetate esterase AS-D and leukocyte alkaline phosphatase (LAP)
d. periodic acid–Schiff and LAP

126. Antibodies against the p24 core protein of the human immunodeficiency virus (HIV) usually develop

a. within 4–6 weeks after infection
b. within 6–8 weeks after infection
c. within 8–12 weeks after infection
d. within 6 months after infection

127. Antibodies that demonstrate dosage react stronger

a. with homozygous rather than with heterozygous cells
b. with heterozygous rather than with homozygous cells
c. at room temperature rather than at 37°C
d. with enzyme-treated cells only

128. An incompatible cross-match with a negative antibody screen and a negative autocontrol may be caused by which one of the following?

a. patient antibody against a high-frequency antigen
b. donor unit with a positive direct antiglobulin test (DAT)
c. cold agglutinins interfering with the cross-match
d. patient warm autoantibody

129. A patient who is seen with petit mal seizures was treated with phenobarbital by his physician. One year later, a different physician prescribed valproic acid in conjunction with the phenobarbital. Which one of the following statements is correct concerning the interaction of these two drugs?

a. valproic acid does not affect the concentration of phenobarbital in the serum
b. the presence of valproic acid in the serum can increase the serum concentration of phenobarbital
c. the presence of phenobarbital in the serum increases the serum concentration of valproic acid
d. phenobarbital concentration in the serum is decreased by the presence of valproic acid

130. Which one of the following inhibits growth of a platelet aggregate?

a. thrombin
b. an increase in blood flow
c. thromboxane A_2
d. heparin

131. A 50-year-old man was admitted to the hospital after complaining to his physician of fatigue, weakness, and abdominal discomfort. His initial complete blood count demonstrated a white blood cell (WBC) count of 125,000/mm³. His blood smear differential was reported as 80% lymphocytes, 10% segmented neutrophils, and 10% band neutrophils. His bone marrow showed an increase in small mature lymphocytes. His reticulocyte count was 3.5%. Based on this information, which one of the following would be the most likely diagnosis?

a. acute lymphocytic leukemia [acute lymphocytic leukemia (ALL)-Ll]
b. chronic lymphocytic leukemia (CLL)
c. Hodgkin's lymphoma
d. prolymphocytic leukemia

132. The Ouchterlony method is a type of which one of the following techniques?

a. radial immunodiffusion
b. countercurrent immunoelectrophoresis
c. double immunodiffusion
d. immunofixation electrophoresis

133. An alternate blood type that a group A individual may receive when no group A blood is readily available is

a. group O, whole blood
b. group B, red blood cells (RBCs)
c. group O, RBCs
d. group AB, RBCs

134. Fy^a, Fy^b, and M antigens are destroyed by which one of the following enhancement techniques?

a. proteolytic enzymes
b. low-ionic-strength saline
c. albumin
d. polybrene

135. The use of phenylethyl alcohol sheep blood agar (PEA) is helpful in anaerobic culturing because PEA

a. inhibits anaerobe growth so that facultative organisms can grow
b. inhibits facultative organisms but allows the growth of anaerobes
c. inhibits gram-negative anaerobe growth
d. inhibits gram-positive anaerobe growth

136. A cerebrospinal fluid (CSF) glucose of 35 mg/dL would indicate which one of the following conditions?

a. a normal value
b. diabetes mellitus
c. bacterial meningitis
d. brain tumor

137. Antibodies in secondary syphilis have which one of the following characteristics?

a. they are mostly immunoglobulin (Ig) M
b. they are usually undetectable
c. they are directed only against treponemal antigens
d. they are mostly IgG

138. Epstein-Barr virus infects which one of the following?

a. B lymphocytes
b. T lymphocytes
c. B and T lymphocytes
d. monocytes

139. Which one of the following antibody systems is most commonly associated with hemolytic disease of the newborn (HDN)?

a. Rh
b. Kell
c. ABO
d. Duffy

140. Which one of the following best describes a genetic disorder that causes a deficiency of certain enzymes in the synthetic pathways leading to cortisol and aldosterone production?

a. Cushing's syndrome
b. Conn's syndrome
c. congenital adrenal hyperplasia
d. Addison's disease

141. Which one of the following substances directly inactivates factors Va and VIII:Ca?

a. thrombin
b. α_2-antiplasmin
c. heparin
d. protein C

142. A gram-negative bacillus from an abdominal abscess is isolated on anaerobic media, but no growth is seen on sheep blood agar incubated aerobically. The isolate is resistant to vancomycin, kanamycin, and colistin. It is indole-negative and grows in thioglycolate with 20% bile. Which one of the following organisms best describes this isolate?

a. *Fusobacterium nucleatum*
b. *Fusobacterium necrophorum*
c. *Prevotella intermedia*
d. *Bacteroides fragilis*

143. Which one of the following is the most widely used test for rubella antibodies?

a. passive latex agglutination
b. immunofluorescent assay
c. radioimmunoassay
d. hemagglutination inhibition (HAI)

144. The results of a Kleihauer-Betke stain indicate a fetomaternal hemorrhage of 35 mL of blood. How many vials of Rh$_0$ (D) immune globulin should be given to the mother?

a. 0
b. 1
c. 2
d. 3

145. A chronic lymphocytic leukemia (CLL) variant characterized by splenomegaly, a proliferation of abnormal lymphocytes in bone marrow and secondary lymphoid organs, and the findings of abnormal lymphocytes with hairlike projections that stain positive with acid phosphatase (even with L-tartrate inhibition) most likely indicates which one of the following conditions?

a. Hodgkin's lymphoma
b. chloroma
c. lymphosarcoma cell leukemia
d. hairy-cell leukemia

146. A false-negative result in a Venereal Disease Research Laboratory (VDRL) test may be caused by which one of the following factors?

a. prozone phenomenon
b. systemic lupus erythematosus (SLE)
c. infectious mononucleosis (IM)
d. old age

147. A low minimum inhibitory concentration can be correlated to what Kirby-Bauer disk diffusion result?

a. large zone of inhibition
b. small zone of inhibition
c. overlapping zones of inhibition
d. no zone of inhibition

148. Acute myelogenous leukemia (AML) patients with severe bleeding problems caused by procoagulant material released from the granules of abnormal cells would most likely have which one of the following conditions?

a. AML-M1
b. AML-M2
c. AML-M3
d. erythroleukemia

149. The antigens used in the Weil-Felix test are prepared from strains of which one of the following genera?

a. *Salmonella*
b. *Rickettsia*
c. *Proteus*
d. *Shigella*

150. Immunofixation electrophoresis is often used in conjunction with immunoelectrophoresis to

a. work up a polyclonal gammopathy
b. work up a monoclonal gammopathy
c. quantitate serum immunoglobulins
d. quantitate circulating immune complexes

Answers and Explanations

1. The answer is c [Chapter 5 I B 2]. Most clinically significant blood group antibodies are immunoglobulin (Ig) G. The remainder are usually IgM, although there are a few rare IgA antibodies against blood group antigens.

2. The answer is a [Chapter 5 I C 2 a]. The prozone phenomenon occurs when antibody molecules are present in excess of available antigenic sites. This results in false-negative reactions. Antigen excess can also cause false-negative reactions.

3. The answer is c [Chapter 1 I B 2 d]. Coefficient of variation is used to compare the variability in sets of values and is expressed as a percentage. It is calculated by multiplying the standard deviation by 100 and then dividing this value by the mean.

4. The answer is c [Chapter 2 II A 1 a (2)]. A vitamin B_{12} deficiency results in a block of cellular mitosis and maturation. Lymphoma (option B) and chronic alcohol consumption (option D) result in a decreased megakaryocyte population and production.

5. The answer is b [Chapter 5 VIII A 4]. The American Association of Blood Banks (AABB) requires that all patient samples be stored between 1°C and 6°C for a minimum of 7 days after transfusion.

6. The answer is d [Chapter 6 I D 3]. Immunoglobulin (Ig) E binds to mast cells and basophils in immediate-type hypersensitivity reactions, and is elevated in parasitic infections and allergic disorders.

7. The answer is b [Chapter 3 IV E 3 d (1), F 4 c]. Intravascular hemolysis results in an increase in unconjugated serum bilirubin. Laboratory methods measure the unconjugated bilirubin fraction as the indirect bilirubin.

8. The answer is a [Chapter 7 I A 1]. Although personnel and instrumentation are included in the quality assurance program, the entire program exists to ensure that results are reliable.

9. The answer is c [Chapter 5 I B 2]. Immunoglobulins (Ig) G1, G2, and G3 are all capable of binding complement, but IgG1 and IgG3 bind complement much more efficiently than does IgG2.

10. The answer is d [Chapter 9 I B 1; Figure 9-1]. The trophozoite of *Entamoeba* is the only protozoan that contains ingested red blood cells (RBCs).

11. The answer is b [Chapter 10 III A 1]. Observations of urine color and transparency should be performed on a well-mixed, unspun specimen.

12. The answer is b [Chapter 8 I A]. The cell membrane serves as a barrier to molecules as well as being the site of action of a limited number of antibiotics. The cell wall (option A), although giving rigidity to the cell, does not serve as an osmotic barrier.

13. The answer is b [Chapter 5 II B 12]. D^u testing is done by incubating patient red blood cells (RBCs) with anti-D reagent at 37°C. This incubation is followed by saline washes and addition of the antihuman globulin (AHG) reagent.

14. The answer is c [Chapter 6 IV A 3]. The second or any subsequent exposure to the same antigen stimulates the secondary antibody response.

15. The answer is c [Chapter 1 I A 1 b,c]. Molarity is a term describing the concentration of a solution. It is expressed as the number of moles per liter of solution. One mole of a substance equals its gram molecular weight.

16. The answer is b [Chapter 2 II A 1 c (2) (a) (iii)]. One of the suspected causes of thrombotic thrombocytopenic purpura (TTP) is a decrease in prostaglandin I_2 (PGI_2), which results in an increase

A, B]. The majority of autoimmune hemolytic anemias (AIHAs) mmon type are cold AIHAs.

II A 1 b (3)]. A yellow-brown urine results from the excretion

B 6 e]. Viruses may be detected by observing a characteristic swellings or inclusions.

III F 1]. The A-negative units of blood are the best choice for -positive (option A) and A-positive (option C) units should not negative. The O-negative units (option D) could be given, but the A-negative units are closer to being type specific.

F 5 c (3) (b)]. The answer should be obtained with the follow-

mm^3

27 ÷ 45) = 8.0%

= RI ÷ 2 (maturation time) = 4 times as many reticulocytes

A 5 a]. Both patient cell suspensions and those of reagent red nking procedures are usually between 3% and 5%.

2 e]. Beer's law states that the concentration of a substance is of light absorbed; therefore, A = *abc*, where *a* is equal to the tance, *b* is the path length of light, and *c* is the concentration

1 c (3) (a)]. Idiopathic thrombocytopenic purpura results from n the circulation and spleen. A loss in circulating platelet mass ryopoiesis in the marrow.

25. The answer is b [Chapter 3 IV D 3 a]. The Embden-Meyerhof (EM) pathway produces the adenosine triphosphate needed to maintain membrane ion pumps and membrane stability. A defect in the EM metabolism pathway results in short-lived red blood cells (RBCs) and a hemolytic anemia.

26. The answer is d [Chapter 5 VII B 2 a]. Proteolytic enzymes can be used to enhance the reactions of antibodies such as Rh and Kidd. M (option A), N (option B), and Duffy (option C) antibodies are denatured by enzyme treatment.

27. The answer is d [Chapter 6 II B 1 d]. The mature B cell has developed surface immunoglobulin (Ig) D and IgM as well as crystallizable fragment (Fc) receptors.

28. The answer is d [Chapter 7 II A 6 a (16)]. The laboratory director must approve all procedures by signature and must also periodically update and review procedures.

29. The answer is d [Chapter 8 II B, C, D, F]. Acridine orange is useful in detecting bacteria in specimens where numbers may be few, such as blood and spinal fluid. Kinyoun acid-fast stain (option A) and methylene blue stain (option B) are not fluorescent stains. Calcofluor white (option C) is a fluorescent stain, but it is used to detect yeast cells and fungal hyphae.

30. The answer is b [Chapter 5 V K 1 c]. Irradiating blood products can help reduce the risk of graft-versus-host disease in patients who are at risk, such as low-birth-weight neonates or patients who are immunosuppressed or immunocompromised because of disease or chemotherapy.

31. The answer is a [Chapter 5 III E 4]. Because heparin has no preservative qualities, blood collected in heparin should be transfused within 24 hours of collection.

32. The answer is a [Chapter 1 IV G 3 b]. Most triglycerides are transported in the serum via chylomicrons and very low density lipoproteins (VLDL). When a serum is extremely high in triglycerides, it appears creamy or milky after incubation at 4°C because of the presence of the chylomicrons and VLDL.

33. The answer is a [Chapter 5 III E 2]. The citrate in citrate-phosphate-dextrose-adenine (CPDA)-1 functions by chelating calcium, which prevents clotting.

34. The answer is c [Chapter 8 III B b]. *Staphylococcus epidermidis* is commonly found on skin surfaces and may contaminate a blood culture during venipuncture. The other choices are not found as normal skin flora but may be seen as transients.

35. The answer is b [Chapter 5 V G 3]. A patient's platelet count should increase by 5 to 10 × 10^9/L for each unit of platelet concentrate transfused.

36. The answer is b [Chapter 1 III D 1 a (1), (2)]. Insulin has the ability to decrease serum glucose by promoting glycogenesis and increasing uptake of glucose by cells. Glucagon and thyroid hormone both increase glucose in the blood by stimulating glycogenolysis. If insulin is present in decreased amounts, serum glucose increases.

37. The answer is b [Chapter 6 XIII D 1]. The Monospot assay differentially absorbs the patient serum to distinguish between Forssman and infectious mononucleosis (IM) heterophile antibodies. In this assay, the IM heterophile antibodies are absorbed by the beef erythrocytes.

38. The answer is a [Chapter 8 IV A 3 g]. Some of the organisms found in meningitis, most notably *Neisseria meningitidis*, are sensitive to environmental changes. Viability decreases rapidly. Immediate processing of the specimen is necessary to minimize this decrease because cold, heat, and drying all adversely affect recovery.

39. The answer is d [Chapter 5 VI B 4 a]. If the red blood cells (RBCs) are not properly washed, the antihuman globulin (AHG) reagent is not able to bind to any antibodies that may be on the cells, and false-negative reactions result.

40. The answer is c [Chapter 5 II A 4, X E 5]. Blood used for exchange transfusion must be negative for the antigen against which the maternal antibody is made. Because the antibody involved must be able to cross the placental barrier, the mother's antibody must be immunoglobulin (Ig) G.

41. The answer is b [Chapter 4 IV C 2 c]. A left shift in a white blood cell (WBC) differential usually indicates an increase in marrow granulopoiesis. This is seen in the peripheral blood as an increase in percent of band neutrophils and other immature myeloid forms.

42. The answer is d [Chapter 5 VII C 1 a]. A cold-reacting autoantibody reacts optimally below 37°C. If panel cells react at room temperature and react less strongly after incubation at 37°C, and if the autocontrol is positive, a cold-reacting autoantibody should be suspected. A warm autoantibody would react more strongly after incubation.

43. The answer is d [Chapter 2 IV B 6]. A prolonged time in both pathways indicates a deficiency in the common pathway. The use of aged serum was able to correct the prolonged activated partial thromboplastin time (APTT) for the missing factor, but the prolonged APTT was not corrected with adsorbed plasma. Factor X is present in aged serum but absent in adsorbed plasma.

44. The answer is a [Chapter 5 VIII E 2]. The most likely cause of the incompatibility is a recipient alloantibody. A recipient autoantibody (option B) would have yielded a positive autocontrol. DAT–positive (option C) donor units would not have resulted in a positive antibody screen. Rouleaux (option D) would have been observed after the 37°C incubation but would have disappeared in the antihuman globulin (AHG) phase after the red blood cells (RBCs) had been thoroughly washed with saline.

45. The answer is b [Chapter 9 I D 14]. *Onchocerca* microfilariae typically encapsulate to form nodules on the head. These microfilariae can be observed in skin snips taken from the nodules.

46. The answer is d [Chapter 10 III C 2]. Urine with a fixed specific gravity equal to 1.010 is termed isothenuric.

47. The answer is b [Chapter 10 III D 1]. A 25-year-old man with a normal food and fluid intake excreted 1400 mL of urine in 24 hours. This urine volume can best be described as normal. The normal range for urine volume in a healthy adult is 400–2000 mL per day.

48. The answer is a [Chapter 5 VII A 3]. Most immunoglobulin (Ig) M antibodies will react on immediate spin in saline. Examples include M, N, Lewis, and P antibodies.

49. The answer is c [Chapter 5 V F 2]. Fresh frozen plasma (FFP) can be stored for up to 1 year after collection, if it is stored at $-18°C$.

50. The answer is d [Chapter 1 III C 1 a (2), IV H 2 b]. Intrinsic factor is a substance in the gastric fluid of humans that makes absorption of vitamin B_{12} possible. Lack of intrinsic factor, because of atrophy of the stomach lining, leads to vitamin B_{12} deficiency and pernicious anemia.

51. The answer is c [Chapter 8 V C 2 c]. *Staphylococcus saprophyticus* is resistant to novobiocin, whereas *S. aureus*, *S. epidermidis*, and *Micrococcus* spp are sensitive to novobiocin.

52. The answer is d [Chapter 6 XII C 1 b]. Although normal values are difficult to establish for the antistreptolysin O (ASO) test, results of greater than 166 Todd units are generally considered to indicate recent infection.

53. The answer is a [Chapter 6 X E]. Fibrinogen is the acute phase protein that is primarily responsible for an increased erythrocyte sedimentation rate (ESR).

54. The answer is c [Chapter 5 V A 1]. A unit of whole blood collected from an adult should contain approximately 450 mL of blood. The bag should contain approximately 63 mL of anticoagulant.

55. The answer is d [Chapter 3 IV E 2 a]. A loss in pliability results in splenic destruction because red blood cells (RBCs) must be flexible enough to pass through splenic red pulp fenestrations.

56. The answer is b [Chapter 1 IV G 6 c (1)]. The classic calculation for determining low density lipoprotein (LDL) concentration is total cholesterol minus the high density lipoprotein (HDL) concentration plus triglycerides divided by 5. In the presented case, this equation is LDL = 210 − [23 + (150/5)], or 157. This calculation, however, has been shown to give false LDL values because of the inclusion of the triglyceride level, which is easily affected by diet.

57. The answer is a [Chapter 5 II D 2 a]. Anti-M antibodies are relatively common, naturally occurring antibodies that can be a mixture of immunoglobulin (Ig) G and IgM.

58. The answer is d [Chapter 5 II A 2 a]. An individual who secretes A and H substances must have A and H genes. However, he or she must also have the Se gene, which enables secretion of the other substances.

59. The answer is d [Chapter 6 VII D 3 d (2)(a)]. The enzyme-linked immunosorbent assay (ELISA) is the most commonly used screening test for the presence of human immunodeficiency virus (HIV) antibodies. Repeatedly positive results are confirmed with a Western blot.

60. The answer is a [Chapter 1 IV C 6 a]. Respiratory acidosis results from hypoventilation that can be caused by alcohol overdose. Hypoventilation causes a decrease in carbon dioxide elimination, thereby causing an increase in blood pH.

61. The answer is c [Chapter 6 XI A]. Hepatitis A is an acute, self-limiting disease transmitted primarily by a fecal-oral route. Infections do not become chronic, and there is no carrier state.

62. The answer is d [Chapter 8 VI B 1 e]. *Streptococcus agalactiae* (option A) and *S. pyogenes* (option B) are beta hemolytic. The viridans streptococci (option C) are alpha hemolytic but are resistant to optochin.

63. The answer is a [Chapter 5 II A 4]. Most ABO antibodies are naturally occurring immunoglobulin (Ig) M antibodies that develop shortly after birth. ABO antibodies that develop as a result of red blood cell (RBC) stimulation are typically IgG.

64. The answer is c [Chapter 1 IV D 6]. Anion gap is the difference between measured cations and measured anions. It is calculated to determine the presence of any unmeasured electrolytes that could have a physiologic effect. The formula is a subtraction of measured anions from measured cations. In the presented case, the equation would be $(148 + 5.8) - (87 + 24) = 42.8$. Normal anion gap is 6–18.

65. The answer is b [Chapter 2 IV A 1 a]. Afibrinogenemia results from a lack of fibrinogen synthesis in the liver. Underlying causes can be genetic or acquired.

66. The answer is b [Chapter 5 II L 2]. Sd^a antigens are high-incidence antigens. Antibodies against them are not usually considered to be clinically significant, but they do yield a characteristic mixed field agglutination reaction that can be useful in identifying the antibody.

67. The answer is a [Chapter 3 IV D 3 a (2) (a)]. Methemoglobin is the oxidized form of oxyhemoglobin. When the heme iron is in the ferric (Fe^{3+}) form, it cannot bind oxygen.

68. The answer is a [Chapter 5 II B 2 c]. The D^u antigen is a weakened form of the D antigen and is clinically significant. D^u-positive recipients should receive D-negative blood.

69. The answer is b [Chapter 6 XI B]. Before the hepatitis B virus (HBV) was identified, the term "Australia antigen" was used to describe the causative agent of the disease.

70. The answer is a [Chapter 6 XIV C 1]. Although both immunoglobulin (Ig) G and IgM antibodies develop during acute rubella, the IgM antibodies disappear within a few weeks, and the IgG antibodies persist for life. These IgG antibodies, when present at a titer of at least 8, are indicative of prior infection and therefore immunity.

71. The answer is a [Chapter 8 VI D 10]. L-pyrrolidonyl-β-naphthylamide (PYR) hydrolysis is specific for *Enterococcus* spp and *S. pyogenes*.

72. The answer is c [Chapter 9 II F 3]. *Coccidioides immitis* is a dimorphic fungus that produces arthroconidia in the mold phase.

73. The answer is b [Chapter 10 IV A; Table 10-2]. An unpreserved urine specimen was at room temperature for 4 hours in an unsterile container. The dipstick reaction that is most likely to be reliable is blood that detects lysed and intact red blood cells (RBCs).

74. The answer is c [Chapter 5 II A 5 c (5)]. This patient forward-typed as an A and reverse-typed as an O. An acquired B phenomenon would not have a positive autocontrol. However, a cold-reacting autoantibody, such as anti-I, would produce these results.

75. The answer is d [Chapter 5 VIII E 2]. A recipient alloantibody to donor red blood cell (RBC) antigens will result in a positive antibody screen, a positive major cross-match, and a negative autocontrol. An autoantibody would have given a positive autocontrol.

76. The answer is b [Chapter 1 IV F 2 e]. The conversion of glucose to lactate or pyruvate to form energy as adenosine triphosphate (ATP) occurs in the Kreb's cycle. This function is referred to as glycolysis.

77. The answer is c [Chapter 8 VII B]. *Haemophilus influenzae* will not grow on blood agar. Susceptibility to penicillin is unusual for the gram-negative coccobacilli and is characteristic of *Pasteurella multocida*.

78. The answer is c [Chapter 5 II G 2]. Anti-Fy^a antibodies are capable of causing hemolytic transfusion reactions (HTR). They are usually immunoglobulin (Ig) G and react best at 37°C. They are denatured by enzyme treatment.

79. The answer is b [Chapter 4 III F 2 e]. Red blood cells (RBCs) that are hypersensitive to complement binding are prone to hemolysis.

80. The answer is d [Chapter 6 VII A 1 a (2)]. The nitroblue tetrazolium (NBT) reductase test is used to evaluate the respiratory burst of neutrophils and to detect impaired neutrophil phagocytosis.

81. The answer is c [Chapter 5 IX A 1]. Acute hemolytic transfusion reactions (HTRs) are rare but can be life threatening. They are usually caused by ABO incompatibilities between the recipient and the donor red blood cells (RBCs). Delayed HTRs are usually caused by recipient alloantibodies against donor RBC antigens.

82. The answer is a [Chapter 5 IX A 3]. Anaphylactic transfusion reactions are severe, acute allergic reactions triggered by antibodies against immunoglobulin (Ig) A.

83. The answer is a [Chapter 9 II H 4 a]. *Epidermophyton floccosum* is a major cause of tinea cruris and produces two-cell to four-cell smooth, club-shaped macroconidia.

84. The answer is d [Chapter 8 VII H]. The absolute requirement for carbon dioxide, yellow-pigmented colonies, gliding motility, and fusiform morphology make this isolate *Capnocytophaga*. *Actinobacillus* (option A) is slow growing. *Kingella* (option B) shows short, plump rods with square ends on Gram's stain. *Cardiobacterium* (option D) is pleomorphic without gliding motility.

85. The answer is c [Chapter 10 IV B 7 a]. The reagent strip method used to detect protein in urine is based on the protein error of indicators.

86. The answer is c [Chapter 5 VIII B 6 a]. The major cross-match will detect any ABO incompatibilities between a donor and a recipient. In this case, the A-positive recipient's serum has antibodies against the donor red blood cells' (RBC) B antigens, which makes the unit incompatible. The Rh incompatibility in option D would not be detected by the major cross-match.

87. The answer is c [Chapter 6 IX E 2 b]. Tests for syphilis can detect nontreponemal antibodies or treponemal antibodies. The microhemagglutination-*Treponema pallidum* (MHA-TP) test uses red blood cells (RBCs) coated with treponemal antigens to detect antibodies.

88. The answer is d [Chapter 6 Table 6-1]. IgG and IgM are the only classes of immunoglobulins that bind complement.

89. The answer is d [Chapter 1 IV D 1 a (1), (2)]. Sodium is regulated in two ways; via the renin-antidiuretic hormone (ADH) system and via the renin-aldosterone system. Renin is a renal hormone, and aldosterone is an adrenal hormone. Both hormones are present during decreased blood pressure and blood volume states. The two hormones act together to retain water and sodium.

90. The answer is c [Chapter 4 III A 2]. In secondary polycythemia, erythrocytosis and increased marrow erythropoiesis are the secondary results of increased plasma erythropoietin levels. Leukocytes and platelet counts are typically normal, as contrasted with absolute primary polycythemia.

91. The answer is c [Chapter 5 IX B 1]. Delayed hemolytic transfusion reactions (HTRs) are most often associated with secondary antibody responses to donor red blood cell (RBC) antigens. Immunoglobulin (Ig) G antibodies such as anti-Rh, anti-MNS, anti-Kell, and anti-Duffy are frequently identified as the cause of delayed HTR.

92. The answer is b [Chapter 5 XIII D]. Donor organ compatibility with the recipient's human leukocyte antigens (HLA)-A, HLA-B, and HLA-DR is important in reducing the risk of rejection after organ transplantation.

93. The answer is a [Chapter 6 Table 6-5]. Autoantibodies are associated with many diseases, and detection of these antibodies can aid in diagnosis. Primary biliary cirrhosis is often associated with the presence of antimitochondrial antibodies.

94. The answer is c [Chapter 6 VII B]. More than half of all immunodeficiencies are associated with defects in B cells and B-cell function.

95. The answer is a [Chapter 10 V C 4]. The number and type of casts found in urine sediment reflect the extent of renal tubular involvement in disease processes.

96. The answer is c [Chapter 8 Table 8-12]. *Klebsiella pneumoniae* (option A) and *Enterobacter cloacae* (option D) are indole negative and citrate positive. *Citrobacter diversus* (option B) is citrate positive.

97. The answer is a [Chapter 5 X]. Erythroblastosis fetalis is another term for hemolytic disease of the newborn (HDN). Rh antibodies are the cause of the most severe forms of HDN.

98. The answer is b [Chapter 4 III C 2 c (1)]. Chronic porphyrias are associated with solar sensitivity of the skin. Erythropoietic porphyria is caused by a defect in the enzyme uroporphyrinogen-III cosynthetase, which results in blood and urine elevations in substrate compounds, coproporphyrin I and uroporphyrin I.

99. The answer is c [Chapter 2 IV A 2 a (2)]. The increase in red blood cell (RBC) fragmentation (i.e., schistocytes) seen in patients who have disseminated intravascular coagulation (DIC) results in a large variation of size in RBCs, which is detected as an increase in the red blood cell distribution width (RDW).

100. The answer is d [Chapter 1 IV C 6 c]. Acidosis is described as a decrease in blood pH and a decreased bicarbonate level. Nonrespiratory acidosis involves reduced excretion of acids by the kidneys or by excess formation of acids, as in diabetic ketoacidosis.

101. The answer is c [Chapter 5 II F 2 a]. Anti-I antibodies are cold-reacting antibodies that can cause cold agglutinin disease or can be associated with infections such as *Mycoplasma pneumoniae*.

102. The answer is a [Chapter 5 II B 1 a, b; Table 5-2]. The five major Rh antigens as defined by the Fisher-Race nomenclature are D, C, E, c, and e, and correspond to Rh_o, rh′, rh″, hr′, and hr″ in the Wiener nomenclature.

103. The answer is a [Chapter 8 XI C 2]. *Acinetobacter* (option B) and *Stenotrophomonas maltophilia* (option C) are oxidase negative. *Flavobacterium* (option D) is not found as a urinary pathogen nor does the colonial morphology or distinct odor of the isolate suggest *Flavobacterium*.

104. The answer is b [Chapter 6 XV B 1]. The Widal reaction is used to diagnose typhoid fever, tularemia, and brucellosis. Q fever (option A) and rickettsial diseases (option C) are detected by the Weil-Felix test. Babesiosis (option D) is not detected by either test.

105. The answer is a [Chapter 6 XI B 3 d]. The presence of the HBe antigen indicates active viral replication. Hepatitis B is most infectious during the time that HBeAg is detectable.

106. The answer is a [Chapter 5 VI B 1]. The antiglobulin reagent in the direct antiglobulin test (DAT) is used to detect the presence of in vivo antibodies or complement. The indirect antiglobulin test is used to detect in vitro antibodies or complement.

107. The answer is b [Chapter 2 IV A 2 c]. Factor VII is the most sensitive indicator of coagulation disorders associated with liver disease because it has the shortest half-life and, therefore, decreases first in the plasma. The prothrombin time (PT) detects abnormalities in factor VII.

108. The answer is b [Chapter 4 III E 3 c]. A lack of vitamin B_{12} or folic acid results in impaired thymidine synthesis, which is one of the deoxyribonucleic acid (DNA) bases needed for DNA replication.

109. The answer is a [Chapter 10 X C 3; Table 10-8]. The prominent neutrophilia, low glucose, and positive culture results indicate an infectious process in the joint. The presence of fibrin clots indicate a damaged synovial plasma membrane.

110. The answer is b [Chapter 5 VI A 2]. Antiglobulin reagents may be monospecific or polyspecific. Polyspecific reagents are made against a combination of immunoglobulins (Ig) and complement components, and they must always contain at least anti-IgG and anti-C3d.

111. The answer is a [Chapter 5 VI B 2 a]. The addition of Coombs' control cells to negative antiglobulin testing confirms that the patient's red blood cells (RBCs) were thoroughly washed before the antihuman globulin (AHG) reagent was added. The Coombs' cells are coated with immunoglobulin (Ig) G antibody or C3d, depending on the specificity of the AHG reagent used. If the cells were properly washed, the IgG or C3d on the Coombs' cells will react with the AHG reagent, which results in agglutination. This confirms that a negative test is valid.

112. The answer is a [Chapter 1 V A 6 c (1) (a)]. Substrate concentration initially influences the rate of an enzymatic reaction until the substrate saturates all enzyme that is available. This is first-order kinetics with regard to enzymatic reactions.

113. The answer is d [Chapter 2 IV A 1]. A prolonged result of both the prothrombin time (PT) and the activated partial thromboplastin time (APTT) indicates a disorder of the common pathway. Because the thrombin time (TT) is prolonged, it would indicate a deficiency of fibrinogen (i.e., factor I). Substitution test results confirm this diagnosis.

114. The answer is c [Chapter 4 IV E 2 a]. The patient is seen with anemia and marked leukocytosis in the myeloid cell line. All stages of maturation are present, with a "bulge" in segmented neutrophils and myelocytes. Very few blasts were found. An acute leukemia is typically characterized by a predominance of blast cells.

115. The answer is b [Chapter 6 V B]. Hemolytic disease of the newborn (HDN) and hemolytic transfusion reactions (HTR) are examples of cytotoxic-type hypersensitivity reactions. Immunoglobulin (Ig) G or M antibodies are directed against the antigens on the red blood cells (RBCs).

116. The answer is d [Chapter 7 II B 4 a]. Laboratory personnel must treat all human blood and body fluids as if they were infected with human immunodeficiency virus (HIV) or hepatitis B virus (HBV). Materials that are contaminated with blood or any body fluid are also included.

117. The answer is c [Chapter 8 XII B 3]. The initial results suggest *Streptococcus agalactiae*. However, *Listeria monocytogenes* gives similar results on blood agar. Both are hippurate hydrolysis and cyclic adenosine monophosphate positive. *L. monocytogenes* is catalase positive, whereas *S. agalactiae* is catalase negative.

118. The answer is b [Chapter 10 XI C 2 b]. A normal sperm count should range between 20 to 200 million per milliliter of semen.

119. The answer is b [Chapter 5 VIII B 6]. Donor red blood cells (RBCs) are tested against patient serum in a major cross-match. A major cross-match effectively identifies ABO incompatibilities between the donor and patient. The minor cross-match tests donor serum against patient cells, but this test has largely been eliminated as part of routine compatibility testing.

120. The answer is d [Chapter 5 VIII A 3]. A sample for cross-match should not have been collected more than 72 hours earlier if the patient has a history of previous transfusion or if the patient has been pregnant within the past 3 months.

121. The answer is c [Chapter 1 VI D 2 a, b]. The only disorder listed that demonstrates decreased levels of thyroid hormones and elevated levels of thyroid-stimulating hormone (TSH) is Hashimoto's thyroiditis. Clinically, Hashimoto's disease is difficult to distinguish from hypothyroidism. Graves' disease (option A) is characterized by increased thyroid hormones and decreased TSH. Pituitary tumors (option B) and thyroid tumors (option D) produce hyperthyroid characteristics.

122. The answer is a [Chapter 6 I E 1 b]. The alternate pathway is not activated by immunoglobulin (Ig) but by the polysaccharides and lipopolysaccharides on the surfaces of certain target cells.

123. The answer is c [Chapter 6 V A]. In immediate-type (Type I) hypersensitivity reactions, antigens complex with immunoglobulin (Ig) E and attach to tissue mast cells and basophils, triggering the release of histamines and leukotrienes.

124. The answer is d [Chapter 8 XVI G; Table 8-24]. *Mycobacterium avium* (option A) is niacin, nitrate, and urease negative. *M. kansasii* (option B) is pigmented as well as niacin negative. *M. bovis* (option C) is niacin and nitrate negative.

125. The answer is b [Chapter 4 IV D 2 c; Table 4-9]. The acute myeloid leukemia (AML)-M1 is primarily a myeloblast leukemia. AML-M4 is characterized by a mixture of both myelocytic and monocytic precursors. AML-M5 is defined as a purely monocytic leukemia. To differentiate, it is best to have two stains to distinguish myelocytic precursors from monocytic precursors. Chloroacetate esterase AS-D primarily stains myeloid precursors. The alpha-naphthyl acetate esterase stain demonstrates the strongest positivity with cells of the monocytic cell line. AML-M1 would demonstrate a positive reaction with the AS-D stain but not the alpha-naphthyl esterase. Blasts of AML-M4 would stain positive with both stains. Monoblastic leukemia (i.e., AML-M5) would stain positive with alpha-naphthyl acetate esterase only.

126. The answer is b [Chapter 6 VII D 3 d (2)]. Within 6–8 weeks after infection by the human immunodeficiency virus (HIV), immunoglobulin (Ig) M antibodies against the p24 core protein develop.

127. The answer is a [Chapter 5 II D 3 b]. Antibodies that react more strongly with homozygous than heterozygous cells demonstrate a dosage effect. Anti-M and anti-N are examples of antibodies that exhibit dosage effect.

128. The answer is b [Chapter 5 VIII E 1 b]. A donor unit with a positive direct antiglobulin test (DAT) will result in an incompatible cross-match. A patient antibody against a high-frequency antigen would also have a positive antibody screen. A warm autoantibody would have a positive antibody screen and a positive autocontrol. If cold agglutinins were present, all cells would agglutinate at room temperature incubations.

129. The answer is b [Chapter 1 VII F 2 a, c]. Valproic acid inhibits phenobarbital metabolism by inhibiting certain hepatic enzymes. Decreased metabolism leads to increased serum concentration of the parent drug.

130. The answer is b [Chapter 2 I C 4 a]. An uninterrupted blood flow past the injured vascular area and platelet aggregate dilutes and washes away coagulation and aggregation-promoting factors.

131. The answer is b [Chapter 4 V D 5 b]. This patient is seen with a marked lymphocytosis and a bone marrow infiltrated by small, mature-appearing lymphocytes. In the absence of immature lymphoblasts, this disorder is best classified as chronic lymphocytic leukemia (CLL).

132. The answer is c [Chapter 6 VIII B 1]. The Ouchterlony method is a double immunodiffusion technique that involves antigen-antibody reactions precipitating in a semisolid medium.

133. The answer is c [Chapter 5 Table 5-11]. Group O red blood cells (RBCs) may be given to a group A recipient. Group O whole blood should not be given to a group A recipient, because the plasma will contain anti-A antibodies.

134. The answer is a [Chapter 5 Table 5-7]. Treating red blood cells (RBCs) with proteolytic enzymes such as papain and ficin will destroy some RBC antigens, such as Fy^a, Fy^b, and M. Other antigens such as Kidd, Lewis, and P antigens are enhanced by enzyme treatment.

135. The answer is b [Chapter 8 XVII C 3]. Phenylethyl alcohol sheep blood agar (PEA) is helpful in culturing anaerobes because the facultative anaerobes (e.g., gram-negative bacilli) are inhibited, whereas most anaerobes grow well.

136. The answer is c [Chapter 10 XII D 2 b]. The normal range for a cerebrospinal fluid (CSF) glucose level is 50–80 mg/dL, or two thirds of plasma levels. Microorganisms in CSF infections consume the CSF glucose, which causes a decreased value.

137. The answer is d [Chapter 6 IX B 2]. Immunoglobulin (Ig) G antibodies against syphilis antigens are detectable in secondary syphilis in untreated patients. Patients treated in this stage of syphilis usually become serologically nonreactive between 12 and 18 months after treatment.

138. The answer is a [Chapter 6 XIII A]. The Epstein-Barr virus infects B lymphocytes.

139. The answer is c [Chapter 5 X]. Although ABO and Rh antibodies are both implicated more frequently than other antibodies, hemolytic disease of the newborn (HDN) caused by ABO antibodies is the most common form of the disease.

140. The answer is c [Chapter 1 VI C 5 a (3)]. Congenital adrenal hyperplasia is a genetic disorder that leads to a deficiency of 21-hydroxylase, an enzyme involved with the synthesis of both cortisol and aldosterone. This disorder is associated with hypocortisolism.

141. The answer is d [Chapter 2 III E 5 b]. Protein C inactivates both factors VIII:Ca and Va in the presence of cofactor protein S.

142. The answer is d [Chapter 8 XVII D 1; Table 8-28]. *Fusobacterium* is resistant to vancomycin but susceptible to kanamycin and colistin. *F. nucleatum*, *F. necrophorum*, *Prevotella intermedia*, and *Bacteroides fragilis* are all indole positive, but none will grow in 20% bile. *P. intermedia* shows the same pattern as *Fusobacterium* spp.

143. The answer is d [Chapter 6 XIV C 1]. The hemagglutination inhibition test is the most widely used test for the determination of immunity against rubella.

144. The answer is c [Chapter 5 X F 2 e]. The number of milliliters of fetal whole blood divided by 30 is the number of vials that should be given. In this case, the calculated number of vials is 1.2. Whole vials are given, so the mother should receive 2 vials of RhIG.

145. The answer is d [Chapter 4 V D 5 c (1)]. Hairy-cell leukemia (HCL) is a clinical variation of chronic lymphocytic leukemia (CLL). Secondary lymphoid organs are involved to a greater extent, and lymphocytes stain positive with the L-tartrate variation of the acid phosphatase stain. Only the abnormal lymphocytes of HCL stain positive with L-tartrate inhibition.

146. The answer is a [Chapter 6 IX E 1 c (2)]. False-negative reactions may occur in nontreponemal syphilis testing and can be caused by prozone, technical error, or low antibody titers. Systemic lupus erythematosus (SLE) [option B], infectious mononucleosis (IM) [option C], and old age (option D) can all cause false-positive reactions in nontreponemal tests for syphilis.

147. The answer is a [Chapter 8 XVIII E]. A low minimum inhibitory concentration is correlated with a large inhibition zone diameter. The concentration of antibiotic decreases with the distance from the disk. The farther the distance from the disk, the lower the antibiotic concentration.

148. The answer is c [Chapter 4 IV E 3 c (4) (a)]. Patients who have promyelocytic leukemia [i.e., acute myelogenous leukemia (AML)-M3] are at high risk for developing disseminated intravascular coagulation (DIC).

149. The answer is c [Chapter 6 XV B 2]. Weil-Felix antigens are prepared from the O antigens of strains of *Proteus vulgaris* and *Proteus mirabilis*.

150. The answer is b [Chapter 6 VIII C 2]. Immunofixation electrophoresis and immunoelectrophoresis are often used in combination in working up monoclonal gammopathies.

Index

Note: *Italic* page numbers indicate figures, page numbers followed by *t* indicate tables, those followed by Q indicate questions, and those followed by E indicate explanations.